LOCAL ANESTHESIA *for the* DENTAL HYGIENIST

Third Edition

Demetra Daskalos Logothetis, RDH, MS

Professor Emeritus and Graduate Program Director
Department of Dental Medicine
University of New Mexico, Albuquerque, New Mexico
Educational Consultant, Albuquerque, New Mexico

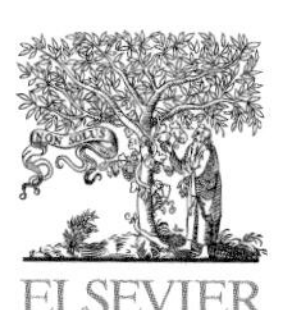

Elsevier
3251 Riverport Lane
St. Louis, Missouri 63043

LOCAL ANESTHESIA FOR THE
DENTAL HYGIENIST, EDITION 3

ISBN: 978-0-323-71856-1

Previous editions copyrighted 2017 and 2012.

Library of Congress Control Number: 2020946267

Content Strategists: Joslyn Dumas and Kelly Skelton
Content Development Specialists: Meghan B. Andress and Laura Klein
Publishing Services Manager: Julie Eddy
Project Managers: Andrew Schubert and Clay S. Broeker
Design Direction: Brian Salisbury

Printed in India

Last digit is the print number: 9 8 7 6 5

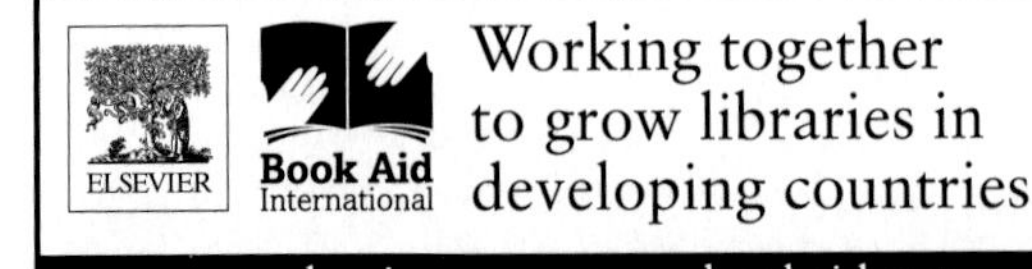

To my husband, Nick, for your unwavering, unconditional support and love of our family; for always reminding me every day of what is really important in life; and for always putting a smile on my face. After 34 years of marriage, you are still the shining light of my world!

To my children, Stacey and Costa, for making my life so worthwhile. I am so proud of all you have already accomplished in life; you both constantly amaze me. To my son-in-law, Travis, who has added so much fun and love to our family. We are so blessed to have you in our lives.

To my granddaughter, Demetra Marie, my heart is bursting with love for you as you bring so much joy and happiness to my life!

REVIEWERS

Randa Colbert, RDH, MS
Program Director
Department of Dental Hygiene
Hiwassee College
Madisonville, Tennessee

Kyle Fraser, RDH, BComm, BEd, MEd
Professor
Department of Dental Hygiene
Fanshawe College
London, Ontario, Canada

Shelley Getty, RDH, BA, MEd
Professor
Department of Dental Hygiene
Fanshawe College
London, Ontario, Canada

Lisa Graciana, RDH, EdM
Associate Professor
Department of Dental Hygiene
Rock Valley College
Rockford, Illinois

Ruth Lunn, Dip DH, RDH, PID (BC), CDA
Second Year Clinical Coordinator and Instructor
Department of Dental Hygiene
Vancouver Community College
Vancouver, British Columbia, Canada

Jennifer S. Sherry, RDH, MSEd
Associate Professor
Department of Dental Hygiene
Southern Illinois University
Carbondale, Illinois

Amber Telander, RDH, BSDH, MA, CDA
Instructor, Dental Hygiene Radiology Coordinator
Department of Dental Hygiene
Laramie County Community College
Cheyenne, Wyoming

Laura J. Webb, MSHSA, RDH, FAADH, CDA-Emeritus
Dental Hygiene Education Program Consultant and Continuing Education Provider
LJW Education Services
Fallon, Nevada

CONTRIBUTORS

Diana Burnham Aboytes, RDH, MS
Associate Professor
University of New Mexico
Department of Dental Medicine
Albuquerque, New Mexico

Margaret Fehrenbach, RDH, MS
Oral Biologist and Dental Hygienist
Adjunct Instructor
Bachelor of Applied Science Degree, Dental Hygiene Program
Seattle Central College, Seattle, Washington
Educational Consultant and Dental Science Technical Writer
Seattle, Washington

Constantine N. Logothetis, MD
Resident Physician
University of South Florida
Morsani College of Medicine
Tampa, Florida

Christine N. Nathe, RDH, MS
Professor and Vice Chair
Department of Dental Medicine
Director
Division of Dental Hygiene
University of New Mexico
Albuquerque, New Mexico

PREFACE

Over the last 50 years, the delivery of local anesthetics has been added to the scope of dental hygiene practice in many states and has been taught in most dental hygiene curriculums. Knowledge of local anesthetics is imperative to the successful administration of pain control agents. Although there are other local anesthetic textbooks available on the market for educating dental hygiene students to administer local anesthetics, none of them have specifically related to the practice of dental hygiene until now! *Local Anesthesia for the Dental Hygienist* is a textbook that is directly related to the uses of local anesthesia in dental hygiene practice. It speaks directly to the dental hygienist and offers examples of local anesthetic use during nonsurgical periodontal therapy. *Local Anesthesia for the Dental Hygienist* is intended to help transform information into knowledge that is essential in both teaching and learning. This textbook will help transform the important information into a manageable knowledge base focusing on the significant information that is truly relevant to the practice of dental hygiene. *Local Anesthesia for the Dental Hygienist* offers comprehensive information on every aspect of the use of local anesthesia in dental hygiene practice.

INTENDED AUDIENCE

The intended audience of this textbook is the student dental hygienist and the practicing dental hygienist who is taking the necessary coursework to become licensed in local anesthesia. In addition, practicing dental hygienists licensed to administer local anesthetics and dentists might find this book useful for a quick reference or review during everyday practice. This textbook will also benefit the dental student as a classroom textbook or an additional resource.

NEW TO THIS EDITION

The third edition of *Local Anesthesia for the Dental Hygienist* includes a new chapter on nitrous oxide/oxygen (N_2O/O_2), more in-depth coverage on the use of the Ultra Safety syringe, information on anesthetic buffering, updated research regarding articaine and paresthesia, and updated information on dosing requirements.

Chapter 8: The U.S. Food and Drug Association (FDA)–approved manufacturer recommended doses (MRDs) will continue to be used in this edition, with an updated change to the anesthetic prilocaine at 3.6 mg/lb and 8.0 mg/kg. The dental hygienist may continue to use the conservative dosages because they offer an additional level of safety while maintaining efficacy and patient comfort and do not exceed the FDA-approved MRDs. The conservative doses are presented in Appendix 8.2. For pediatric doses, this edition will continue to use the doses approved by the Academy of Pediatric Dentistry.

Chapter 9: This chapter includes more in-depth coverage of the Ultra Safety syringe because many dental and dental hygiene programs across the United States and Canada are using this syringe exclusively. In addition, a new procedure box on the assembly and disassembly of the Ultra Safety syringe, along with new images to facilitate learning, is included in this chapter. Information regarding the use of the *Safe-D-Needle* as a training needle is also included in this chapter to be used as an effective teaching aid for clinical instruction of the administration of local anesthesia. More in-depth information on anesthetic buffering and the use of the Onset Mixing Pen has been added to this chapter, along with a new procedure table and new images on how to buffer local anesthetics using the Onset Mixing Pen.

Chapter 15: A new chapter on N_2O/O_2 is included in this third edition to be used as a reference regarding N_2O/O_2 administration and as an adjunct alongside the administration of local anesthetics by increasing a patient's pain threshold and overall tolerance to the local anesthesia injections. In addition, several written regional local anesthesia board examinations include N_2O/O_2 administration questions as part of the overall assessment, and this chapter will serve as an excellent review to prepare students for their board examinations.

ORGANIZATION

The material is divided into five parts to provide a clear and consistent organization of the content:

Part 1: Introduction to Pain Control includes important general information on the history of local anesthetics and pain control based on the human-needs paradigm. Basic neurophysiology content is used for the dental hygienist to fully understand the generation and conduction of nerve impulses and the mode of action of local anesthetic agents.

Part 2: Local and Topical Anesthetic Agents includes pharmacology of local anesthetic and vasoconstrictor agents. This section provides detailed information on all local anesthetic agents and offers color-coded local anesthetic tables to help in distinguishing among specific categories of agents and match the color codes of the American Dental Association (ADA). In addition, these tables offer helpful hints to local anesthetic selection. An entire chapter is devoted to topical anesthetics and their uses in dental hygiene practice. Local anesthetic and vasoconstrictor reference tables are included as an appendix for quick reference information.

Part 3: Patient Assessment offers comprehensive information on the importance of preanesthetic patient assessment using the patient's medical history. In addition, an entire chapter is devoted to determining individual patient drug doses for local anesthetics and vasoconstrictors with sample drug calculations and several practice problems.

Part 4: Pain Control Techniques includes a complete review of the anatomic considerations for administration of topical anesthetics, local anesthetics, and N_2O/O_2. In addition, this section provides step-by-step instruction on how to set up the local anesthetic armamentarium, and technique/procedure boxes provide step-by-step instructions on how to perform specific injections for both the maxillary and mandibular arches with syringe stabilization examples for each injection. These technique/procedure boxes are helpful tools for students to use during the clinical practice section of their course or for practicing dental hygienists during everyday practice. In addition, a new chapter on N_2O/O_2 is included in the third edition to be used as a reference regarding N_2O/O_2 administration and as an adjunct alongside the administration of local anesthetics. Appendices include a summary of the maxillary and mandibular injections, as well as a special appendix perfect for chairside use that summarizes the maxillary and mandibular injection techniques, needle selections, and amount and distribution of anesthesia.

Part 5: Complications, Risk Management, and Exposure Prevention offers comprehensive material on how to prevent local and systemic anesthetic complications and management of common local anesthetic and general medical emergencies. Risk management and its importance to the administration of local anesthetics by dental hygienists is addressed. In addition, this section includes information on needlestick exposure prevention and postexposure management.

KEY FEATURES

Several key features are included in this book to assist the dental hygiene student studying and learning the fundamentals of local anesthesia:

- ***Dental Hygiene Focus:*** Although the focus of this textbook is on administration of local anesthesia, the information is tailored to the specific role and needs of a dental hygienist administering local anesthetics.
- ***Key Terminology:*** Key terms are colored and bolded throughout the chapter to help students learn new terminology. Local anesthesia terminology might be new to many dental hygiene students, and this will help draw attention to important key terms. These terms, along with other important concepts, are combined into a glossary at the end of the book.
- ***Summary Tables and Boxes:*** Throughout the text, important concepts are organized in summary tables and boxes to assist visual learners and are useful in studying and learning the material.
- ***Procedure Tables and Boxes:*** Procedure boxes for each injection are included that can be used as a guide in clinical situations. Tables are used for each injection to assist in the organization of information for each injection. Photos are placed in each relevant table for easy visualization of techniques and written material.
- ***Consistent Presentation:*** All injection techniques include detailed instructions and full-color photographs. All technique photos were taken by the author to maintain consistency and include examples of patient operator positioning and syringe stabilization.
- ***Dental Hygiene Considerations:*** At the end of each chapter, important dental hygiene considerations are presented, summarizing the important concepts presented in the chapter and discussing their clinical relevance.
- ***Case Studies:*** Numerous case studies make it easier for students to apply knowledge to real-life situations and develop essential problem-solving skills. In addition, case-based examination questions have been included in regional local anesthesia written board examinations.
- ***Chapter Review Questions:*** Twenty chapter review questions are presented at the end of each chapter to provide an opportunity for students to assess their knowledge.

EVOLVE COMPANION WEBSITE

A companion Evolve website has been specifically created for *Local Anesthesia for the Dental Hygienist* and can be accessed from http://evolve.elsevier.com/Logothetis/anesthesia/. The website has been revised to support the content of the book and enhance the faculty's instruction and student learning.

EVOLVE FOR THE INSTRUCTOR

TEACH Instructor's Resource

Instructors who adopt the textbook will also receive access to the TEACH Instructor's Resource, which links all parts of the Logothetis educational package with customizable lesson plans based on objectives drawn from the text. The instructor's resource is designed around standard 50-minute classes and includes the following assets: TEACH Lesson Plans, TEACH PowerPoints, TEACH Student Handouts, and TEACH Answer Keys. TEACH simplifies instructor preparation with detailed lesson plans and lecture notes with talking points, all mapped to chapter objectives to ensure coverage of all curricular content. The TEACH Answer Keys provide answers and rationales for the end-of-chapter questions and cases. The instructor can decide whether to provide the answer keys and rationales to their students.

Competency Skill Sheets

Evaluation forms that correlate to each injection technique are available for instructor assessment.

Test Question Bank

An updated test bank of approximately 600 questions is provided, with accompanying rationales for correct and incorrect answers and page number references. Cognitive leveling based on Bloom's Taxonomy is also included along with National Board Dental Hygiene Exam (NBDHE) tracking. These questions easily can become part of an educator's overall assessment plan and for student preparation for national or regional written examinations.

Image Collection

An electronic image collection organized by chapters with correlating figure numbers to the textbook can be downloaded for PowerPoint presentations, handouts, and examinations.

EVOLVE FOR STUDENTS

Board Preparation

A mock board examination assists students who will be taking the Western Regional Examining Board (WREB); Commission on Dental Competency Assessments (CDCA), formerly the NERB; Central Regional Dental Testing Services (CRDTS); or other regional or state local anesthesia examinations. In addition, test-taking tips and strategies are available to assist the local anesthesia licensure candidate. Moreover, Appendix 8.3 offers drug dosage calculations to assist the local anesthesia licensure candidate who will be taking written board examinations that require dosage calculations based on 1.7 mL of solution per cartridge rather than the recommended 1.8 mL of solution per cartridge.

Practice Quizzes

Approximately 320 questions are provided in an instant-feedback format to allow students to assess their understanding of the content and to help prepare them for examinations. Rationales and page number references are also provided.

Sincerely, Demetra Daskalos Logothetis

ACKNOWLEDGMENTS

I would like to express my sincere gratitude to the many individuals who assisted in making this book a success. First, I would like to sincerely thank the contributors of this book, Diana Aboytes, Margaret Fehrenbach, Constantine Logothetis, and Christine Nathe, for their hard work, perseverance, and attention to detail. A special thank you to Cynthia Guillen, who worked so hard to get me the images I needed for this book, and Gloria Lopez, who spent hours in the dental chair allowing me to administer many local anesthetic injections to her for the photographs used in this book.

I would like to thank my husband, Nick, for his outstanding photography skills and for spending countless hours with me taking and retaking photographs to get them just right. Thank you to my children, Costa and Stacey, and son-in-law, Travis, who supported and encouraged me throughout the work on this book. Thank you to my clinical anesthesia instructors-Sandy Bartee, RDH, BS; Kirstin Peterson, RDH, BS; Diana Aboytes, RDH, MS; and Justine Ponce, RDH, MS-for assisting in the technique photographs and/or for all their feedback. A special thank you to Sandra Arill, CRDH; Jackie Podboy-Navarro, CRDH; and Alina Guasch, CRDH for their time in helping me take some photographs for Chapter 12, and to Donna Low, CRDH, MS for developing the special appendix for Chapter 13. In addition, I would like to thank all the reviewers for offering wonderful feedback and advice.

Thank you to my students for always challenging knowledge and for your love of learning. Thank you for your recommendations and advice that assisted in making this textbook so valuable to your learning process.

I am very grateful to the Elsevier developmental team for their support and encouragement throughout this project. This incredible team was amazing to work with, and I cannot thank all of you enough for making this experience so enjoyable. A special thank you to Kelly Skelton, Content Strategist, who was so wonderful to work with. Her continued support of this project, good advice, and encouragement was invaluable. Thank you to Meghan Andress, Content Development Specialist, for her understanding of the needs of an author and her willingness to help whenever I needed her. A special shout out to Laura Klein, Senior Content Development Specialist, who jumped in to cover for Meghan while she was on maternity leave; I appreciate all of your help. Thank you for making the transition so easy for me. Thank you to Andrew Schubert, Project Manager, and Clay Broeker, Book Production Specialist, for their assistance throughout the production phase of the textbook and for their willingness to accommodate the multiple changes throughout the project. You were both wonderful to work with.

In addition, I would like to thank the companies who provided their information and photographs as a contribution to this book. Thank you to Carestream Health Inc., Dentsply Pharmaceuticals, Septodont USA, BING Innovations LLC, Milestone Scientific Inc., and Onpharma Inc.

CONTENTS

Part 1 Introduction to Pain Control

1 **Local Anesthesia in Dental Hygiene Practice: An Introduction**, 2
Christine N. Nathe, RDH, MS

2 **Neurophysiology**, 12
Constantine N. Logothetis, MD

Part 2 Local and Topical Anesthetic Agents

3 **Pharmacology of Local Anesthetic Agents**, 29
Demetra Daskalos Logothetis, RDH, MS

4 **Pharmacology of Vasoconstrictors**, 43
Demetra Daskalos Logothetis, RDH, MS

5 **Local Anesthetic Agents**, 53
Demetra Daskalos Logothetis, RDH, MS
Appendix 5.1: Summary of Amide Local Anesthetic Agents and Vasoconstrictors, 79

6 **Topical Anesthetic Agents**, 80
Diana Burnham Aboytes, RDH, MS

Part 3 Patient Assessment

7 **Preanesthetic Assessment**, 94
Demetra Daskalos Logothetis, RDH, MS
Appendix 7.1: Sample Medical History Form in English/Spanish, 111

8 **Determining Drug Doses**, 114
Demetra Daskalos Logothetis, RDH, MS
Appendix 8.1: Summary of Local Anesthetic Agents and Vasoconstrictors, 126
Appendix 8.2: Comparison of Previous and Current Maximum Recommended Doses of Anesthetic Drugs per Appointment for Healthy Patients, 127
Appendix 8.3: Dosing Information for Regional Local Anesthesia Board Examinations Requiring Calculations Based on 1.7 mL of Solution, 128

Part 4 Pain Control Techniques

9 **Armamentarium/Armamentarium Preparation, 131**
Demetra Daskalos Logothetis, RDH, MS

10 **Anatomic Considerations for Local Anesthesia Administration**, 184
Margaret Fehrenbach, RDH, MS

11 **Basic Injection Techniques**, 209
Demetra Daskalos Logothetis, RDH, MS
Appendix 11.1: Sharps Management: Centers for Disease Control and Prevention Guidelines for Infection Control in the Dental Health Care Setting, 229
Appendix 11.2: Safe and Unsafe Needle Recapping Techniques, 230

12 **Maxillary Anesthesia**, 233
Margaret Fehrenbach, RDH, MS and Demetra Daskalos Logothetis, RDH, MS
Appendix 12.1: Summary of Maxillary Injections, 277

13 **Mandibular Anesthesia**, 280
Margaret Fehrenbach, RDH, MS and Demetra Daskalos Logothetis, RDH, MS
Appendix 13.1: Summary of Mandibular Injections, 321
Special Appendix: Summary of Maxillary and Mandibular Injection Techniques With Distribution of Anesthesia, 325

14 **Local Anesthesia for the Child and Adolescent**, 326
Demetra Daskalos Logothetis, RDH, MS

15 **Nitrous Oxide/Oxygen Administration**, 335
Diana Burnham Aboytes, RDH, MS

Part 5 Complications, Risk Management, and Exposure Prevention

16 **Local Complications**, 347
Demetra Daskalos Logothetis, RDH, MS

17 **Systemic Complications and Emergency Management**, 362
Constantine N. Logothetis, MD

18 **Risk Management and Exposure Prevention**, 377
Demetra Daskalos Logothetis, RDH, MS

Glossary, 386
Index, 391

PART 1

Introduction to Pain Control

CHAPTER 1 Local Anesthesia in Dental Hygiene Practice: An Introduction, 2

CHAPTER 2 Neurophysiology, 12

1

Local Anesthesia in Dental Hygiene Practice: An Introduction

Christine N. Nathe, RDH, MS

LEARNING OBJECTIVES

1. Describe the history of pain control in health care and specifically to the practice of dental hygiene.
2. Describe how anesthesia is practiced by dental hygienists.
3. List state requirements for local anesthesia provided by dental hygienists.
4. Discuss patients' perceptions of anesthesia and pain control.
5. Describe the human-needs paradigm as it relates to pain control.

INTRODUCTION

Pain is an unpleasant sensory and emotional experience and can be thought of as one of the oldest of all dental problems. In fact, the control of pain during routine dental procedures is an important part of dental care delivery. Pain relievers are routinely referred to as analgesics. Specifically, the use of topical and local anesthetics provided by the dental hygienist is necessary for many dental hygiene appointments. Local anesthesia creates a numbing feeling that eliminates the feeling of sensation in a specific area without loss of consciousness. Although pain is seemingly associated with dental care, dental providers have the ability to control and alleviate pain during and after procedures. This chapter details the history of pain control and anesthetics in general, introduces the concept of anesthesia in dental hygiene practice, and discusses pain control in clinical practice.

HISTORY OF PAIN CONTROL

Pain is the oldest medical problem, and historically, the physician valued pain as a symptom, a sign of the patient's vitality, and a sign of a prescription's effectiveness.[1] Pain control is the mechanism that alleviates pain. Although some methods of pain control have probably always existed, historical evidence suggests that modern anesthetics can be traced to medieval times.[2] Early on, plants and herbs, including roots, berries, and seeds, became the prominent method for treating pain.[2] Interestingly, many drugs are still derived from plant-based substances.

The use of narcotics to reduce pain was a universally accepted practice and involved the use of cannabis, opium, and alcohol[3] (Box 1.1). However, the drugs used were not completely effective at altering pain, caused side effects, and were addictive. Opium was most useful for pain control. In fact, opium proved even more effective when converted into a more potent form, morphine, and injected into the bloodstream.[4] Currently, research is being conducted on the use of different pain medication regimens for patients after invasive dental procedures because of the issues with opium addiction.

Interestingly, chemists also prepared acetylated salicylic acid, a plant compound used in headache powder, which often left the patient with severe gastric distress. A new compound containing salicylic acid introduced as aspirin in 1899 was highly effective as an analgesic and antipyretic and proved to be remarkably safe and well tolerated by patients.[1] However, for severe pain, more pain reducers and controllers were still in need.

BOX 1.1 Drugs Used in the Past to Reduce Pain

Alcohol: a psychoactive drug that is the active ingredient in alcoholic beverages.
Cannabis: a psychoactive drug that comes from a plant.
Henbane: a psychoactive drug that comes from a plant that was used in combination with other plants.
Mandragora: a plant that has been used for sedative and pain-killing effects.
Opium: a plant, related to opiates, known for psychoactive and pain-killing effects.

The chemical that finally proved to be an effective surgical anesthetic was ether.[3] Several individuals were involved in the development of the concept of gas inhalation for anesthesia. In 1842 it was reported that William Clarke administered ether, via a towel, to a woman as one of her teeth was extracted by a dentist.[4] Horace Wells, a dentist, first tried nitrous oxide for dental pain control after attending several "laughing gas" parties. He practiced on himself by using nitrous oxide, which he considered safer than ether, and had a fellow dentist extract his tooth. He felt nothing during the extraction and discovered nitrous oxide to be an effective anesthetic (see Chapter 15). Halothane, a safe and stable chemical for inhalation anesthesia, was introduced in 1956. Short-acting anesthetics have also been introduced and are generally administered intravenously.[5]

During the 1800s, in both Europe and the United States, there was an extended debate over the ethics of operating on an unconscious patient and whether or not the relief from pain might actually retard the health process. Physicians used a calculus (measurement benchmark) to determine which patients were of the correct sensibility (exhibiting overall health) and who needed to benefit from the use of anesthesia.[1,6,7]

BOX 1.2 History of Local Anesthetics

Cocaine: 1884
Procaine: 1905
Lidocaine: 1943
Bupivacaine: 1957
Mepivacaine: 1957
Prilocaine: 1959
Articaine: 1969; available in the United States in 2000
Tetracaine HCl and oxymetazoline HCl Nasal Spray: 2016

During World War II, Dr. Henry Beecher observed that seriously wounded soldiers reported much lower levels of pain than his civilian patients. Based on his inference that clinical pain was a compound of the physical sensation *and* a cognitive and emotional reaction component, he challenged laboratory studies in healthy volunteers and argued that pain could only be legitimately studied in a clinical situation. These observations formed the basis for real clinical research trials on pain control.[1,8–11] Eventually, in 1956, the gate control theory was published. The classic articles proposed a spinal cord mechanism that related the transmission of pain sensations between the peripheral nervous system and the brain.[12]

History of Local Anesthetics

The first local anesthetic, cocaine, was isolated from coca leaves by Albert Niemann and Francesco Di Stefano in Germany in the 1860s.[13] Cocaine was first used as a local anesthetic in 1884 by Karl Koller, who demonstrated the use during painless ophthalmologic surgery.[14,15] Although effective as an anesthetic, it was addictive, and many of those pioneer researchers who first studied cocaine's effects on themselves became addicted.[3]

In 1905, the ester procaine (Novocaine) was created in Germany and, when mixed with a proportion of epinephrine, was found to be effective and safe (Box 1.2).[2] Procaine took a long time to produce the desired anesthetic result, wore off quickly, and was not as potent as cocaine. Additionally, many patients were allergic to procaine because procaine is an ester that has a high potential for allergic reactions.

In the 1940s, a new group of local anesthetic compounds, the amides, were introduced. The initial amide local anesthetic, lidocaine, was synthesized by the Swedish chemist Nils Lofgren in 1943. Lidocaine revolutionized pain control in dentistry worldwide because it was both more potent and less allergenic than procaine. In the succeeding years, other amide local anesthetics (prilocaine in 1959, bupivacaine and mepivacaine in 1957) were introduced. These new amide local anesthetics provided the dental practitioner with an array of local anesthetics for pulpal anesthesia that could last from 20 minutes (mepivacaine plain) to 3 hours (bupivacaine with epinephrine). In 1969 Rusching and colleagues prepared a new drug, carticaine, which differed from the previous amide local anesthetics. Renamed *articaine* in 1984, the drug was derived from thiophene and thus contained a thiophene ring in its molecule instead of the usual benzene ring. Articaine became available in 2000 for marketing in the United States in a 4% 1:100,000 epinephrine formulation. Today, lidocaine remains the most popular anesthetic used in dentistry in the United States; however, articaine is increasing in popularity and is a close second to lidocaine. Many patients do not understand the distinction among the agents and still ask for Novocaine, which is no longer available in dentistry.

ANESTHESIA IN DENTAL HYGIENE PRACTICE

Dental hygienists often treat patients with periodontal infections or dentinal hypersensitivity, which is why it is paramount for dental hygienists to be able to reduce and control pain while treating patients. Local anesthetics work by blocking the travel of the pain signal to the brain.[16] In addition to pain control, local anesthetics can provide vasoconstriction if vasoconstricting drugs, such as epinephrine or levonordefrin, are added to the anesthetic. During the course of treatment, patients may have gingival inflammation and bleeding. Hemostasis is achieved via the vasoconstrictor in the anesthetic. By controlling the bleeding, proper visualization of the tissues and the working end of the instrument can be achieved.[17]

Many dental practices will hire a dental hygienist with certification in local anesthesia to provide local anesthesia for all dental and dental hygiene patients in the practice. Just as a nurse anesthetist or anesthesiologist focuses his or her nursing or medical specialization in the provision of anesthetics, many dental hygienists exclusively provide local anesthesia without providing any traditional dental hygiene services.

The delivery of local anesthetic and nitrous oxide has been added to the scope of dental hygiene practice over the past 50 years (Table 1.1 and Fig. 1.1). Washington State added the provision of local anesthesia to state law in 1971, followed by New Mexico in 1972 and Missouri in 1973. Currently, 46 states allow dental hygienists to deliver local anesthetics. New York and South Carolina are states where dental hygienists may provide supraperiosteal injections but not block anesthesia (see Chapter 11).[18]

Proficiency is determined by coursework during the dental hygiene program or completion of appropriate training in an accredited continuing education setting. States vary in the amount of coursework, required minimal education, and necessity of examination before certification. Additionally, some states govern anesthetic practices by statutes, and some govern by rules.[17]

Thirty-three states permit the administration of nitrous oxide by dental hygienists. The first state to enact this increase in the scope of practice for dental hygienists was Washington in 1971.[19] Seven states may allow dental hygienists to monitor nitrous oxide but not actually administer the drug. This simply means that the dental hygienist may not turn on the nitrous oxide but may change settings during the dental hygiene appointment as needed. More states are permitting this pain control modality for dental hygienists, which increases the need for educational preparation of the dental hygienist in nitrous oxide fundamentals (see Chapter 15).

A recent study of dental hygienists mirrored past results, which revealed that the majority of dental hygienists reported a perceived need and use for pain control in practice.[20] Moreover, a review study confirmed patient and dentist satisfaction with dental hygienists providing local anesthesia. This review also reported on safety issues[21] (Table 1.2). A recent study that reviewed local anesthesia programs for dental hygiene students compared with those for dental students reported that the majority interviewed felt that dental hygiene students had more educational preparation in local anesthesia than their dental student cohorts.[22] These research studies suggest acceptance and advancement in the practice of dental hygiene pain control modalities.

Some educators have questioned students on student learning models, specifically related to the administration of local anesthesia. Researchers found that students preferred learning on one another (student-on-student) before practicing on patients.[23] Another study assessed a training needle for practice before local anesthesia administration in student-on-student learning and found that anxiety was decreased with the training needle or control device practice before application (see Chapters 9 and 11).[24]

PATIENT PERCEPTION OF LOCAL ANESTHESIA

Patients often present to the dental office with pain. By definition, pain is the sensation of discomfort and can range from mild to severe. It is well recognized that patients react differently to painful stimuli, and

TABLE 1.1 Local Anesthesia Administration by Dental Hygienists State Chart

State & Year Implemented	Supervision Required	Block and/or Infiltration	Education Required	Exam Required	Authorized by Statute or Rule	Legal Requirements for Local Anesthesia Courses
AL 2018	Direct	Infiltration	Board approved	No	Statute	32 h
AK 1981	General	Both	Specific	Yes – WREB	Statute	16 h didactic; 6 h clinical; 8 h lab
AZ 1976	General	Both	Accredited	Yes – WREB	Statute	36 h; 9 types of injections
AR 1995	Direct	Both	Accredited/ board approved	No	Statute	16 h didactic; 12 h clinical
CA 1976	Direct	Both	Course taken as part of a DH program/ approved by the Dental Hygiene Committee of CA	No	Rules	At least 15 h didactic; preclinical & clinical; 14 injection sites
CO 1977	General	Both	Accredited	No	Statute	12 h didactic; 12 h clinical
CT 2005	Direct	Both	Accredited	No	Statute	20 h didactic; 8 h clinical
DC 2004	Direct	Both	Board approved	No	Rules	20 h didactic; 12 h clinical
FL 2012	Direct	Both	Accredited/ board approved	No	Statute	30 h didactic; 30 h clinical
HI 1987	Direct	Both	Accredited	Yes – Exam given by course	Statute	39 h didactic and clinical; 50 injections
ID 1975	General	Both	Accredited	Yes – Board approval	Statute	No
IL 2000	Direct	Both	Accredited	No	Statute	24 h didactic; 8 h clinical
IN 2008	Direct	Both	Accredited	Yes – CDCA (formerly NERB) Local anesthesia exam or equivalent state or regional exam	Rules	15 h didactic; 14 h clinical; permit required
IA 1998	Direct	Both	Accredited	No	Rules	No
KS 1993	Direct	Both	Accredited/ board approved	No	Statute	12 h
KY 2002	Direct	Both	Accredited/ board approved	Yes – Written exam given by course	Statute	32 h didactic; 12 h clinical
LA 1998	Direct	Both	Accredited	Yes – Board approved	Rules	72 h; Minimum of 20 injections
ME 1997	Direct	Both	Accredited	Yes – Board administered	Rules	40 h; minimum of 50 injections
MD 2009	Direct	Both	Accredited/ board approved	Yes – CDCA (formerly NERB)	Rules	20 h didactic; 8 h clinical
MA 2004	Direct	Both	Accredited	Yes – CDCA (formerly NERB) written exam	Statute	35 h; No less than 12 h clinical
MI 2002	Direct	Both	Accredited	Yes – State or regional board administered written exam (CDCA [formerly NERB])	Statute	15 h didactic; 14 h clinical
MN 1995	General	Both	Accredited	No	Rules	No
MO 1973	Indirect	Both	Accredited/board approved	No	Rules	No
MT 1985	Direct	Both	Accredited	Yes – WREB	Statute	No
NE 1995	Direct	Both	Board approved	No	Statute	12 h didactic; 12 h clinical; 10 types of injections
NV 1982	Direct/general	Both	Accredited/board approved	No	Rules	No
NH 2002	Direct	Both	Accredited	Yes – CDCA (formerly NERB) local anesthesia exam	Statute	20 h didactic; 12 h clinical
NJ 2008	Direct	Both	Accredited/board approved	Yes – CDCA (formerly NERB) local anesthesia	Rules	20 h didactic; 12 h clinical; Minimum of 20 h monitored administration of local anesthesia

TABLE 1.1 Local Anesthesia Administration by Dental Hygienists State Chart (*Cont.*)

State & Year Implemented	Supervision Required	Block and/or Infiltration	Education Required	Exam Required	Authorized by Statute or Rule	Legal Requirements for Local Anesthesia Courses
NM 1972	Direct/general	Both	Accredited/board approved	Yes – WREB	Statute	24 h didactic; 10 h clinical
NY 2001	Direct	Infiltration	Accredited	No	Statute	30 h didactic; 15 h clinical & lab
ND 2003	Direct	Both	Accredited	No	Rules	Course must include clinical and didactic
OH 2006	Direct	Both	Accredited	Yes – Written regional or state exam	Statute	15 h didactic; 14 h clinical
OK 1980	Direct	Both	Board approved	No – Exam given by course	Rules	20.5 h
OR 1975	General/ unsupervised	Both	Accredited/board approved	No	Rules	No
PA 2009	Direct	Both	Accredited/board approved	No	Rules	30 h didactic and clinical permit, must renew
RI 2005	Direct	Both	Accredited	Yes - CDCA (formerly NERB)	Statute	20 h didactic; 12 h clinical
SC 1995	Direct	Infiltration	Board approved	Yes - Board	Statute	No
SD 1992	Direct	Both	Accredited/board approved	No	Statute	No
TN 2004	Direct	Both	Accredited/board approved	No	Rules	24 h didactic; 8 h clinical
UT 1983	Direct	Both	Accredited	Yes - WREB	Statute	No
VT 1993	Direct	Both	Accredited	Yes – Board administered	Statute	24 h
VA 2006	Direct	Both (only on patients over 18)	Accredited	Yes – Accredited program; board of another jurisdiction accepted	Statute	36 h didactic-clinical
WA 1971	General	Both	Board approved	Yes – WREB	Statute	10 injections
WI 1998	Indirect	Both	Accredited	No	Statute	10 h didactic; 11 h clinical
WV 2003	Direct	Both	Board approved	CDCA (formerly NERB) local anesthesia exam or equivalent state or regional exam	Statute	12 h didactic; 15 h clinical
WY 1991	Direct	Both	Board approved	Yes	Rules	None

CDCA, Commission on Dental Competency; *DH,* dental hygiene; *NERB,* North East Regional Board; *WREB,* Western Regional Examining Board.
Modified from https://www.adha.org/resources-docs/7514_Local_Anesthesia_Requirements_by_State.pdf.

the same patient may react differently to painful stimuli depending on a variety of environmental, social, emotional, or physical factors. The term *pain threshold* is often used when discussing pain. Pain threshold pertains to the point at which a sensation starts to be painful and discomfort results. This threshold varies among individuals and may be altered by some drugs such as local anesthesia. Pain perception is a neurologic experience of pain. Pain is perceived when painful stimuli are received and transmitted to the brain; pain perception differs little among individuals. Pain reaction is the personal interpretation and response to the pain message and is highly variable among individuals.[25] Pain reaction threshold is the moment when pain crosses the threshold of tolerance and at which point a reaction may occur. It may be influenced by the patient's emotional state, fatigue, age, culture, and fear and apprehension[25,26] (Table 1.3).

The fear of pain is associated not only with dental problems but also with the administration of local anesthesia.[26] Many patients fear the dental provider because they are apprehensive about a "dental shot." Dental hygienists must be cognizant of the common fear associated with local anesthesia and communicate sincerely and empathetically to patients about the provision of pain control.

A tool used to help a person rate the intensity of certain sensations and feelings such as pain is the Visual Analog Scale (VAS). A VAS is a measurement instrument that attempts to measure pain believed to range across a continuum of values that cannot easily be directly measured. For example, the amount of pain that a patient feels ranges across a continuum from none to an extreme amount of pain. Operationally, a VAS is usually a horizontal line, 100 mm in length, anchored by word descriptors at each end as illustrated in Fig. 1.2. The patient marks on the line the point that they feel represents their perception of their current state. The VAS score is determined by measuring in millimeters from the left-hand end of the line to the point that the patient marks. Pain scales are subjective but nonetheless useful for clinicians. The VAS scale will be used in Chapters 12 and 13 to describe the average level of pain associated with maxillary and mandibular injections.

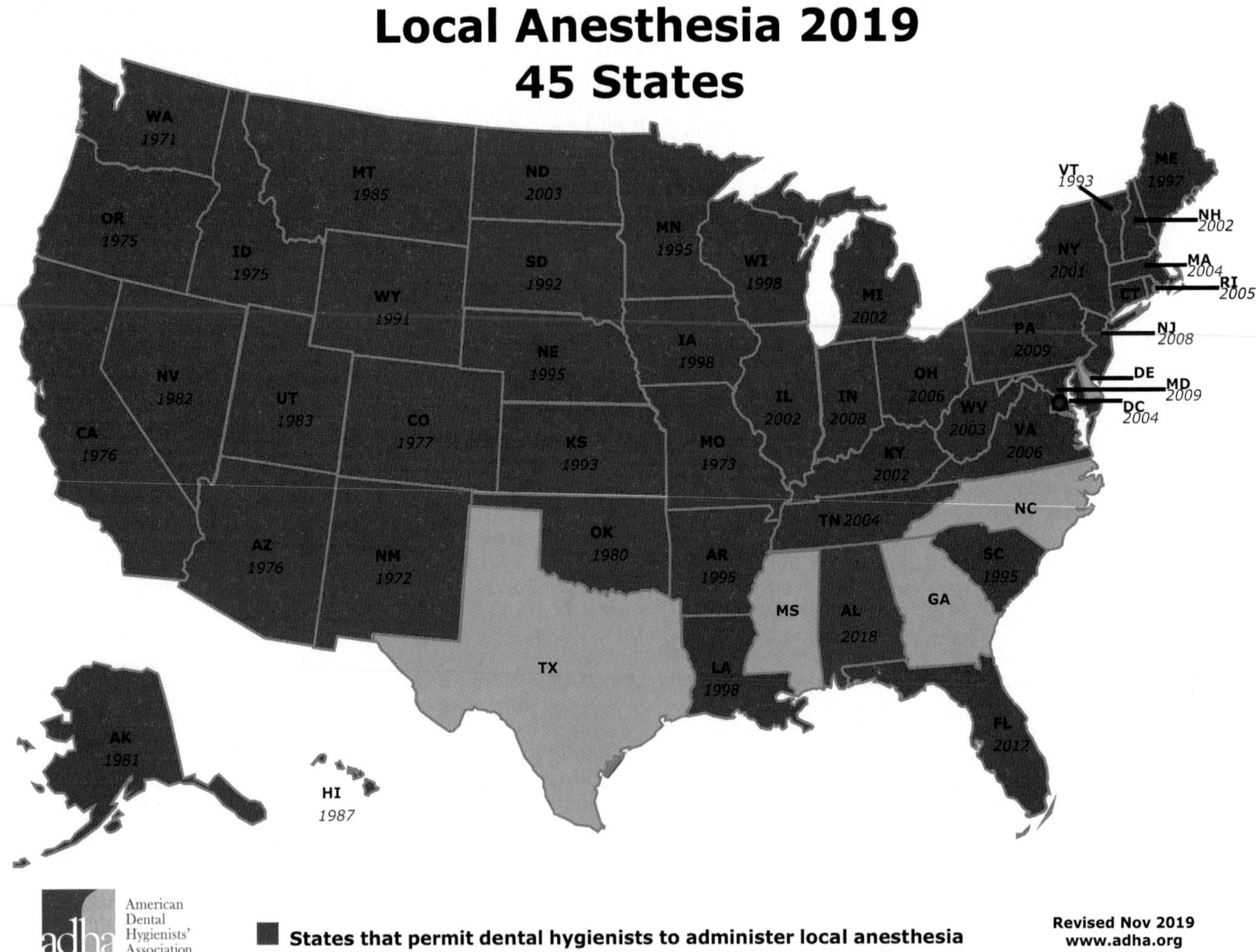

Fig. 1.1 States where dental hygienists may administer local anesthesia. (From American Dental Hygienists' Association. https://www.adha.org/resources-docs/7521_Local_Anesthesia_by_State.pdf. For Canadian data, please visit https://www.cdha.ca/pdfs/profession/RegulatoryComparisonCharts_final.pdf.)

HUMAN-NEEDS PARADIGM

Dental hygiene care promotes health and prevents oral disease over the human life span through the provision of educational, preventive, and therapeutic services.[27] The human-needs paradigm helps dental hygienists understand the relationship between human-need fulfillment and human behavior. A human need is a tension within a person. This tension expresses itself in some goal-directed behavior that continues until the goal is reached.[28] The human-needs theory explains that need fulfillment dominates human activity and that behavior is organized in relation to unsatisfied needs (Fig. 1.3). Dental pain can be an unsatisfied need because pain can be such an overwhelming force. Treating the cause of and alleviating dental pain using local anesthesia can be a welcome asset for the dental hygienist.

Interestingly, Darby proposed eight human needs related to dental hygiene that have many implications for pain control in dental hygiene[28] (Box 1.3). The human-needs theory emphasizes the use of a patient-centered approach and relates to pain control and prevention, which may include the provision of dental anesthesia.

Most of these needs relate directly to the need for and use of local anesthesia for dental patients. Specifically, two of these needs relate to the provision of stress reduction principles and the use of local anesthesia. Freedom from fear and stress is the need to feel safe and to be free from emotional discomfort in the oral health care environment and to receive appreciation, attention, and respect from others. Freedom from pain is the need to be exempt from physical discomfort in the head and neck area. Once again, the use of local anesthesia by the dental hygienist can help attain these human needs.

Management of Fearful Patients

Fear prevents many patients from obtaining dental care, whether it is fear of dental treatment, local anesthesia, or past experiences. Studies have revealed that from 50% to 85% of patients who report dental anxiety had the onset of fear during their childhood or adolescence and the remainder became fearful of dental care during adulthood.[29] Patients who are anxious may have had unpleasant experiences in the past or may have a learned fear of dental care. Interestingly, the majority of studies confirmed a relationship between parental and child dental fear.[30] It is important to discuss this anxiousness with patients so that the dental hygienist can respond effectively to help alleviate fear.

Many patients do present to the dental provider when they are anxious and nervous. Although significant fear may be termed *dental phobia*, many patients are anxious about dental treatment, and all

TABLE 1.2 Synopsis of Local Anesthesia Administration Safety and Efficacy Studies With Dental Hygienists

Category	Subject	Findings
Anderson safety	Aspiration safety protocol	86% of responding hygienists reported the use of consistent aspiration before injection, 7% reported the use of aspiration most of the time, and 3% reported infrequently aspirating before injection
Anderson safety	Complication rates	87.8% of dental hygienists signified no complications when administering local anesthesia injections
Anderson efficacy	Self-reporting of success	76% of surveyed dental hygienists reported successful anesthetization 90%–100% of the time and 16% reported success 75%–89% of the time
Cross-Poline et al. efficacy	Employer/dentist observer ratings	Dentists (n = 57) identified a benefit to both their practices and their patients as a result of the administration of local anesthesia by their dental hygiene employees; the mean percentage of agreement with this statement was reported at 80.4%
DeAngelis and Goral efficacy	Employer/dentist observer ratings	92% of dentist employers were satisfied with their dental hygienists' ability in administering local anesthesia injections
Lobene safety	Complication rates	Out of 19,849 anesthetizations by dental hygienists, only three cases of temporary paresthesia were identified
Lobene efficacy	Success rates	Out of 19,849 injections performed by dental hygienists, a success rate of 96.7% with supraperiosteals and an 85.7% success rate with nerve block techniques were found with dental hygienists
Rich and Smorang safety/efficacy	Continued delegation of anesthesia administration to hygienists	100% of periodontists and 86% of general dentists delegated the administration of local anesthesia to dental hygienists based on this survey of California dental hygiene graduates
Scofield et al. safety	Disciplinary reports	No formal complaints associated with local anesthesia administration against dental hygienists were known to state dental boards or American Dental Hygienists' Association constituent presidents based on surveys reported in 1990 and again in 2005
Sisty-LePeau et al. efficacy	Adequacy of anesthesia with dental hygiene students	Through evaluations completed by restorative dentistry and periodontics faculty, it was determined that out of 3926 injections administered by dental hygiene students, adequate anesthesia was achieved 95% of the time

From Boynes SG, Zovko J, Peskin RM: Local anesthesia administration by dental hygienists. *Dent Clin North Am.* 2010;54(4):769–778.

TABLE 1.3 Influences of Pain Reaction Threshold

Influence	Clinical Relevance
Emotional state	Personal pain interpretation may vary within an individual based upon their emotional state at the time of dental treatment. Patients who are in a difficult emotional condition generally have a lower pain reaction threshold.
Fatigue and stress	Personal pain interpretation may vary within an individual based upon their level of fatigue and stress. Patients who are overly tired or stressed at the time of their appointment will generally have a lower pain reaction threshold.
Age	Older patients generally have higher pain reaction thresholds compared with younger patients, as they have accepted pain as part of life.
Cultural characteristics	Individuals from different cultures will react to pain differently as influenced by what is considered an appropriate reaction to convey within their culture.
Fear and apprehension	The more fear and apprehension patients have regarding their dental appointment, the lower the pain reaction threshold. These are patients who frequently miss dental appointments.

From Bowen DM, Pieren JA: *Darby and Walsh dental hygiene theory: and practice*, ed 5, St Louis, 2020, Elsevier.

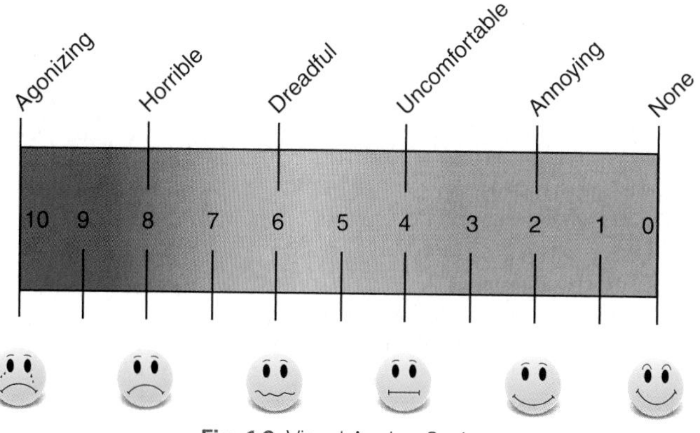

Fig. 1.2 Visual Analog Scale.

dental hygienists can expect to treat many anxious patients.[28] A patient with dental phobia may not be a regular (recall) dental patient, based on the extreme fearfulness toward dental care in general.

The effects of fear on the body can physiologically evoke the stress response. **Stress** is a physical and emotional response to a particular situation. The response to stress is often termed *fight or flight* and occurs automatically (see Chapter 4). Studies suggest that patients who are fearful of dental treatment may have elevated blood pressure, heart rate, and salivary cortisol levels immediately before dental checkups and treatment, although not all studies confirm this.[30,31] Dental hygienists must be cognizant of the important role patient fear plays in the provision of dental care.

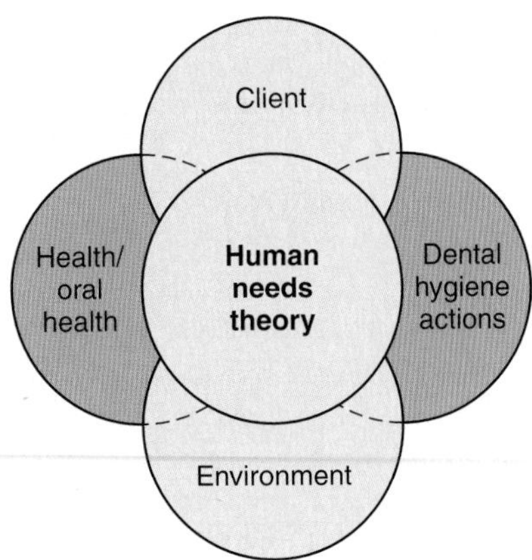

Fig. 1.3 Human-needs paradigm in relation to dental hygiene. (From Bowen DM, Pieren JA: *Darby and Walsh dental hygiene: theory and practice,* ed 5, St Louis, 2020, Elsevier.)

BOX 1.3 Eight Human Needs Related to Dental Hygiene Care

Protection from health risks
Freedom from fear and stress
Freedom from pain
Wholesome facial image
Skin and mucous membrane integrity of the head and neck
Biologically sound and functional dentition
Conceptualization and problem solving
Responsibility for oral health

From Bowen DM, Pieren JA: *Darby and Walsh dental hygiene: theory and practice,* ed 5, St Louis, 2020, Elsevier.

Stress Reduction Principles

Prevention is the best method to manage an anxious patient. Basically, the dental hygienist should look for symptoms of stress immediately so that stress reduction principles are enacted before stress levels elevate. Box 1.4 lists signs of moderate anxiety, including patients' discussions with the receptionists or other patients in the waiting room about their fear, cold or sweaty palms, or unnaturally stiff posture. An astute practitioner looks for signs of anxiousness.

During the health and dental history review, dental hygienists should determine whether or not the patient is anxious. Some patients will express their apprehension and stress immediately, directly to the provider, whereas other patients may need questioning or persistent listening by the provider to find out about anxiousness. Ensuring a complete health history review at each appointment is important to recognize stressors and health conditions that may complicate procedures. Even a patient who is feeling fatigued or "under the weather" may be more anxious and stressed during dental appointments. Obtaining the patient's vital signs is also important to understand a patient's total health history.

BOX 1.4 Signs of Dental Anxiety

- Cold, sweaty palms
- High blood pressure and pulse rate
- History of canceled appointments for nonemergency treatments
- History of emergency dental care only
- Muscle tightness
- Nervous conversations with others in the reception area
- Nervous play with tissue or hands
- Perspiration on forehead and hands
- Questioning the receptionist regarding injections or the use of sedation
- Quick answers
- Restlessness
- Unnaturally stiff posture
- White-knuckle syndrome

From Bowen DM, Pieren JA: *Darby and Walsh dental hygiene: theory and practice,* ed 5, St Louis, 2020, Elsevier.

BOX 1.5 Stress-Reduction Protocols

General:
- Build patient rapport to evaluate and relieve anxiety.
- Maintain communication with the patient about fears and anxiety.
- Minimize waiting time.
- Schedule short, preferably morning, appointments.

Pharmacologic options as needed:
- Use adequate pain control medications during and after the procedure.
- Prescribe preappointment sedation (e.g., a short-acting benzodiazepine drug).
- Offer sedation during the appointment (e.g., nitrous oxide sedation).
- Administer profound local anesthesia.
- Follow up with the patient after treatment.

From Bowen DM, Pieren JA: *Darby and Walsh dental hygiene: theory and practice,* ed 5, St Louis, 2020, Elsevier.

Considering shorter appointments, even though more appointments may be needed, may help some patients reduce stress levels, as can scheduling patients during specific time periods of the day. For example, some patients may do better in the morning, whereas others may do better later in the day. However, most patients are more rested and less fatigued in the mornings and are better able to handle the stressful dental appointment if scheduled before lunch. Patients who are fearful of dental pain may be better served by appointments in the middle of the week so they can be assured of seeing a provider the next day if needed. Telephone calls after treatment may be welcomed by some patients to ensure comfort and adequate care. The use of anesthesia as needed is an important key to prevention of fear associated with pain, which is discussed throughout this text. See Box 1.5 for stress-reduction protocols.

SUMMARY

Dental hygienists have the unique responsibility and opportunity to alleviate pain for many patients. The history of pain control focuses on the use of different substances that help individuals endure pain. Anesthesia has been used in dentistry for more than a century and continues to improve. The dental hygienist may need to use anesthesia while treating infections that result in pain or while treating patients who perceive pain during regular procedures. Using the patient-centered approach to stress reduction and pain control in conjunction with the correct use of anesthesia can be advantageous to dental hygiene treatment.

DENTAL HYGIENE CONSIDERATIONS

- Fear and anxiety during dental treatment is not uncommon and affects approximately three-fourths of the population.
- Fear, anxiety, emotional distress, and fatigue lower the pain reaction threshold.
- Patients who are anxious or fear dental treatment are more likely to refuse local anesthesia for dental hygiene procedures. Explain that when local anesthetics are administered, the patient can relax during the treatment and will feel less pain.
- The attitude and demeanor of the dental hygienist will significantly influence the confidence and comfort of the patient and overall success of the administration of the local anesthetic.
- Although the patient may be fearful of receiving a local anesthetic injection, once the injection is administered, the anesthesia will help attain the human need for comfort.
- Not all patients will inform the dental hygienist of their fear of dental treatment. The dental hygienist must recognize stress and health conditions that may complicate treatment through dialogue and a complete health history.
- The best time of day for dental treatment of apprehensive patients should be determined on an individual basis. For many patients, shorter, morning appointments in the middle of the week may better serve the apprehensive and fatigued patient.

CASE STUDY 1.1 A Patient Experiencing Emotional Distress

Your recall patient is a single parent of two children 12 and 14 years of age. She is returning to the office for treatment on her third quadrant of nonsurgical periodontal therapy with local anesthesia. The dental hygienist is happy to see that this patient is on the schedule for today because she is a delightful person who is excited about the results she is seeing with her periodontal treatment. Her treatment has been progressing very nicely, and she is an ideal patient.

Unfortunately, the patient is informed on the day of her dental visit that she will be laid off from her job in a month because of cutbacks in the company's budget. She, of course, is devastated when she hears the news and considers rescheduling her dental appointment, but she is unsure how much longer she will have dental insurance provided to her by the company.

The patient decides to keep her dental appointment, and because she does not like to burden others with her problems, she decides not to tell the dental hygienist about her bad news.

Critical Thinking Questions

- How can the patient's bad news affect her pain reaction threshold?
- How can the patient's decision not to inform the dental hygienist of her emotional state affect the treatment scheduled for today?

CHAPTER REVIEW QUESTIONS

1. What potent drug used for pain control was derived from opium?
   A. Lidocaine
   B. Novocaine
   C. Morphine
   D. Codeine
2. What drug did Horace Wells first introduce into dentistry for pain control?
   A. Nitrous oxide
   B. Local anesthetics
   C. Topical anesthetics
   D. Morphine
3. All of the following are reasons why procaine was NOT as desirable as lidocaine for pain control EXCEPT one. Which one is the EXCEPTION?
   A. Difficult to produce the desired anesthetic result
   B. It causes allergic reactions
   C. It was not as potent
   D. It was addictive
4. Injectable amides are recommended over esters because there is:
   A. Less risk of allergic reactions
   B. Increased potency
   C. Decreased mechanism of action
   D. Both A and B
5. What is the most popular local anesthetic used in the United States today?
   A. Procaine
   B. Novocaine
   C. Epinephrine
   D. Lidocaine
6. What is the definition of *pain threshold*?
   A. A neurologic experience of pain related to the process of receiving pain stimuli and transmission of this pain to the brain that differs little among individuals
   B. The point at which a sensation starts to be painful and discomfort results
   C. Personal interpretation and response to the pain message that is highly variable among individuals
   D. The sensation of discomfort that the patient feels, ranging from mild to severe
7. What is pain perception?
   A. A neurologic experience of pain related to the process of receiving pain stimuli and transmission of this pain to the brain that differs little among individuals
   B. The point at which a sensation starts to be painful and discomfort results
   C. Personal interpretation and responses to the pain message that is highly variable among individuals
   D. The sensation of discomfort that the patient feels, ranging from mild to severe
8. What is pain?
   A. A neurologic experience of pain related to the process of receiving pain stimuli and transmission of this pain to the brain that differs little among individuals
   B. The point at which a sensation starts to be painful and discomfort results
   C. Personal interpretation and responses to the pain message that is highly variable among individuals
   D. The sensation of discomfort that the patient feels, ranging from mild to severe
9. What is pain reaction?
   A. A neurologic experience of pain related to the process of receiving pain stimuli and transmission of this pain to the brain that differs little among individuals
   B. The point at which a sensation starts to be painful and discomfort results

C. Personal interpretation and responses to the pain message that is highly variable among individuals
D. The sensation of discomfort that the patient feels, ranging from mild to severe

10. Pain can be influenced by all of the following EXCEPT one. Which one is the EXCEPTION?
A. Fear
B. Fatigue
C. Culture
D. Positive attitude

11. What theory helps dental hygienists understand the relationship between human-need fulfillment and human behavior?
A. Pain-threshold theory
B. Human-needs theory
C. Human-fulfillment theory
D. Behaviorism theory

12. What is the definition of stress?
A. The sensation of discomfort that the patient feels, ranging from mild to severe
B. A physical and emotional response to a particular situation
C. Being anxious or nervous
D. Having an unrealistic phobia

13. Which of the following may negatively influence the pain reaction threshold?
A. Fear
B. Overeating
C. Positive communication
D. Explaining each procedure in advance

14. What is a visual analog scale (VAS)?
A. A measurement instrument that attempts to measure stress
B. A measurement instrument that attempts to measure fear
C. A measurement instrument that attempts to measure anxiety
D. A measurement instrument that attempts to measure pain

15. Which of the following is the personal interpretation and response to the pain message and is highly variable among individuals?
A. Pain threshold
B. Pain perception
C. Pain reaction
D. Pain reaction threshold

16. In what year was the first local anesthetic introduced?
A. 1884
B. 1904
C. 1943
D. 1957

17. It is best to schedule apprehensive patients for long appointments to complete as much work as possible. It is best to schedule these appointments in the morning.
A. Both statements are correct.
B. Both statements are NOT correct.
C. The first statement is correct; the second statement is NOT correct.
D. The first statement is NOT correct; the second statement is correct.

18. What percentage of patients have reported to have had onset of dental anxiety by adolescence?
A. 5% to 20%
B. 20% to 40%
C. 40% to 50%
D. 50% to 85%

19. Which of the following are signs of moderate anxiety?
A. Slow to answer questions
B. History of frequently missed appointments
C. History of emergency appointments only
D. B and C only
E. Relaxed posture

20. What is the best method of managing an anxious patient?
A. Prevention
B. Administering local anesthesia
C. Administering general anesthesia
D. Not telling the patient what is about to happen

REFERENCES

1. Meldrum ML. A capsule history of pain management. *JAMA*. 2003;290(18):2470–2475.
2. Goldie MP. The evolution of analgesia and anesthesia in oral health care. *RDH*. 2009;29(9):58–64.
3. Gallucci JM. Who deserves the credit for discovering ether's use as a surgical anesthetic? *J Hist Dent*. 2008;56(1):38–43.
4. Keys TE. *The history of surgical anesthesia*. New York: Dover; 1963.
5. Fenster JM. *Ether day: the strange tale of American's greatest medical discovery and the haunted men who made it*. New York: HarperCollins; 2001.
6. Pernick MS. *A calculus of suffering: pain, professionalism and anesthesia in nineteenth-century America*. New York: Columbia University Press; 1985.
7. Rey R. *The history of pain*. Cambridge, MA: Harvard University Press; 1993.
8. Beecher HK. Pain in men wounded in battle. *Ann Surg*. 1946;123:96–105.
9. Beecher HK. *Measurement of subjective responses: quantitative effects of drugs*. New York: Oxford University Press; 1959.
10. Modell W, Houde RW. Factors influencing the clinical evaluation of drugs, with special reference to the double-blind technique. *JAMA*. 1958;167:2190–2199.
11. Meldrum ML. Each patient his own control: James Hard and Henry Beecher on ten problems of pain measurement. *Am Pain Soc Bull*. 1999;9:3–5.
12. Melzack R, Wall PD. Pain mechanisms: a new theory. *Science*. 1965;150:971–979.
13. Gootenberg P. *Cocaine: global histories*. New York and London: Routledge; 1999.
14. Schulein TM. Significant events in the history of operative dentistry. *J Hist Dent*. 2005;53(2):69.
15. Dos RA. Sigmund Freud (1856–1939) and Karl Koller (1857–1944) and the discovery of local anesthesia. *Rev Bras Anestesiol*. Mar–Apr 2009; 2009;59(2): 244–257.
16. Overman P. Controlling the pain. *Dimens Dent Hyg*. 2004;2(11):10, 12, 14.
17. Doniger SB. Delivering local anesthetic. *RDH*. 2005;25(4):68–73.
18. Local anesthesia by dental hygienists. 2015. American Dental Hygienists' Association, Chicago. https://www.adha.org/resources-docs/7514_Local_Anesthesia_Requirements_by_State.pdf.
19. Nitrous oxide administration by dental hygienists. 2018. American Dental Hygienists' Association, Chicago. https://www.adha.org/resources-docs/7522_Nitrous_Oxide_Requirements_by_State.pdf.
20. Boynes SG, Zovko J, Bastin MR, Grillo MA, Shingledecker BD. Dental hygienists' evaluation of local anesthesia education and administration in the United States. *J Dent Hyg*. 2011;85(1):67–74.
21. Boynes SG, Zovko J, Peskin RM. Local anesthesia administration by dental hygienists. *Dent Clin North Am*. 2010;54(4):769–778.

22. Teeters AN, Gurenlian JR, Freudenthal J. Educational and clinical experiences in administering local anesthesia: a study of dental and dental hygiene students in California. *J Dent Hyg.* 2018;92(3): 40–46.
23. Aboytes D, Calleros C. Learners' perceptions of local anesthesia education. *Can J Dent Hyg.* 2017;51(2):75–79.
24. Aboytes D, Calleros C. Training needle effects on dental hygiene student anxiety. *J Dent Hyg.* 2018;92(2):57–61.
25. Wilkins EM. *Clinical practice of the dental hygienist.* ed 12. Philadelphia: Lippincott Williams & Wilkins; 2016.
26. Milgrom P, Coldwell SE, Getz T, et al. Four dimensions of fear of dental injections. *J Am Dent Assoc.* 1997;128:756–766.
27. American Dental Hygienists' Association. 2004–2005. Dental hygiene: focus on advancing the profession. Position paper. http://wsdha.com/clientuploads/pdfs/ADHA%20pdf/ADHA_Focus_on_Advancing_Profession.pdf.
28. Bowen DM, Pieren JA. *Darby and Walsh dental hygiene: theory and practice.* ed 5. St Louis: Elsevier; 2020.
29. Locker D, Liddell A, Depster L, Shapiro D. Age of onset of dental anxiety. *J Dent Res.* 1999;78:790.
30. Lahti S, Luoto A. Significant relationship between parental and child fear. *Evid Based Dent.* 2010;11(3):77.
31. Sadi H, Finkelman M, Rosenberg M. Salivary cortisol, salivary alpha amylase, and the dental anxiety scale. *Anesth Prog.* 2013;60(2):46–53.

2

Neurophysiology

Constantine N. Logothetis, MD

LEARNING OBJECTIVES

1. Discuss the organization of the nervous system.
2. Name the functional unit of a nerve system and explain its main function.
3. Discuss the structure and classification of neurons and differentiate between afferent and efferent nerves.
4. Describe the basic structures and functions of a sensory neuron:
   - Dendritic (input) zone
   - Cell body (soma)
   - Axon hillock (summation zone)
   - Axon
   - Output zone (synaptic knobs)
5. Discuss peripheral nerve anatomy and discuss the speed of impulse propagation with myelinated versus nonmyelinated nerves.
6. Differentiate between type A, B, and C fibers in terms of their function, size, and relative speed of impulse transmission.
7. Discuss neurophysiology and action potential.
8. Compare the ions in nerve transmission in regard to their functional element, relative concentrations and location during the resting stage, depolarization, and repolarization.
9. Discuss the mode of action of local anesthetic agents on nerves.

INTRODUCTION

A local anesthetic is a drug that causes reversible local anesthesia and a loss of nociception (also called a *pain receptor*) as a result of depression of excitation in nerve endings or inhibition of the conduction process in peripheral nerves. Local anesthetic agents used in dental practice prevent both the generation and conduction of a nerve impulse. When it is used on specific nerve pathways (nerve block), effects such as analgesia (loss of pain sensation) can be achieved. Basically, local anesthetics provide a chemical roadblock between the source of the impulse and the brain. The impulse therefore is unable to reach the brain.[1,2]

Local anesthetics are known as membrane-stabilizing drugs, which work by decreasing the rate of depolarization (see Generation and Conduction of Nerve Impulses) when a membrane potential is initiated. Local anesthetic drugs work essentially by inhibiting sodium influx through stimulus-gated sodium ion channels in the neuronal cell membrane. When the local anesthetic binds to the sodium channels, the influx of sodium is interrupted, the action potential cannot rise, and the signal conduction is inhibited. The receptor site is located at the cytoplasmic (axoplasmic, inner) portion of the sodium channel. When neurons are firing quickly, causing sodium channels to be in their activated state, the local anesthetic drugs bind easier to the sodium channels, increasing the onset of neuronal blockade. This phenomenon is called *state dependent blockade.*[2]

To fully understand how local anesthetics work, the dental hygienist must understand the inner working of the nervous system and its components.

ORGANIZATION OF THE NERVOUS SYSTEM

The nervous system is organized to detect changes (stimuli) from the environment, either internal or external, by processing and responding to the information received.

Central and Peripheral Nervous Systems

The central and peripheral nervous systems are divisions of the nervous system that are based upon location and direction of nerves (Fig. 2.1).

The central nervous system (CNS) is the structural and functional center of the entire nervous system that includes the brain, contained within the skull, and the spinal cord, contained within the vertebral canal. The CNS is responsible for receiving sensory information, processing the information, and initiating an outgoing response.[3,4]

The peripheral nervous system (PNS) includes nerve tissues that lie in the periphery, or "outer regions," of the nervous system, consisting of 31 pairs of spinal nerves arising from the spinal cord and 12 pairs of cranial nerves arising from the brain.[3,4]

Nerve fibers that extend from the cell body toward the CNS are termed central fibers, and nerve fibers that extend from the cell body away from the CNS are termed peripheral fibers. Fig. 2.2 illustrates the divisions and relationship between the CNS and PNS.

Afferent and Efferent Divisions

Afferent and efferent divisions of the CNS and PNS are categorized according to the direction in which they carry information. The afferent division consists of all *incoming* information traveling along *sensory or afferent pathways.* The efferent division consists of all *outgoing* information along *motor or efferent pathways.* Fig. 2.2 illustrates the afferent and efferent pathways.

Somatic and Autonomic Nervous Systems

Another way to organize the nervous system is based on function. The somatic nervous system is a subdivision of the efferent division of the PNS and controls the body's voluntary and reflex activities through somatic sensory and somatic motor components. External sense organs (including skin) are receptors. Somatic effectors are skeletal muscles and gland cells. The autonomic nervous system pathways

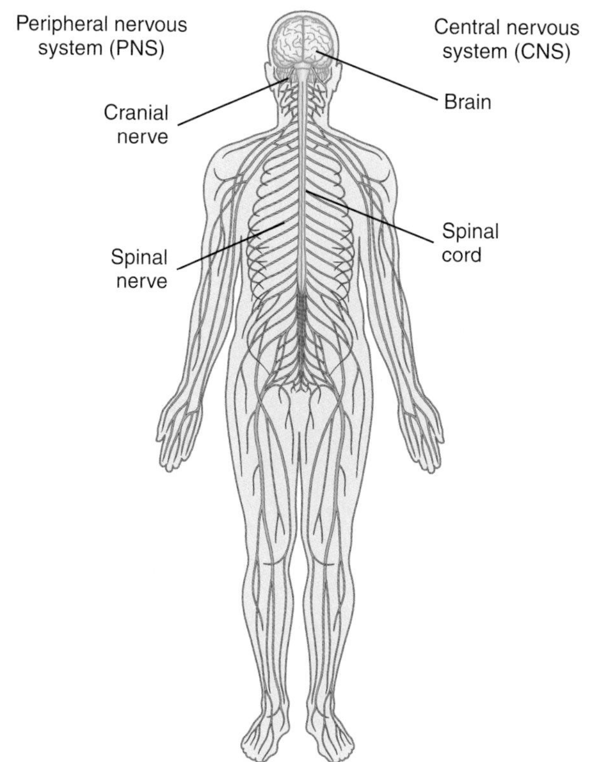

Fig. 2.1 The nervous system includes the brain and spinal cord (CNS) and the peripheral nerves and its branches (PNS). (From Drake RL, Vogl AW, Mitchell AWM: *Gray's anatomy for students*, ed 4, St Louis, 2020, Elsevier.)

carry information to the autonomic or visceral effectors that control involuntary (without conscious control) smooth muscle, cardiac muscle, glandular tissue, and other involuntary tissue. The motor component controls smooth muscle contractions of viscera and blood vessels and the secretion of glands (e.g., salivary glands). The autonomic nervous system is further divided into the sympathetic and the parasympathetic divisions. The sympathetic division prepares the body to deal with an emergency situation and is involved with the "fight-or-flight" response. The parasympathetic division coordinates the body's normal resting activities and is known as the "rest or digest" response.[3] Fig. 2.2 summarizes the various ways in which the nervous system is subdivided and combines these approaches into a single "big picture."

NEUROANATOMY

Nerve cells (neurons) are the basic functional units of the nervous system that manipulate information and respond to either excitation or inhibition. Doing so involves changes in the bioelectric or biochemical properties of the cell that require a vast expenditure of energy for each cell. The nervous system, compared with other organs, is the greatest consumer of oxygen and glucose. These energy requirements arise directly from the metabolic demand placed on cells, which have a large surface area and concentrate biomolecules and ions against an energy gradient. In addition to maintaining its metabolism, each neuron receives information from the environment or from other nerve cells, processes information, and sends information to other neurons.[5-7]

For neurons to carry out the three tasks of receiving, processing, and sending information, they must have specialized structures. These structures conduct electrical impulses and communicate with other neurons through long cellular extensions (called *axons*) and synapses.

The basic parts of a neuron are illustrated in Fig. 2.3. Additionally, specialized mechanisms and structures exist for neurons to maintain a difference in the concentration of ions across their membranes. First, the mix of ions inside neurons is different from the mix of ions outside the cell. Maintaining this difference requires huge amounts of energy because ions must be pumped against electrical and diffusion gradients. The large surface area of neurons compounds this problem. Second, those neurons that send information over long distances must have a way to supply these distant sites with macromolecules and energy. To fully understand the cell biology of neurons, the biochemical, anatomic, and physiologic properties of neurons should be viewed as part of an integrated whole; the machinery that permits the neuron to do its specialized functions.[5–7]

Structure of Neurons

The neuron is an excitable cell that is the basic functional unit of the nervous system, specialized in sending impulses and making all nervous system functions possible. Simply explained, neurons are the functional unit for communication between the CNS and all parts of the body. A nerve contains many cable-like bundles of peripheral axons (the long, slender projections of neurons), which are encapsulated together. The nerve provides a pathway for the electrochemical nerve impulses to be transmitted along each of the axons. Nerves are found only in the PNS. In the CNS, the analogous structures are known as *tracts.*

Each nerve is a cordlike structure containing many axons. These axons are often referred to as *nerve fibers.* Within a nerve, each axon is surrounded by a layer of connective tissue called the *endoneurium.* The nerve fibers are bundled together into groups called *fascicles,* and each fascicle is wrapped in a layer of connective tissue called the *perineurium.* Finally, the entire nerve is wrapped in a layer of connective tissue called the *epineurium* (Fig. 2.4).

Fasciculi located in the mantle region are called *mantle bundles,* and fasciculi located in the core region are called *core bundles.* Mantle bundles are located near the outside of the nerve, and core bundles are located closer to the center of the nerve. The location of the bundles in larger nerves has an effect on which bundles are affected by the local anesthetic first. When administered, the local anesthetic diffuses through the nerve to the mantle bundles (outer core) initially at a higher concentration and then to the core bundles (inner core) at a more diluted concentration because some anesthetic is absorbed by capillaries and lymphatics. Because the mantle bundles are affected by the local anesthetic first, these bundles also begin to lose anesthesia before the core bundles. This allows the anesthetic within the core bundles to diffuse into the mantle bundles and the innermost core fibers will be the first to recover. The mantle bundles will retain the local anesthetic the longest and will be the last fibers to completely recover (Fig. 2.5 and Chapter 3).[1,8]

Classification of Neurons

Nerves are categorized into three groups classified according to the direction of the conducted signals: Afferent nerves conduct signals from sensory neurons to the spinal cord or brain *(carry toward).* Efferent nerves conduct signals away from the brain or spinal cord along motor neurons to their target muscles and glands (*carry away*). *Mixed nerves* contain both afferent and efferent axons, and thus conduct both incoming sensory information and outgoing muscle commands in the same bundle. Although sensory and motor nerves are slightly different in structure, their main components of the neuron are the same: the cell body with a nucleus, axon, dendritic zone with free nerve endings (where stimulus is picked up), and terminal arborization (where the impulse is sent toward the CNS). The location of the cell body along the axon is the main difference between motor (efferent) neurons and

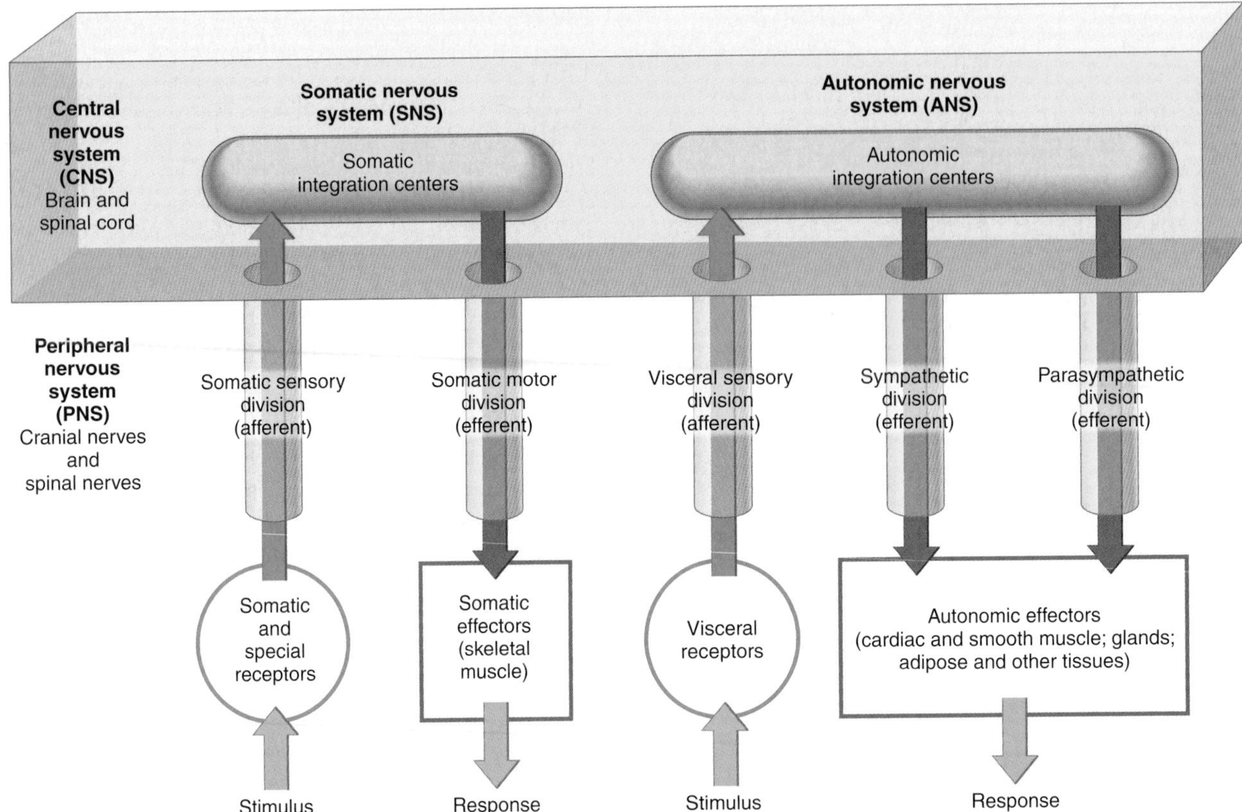

Fig. 2.2 Organizational plan of the nervous system. Diagram summarizes the scheme used by most neurobiologists in studying the nervous system. Both the somatic nervous system (SNS) and the autonomic nervous system (ANS) include components in the central nervous system (CNS) and peripheral nervous systems (PNS). Somatic sensory pathways conduct information toward integrators in the CNS, and somatic motor pathways conduct information toward somatic effectors. In the ANS, visceral sensory pathways conduct information toward CNS integrators, whereas the sympathetic and parasympathetic pathways conduct information toward autonomic effectors. (From Patton K, Thibodeau G: *Anthony's textbook of anatomy and physiology*, ed 21, St Louis, 2019, Elsevier.)

sensory (afferent) neurons. The cell body of the motor neuron participates in impulse conduction and is therefore located at the terminal arborization (Fig. 2.6A). The cell bodies of sensory neurons do not participate in nerve conduction and, therefore, are located off the axon (Fig. 2.6B).

Functional Regions of a Sensory Neuron

There is a wide variation in the shape of sensory neurons, but they all have the same basic structures and functions (Fig. 2.7).

Dendritic (Input) Zone

The dendritic zone is the most distal section of the neuron and is an arborization of nerve endings. These free nerve endings respond to stimulation (e.g., bradykinin, a "pain mediator" produced during cellular injury) produced in the tissue in which they lie, initiating nerve conduction. The dendrites of a neuron are cellular extensions with many branches, and metaphorically this overall shape and structure is referred to as a *dendritic tree.* This is where the majority of input to the neuron occurs.[3]

Cell Body (Soma)

The cell body is located at a distance from the axon in a sensory neuron and is not involved in impulse transmission. The cell body is responsible for protein synthesis and provides metabolic support for the neuron (see Fig. 2.6B).

Axon Hillock (Summation Zone)

The part of the axon where it emerges from the soma is called the *axon hillock.* The axon hillock decides whether or not to send the impulse further down the axon. If the total strength of the signal exceeds the threshold potential (see Box 2.1) of the axon hillock, the structure will fire a signal. Besides being an anatomic structure, the axon hillock is also the part of the neuron that has the greatest density of voltage-dependent sodium channels. This makes it the most easily excitable part of the neuron and the spike initiation zone for the axon: In neurologic terms, it has the most negative action potential threshold. Whereas the axon and axon hillock are generally involved in information outflow, this region can also receive input from other neurons.[3]

Axon

If the axon hillock continues the impulse, it is then relayed from the periphery to the CNS by a thin, cable-like structure called the *axon,* which is made up of cytoplasm, or *axoplasm,* and is surrounded by a multilayer lipid membrane. Terminal branches of the axon distribute incoming signals to various CNS nuclei, which are responsible for their processing, similar to that seen in the dendritic zone, and form synapses. The axon is a finer, cable-like projection that can extend tens, hundreds, or even tens of thousands of times the diameter of the soma in length. The axon carries nerve signals away from the soma and also carries some types of information back to it. Many neurons have only one axon, but this axon may undergo extensive branching, enabling

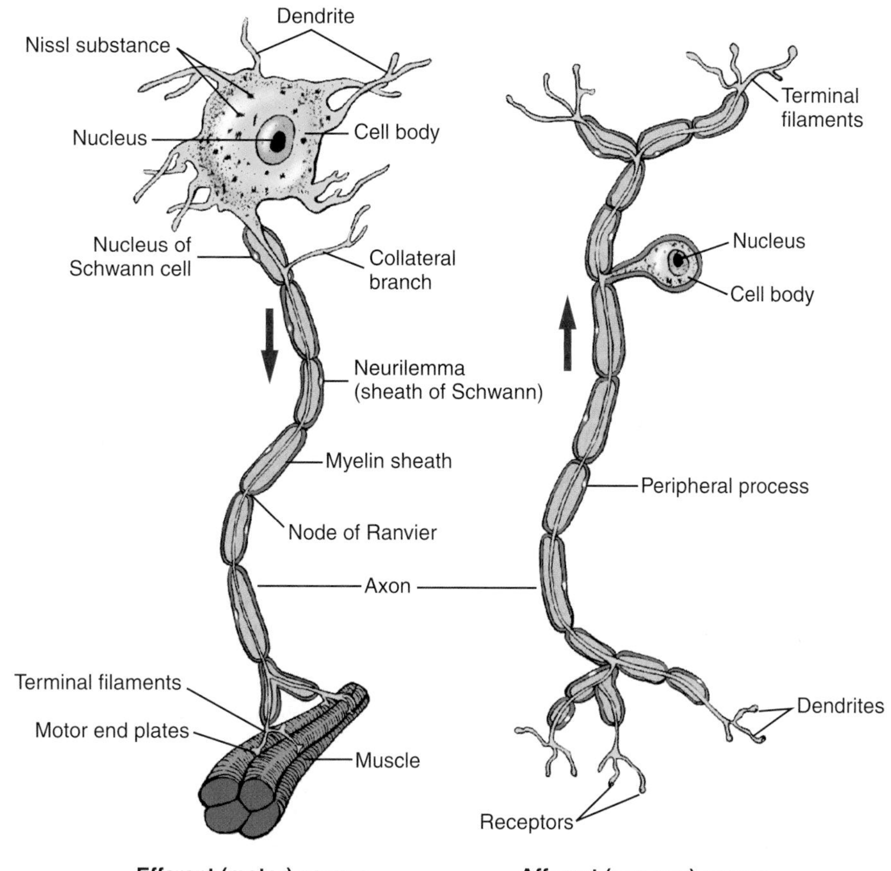

Fig. 2.3 Diagram of a typical efferent (motor) neuron and afferent (sensory) neuron. (From Linton AD: *Introduction to medical-surgical nursing,* ed 6, St Louis, 2016, Elsevier.)

communication with many target cells. A single axon, with all its branches taken together, can innervate multiple parts of the brain and generate thousands of synaptic terminals.[3]

Output Zone (Synaptic Knobs)

The axon terminal contains synapses, or specialized structures where neurotransmitter chemicals are released for possible reception by a nearby neuron. At a synapse, the membrane of the axon closely adjoins the membrane of the target cell, and special molecular structures transmit electric or electrochemical signals across the gap.[3]

Peripheral Nerve Anatomy

The axon of a neuron is a single process and is the primary transmission line of the nervous system, and, as bundles, they help make up nerves. Each individual axon is microscopic in diameter (typically about 1 μm across) and varies in both length and diameter. Some can be a meter long, whereas others measure only a few millimeters. In general, the larger the diameter of the axon, the faster the speed of the impulse will travel across the nerve fiber. In vertebrates, the axons of many neurons are sheathed in myelin, which increases the speed of impulse conduction.

Myelinated Nerve

Myelin (lipoprotein sheath) is composed of about 75% lipid, about 20% protein, and about 5% carbohydrates. Myelin is made up primarily of a glycolipid called *galactocerebroside* and almost completely insulates the axon from the outside. Myelin is formed by either one of two types of glial cells (which serve various roles in supporting the function of neurons): Schwann cells ensheathing peripheral neurons (Fig. 2.8) and oligodendrocytes insulating those of the CNS (Fig. 2.9). The myelin sheath of peripheral neurons is formed by many layers of thick Schwann cell membranes, which contain a fatty phospholipid myelin called *myelinated fibers* or white fibers (Fig. 2.10). Along myelinated nerve fibers, gaps in the sheath between adjacent Schwann cells are called nodes of Ranvier (Box 2.2) and occur at evenly spaced intervals (see Figs. 2.8 and 2.9). Only at the nodes of Ranvier, where the Schwann cells abut one another and the sheath is interrupted, does the myelinated axon have any direct contact with the extracellular space.

When a peripheral fiber is severed, the myelin sheath provides a track along which regrowth can occur. Unmyelinated fibers and myelinated axons of the CNS do not regenerate. The demyelination of axons is the cause of the multitude of neurologic symptoms seen in multiple sclerosis.[2,3]

Nonmyelinated Nerve

The nonmyelinated nerve fibers are long cylinder fibers with high-electrical resistance cell membranes that have no myelin sheath (Fig. 2.11). These nonmyelinated nerve fibers are surrounded by low-resistance extracellular fluid. Typically these are free nerve endings; the smallest nerve fibers, which are also known as *C fibers.* C fibers are the most numerous fiber type in the PNS.

Classification of Nerve Fibers

Peripheral nerve fibers differ substantially and can be classified based on axonal conduction velocity, frequency of firing, degree of myelination, and fiber diameter. For example, there are slow-conducting

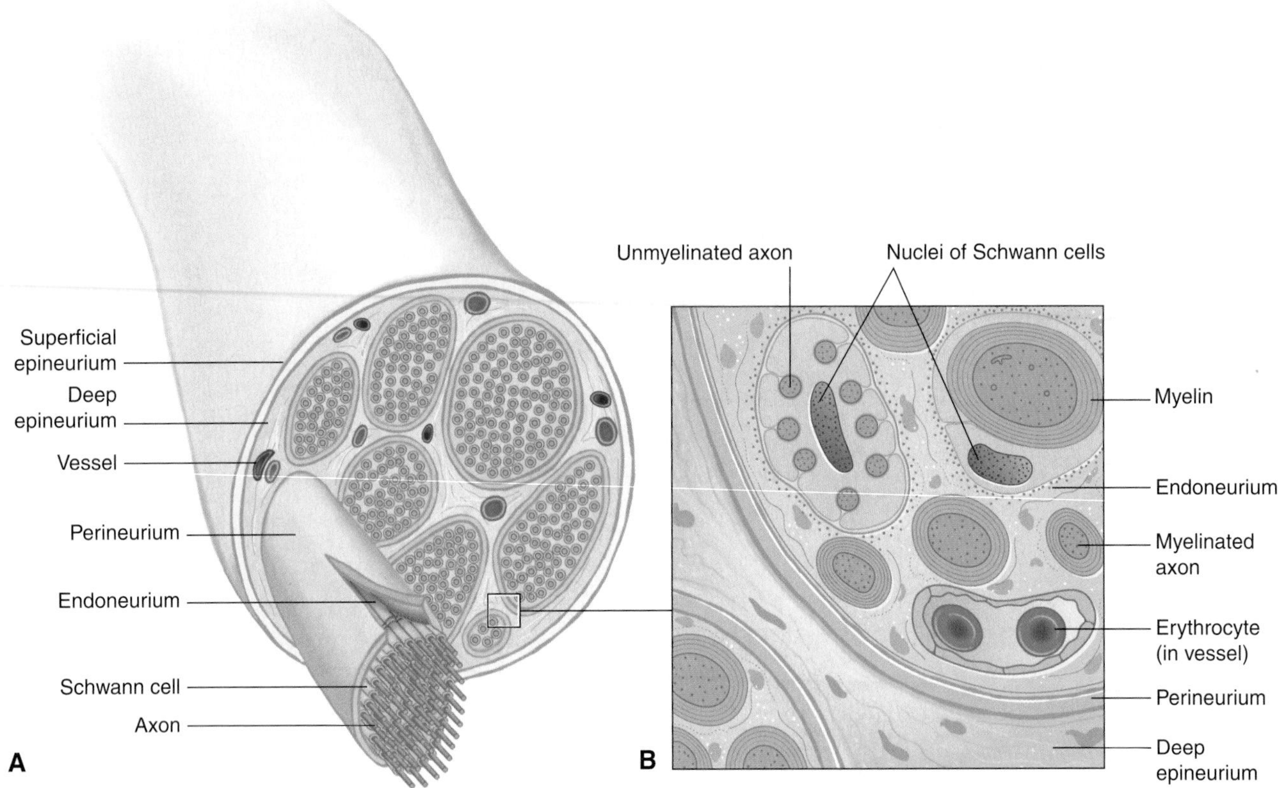

Fig. 2.4 The nerve. (A) Each nerve contains axons bundled into fascicles. A fibrous endoneurium surrounds each axon and its Schwann cells within a fascicle. A perineurium surrounds each fascicle, forming a blood–nerve barrier. A dense connective tissue epineurium wraps the entire nerve. (B) Inset showing magnified view of individual neurons within a fascicle. (From Patton K, Thibodeau G: *Anatomy and physiology,* ed 21, St Louis, 2019, Elsevier.)

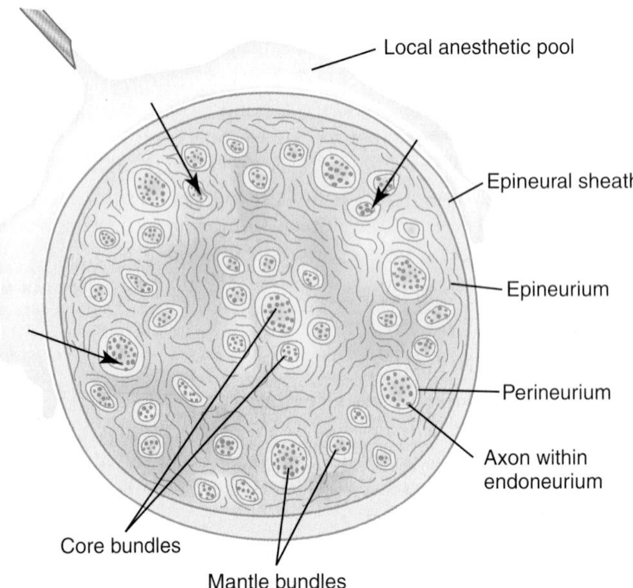

Fig. 2.5 A schematic cross section of a large peripheral nerve illustrating the composition of nerve fibers and bundles and how the deposited local anesthetic solution near the nerve sheath must diffuse inward toward the core fibers, reaching the mantle fibers first.

unmyelinated C fibers and faster-conducting myelinated Aδ fibers. All these factors influence the ability of the local anesthetic to block the nerve conduction.

Type A fibers are the largest fibers present in mammalian nerves, and with the rate of impulse transmission directly proportional to fiber diameter, this group comprises the most rapidly conducting axons. They are responsible for conducting pressure and motor sensations. Type A fibers are further divided into four groups, α through δ. Aδ fibers are distributed primarily in the skin and mucous membranes and are responsible for the conduction of sharp, bright dental pain. Type B fibers are myelinated and moderate in size and are almost indistinguishable from Aδ fibers but are not responsible for dental pain. Type C fibers are unmyelinated and the most numerous fibers in the PNS. They are responsible for carrying the sensations of dull or burning dental pain. As a result, in the lack of a myelin sheath, anesthetics block type C fibers more easily than they do type A fibers. Therefore patients who are adequately anesthetized still feel pressure and have mobility because of the unblocked type A fibers.[1,2,9,10]

Nerve fibers are classified as the following (Fig. 2.12):

A Fibers: A fibers are the largest nerve fibers and can be either motor or sensory. In addition, these large fibers may require a stronger minimal stimulus compared with smaller C fibers. They are myelinated and have the fastest conduction velocity. A fibers, primarily delta fibers (Aδ), are responsible for sharp pain.

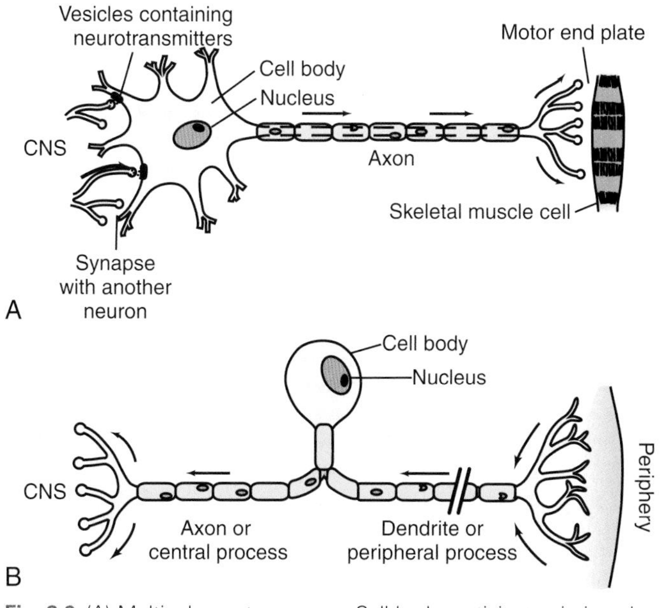

Fig. 2.6 (A) Multipolar motor neuron: Cell body participates in impulse conduction and is therefore located at the terminal arborization. (B) Unipolar sensory neuron: Cell body does not participate in nerve conduction and is therefore located off the axon. *CNS,* Central nervous system. (From Liebgott B: *The anatomical basis of dentistry,* ed 4, St Louis, 2018, Elsevier.)

- *Alpha* (α)*:* Largest, fastest; responsible for muscle movement and light touch
- *Beta* (β)*:* Proprioception (awareness of position/equilibrium)
- *Gamma* (γ)*:* Touch, pressure
- *Delta* (δ)*:* Pain, temperature

B Fibers: These fibers have medium diameters, and they are lightly myelinated motor fibers.

C Fibers: These fibers are the most numerous and the smallest, they are usually unmyelinated, and they are primarily responsible for dull, aching pain.

Both A and C fibers are found abundantly in the oral cavity, with C fibers in greater distribution.[1,2,9,10] Larger-diameter A fibers require more anesthetic volume than smaller C nerve fibers to provide complete nerve blockade.

GENERATION AND CONDUCTION OF NERVE IMPULSES

Ions in Nerve Transmission and Resting Membrane Potentials

Polarization of the neuron's membrane: All living cells, which include neurons, maintain a difference in the ion concentration across their membranes. Sodium (Na^+) ions are predominantly in the extracellular fluid, and potassium (K^+) ions are predominantly in the intracellular fluid. In addition to the K^+ ions intracellularly, negatively charged protein and nucleic acid molecules are synthesized within the cell and, because of their large size and solubility, do not diffuse across the resting membrane, causing the inside of the cell to be negatively charged in relation to the outside. This difference in the electrical charge on the outside of the cell versus the inside of the cell is called the membrane potential. Chloride (Cl^-) ions assist in maintaining the membrane

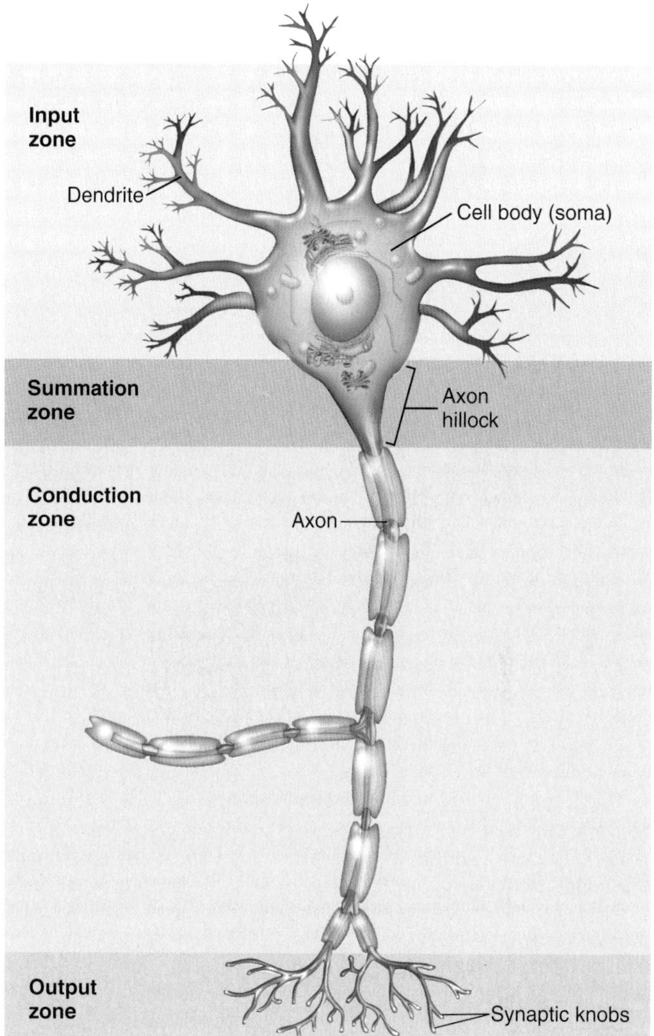

Fig. 2.7 Functional regions of the neuron's plasma membrane. The input zone receives input from other neurons or from sensory stimuli (stimulus-gated ion channels present). The summation zone serves as the site where the nerve impulses combine and possibly trigger an impulse that will be conducted along the axon, or conduction zone. Both the summation (trigger) zone and conduction zone have many voltage-gated sodium (Na^+) channels and potassium (K^+) channels imbedded in the plasma membrane. The output zone (distal end of axon) is where the nerve impulse triggers the release of neurotransmitters. The output zone includes many voltage-gated calcium (Ca^{++}) channels in the membrane. (From Patton K, Thibodeau G: *Anatomy and physiology,* ed 21, St Louis, 2019, Elsevier.)

BOX 2.1 Threshold Potential

The threshold potential is the minimum magnitude a voltage fluctuation in the summation or conduction zone must have to initiate an action potential (impulse) that will trigger the opening of a voltage-gated ion channel to cause depolarization. For example, if the magnitude of slow depolarization surpasses the limit of the threshold potential of −55 mV, the action potential will be initiated to stimulate voltage-gated sodium (Na^+) channels to open, causing rapid depolarization. There are many voltage-gated Na^+ channels and potassium (K^+) channels in the membrane of the neuron's summation zone (axon hillock) and conduction zone (axon) (see Fig. 2.7). Each axon, depending on its size, will have a different threshold potential.

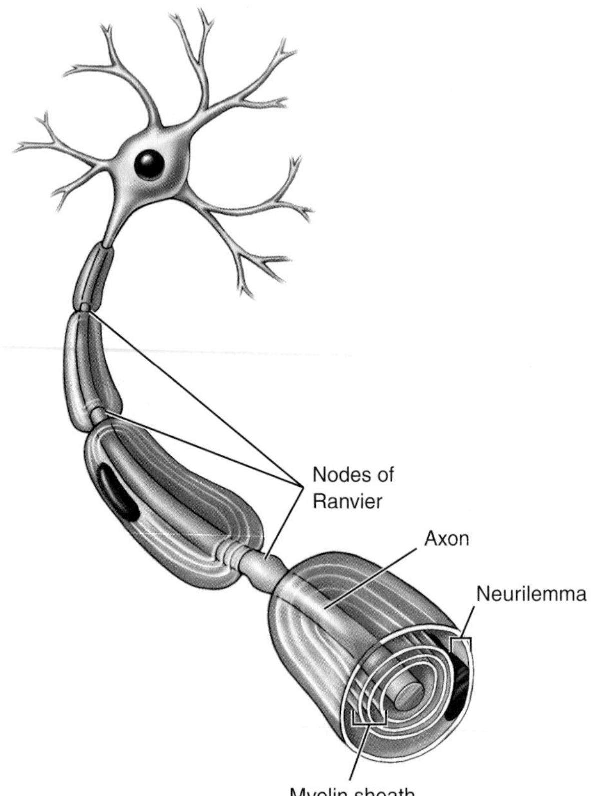

Fig. 2.8 Structure of a myelinated neuron of the peripheral nervous system. Structure surrounding the axon, showing the myelin sheath, the nodes of Ranvier, and the neurilemma (sheath of Schwann cell). (From Herlihy B: *The human body in health and illness,* ed 6, St Louis, 2018, Elsevier.)

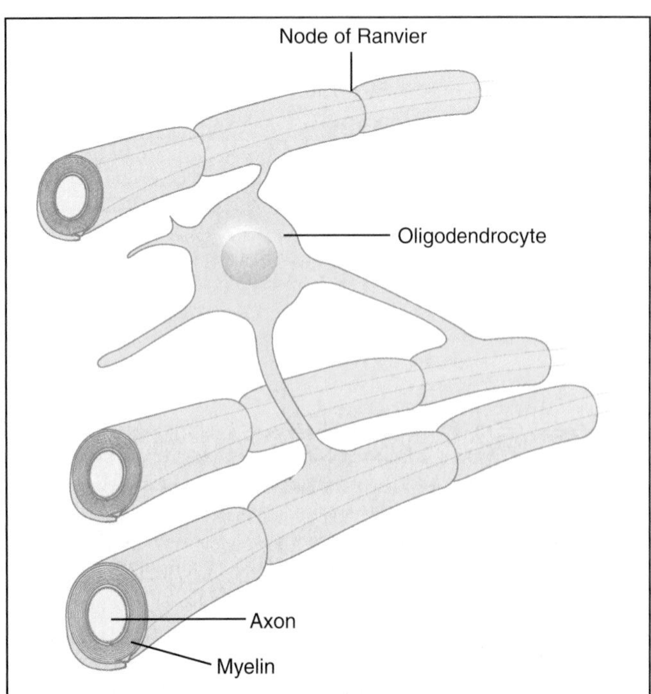

Fig. 2.9 Formation of central nervous system myelin sheath by an oligodendrocyte. (From Nolte J: *Elsevier's integrated neuroscience,* St Louis, 2007, Mosby.)

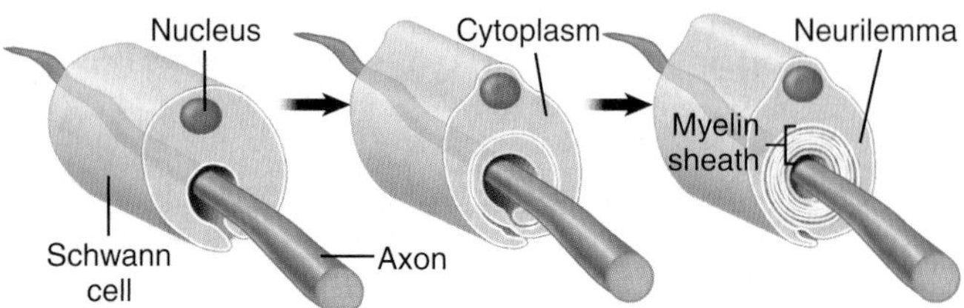

Fig. 2.10 Development of the myelin sheath. A Schwann cell (neurolemmocyte) migrates to a neuron and wraps around an axon. The Schwann cell's cytoplasm is pushed to the outer layer, leaving a dense multilayered covering of plasma membrane around the axon. Because the plasma membrane of the Schwann cell is mostly the phospholipid myelin, the dense wrapping around the axon is called a *myelin sheath.* The outer layer of cytoplasm is called the *neurilemma.* The extensions of oligodendrocytes also wrap around axons to form a myelin sheath. (From Patton K, Thibodeau G: *Anatomy and physiology,* ed 21, St Louis, 2019, Elsevier.)

BOX 2.2 Nodes of Ranvier and Myelin Sheath

Nodes of Ranvier are the gaps (approximately 1 μm in length) formed between the myelin sheaths generated by different cells. A myelin sheath is a many-layered coating, largely composed of a fatty substance called *myelin* that wraps around the axon of a neuron and very efficiently insulates it. At nodes of Ranvier, the axonal membrane is uninsulated and therefore capable of generating electrical activity.

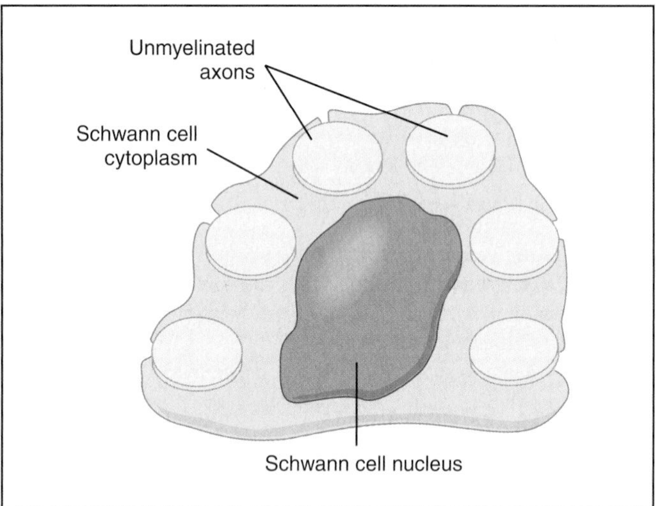

Fig. 2.11 Schwann cell and unmyelinated peripheral nervous system axons. (From Nolte J: *Elsevier's integrated neuroscience,* St Louis, 2007, Mosby.)

potential and are concentrated in the extracellular fluid with the Na^+ ions. When a neuron is not stimulated, it is sitting with no impulse to carry or transmit, and its membrane is considered polarized and in its **resting state**, also called the *resting membrane potential (RMP).* The magnitude of the potential difference between the extracellular verses the intracellular sides of the polarized membrane is measured in millivolts (mV). The electrical potential of nerve axoplasm in the resting state is approximately −70 mV with a range of −40 to −95 mV, and it will remain this way until a stimulus comes along (see Action Potentials). **Polarization** (resting state) means that the electrical charge on the outside of the membrane is positive while the electrical charge on the inside of the membrane is negative. The outside of the cell

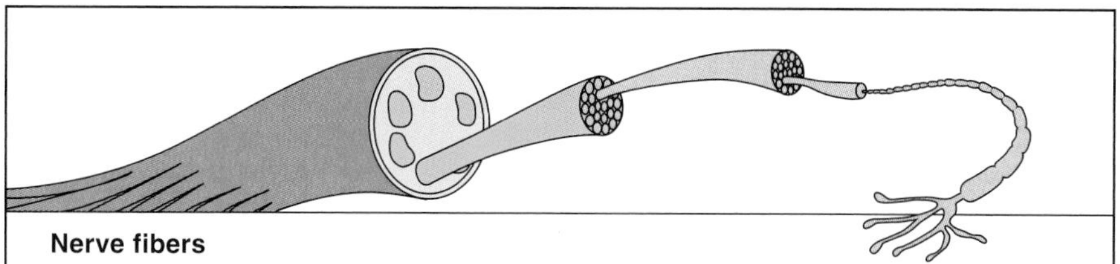

Nerve fibers			
Fiber type	A	B	C*
Diameter μm	2–20	<3	<1.5
Conduction velocity (m/sec)	5–100	3–15	0.1–2.5
Myelinated	Yes	Yes	No
		Preganglionic, autonomic, vascular smooth muscle	Pain, temperature, postganglionic, autonomic

Subtypes of A fibers	Aα	Aβ	Aγ	Aδ*
	Efferent, motor, somatic, reflex activity	Afferent, innervate muscle, touch sensation, pressure sensation	Efferent, muscle spindle tone	Afferent, pain, cold, temperature, tissue damage indication*

* Pain transmission fibers.

Fig. 2.12 Nerve fibers according to anatomic type. (From Wecker L, Taylor DA, Theobald RJ: *Brody's human pharmacology mechanism-based therapeutics,* ed 6, Philadelphia, 2019, Elsevier.)

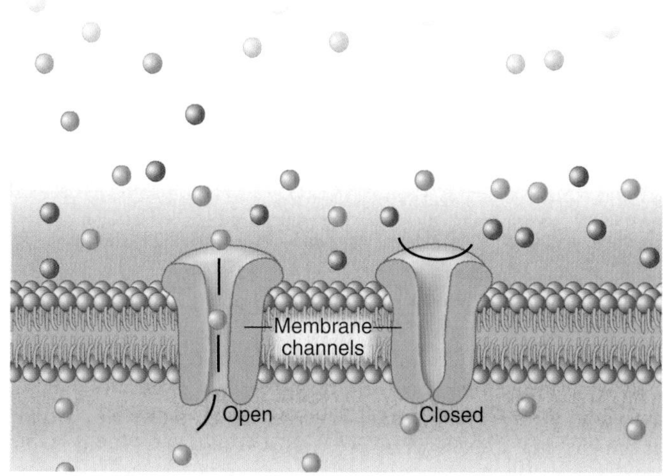

Fig. 2.13 Membrane channels. Gated channel proteins form tunnels through which only specific ions or molecules may pass, as long as the "gates" are open. Ions or molecules that do not have a specific shape and charge are never permitted to pass through the channel. Note that the transported ions or molecules move from an area of higher concentration to an area of lower concentration. The cell membrane is said to be permeable to the type of particle in question. (From Patton K, Thibodeau G: *Anthony's textbook of anatomy and physiology,* ed 21, St Louis, 2019, Elsevier.)

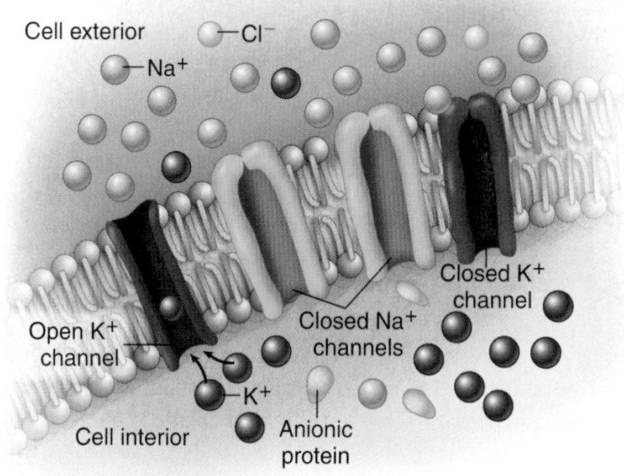

Fig. 2.14 Role of ion channels in maintaining the resting membrane potential (RMP). Some potassium (K^+) channels are open in a "resting" membrane, allowing the K^+ to diffuse down its concentration gradient (out of the cell) and thus add to the excess of positive ions on the outer surface of the plasma membrane. Diffusion of sodium (Na^+) in the opposite direction would counteract this effect but is prevented from doing so by closed Na^+ channels. (From Patton K, Thibodeau G: *Anatomy and physiology,* ed 21, St Louis, 2019, Elsevier.)

contains excess Na^+ ions at a ratio of 14:1; the inside of the cell contains excess K^+ ions.[3,11,12]

Neurons possess protein "tunnels" known as membrane channels through which specific ions such as Na^+ and K^+ can pass. Na^+ ions pass only through Na^+ channels, and K^+ ions pass only through K^+ channels (Fig. 2.13). When a neuron is in its resting state, some of the K^+ ion channels are opened, but most of the Na^+ channels are closed, allowing some intracellular K^+ ions to diffuse out of the cell in an attempt to equalize the concentration gradient (Fig. 2.14). The RMP is maintained by the cell with the operation of the Na^+/K^+ pump, which is an active transport mechanism. The Na^+/K^+ pump in the plasma membrane transports the Na^+ back outside and the K^+ back inside against resistance (Fig. 2.15). The use of adenosine triphosphate (ATP) energy is required for the pump to be fueled. The RMP is altered when either of these two mechanisms is altered.[3]

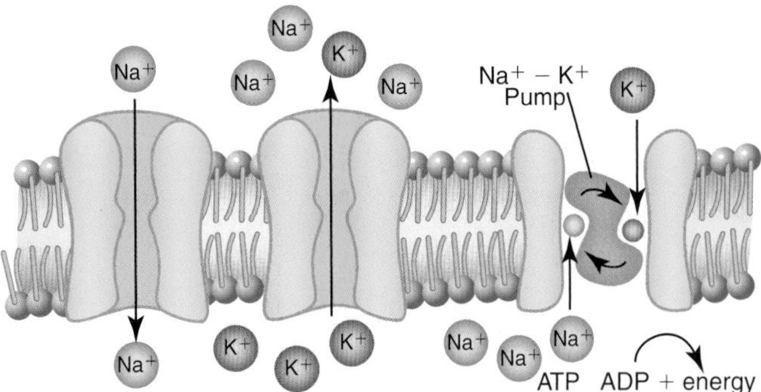

Fig. 2.15 Sodium (Na^+)/potassium (K^+) pump. In this mechanism, the plasma membrane actively pumps Na^+ ions out of the neuron and K^+ ions into the neuron at an unequal (3:2) rate. Because very little Na^+ reenters the cell via diffusion, this maintains an imbalance in the distribution of ions and thus maintains the resting potential.

Action Potentials

As discussed previously, all neurons are electrically excitable, maintaining voltage gradients across their resting membranes by Na^+/K^+ pumps, which combine with ion channels embedded in the membrane to generate intracellular-versus-extracellular concentration differences of ions such as sodium, potassium, chloride, and calcium. The relationship between the relative amounts of ions inside and outside the nerve membrane is known as the *concentration gradient* (Fig. 2.14).

Changes in the voltage across the nerve membrane can alter the RMP and the function of the voltage-dependent ion channels. If the voltage changes by a large enough amount (threshold potential; see Box 2.1), an electrochemical pulse called an action potential (synonym: nerve impulse; Box 2.3) is generated, which travels rapidly along the cell's axon and activates synaptic connections with other cells when it arrives (see Synaptic Transmission). Na^+ channels at each point of stimulation open, and Na^+ rapidly diffuses into the cell producing depolarization (discussed next).[3,11,12]

Depolarization and Firing Thresholds

Action potential: The action potential (see Box 2.3) is the membrane potential of an active nerve conducting an impulse. Excitation of a neuron occurs when a stimulus triggers the opening of a stimulus-gated channel, many of which are located in the membrane of the neuron's input zone (see Fig. 2.7). Na^+ ions move inside the membrane when a stimulus reaches the resting neuron. The gated Na^+ ion channels, on the resting neuron's membrane, release and open suddenly and allow the Na^+ in the extracellular fluid to influx into the cell. As this happens, the resting neuron goes from being polarized to being depolarized (see Fig. 2.16A–B).[3,11,12]

The depolarization process begins with slow depolarization until the axoplasm has depolarized approximately 15 to 20 mV, from −70 to −55 mV, which is necessary to reach the threshold potential (see Box 2.1 and Fig. 2.16B). If the threshold potential of that neuron is not achieved during the slow depolarization phase, no impulse will be generated, causing insufficient Na^+ ion influx to completely depolarize the membrane. In response, the membrane simply recovers back to the resting potential of −70 mV and the action potential is not generated.

If the threshold potential is achieved, more positive ions go charging inside the membrane, and the inside becomes positive as well; polarization is removed, and the threshold is reached. Each neuron has a threshold level, or the point at which there is no holding back, called the all-or-none principle (Box 2.4). After the stimulus goes above the threshold potential, more gated Na^+ ion channels are stimulated to open and allow more Na^+ ions to charge inside the cell. This causes rapid depolarization of the neuron and an action potential is created. In this state, the neuron continues to open Na^+ channels in response to voltage fluctuations all along the membrane (see Fig. 2.16C). Complete depolarization occurs and conduction of the action potential is transmitted along the neuron (see Propagation of Action Potential).

Repolarization

Repolarization occurs once the peak of the action potential is reached and the membrane potential begins to move back toward the resting potential (−70 mV). Surpassing the minimal threshold potential not only opens the Na^+ channels but also triggers the opening of the K^+ channels, which are slower to respond and do not begin to open until the inside of the cell becomes flooded with Na^+ ions and the nerve has reached a potential of approximately +30 mV (see Fig. 2.16D). Repolarization results from the rapid efflux of K^+ ions to an area of lower concentration out of the cell. The gated ion channels on the inside of the membrane open to allow the reversal process to begin repolarization and restoring electrical balance.

The *refractory period* (Box 2.5) is when the Na^+ and K^+ ions are returned to their original sides: Na^+ on the outside and K^+ on the inside. While the neuron is busy returning everything to normal, it resists any additional incoming stimuli. The interval during which a second action potential absolutely cannot be initiated to restimulate the membrane, no matter how large a stimulus is applied, is known as the absolute refractory period, which coincides with nearly the entire duration of the action potential. In neurons, it is caused by the inactivation of the Na^+ channels that originally opened to depolarize the membrane. These channels remain inactivated until the membrane repolarizes, after which they close, reactivate, and regain their ability to open in response to stimulus. The relative refractory period is the interval immediately after the absolute refractory period and before complete reestablishment to the resting state, during which initiation of a second action potential is *inhibited* but not impossible if a larger stimulus is achieved to produce successful firing. The return to the resting potential marks the end of the relative refractory period[3] (Fig. 2.17).

Return to Resting State

After the Na^+/K^+ pumps (see Fig. 2.15) return the ions to their rightful side of the neuron's cell membrane, the neuron is back to its normal polarized state of approximately −70 mV; the nerve is fully recovered and stays in the resting potential until another impulse comes along.

BOX 2.3 Action Potential

An *action potential,* also known as a *nerve impulse,* is a spike of positive and negative ionic discharge that travels along the membrane of a cell. The creation and conduction of action potentials represent a fundamental means of communication in the nervous system. Action potentials represent rapid reversals in voltage across the plasma membrane of axons. These rapid reversals are mediated by voltage-gated ion channels found in the *plasma membrane.* The action potential travels from one location in the cell to another, but *ion flow* across the membrane occurs only at the nodes of Ranvier. As a result, the action potential signal jumps along the axon, from node to node, rather than propagating smoothly, as it does in axons that lack a myelin sheath. The clustering of voltage-gated sodium and potassium ion channels at the nodes permits this behavior.

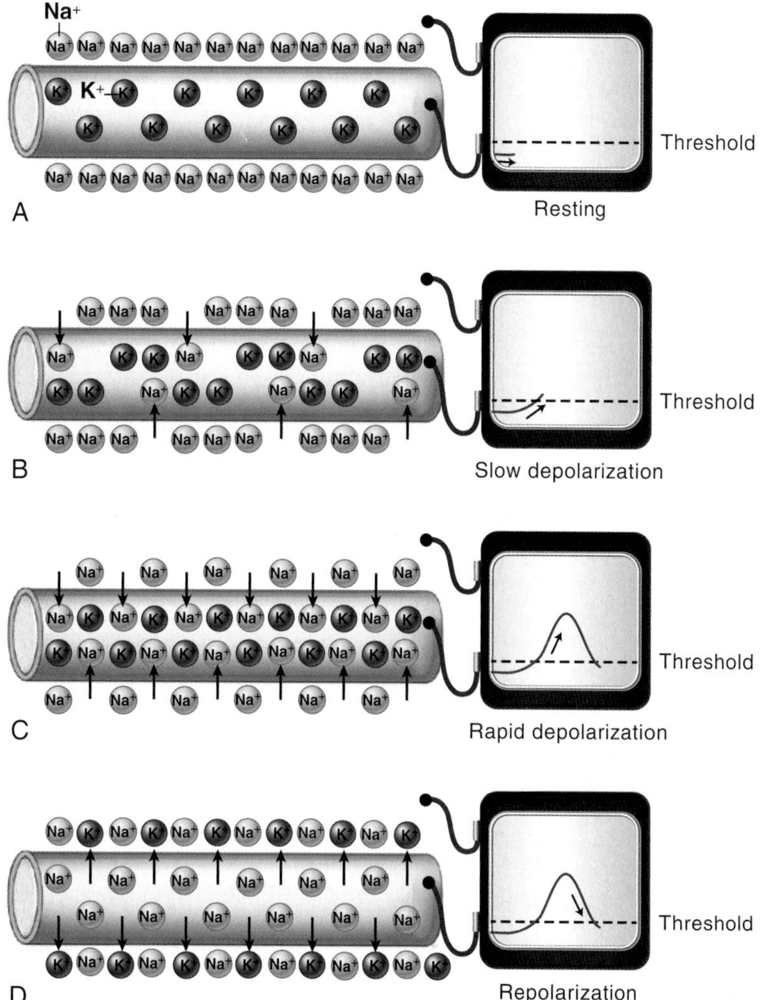

Fig. 2.16 Depolarization and repolarization. (A) Resting membrane potential results from an excess of positive ions on the outer surface of the plasma membrane while the electrical charge on the inside of the membrane is negative. More sodium (Na^+) ions are on the outside of the membrane than potassium (K^+) ions are on the inside of the membrane. (B) Slow depolarization of a membrane occurs when a stimulus triggers the opening of Na^+ channels, allowing the Na^+ ions to slowly move to an area of lower concentration (and more negative charge) inside the cell. Slow depolarization will continue until the minimal firing threshold is achieved. (C) If the minimal firing threshold is achieved, more Na^+ channels open and more positive ions go charging inside the membrane reversing the polarity to an inside-positive state. (D) Repolarization of a membrane occurs when K^+ channels then open, allowing K^+ to move to an area of lower concentration (and more negative charge) outside of the cell. This begins the process of reversing the polarity back to an inside-negative state. (From Patton K, Thibodeau G: *Anatomy and physiology,* ed 21, St Louis, 2019, Elsevier.)

BOX 2.4 All-or-None Principle

Once a nerve is excited by the minimal threshold level (stimulus of sufficient magnitude to stimulate the nerve impulse), the impulse travels the full length of the fiber without additional stimulus. Impulse travels at the same speed from any stimulus that exceeds minimum threshold level. The conduction of nerve impulses is an example of an all-or-none response. In other words, if a neuron responds at all, then it must respond completely and will be no longer dependent on the stimulus to continue. Conduction of an impulse is self-propagating energy. Greater intensity of stimulation does not produce a stronger signal but can produce *more* impulses per second.

BOX 2.5 Refractory Periods

Absolute refractory period is the interval during which a second action potential absolutely cannot be initiated, no matter how large a stimulus is applied.

Relative refractory period is the interval immediately after the absolute refractory period, during which initiation of a second action potential is *inhibited* but not impossible if a larger stimulus is applied.

Fig. 2.16 illustrates the depolarization and repolarization mechanisms, and Table 2.1 describes the steps of the mechanism that produce an action potential. Nerve conduction requires only 1 ms to respond to a minimal threshold stimulus and recover (Fig. 2.18).

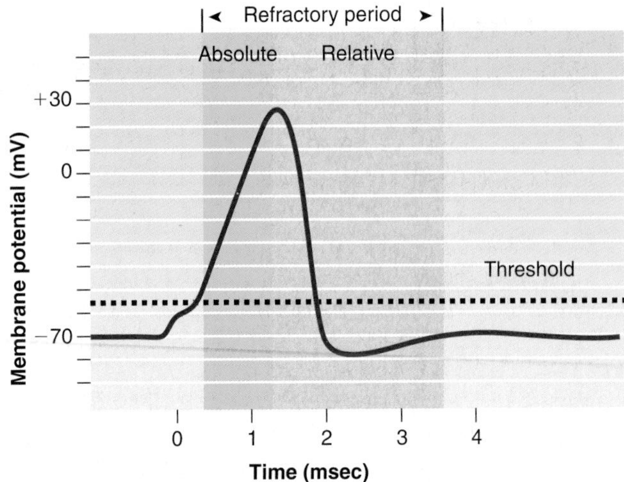

Fig. 2.17 Refractory period. During the absolute refractory period, the membrane will not respond to any stimulus. During the relative refractory period, however, a very strong stimulus may elicit a response in the membrane. (From Patton K, Thibodeau G: *Anatomy and physiology*, ed 21, St Louis, 2019, Elsevier.)

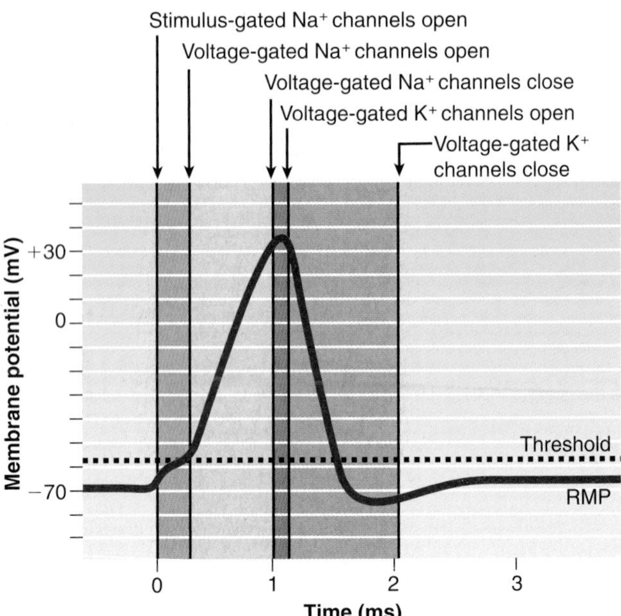

Fig. 2.18 Action potential in a neuron. Schematic of an electrophysiologic recording of an action potential showing the various phases that occur as the wave passes a point on the cell membrane. Each voltmeter records the changing membrane potential as a redline. *RMP,* Resting membrane potential. (Modified from Patton K, Thibodeau G: *Anatomy and physiology*, ed 21, St Louis, 2019, Elsevier.)

TABLE 2.1 Steps to the Mechanism That Produces an Action Potential

Steps	Description
1	The membrane is in its resting state and is polarized. Na^+ ions are predominately in the extracellular fluid, and K^+ ions are predominately in the intracellular fluid. The electrical potential of the nerve axoplasm is approximately −70 mV.
2	A stimulus triggers stimulus-gated Na^+ channels in axonal membrane to open and allows inward Na^+ diffusion. This causes the membrane to begin slow depolarization.
3	As the threshold potential is reached, it triggers an action potential (impulse), causing more voltage-gated Na^+ channels to open.
4	As more Na^+ enters the cell through voltage-gated Na^+ channels, the membrane rapidly depolarizes even further.
5	The magnitude of the action potential peaks (at +30 mV) when voltage-gated Na^+ channels close.
6	Repolarization begins when voltage-gated K^+ channels open, allowing outward diffusion of K^+.
7	After the absolute and relative refractory periods that occur during repolarization, the resting potential is restored by the Na^+/K^+ pump.

K^+, Potassium; *Na^+*, sodium.

Propagation of Action Potential

After a stimulus meets the threshold potential (see Box 2.1) and produces an action potential causing a reversal of polarity of the RMP, the current flow triggers the voltage-gated Na^+ channel in the next segment of the membrane to open and depolarize. As Na^+ ions rush inward, the next segment receives the action potential. Because an action potential is an all-or-none response (see Box 2.4), the height of each nerve impulse is the same as it depolarizes the next segment of the membrane, and so on. This ensures that the nerve impulse will travel the full length of the nerve fiber at its initial strength and will not weaken. The action potential always moves forward on an axon in a one-way movement and is never able to move backward to restimulate the region from which it just came. It is prevented from moving backward because the previous segment of the membrane remains in the refractory period for too long to allow restimulation[3] (Fig. 2.19).

When an impulse travels down an axon covered by a myelin sheath, the action potential (impulse) must move between nodes of Ranvier (uninsulated gaps; see Box 2.2) that exist between each Schwann cell (Fig. 2.20A). The myelination and its nodes of Ranvier enable an especially rapid mode of electrical impulse propagation called *saltatory conduction* (Fig. 2.20B and Box 2.6). Saltatory conduction (from the Latin *saltare,* to hop or leap) is the propagation of action potentials along myelinated axons from one node of Ranvier to the next node, opening the stimulus-gated channels and allowing Na^+ ions to rush into the cell, causing depolarization. This process increases the conduction velocity of action potentials without needing to increase the diameter of an axon[1-3] (Fig. 2.21A).

When an impulse travels down an axon with unmyelinated fibers, impulses move continuously as waves called *action potential conduction.* Action potential conduction moves impulses at a much slower rate compared with myelinated nerve fibers. Ion diffusion occurs all along the nerve fiber through minute pores in the nerve sheath. Therefore diffusion of electrolytes must occur all along the nerve cell membrane instead of jumping from node to node, causing these impulses to travel much slower than those traveling along a myelinated nerve sheath (Fig. 2.21B).

How fast does a nerve fiber conduct an impulse? It depends on the presence or absence of a myelin sheath and the diameter of the nerve

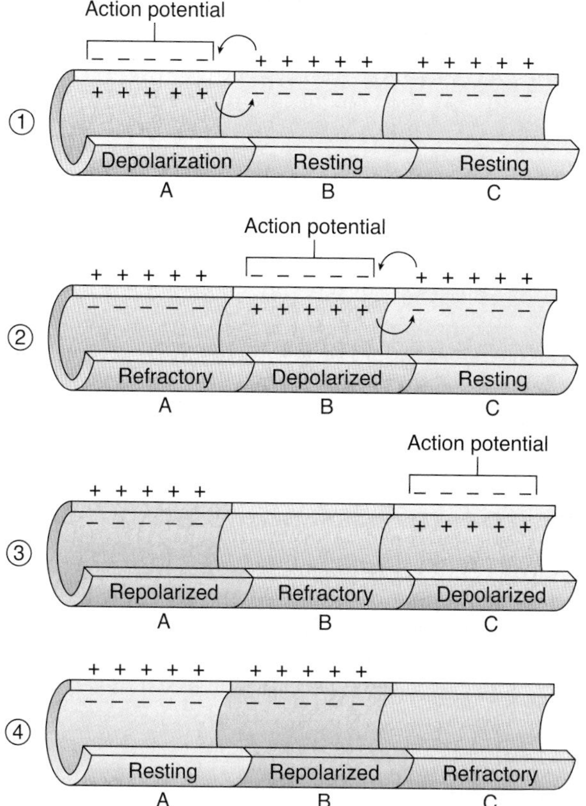

Fig. 2.19 Impulse propagation. This image shows the four stages of nerve conduction, and how the all-or-none firing (see Box 2.4) moves the nerve impulse at the same height as it depolarizes the next segment of the membrane without an additional stimulus. (1A) Action potential (nerve impulse) moves between active (*depolarized*) segment and resting (*polarized*) segment (1B) because depolarization reverses the membrane potential. (2) The previously resting membrane segment (1B) is now depolarized (2B), setting up new current flows between it and the next membrane segment. The previously depolarized nerve segment (1A) is on the road back to repolarization, leaving it refractory (2A). The impulse can only move forward, as retrograde propagation is prevented by inexcitable (*refractory*) membrane. (3) The wave of depolarization has advanced to another segment (3C) always trailed by a refractory membrane segment (3B). The left-most membrane segment (3A) has repolarized and is once again in its resting state (4A) ready to conduct a fresh impulse. (Modified from de Jong RH: *Local anesthetics*, St Louis, 1994, Mosby.)

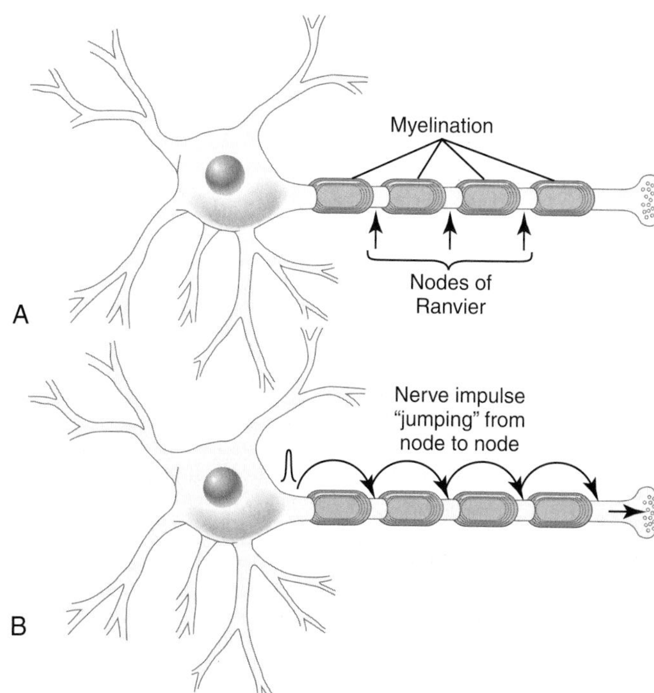

Fig. 2.20 Saltatory conduction. These diagrams show the insulating nature of the myelin sheath preventing ion movement everywhere but at the nodes of Ranvier (A). (B) The action potential at one node triggers current flow *(arrows)* across the myelin sheath to the next node, producing an action potential there. The action potential thus seems to "leap" rapidly from node to node.

BOX 2.6 Saltatory Conduction

Because an axon can be unmyelinated or myelinated, the action potential has two methods to travel down the axon. These methods are referred to as *action potential conduction* for unmyelinated axons and *saltatory conduction* for myelinated axons. Saltatory conduction is defined as an action potential moving in discrete jumps down a myelinated axon. This process is outlined as the charge passively spreading to the next node of Ranvier to depolarize it to threshold, which will then trigger an action potential in this region and then passively spread to the next node and so on. Saltatory conduction provides two advantages over action potential conduction that occurs along an axon without myelin sheaths. First, it saves energy by decreasing the use of sodium/potassium pumps in the axonal membrane. Second, the increased speed afforded by this mode of conduction ensures faster interaction among neurons.

fiber. In general, the larger the diameter of the nerve fiber, the faster it conducts impulses. Moreover, myelinated nerve fibers conduct faster impulses because salutatory conduction is more rapid than continuous conduction of unmyelinated nerves.

Synaptic Transmission

A nerve conveys information, carried by neurons, in the form of electrochemical impulses (known as nerve impulses or action potentials). The impulses rapidly travel from one neuron to another by crossing a synapse; the message is converted from electrical to chemical and then back to electrical (Fig. 2.22).

For the impulse to cross the synapse to another cell, it requires the actions of either electrical synapses or chemical synapses. Electrical synapses occur where two cells are joined end-to-end by gap junctions (Fig. 2.23A).[2,3] Action potentials can easily continue along the postsynaptic membrane because the plasma membrane and cytoplasm are functionally continuous in this type of junction.

Chemical synapses use chemical transmitters called **neurotransmitters**, which are packaged into synaptic vesicles that cluster beneath the membrane on the presynaptic side of a neuron. The neurotransmitters are discharged with the arrival of the action potential to send a signal from the presynaptic cell to the postsynaptic cell (Fig. 2.23B). These endogenous neurotransmitters transmit signals from a neuron to a target cell across the synapse. Neurotransmitters cause ion channels to open or close in the second cell, prompting changes in the excitability of that cell's membrane. Excitatory neurotransmitters such as acetylcholine and norepinephrine (in most organs) make it more likely that an action potential will be triggered in the second cell, causing depolarization (Fig. 2.24). Neurotransmitters are either destroyed by specific enzymes, diffused away, or reabsorbed by the neuron.

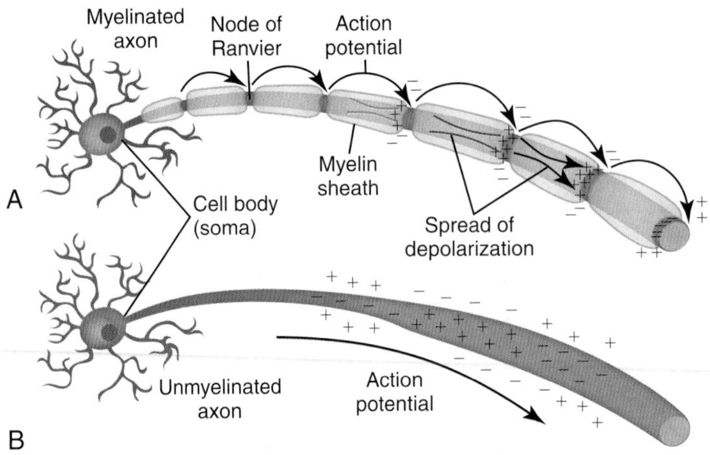

Fig. 2.21 Impulse propagation along a myelinated axon compared with an unmyelinated axon. (A) Myelinated axon allows a rapid propagation of the action potential by leaping from one node of Ranvier to the next node (called saltatory conduction). (B) Unmyelinated axon provides a much slower propagation of the action potential all along the nerve fiber (called action potential conduction).

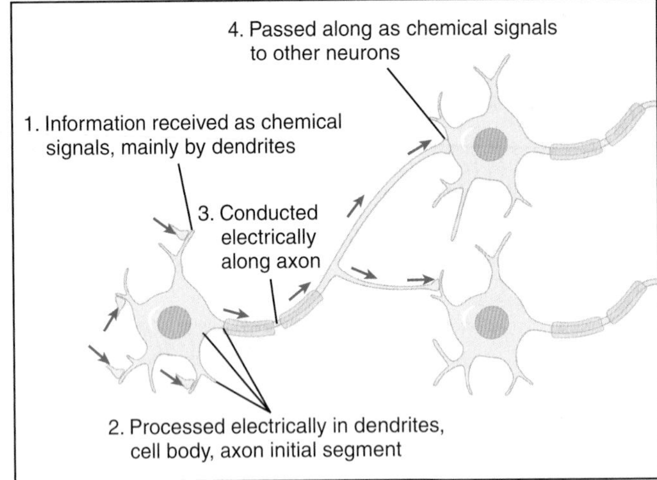

Fig. 2.22 Spread of electrical signals within a neuron and the use of chemical signals to transfer information from one neuron to another. (From Nolte J: *Elsevier's integrated neuroscience*, St Louis, 2007, Mosby.)

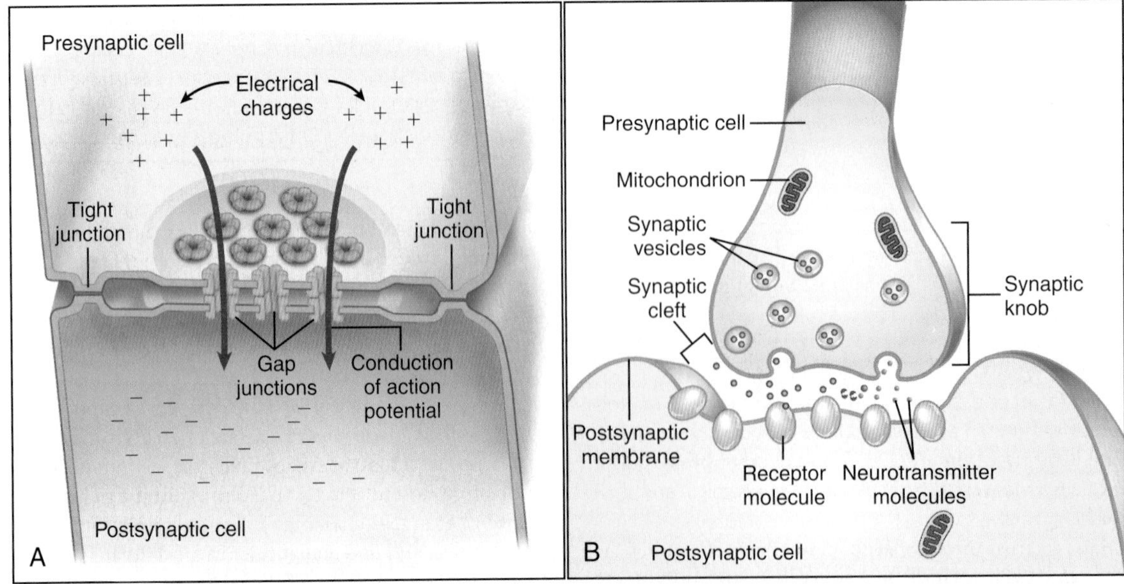

Fig. 2.23 Electrical and chemical synapses. (A) Electrical synapses involve gap junctions that allow action potentials to move from cell to cell directly by allowing electrical current to flow between cells. (B) Chemical synapses involve transmitter chemicals (neurotransmitters) that signal postsynaptic cells, possibly inducing an action potential. (From Patton K, Thibodeau G: *Anatomy and physiology*, ed 21, St Louis, 2019, Elsevier.)

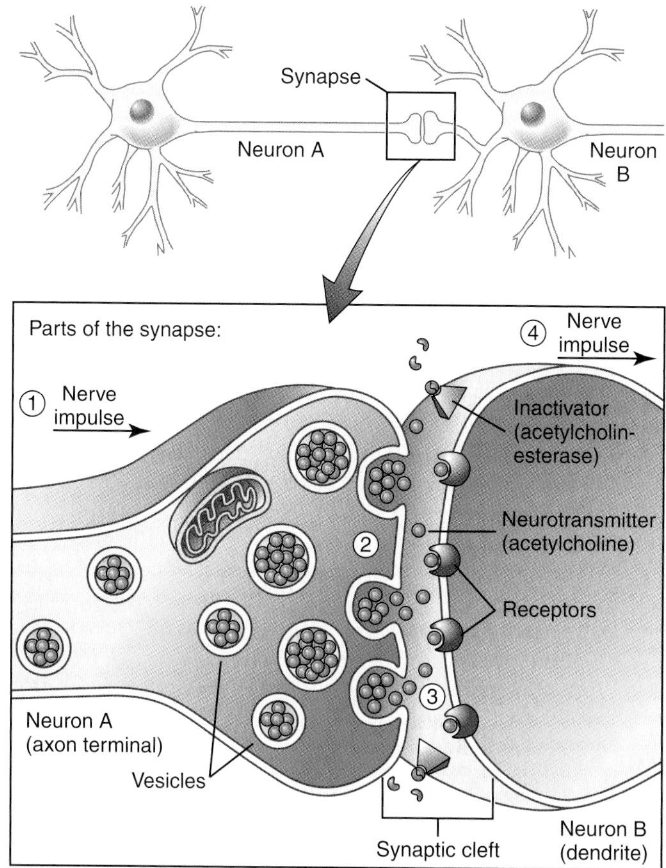

Fig. 2.24 Chemical synapse. Diagram shows detail of synaptic knob, or axon terminal, of presynaptic neuron, the plasma membrane of a postsynaptic neuron, and a synaptic cleft. On the arrival of an action potential at a synaptic knob, voltage-gated calcium (Ca^{++}) channels open and allow extracellular Ca^{++} to diffuse into the presynaptic cell (step 1). In step 2, the Ca^{++} triggers the rapid exocytosis of neurotransmitter molecules from vesicles in the knob. In step 3, neurotransmitter diffuses into the synaptic cleft and binds to receptor molecules in the plasma membrane of the postsynaptic neuron. In step 4, the local potential may move toward the axon, where an action potential may begin. (From Herlihy B: *The human body in health and illness*, ed 6, St Louis, 2018, Elsevier.)

MODE OF ACTION OF LOCAL ANESTHETICS

Local anesthetic drugs act mainly by inhibiting Na^+ influx through Na^+ specific ion channels in the neuronal cell membrane; in particular the so-called *voltage-gated sodium channels.* When the influx of Na^+ is interrupted, an action potential cannot arise, and signal conduction is inhibited. The receptor site is thought to be located at the cytoplasmic (axoplasmic, inner) portion of the Na^+ channel. Local anesthetic drugs bind more readily to Na^+ channels in an activated state; thus onset of neuronal blockade is faster in neurons that are rapidly firing. This is referred to as state dependent blockade (see Chapter 3 and Fig. 3.8).[2]

All nerve fibers are sensitive to local anesthetics, but generally, those with a smaller diameter tend to be more sensitive than larger fibers. Local anesthetics block conduction in the following order: small myelinated axons (e.g., those carrying nociceptive impulses), nonmyelinated axons, and then large myelinated axons. Thus a differential block can be achieved (i.e., pain sensation is blocked more readily than other sensory modalities). In myelinated nerves, the local anesthetic blocks only at the nodes of Ranvier. Because of the excess current available in saltatory conduction (10 times more), at least two to three adjacent nodes must be blocked to ensure total block to the nerve. The larger the diameter of the nerve fiber, the greater the amount of local anesthetic needed to prevent depolarization (inferior alveolar [IA] and posterior superior alveolar [PSA] blocks require more anesthetic for successful nerve blockage than supraperiosteal injections).[2] In-depth discussion on the mode of action of local anesthetics will be presented in Chapter 3.

DENTAL HYGIENE CONSIDERATIONS

- When a local anesthetic is administered, it diffuses through the nerve to the mantle bundles (outer core) at a higher concentration first and then to the core bundles (inner core) at a more diluted concentration. Because the mantle bundles are affected by the local anesthetic first, these bundles also begin to lose anesthesia before the core bundles. However, as the local anesthetic from the core bundles diffuses to the mantel bundles, this causes the mantel bundles to remain anesthetized the longest (see Chapter 3).
- Large nerve trunks (such as the inferior alveolar [IA] and posterior superior alveolar [PSA] nerves) are myelinated A fibers and require more local anesthetic volume to successfully block the core fibers.

CASE STUDY 2.1 A Patient Complains of Inadequate Anesthesia

A patient is in the office for nonsurgical periodontal therapy of the mandibular right quadrant. The dental hygienist anesthetizes the mandibular right quadrant using an inferior alveolar block and buccal block, and she administers one cartridge of anesthetic. When the dental hygienist begins scaling, the patient informs her that he feels numb in general, but not completely numb, especially on the anterior teeth and soft tissue.

Critical Thinking Questions

- What could be the reason for the patient not feeling completely numb?
- Why does the patient feel more sensitivity on the anterior teeth and adjacent soft tissue?
- How should the dental hygienist respond to this situation?

CHAPTER REVIEW QUESTIONS

1. The threshold potential is the minimum magnitude needed to initiate an action potential. An action potential will trigger the opening of the voltage-gated sodium (Na^+) ion channel to cause rapid depolarization.
   A. Both statements are correct.
   B. Both statements are NOT correct.
   C. The first statement is correct; the second statement is NOT correct.
   D. The first statement is NOT correct; the second statement is correct.

2. Which fibers are the principle fibers in the transmission of sharp, bright dental pain?
   A. Aδ fibers
   B. B fibers
   C. C fibers
   D. Aβ fibers
   E. Aγ fibers
3. Local anesthetics work by:
   A. Penetrating the nerve to inhibit Cl^- influx
   B. Penetrating the nerve to inhibit Na^+ influx
   C. Penetrating the nerve to inhibit K^+ efflux
   D. Penetrating the nerve to inhibit Na^+ efflux
   E. Penetrating the nerve to inhibit K^+ influx
4. Local anesthetics mostly have their effect on myelinated nerves in which way?
   A. All along the nerve membrane
   B. Mostly at the synapse
   C. Mostly at the cell bodies
   D. Mostly at the node of Ranvier
5. Type A fibers comprise the most rapidly conducting axons. The minimal threshold stimulus required to excite a C fiber will also be sufficient to stimulate an A fiber.
   A. Both statements are correct.
   B. Both statements are NOT correct.
   C. The first statement is correct; the second statement is NOT correct.
   D. The first statement is NOT correct; the second statement is correct.
6. When energy for conduction is derived from the nerve cell membrane itself and is no longer dependent on the stimulus for continuance, the conduction is considered to be:
   A. Below the minimal threshold level
   B. Above the minimal threshold level
   C. Self-propagating
   D. In the absolute refractory period
7. The absolute refractory period occurs during the fraction of a millisecond when a nerve fiber can be excited only by a much stronger stimulus than the initial stimulus. The relative refractory period is the interval during which a second action potential absolutely cannot be initiated to restimulate the membrane, no matter how large a stimulus is applied.
   A. Both statements are correct.
   B. Both statements are NOT correct.
   C. The first statement is correct; the second statement is NOT correct.
   D. The first statement is NOT correct; the second statement is correct.
8. Saltatory conduction refers to:
   A. Rapid transmission of nerve impulses along a myelinated nerve fiber
   B. Diffusion of sodium chloride into the nerve cell during impulse conduction
   C. Conduction of an impulse along a nonmyelinated nerve at the nodes of Ranvier
   D. The movement of continuous waves along a nerve fiber
9. What is the type of glial cell located in the peripheral nervous system?
   A. Astrocyte
   B. Microglia
   C. Ependymal
   D. Oligodendrocyte
   E. Schwann
10. Myelin (lipoprotein sheath) is composed of:
    A. Approximately 75% lipid, 20% protein, and 5% carbohydrate
    B. Approximately 60% lipid, 35% protein, and 5% carbohydrate
    C. Approximately 65% lipid, 30% protein, and 5% carbohydrate
    D. 100% lipid
11. The sympathetic division is involved with the "rest or digest" response. The parasympathetic division is known as the "fight-or-flight" response.
    A. Both statements are correct.
    B. Both statements are NOT correct.
    C. The first statement is correct; the second statement is NOT correct.
    D. The first statement is NOT correct; the second statement is correct.
12. The afferent division consists of all *incoming* information traveling along sensory or afferent pathways. The efferent division consists of all *outgoing* information along motor or efferent pathways.
    A. Both statements are correct.
    B. Both statements are NOT correct.
    C. The first statement is correct; the second statement is NOT correct.
    D. The first statement is NOT correct; the second statement is correct.
13. What is the term for the outer layer of the myelin sheath that wraps the entire nerve?
    A. Endoneurium
    B. Schwann cell
    C. Epineurium
    D. Perineurium
14. The axon hillock:
    A. Is where the majority of input to the neuron occurs
    B. Is not involved in impulse transmission
    C. Is where neurotransmitter chemicals are released for possible reception by a nearby neuron
    D. Decides whether to send the impulse further down the axon
15. In a resting neuron, what positive ion is most abundant *outside* the plasma membrane?
    A. Potassium
    B. Sodium
    C. Calcium
    D. Chloride
16. In a resting neuron, what positive ion is most abundant *inside* the plasma membrane?
    A. Potassium
    B. Sodium
    C. Calcium
    D. Chloride
17. The electrical potential of nerve axoplasm in the resting state is approximately:
    A. -70 mV
    B. -30 mV
    C. Zero
    D. +30 mV
    E. +70 mV
18. Mantle bundles are located near the outside of the nerve and will be anesthetized first by a local anesthetic compared with core bundles that are located closer to the center of the nerve.
    A. Both statements are correct.
    B. Both statements are NOT correct.
    C. The first statement is correct; the second statement is NOT correct.
    D. The first statement is NOT correct; the second statement is correct.

19. Chemical synapses use chemical transmitters called:
    A. Neurotransmitters
    B. Chemical transmitters
    C. Synaptic transmitters
    D. Endogenous transmitters

20. The "all-or-none" principle occurs:
    A. With a spike of positive and negative ionic discharge
    B. In the interval during which a second action potential absolutely cannot be initiated
    C. Once a nerve is excited by the minimal threshold level
    D. Once a nerve is excited by a stimulus greater than the first stimulus

REFERENCES

1. Malamed S. *Handbook of local anesthesia.* ed 7. St Louis: Elsevier; 2020.
2. de Jong RH. *Local anesthetics.* St Louis: Mosby; 1994.
3. Patton K, Thibodeau G. *Anatomy and physiology.* ed 21. St Louis: Elsevier; 2019.
4. Liebgott B. *The anatomical basis of dentistry.* ed 4. St Louis: Mosby; 2018.
5. Nolte J. *Elsevier's integrated neuroscience.* St Louis: Mosby; 2007.
6. Castro A, Merchut MP, Neafsey E, Wurster R. *Neuroscience: an outline approach.* St Louis: Mosby; 2002.
7. Haines D. *Fundamental neuroscience for basic and clinical applications.* ed 3. St. Louis: Churchill Livingstone; 2006.
8. Hargreaves KM, Berman LH. *Cohen's pathways of the pulp.* ed 11. St Louis: Elsevier; 2016.
9. Daniel SJ, Harfst SA, Wilder RS. *Mosby's dental hygiene: concepts, cases and competencies.* ed 2. St Louis: Mosby; 2008.
10. Jastak T, Yagiela J, Donaldson D. *Local anesthesia of the oral cavity.* St Louis: Saunders; 1995.
11. Tasaki I. The electro-saltatory transmission of the nerve impulse and the effect of narcosis upon the nerve fiber. *Am J Physiol.* 1939;127:211–227.
12. Huxley AF, Stämpfli R. Evidence for saltatory conduction in peripheral myelinated nerve fibres. *J Physiol.* 1949;108:315–339.

ADDITIONAL RESOURCES

Bahl R. Local anesthesia in dentistry. *Anesth Prog.* 2004;51:138–142.

Becker D, Reed K. Essentials of local anesthetic pharmacology. American Dental Society of Anesthesiology. *Anesth Program.* 2006;53:98–109.

Haveles B. *Applied pharmacology for the dental hygienist.* ed 8. St Louis: Elsevier; 2020.

PART 2

Local and Topical Anesthetic Agents

CHAPTER 3 Pharmacology of Local Anesthetic Agents, 29

CHAPTER 4 Pharmacology of Vasoconstrictors, 43

CHAPTER 5 Local Anesthetic Agents, 53

APPENDIX 5.1 Summary of Amide Local Anesthetic Agents and Vasoconstrictors, 79

CHAPTER 6 Topical Anesthetic Agents, 80

3

Pharmacology of Local Anesthetic Agents

Demetra Daskalos Logothetis, RDH, MS

LEARNING OBJECTIVES

1. Define local anesthetics.
2. Describe the mechanism of actions of local anesthetics.
3. Describe the structure of local anesthetics.
4. Discuss the difference between esters and amides.
5. Discuss the properties and ionization factors of local anesthetics.
6. Discuss the two major routes of delivery of local anesthetics.
7. Describe pH and the dissociation constant (pK_a), as well as their effects on the onset of action of local anesthetics.
8. Discuss how infection in the area of local anesthetic administration decreases its efficiency.
9. Discuss the advantages of buffering local anesthetics prior to injection.
10. Discuss the buffering process of local anesthetics.
11. Describe the differences between the membrane expansion theory and the specific protein receptor theory.
12. Discuss the pharmacokinetics of local anesthetics, including onset of action, induction, duration, absorption, distribution, metabolism (biotransformation) of both esters and amides, and excretion.
13. Discuss the systemic effects of local anesthetic drugs on the central nervous system and cardiovascular system.

INTRODUCTION

Local anesthetics are agents that block the sensation of pain by reversibly blocking nerve conduction when applied to a circumscribed area of the body. Local anesthetics interrupt neural conduction by interfering with the propagation of peripheral nerve impulses, thus inhibiting the influx of sodium ions during depolarization.

In most cases, this follows the anesthetic's diffusion through the neural membrane into the axoplasm, where the ionized RNH^+ anesthetic molecules enter sodium channels and prevent them from assuming an active or "open" state. Local anesthetics block the conduction of a nerve impulse by preventing the nerve from reaching its firing potential. Local anesthetics bind to specific receptors in the nerve membrane to prevent the influx of sodium ions through the cell membrane. As long as the anesthetic remains bound to the receptor sites, the conduction of nerve impulses is prevented. If this process can be inhibited for just a few nodes of Ranvier along the axon, then nerve impulses generated further down on the axon from the blocked nodes cannot propagate to the ganglion. To accomplish this process, the anesthetic molecules must enter through the cell membrane of the nerve and are dependent on the potency, time of onset, and duration of the local anesthetic agent.

The use of reversible local anesthetic chemical agents is the most common method to secure pain control in dental practice. Box 3.1 describes the properties of ideal local anesthetics. None of the local anesthetics that are available for use in dentistry today meet all of these properties, although they are clinically acceptable.

CHEMISTRY

Local anesthetic agents are divided chemically into two major groups: the esters and the amides. The clinical significance of the two major groups is the potential for allergic reactions and the route of biotransformation. **Ester local anesthetics** have a high probability of producing an allergic reaction compared with amide local anesthetics. With ester local anesthetics, a patient who has an allergic reaction to one ester agent is likely to experience hypersensitivity to all ester anesthetics. This is less likely to occur within the **amide local anesthetic** group. Cross-hypersensitivity between esters and amides is unlikely. As a result of the high degree of hypersensitivity to injectable esters, all injectable local anesthetics manufactured for dentistry today are in the amide group. Ester local anesthetics are hydrolyzed in the plasma by the enzyme pseudocholinesterase, and amide local anesthetics are biotransformed generally in the liver. Topical anesthetics are available in both the esters and amides (see Chapter 6).

The local anesthetic molecule consists of three components: (1) the **lipophilic aromatic ring**, (2) **intermediate hydrocarbon** ester or amide chain, and (3) **hydrophilic terminal amine** (Fig. 3.1). The lipophilic aromatic ring improves the lipid solubility of the molecule, which facilitates the penetration of the anesthetic through the lipid-rich membrane where the receptor sites are located. The greater the lipid solubility of the anesthetic molecule, the greater the potency of the drug. For example, the local anesthetic bupivacaine is more lipid-soluble than lidocaine, and it is therefore more potent because more of the anesthetic dose can enter the neurons. Because bupivacaine is more lipid-soluble and is more potent than lidocaine, it is prepared as a 0.5% concentration (5 mg/mL) rather than a 2% concentration of lidocaine (20 mg/mL).

The intermediate hydrocarbon chain determines whether the molecule is an ester or amide, and this chain is important because it predetermines the course of biotransformation. Ester local anesthetics are hydrolyzed by appropriate esterases, and amide local anesthetics generally require enzymatic breakdown by the liver.

The hydrophilic terminal amine may exist in a tertiary form (three bonds) that is uncharged and lipid-soluble (or base **anion** form) or as a quaternary form (four bonds) that is positively charged and renders

BOX 3.1 Properties of the Ideal Local Anesthetic

Potent local anesthesia
Reversible local anesthesia
Absence of local reactions
Absence of systemic reactions
Absence of allergic reactions
Rapid onset
Satisfactory duration
Adequate tissue penetration
Low cost
Stability in solution (long shelf life)
Ease of metabolism and excretion

the molecule water-soluble (or acid cation form), which is how it is delivered from the dental hygienist's syringe into the patient's tissue. As explained earlier, the aromatic ring determines the actual degree of lipid solubility, but the terminal amine acts as an "on-off" switch, allowing the local anesthetic to exist in either lipid-soluble or water-soluble configurations. Once the anesthetic is injected into the tissue of normal pH, the quaternary amine with its four hydrogen bonds dissociates into an uncharged tertiary amine base (three hydrogen bonds) and a hydrogen ion to penetrate the lipid-rich nerve membrane. The tertiary amine, after penetration of the nerve membrane, will once again gain a hydrogen ion found within the axoplasm to convert back to its ionized form (quaternary amine) that will successfully bind to the receptor sites. The tertiary and quaternary forms exhibit vital roles in the sequence of events leading to the conduction block[1] (discussed later; see Pharmacodynamics of Local Anesthetic Drugs and Fig. 3.1).

ROUTES OF DELIVERY

There are two major routes of delivery of local anesthetic drugs, topical and submucosal injection. Topical anesthetics are drugs applied to the surface of mucosal tissue that produce local insensibility to pain. Topical anesthetic agents are prepared in higher concentrations than injectable anesthetics to facilitate diffusion of the drug through the mucous membranes. Because of this, there is a risk for toxicity if large amounts of topical anesthetics are applied to limited areas (see Chapter 6). In contrast, submucosal injections of local anesthetics are more effective than topical routes of administration because the local anesthetic solution is injected and placed in close proximity to the nerve trunk of the area to be anesthetized. This allows the solution to more effectively reach the nerve.

PHARMACODYNAMICS OF LOCAL ANESTHETIC DRUGS

Pharmacodynamics refers to the physiologic effects of drugs on the body and the mechanisms of drug action and the relationship between drug concentration and effect. Synthetic local anesthetics are prepared

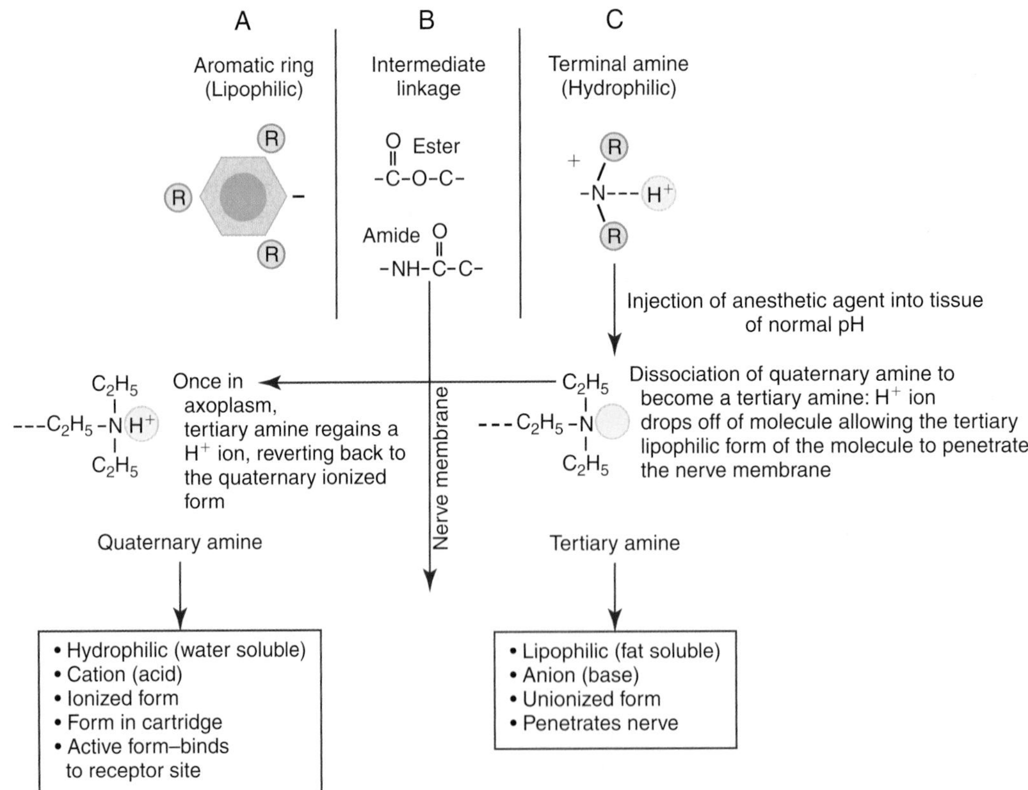

Fig. 3.1 Local anesthetic structure. All local anesthetics consist of three principal components. (A) The aromatic ring is the lipophilic (base) portion of the molecule that improves the lipid solubility and facilitates penetration of the anesthetic through the lipophilic nerve and determines the anesthetic potency. (B) The intermediate chain determines whether the local anesthetic is an ester or an amide. (C) The terminal amine is the hydrophilic (acid) portion of the molecule; it is the active form in the cartridge and binds to the receptor sites on the nerve membrane. To bind to the receptor sites, it must first dissociate (H^+ ion drops off) to a tertiary amine after injection into the tissue, of normal pH, to become lipid soluble and penetrate the nerve membrane. Upon nerve penetration, it will regain a H^+ ion found within the axoplasm, creating the ionized form necessary to bind to the receptor sites.

$$C_6H_5-NHC(=O)-R-N< + H^+ \rightleftharpoons C_6H_5-NHC(=O)-R-N^+- \quad (pK_a,\ pH)$$

or written simply as

$$RNH^+ \rightleftharpoons RN + H^+$$

Salt	Free base
• Crystalline solids	• Viscid liquids or amorphous solids
• Water soluble (hydrophilic)	• Fat soluble (lipophilic)
• Stable	• Unstable
• Acidic	• Alkaline
• Charged, cation (ionized)	• Uncharged, nonionized
• Active form at site of action	• Penetrates nerve tissue
• Form present in dental cartridge (pH 3.3–6.0)	• Form present in tissue (pH 7.4)

Fig. 3.2 Properties of base and salt forms of local anesthetics. (Modified from Haveles B: *Applied pharmacology for the dental hygienist,* ed 6, St Louis, 2017, Elsevier.)

as weak bases and, during manufacturing, precipitate as powdered unstable solids that are poorly soluble in water. They are combined with an acid to form a salt (hydrochloride salt) to render them water-soluble; these can be dissolved in sterile water or saline, creating a stable, injectable anesthetic solution. The molecules exist primarily in a quaternary water-soluble state in the cartridge. In the cartridge, the solution contains an equilibrium of positively charged (ionized) molecules, the acid or cation (RNH^+)[1,2] and uncharged (unionized) molecules, the base or anion (RN).[1,2] The formula $RNH^+ \leftrightarrow RN + H^+$ represents the equilibrium between the two ions and H^+ as the hydrogen ion[1-3] (Fig. 3.2). The equilibrium is dependent on the pH of the solution and the dissociation constant (pK_a)(how easily the compound becomes charged) (discussed next; also see Box 3.2).

When the pK_a equals the pH, there is an equal distribution of charged cations (acidic) and uncharged anions (basic) molecules. If there is a high presence of H^+ ions, the equilibrium shifts to the left and the anesthetic solution will have higher concentrations of the ionized (charged) cationic form (water-soluble), which is the active form of the molecule ($RNH^+ > RN + H^+$). In contrast, if the presence of H^+ ions is decreased, the equilibrium shifts to the right and the anesthetic solution will have a higher concentration of unionized (uncharged) free base form (fat-soluble), which is the form that penetrates the nerve membrane ($RNH^+ < RN + H^+$).

The pH (the acid-base balance) of the solution is manipulated by the manufacturer to complement the specific molecular structure of each anesthetic. However, all local anesthetic solutions are acidic prior to injection. The lower the pH, the more acidic the solution, and the higher the pH, the more alkaline (basic) the solution. Local anesthetic solutions without vasoconstrictors have a pH of approximately 6.5; generally, preparations with vasoconstrictors are more acidic than plain formulations because of the presence of the preservative (antioxidant) sodium bisulfite (see Chapter 4), and the pH ranges from approximately 3.0 to 5.5.[4] Once injected, the hydrophilic (ionized) cation component, which is acidic, facilitates diffusion through the extracellular fluid to the nerve. However, the cation form will not penetrate the nerve. Therefore the time of onset of the local anesthetic is based on the proportion of the molecule that converts to the tertiary, lipid-soluble (unionized) base structure when exposed to the normal physiologic pH (7.4) of the body. Once injected into the tissue (pH 7.4), the amount of local anesthetic in the free base unionized form will increase to provide greater lipid penetration of the nerve. The increase in the base molecules is caused by the dissociation of the H^+ ion from the quaternary molecule, now rendering it a tertiary-base molecule that can penetrate the nerve. The dissociation constant (pK_a) for the anesthetic predicts the proportion of molecules that exist in each of these states. By definition, the pK_a of a molecule represents the pH at which 50% of the molecules exist in the lipid-soluble tertiary anionic (uncharged base) form and 50% in the quaternary water-soluble cationic (charged acid) form[3] (see Box 3.2). As the pH of the tissue differs from the pK_a of the specific drug, more of the drug exists either in its charged or uncharged form. This is expressed in the Henderson-Hasselbalch equation: $pK_a - pH = \log [RH^+] / [R]$ where [R] is the concentration of unionized (uncharged) drug and $[RH^+]$ is the concentration of ionized (charged) drug. This is important because the molecular form of the anesthetic that allows diffusion through the lipid-rich nerve membrane is the free base (RN, anionic) portion of the molecule. Once the free base of the molecule reaches the axoplasm inside the nerve membrane, the amine gains a hydrogen ion and reverts back to the ionized quaternary (cationic) form (RNH^+), the active form of the molecule that binds to the receptor site, preventing the influx of sodium during depolarization (see Figs. 3.1 and 3.3).

Because the pH of the body tissue is 7.4, the ideal pK_a of an anesthetic should be 7.4, indicating that 50% of the molecules are uncharged base, and quick diffusion through the lipid membrane would occur. However, the pK_a of all local anesthetics has values greater than 7.5 (except topical benzocaine, which is 3.5), and has a pH of approximately 6.5 in plain solutions and lower with vasoconstrictors; therefore a greater proportion of the molecules exists in the quaternary water-soluble form when injected into tissue having normal pH of 7.4.[1,2] The higher the pK_a of the anesthetic, the lower the concentration of uncharged base molecules. This causes slower diffusion into the nerve cell and a slower onset of action of the local anesthetic. Table 3.1 lists

BOX 3.2 Dissociation Constant (pK_a)

The pK_a of a molecule represents the pH at which 50% of the molecules exist in the lipid-soluble tertiary form and 50% in the quaternary, water-soluble form. It is the proportion of cation to base molecules when manufactured.

Higher pK_a = Fewer base molecules = Slower onset of action
Lower pK_a = More base molecules = Rapid onset of action

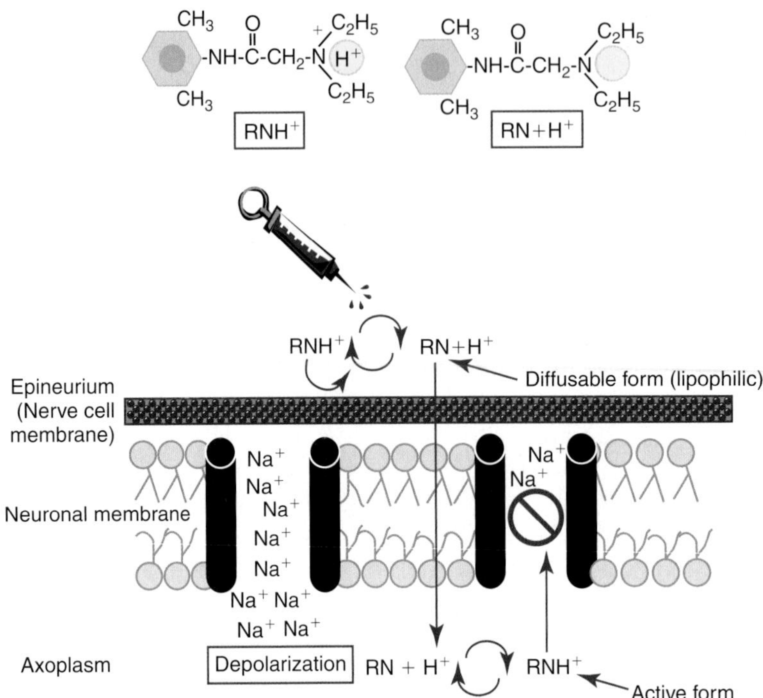

Fig. 3.3 Local anesthetic action. A local anesthetic exists in equilibrium as a quaternary salt (RNH^+) and tertiary base (RN). The proportion of each is determined by the pK_a of the anesthetic and the pH of the tissue. The lipid-soluble tertiary form (RN) is essential for penetration of both the epineurium and neuronal membrane. Once the molecule reaches the axoplasm of the neuron, the amine gains a hydrogen ion, and this ionized quaternary form (RNH^+) is responsible for the actual blockade of the sodium channel. Presumably, it binds within the sodium channel near the inner surface of the neuronal membrane, preventing depolarization.

factors affecting local anesthetic induction time and action, and Table 3.2 lists pK_a of commonly used local anesthetic drugs. As a consequence, the proportion of cations and base molecules are determined by the pH of the anesthetic, the pK_a of the anesthetic, and the pH of the tissue. In addition, the uncharged tertiary amine base and the positively charged quaternary amine cation each have different important biophysical characteristics that influence the ability of the local anesthetic to block the nerve impulse.

Infection in the Area of Injection

Tissue acidity, a result of many dental diseases, can impede the development of local anesthesia. The normal pH of the tissue is 7.4, and the solution in the cartridge is predominantly cationic (acidic). When the solution is injected into the tissue, the alkalinity of the tissue liberates the free base, allowing penetration of the local anesthetic molecule into the lipid-rich nerve. The acidic environment associated with an active infection causes a much lower tissue pH in the vicinity of 5 to 6,

TABLE 3.1 Characteristics Affecting Local Anesthetic Induction and Action

Characteristics	Action Affected	Explanation
Concentration of local anesthetic	Diffusion and onset	Higher concentration = molecules diffuse more readily through the nerve = rapid onset.
Dissociation constant (pK_a)	Onset	Determines the portion of administered dose in the lipid-soluble state (RN). Lower pK_a = more rapid the onset of action. More RN molecules are present to diffuse through the nerve, decreasing the time of onset. Higher pK_a = slower the onset of action. Less RN molecules are present to diffuse through the nerve, increasing the time of onset.
Lipid solubility	Potency	Greater lipid solubility enhances diffusion through the nerve, allowing a lower effective dose.
Protein binding	Duration	Increased protein binding allows more cations (RNH^+) to bind to the receptor sites within the sodium channels, prolonging the presence of anesthetic at the site of action. Bupivacaine is a good example of this characteristic.
Perineurium thickness	Onset	Perineurium binds individual neurons together to form fasciculi. The thicker the perineurium, the slower the rate of diffusion and onset of action.
Nonnervous tissue diffusibility	Onset	Increased diffusibility = decreased time of onset.
Vasodilator activity	Anesthetic potency and duration	Greater vasodilator activity = increased blood flow to region = rapid removal of anesthetic molecules from injection site; thus decreased anesthetic potency and decreased duration.

TABLE 3.2 Dissociation Constants (pK_a) of Commonly Used Local Anesthetic Drugs

Agent	pK_a	Percent Base (RN) at pH 7.4	Approximate Onset of Action (Min)
Lidocaine	7.7	29	3–5
Mepivacaine	7.6	33	3–5
Prilocaine	7.7 plain 7.9 w/VC	25	3–5
Articaine	7.8	29	1-3
Bupivacaine	8.1	17	6–10
Procaine	9.1	2	6–10
Topical benzocaine	3.5	100	>1
Topical tetracaine	8.6	7	10–15

Note: pK_a values for commonly used local anesthetics may differ slightly in different studies.

which favors the quaternary water-soluble configuration, and the amount of free base is reduced even further, leaving fewer base molecules to penetrate the nerve. This is one reason why it is difficult to achieve dental anesthesia when infection is present. Other factors for failure of anesthesia are edema and the increase in inflammation associated with infections. The selection of an anesthetic with a lower pK_a that has more base molecules in the cartridge, such as mepivacaine (pK_a, 7.7), would most likely provide more effective anesthesia than bupivacaine (pK_a, 8.1) (see Fig. 3.4).

Buffering of Local Anesthetics

As discussed previously, local anesthetics are combined with an acid to form a salt (hydrochloride salt) to render them water-soluble, causing all local anesthetic solutions to be acidic before injection. This causes a slower than desired onset of pulpal anesthesia. Amide anesthetics have an onset of action between 3 and 5 minutes for soft tissue anesthesia; however, pulpal anesthesia develops more slowly.[5-7] Lai et al.[7] found that at 4 minutes after an inferior alveolar (IA) block with 2% lidocaine 1:100,000 epinephrine, 70% of patients achieved soft tissue anesthesia, and only 25% of patients achieved pulpal anesthesia. At 6 minutes, 85% achieved soft tissue anesthesia, and 40% achieved pulpal anesthesia. Another study by Kanaa et al.[8] found that after an IA block with 2% lidocaine 1:100,000 at 8 minutes, 93% had lip anesthesia, 52% had pulpal anesthesia of the first molar and first premolar, and only 27% had pulpal anesthesia of the lateral incisor. These studies demonstrate that the achievement of soft tissue anesthesia within a specific time frame does not assure pulpal anesthesia. Several clinical trials[8,9] studying the amount of time necessary to achieve profound pulpal anesthesia after an IA block with 2% lidocaine 1:100,000 determined that 60% of patients achieved pulpal anesthesia at 10 minutes with an increase to 67% at 15 minutes. These studies demonstrate that it is reasonable for a clinician to wait 10 to 15 minutes after the local anesthetic injections to assess the patient's level of anesthesia utilizing the standard method of delivery. Moreover, because of the acidic nature of the local anesthetic, there are several disadvantages, such as stinging or burning sensation on injection, postinjection tissue injury, and the reliability of local anesthetic action in the presence of infection and inflammation. The pH of the solution is important because it affects the way anesthetics work. After injection, tissue buffering raises the pH and a percentage of the drug dissociates to become free bases, the amount depending on the pK_a of the individual anesthetic, allowing the free base to penetrate the lipid-cell membrane to reach the interior of the axon where a portion of the anesthetic molecules reionizes. The reionized portion enters and plugs the sodium channels so that sodium ions cannot depolarize. As a result, action potentials are neither generated nor propagated and conduction block occurs.

Reasons for Anesthetic Buffering

Anesthetic buffering in dentistry is accomplished by using sodium bicarbonate, which has a basic pH, as a buffer to be added to a local anesthetic solution, which has an acidic pH, to raise the pH of the anesthetic to that of the sodium bicarbonate. For example, buffering lidocaine with epinephrine raises the pH from 3.5 to 7.4 and produces a 6000-fold increase in active deionized anesthetic.[10] This method provides the practitioner a possible solution to the issues described in the previous section as a way to neutralize the anesthetic

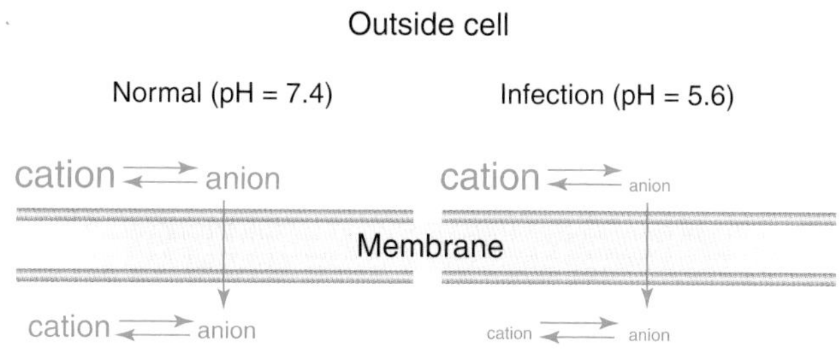

Fig. 3.4 Effect of hydrogen ion concentration (pH) on local anesthetic drug action. In the normal extracellular environment (pH 7.4, *left side of the diagram*), the anion form of the local anesthetic drug exists in sufficient numbers to make anesthesia possible. In infection (pH 5.6, *right side of diagram*), the lower pH reduces the number of anesthetic anions available to penetrate the nerve membrane, and the number of these base molecules needed for anesthesia may not be sufficient to be rendered effective.

immediately before the injection in vitro (outside the body) rather than the in vivo buffering process, which relies on the patient's physiology to buffer the anesthetic. Some authors suggest that bringing the pH of the anesthetic toward physiologic values before injection may improve patient comfort by eliminating the sting, may reduce tissue injury and anesthetic latency, and may provide more effective anesthesia in the area of infection.[10-13] Malamed et al.[14] compared anesthetic latency and injection pain for alkalinized versus nonalkalinized anesthetic in IA blocks. The study buffered the anesthetic directly in the cartridges using a mixing pen device (Fig. 3.5A). Twenty participants each received one control IA block (nonalkalinized 2% lidocaine 1:100,000 at pH 3.85) and one test IA block (2% lidocaine 1:100,000 alkalinized to pH 7.31). Latency was measured using endodontic ice, confirmed with an electric pulp tester (EPT), and injection pain was measured using a Visual Analog Scale (VAS). The onset time for the alkalinized anesthetic revealed that 71% of participants achieved pulpal analgesia within 2 minutes. The onset time for the nonalkalinized anesthetic revealed that 12% achieved pulpal analgesia within 2 minutes ($P = 0.001$). The average time to pulpal analgesia for the nonalkalinized anesthetic was 6:37 (range 0:55–13:25). Average time to pulpal analgesia for alkalinized anesthetic was 1:51 (range 0:11–6:10) ($P = 0.001$). The injection pain results revealed that 72% of the participants rated the alkalinized injection as more comfortable, 11% rated the nonalkalinized injection as more comfortable, and 17% reported no preference ($P = 0.013$). Forty-four percent of the patients receiving alkalinized anesthetic rated the injection pain as zero ("no pain") on a 100-mm VAS, compared with 6% of the patients who received nonalkalinized anesthetic ($P = 0.056$).

Davies[15] conducted a meta-analysis of 22 prospective, randomized, controlled human trials to evaluate the degree to which anesthetic buffering decreases the anesthetic injection pain. It was concluded that anesthetic buffering provided significantly more comfortable injections. In addition, Cochrane et al.[16] revealed that patient satisfaction was significantly improved after the review of 23 clinical trials. Other authors were unable to demonstrate any improvement.[17,18] Anesthetic buffering is well documented in medicine,[11-13,15,19] and was first available as an option for use in dentistry by Onpharma (Carson City, Nevada), using a mixing pen (Fig. 3.5A) and cartridge connectors (Fig. 3.5B) to provide an automated way to adjust the pH of local anesthetics cartridges, at chair side, immediately before injection (see Chapters 9 and 11 for assembly and use of the mixing pen device). Other buffering systems were subsequently introduced (e.g., Anutra Medical Inc., Morrisville, North Carolina).

Buffering Process

The buffering process uses a sodium bicarbonate solution that can be mixed with any type of local anesthetic solution with the exception of bupivacaine, which is not recommended. It can be a plain anesthetic solution, or it can contain a vasoconstrictor. The interaction between the sodium bicarbonate ($NaHCO_3$) and the hydrochloric acid (HCL) in the local anesthetic creates water (H_2O) and carbon dioxide (CO_2).[20] The CO_2 diffuses out of solution immediately and continues after the solution has been injected.[20] Catchlove[13] concluded that the CO_2 in combination with the anesthetic potentiates the action of the anesthetic by a direct depressant effect of CO_2 on the axon, concentrating the local anesthetic inside the nerve trunk through ion trapping, thus changing the charge of the local anesthetic inside the nerve axon. This is of great clinical significance as buffering reduces the onset of pulpal anesthesia and allows clinicians to start the dental procedures more promptly. Dental hygienists are encouraged to periodically review the companion Evolve website for updated information on this product and others in the *content update* section.

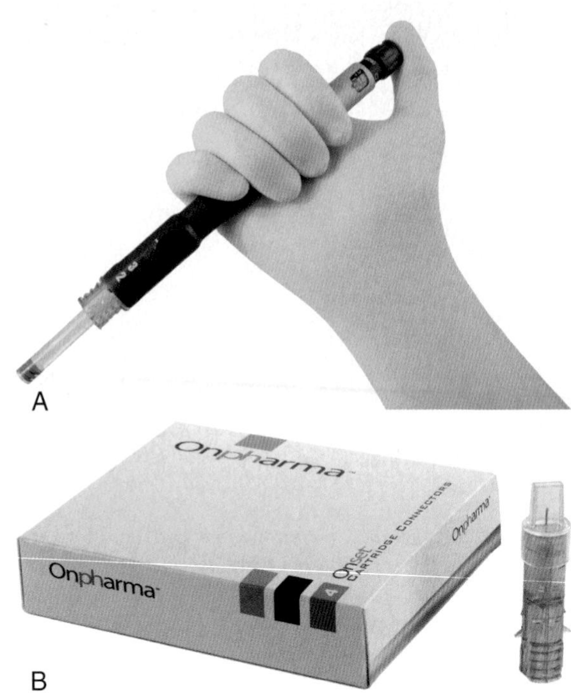

Fig. 3.5 (A) Assembled mixing pen is a compounding and dispensing device used to mix two solutions together. Once assembled, the pen enables the precise transfer of fluid of sodium bicarbonate from a standard 3 mL size cartridge into the 1.8 mL anesthetic cartridge, allowing the two solutions to be mixed. (B) The cartridge connector is used for the transfer of sterile solutions from one sealed container into a second sealed container and provides a reservoir for collecting excess solution displaced from the second sealed container during the transfer process. (Images courtesy Onpharma Inc., Los Gatos, CA.)

MECHANISM OF ACTION OF LOCAL ANESTHETIC AGENTS

As discussed in Chapter 2, the primary effects of local anesthetics is to inhibit the depolarization of the nerve membrane by interfering with both sodium (Na^+) and potassium (K^+) currents. The action potential is not propagated because the local anesthetic blocks the influx of sodium during the slow depolarization stage, and the threshold potential is never attained (see Box 3.3 and Chapter 2). Although the exact mechanism by which local anesthetics retard the influx of Na^+ ions into the cell is unknown, two theories have been proposed: the specific protein receptor theory, which is more widely accepted, and the membrane expansion theory.

Specific Protein Receptor Theory

Several theories have been proposed concerning the action of anesthetics on nerves. However, the specific receptor theory is the most widely accepted theory. One proven fact is that the anesthetic interferes with how the impulses travel down the length of the nerve. This is done by interfering with the influx of Na^+ ions across axonal membranes of peripheral nerves. The local anesthetic diffuses across the cell membrane and binds to a specific receptor at the opening of the voltage-gated Na^+ channel. The local anesthetic's affinity to the voltage-gated Na^+ channel increases significantly with the excitation rate of the neuron. Local anesthetics act during the depolarization phase of the nerve impulse generation by binding to the structural proteins known as *specific receptors* on the Na^+ channel.[3] The rate of depolarization is reduced, and the nerve never reaches the firing potential.

BOX 3.3 Mechanism of Action = Blockade of Voltage-Gated Sodium Channels

Polarized membrane potential = − 70 mV (range −40 to −95 mV)
Excitatory stimulus produces slow depolarization
***Axoplasm slowly depolarizes, reaching the threshold potential initiating an action potential.**
More sodium (Na^+) channels open causing rapid depolarization
Na^+ rapidly influxes in (depolarizes membrane to +40 mV)
Na^+ channels close
Potassium (K^+) channels open
K^+ efflux out
K^+ channels close
Na^+/K^+ exchange (via Na^+/K^+ pump)
Repolarizes membrane (−70 mV)
***Local anesthetics work by blocking the influx of Na^+ during the slow depolarization stage by stopping the threshold potential; therefore an action potential is never achieved.**

Different anesthetics bind at different sites in the membrane. In myelinated nerves, local anesthetics have access to the nerve membrane only at the nodes of Ranvier where Na^+ channels are located. The anesthetic must permeate 8 to 10 mm of the nerve's length, approximately three to four nodes, to profoundly block the generation of the nerve impulse because an impulse can be strong enough to skip over one or two of the blocked nodes. The thickness of the nerve also has an effect on how much local anesthesia is needed to cover three to four nodes to achieve profound anesthesia. Therefore thicker nerve sheaths, such as those found in the IA nerve, will require more anesthetic to achieve adequate nerve blockage (Figs. 3.6 and 3.7).[21]

During the resting stage of nerve conduction, calcium (Ca^{++}) ions are bound to receptor sites within the ion channels of cell membranes. During depolarization, Ca^{++} ions are displaced and are thought to be the most significant factor responsible for the influx of Na^+ into the nerve. Local anesthetics work by competing with Ca^{++} ions to bind to these ion channels during slow depolarization and close (block off) these channels[3] (Fig. 3.8).

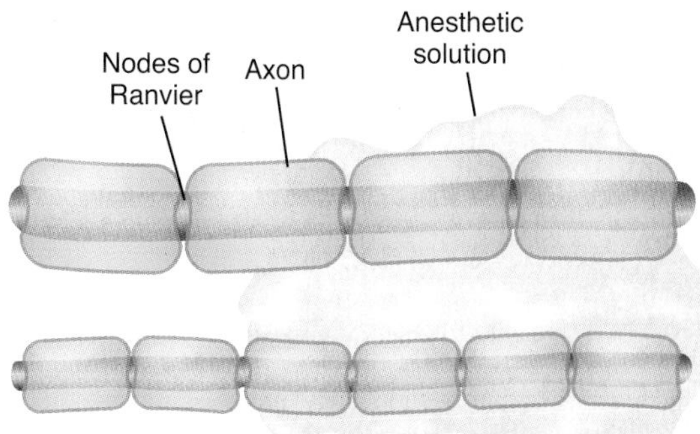

Fig. 3.6 Comparison of nodal interval nerve block between thin and thick axons. Two side-by-side axons (one thin, one thick) are bathed in a puddle of local anesthetic. The nodes of Ranvier interval of the thick fiber is twice that of the thin one. The local anesthetic solution covers four successive nodes of the thin axon (*bottom*) to ensure solid impulse block. At the top, the impulses can easily skip one or even two unexcitable nodes, hence conduction along the thick axon continues uninterrupted, and profound anesthesia is not achieved. (Modified from de Jong RH: *Local anesthetics*, St Louis, 1994, Mosby.)

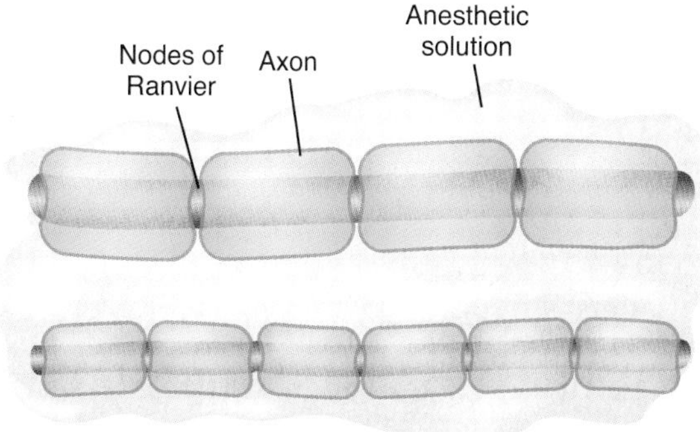

Fig. 3.7 Nodal interval nerve block between thin and thick axons when enough anesthetic is deposited. Both thick (*top*) and thin (*bottom*) axons have more than three nodes covered by local anesthetic solution. Conduction block will be complete in either group. (Modified from de Jong RH: *Local anesthetics*, St Louis, 1994, Mosby.)

The Membrane Expansion Theory

The membrane expansion theory is not as readily accepted as the specific receptor theory and suggests that the local anesthetic agents that are highly lipid-soluble (e.g., benzocaine) insert themselves into the lipid bilayer of the cell membrane, causing three-dimensional changes in the configuration of the lipoprotein matrix by expanding the membrane. Local anesthetic agents that are highly lipid-soluble are able to easily penetrate the lipid-rich cell membrane. This leads to narrowing of the Na^+ channels, thus preventing depolarization by decreasing the diameter of the Na^+ channels[3] (Fig. 3.9). It has not been determined as to how much of the membrane expansion contributes to impulse blockade of excitable tissue. Therefore this theory remains speculative.

PHARMACOKINETICS OF LOCAL ANESTHETIC DRUGS

Pharmacokinetics is the study of the action of drugs within the body. These actions include mechanisms of drug absorption, distribution, metabolism, and excretion; onset of action; duration of effect; biotransformation; and effects and routes of excretion of the metabolites of the drug.

Onset of Action

The onset of action of local anesthetics, the period from local anesthetic deposition near the nerve trunk to profound conduction block, is determined by several factors. The pK_a is the primary factor determining the onset of action. The pK_a of a local anesthetic determines the amount of drug that exists in an ionized (acidic) form at any given pH. The lower pK_a levels increase tissue penetration and shorten onset of action because of more lipid-soluble unionized (base) particles. In contrast, the higher pH level optimizes the dissociation of these base molecules and shortens the onset of action. This theory explains why local anesthetics often do not work in infected tissue. The infected tissue tends to be a more acidic environment and reduces the pH of the tissue, consequently reducing the number of unionized local anesthetic particles, causing a delay in the onset of action, or ineffective anesthesia. Anesthetics that have a high degree of lipid solubility and are in the base unionized form will readily cross the nerve membrane and attach to the sodium receptors, resulting in a rapid onset of action. Anesthetics that have a low degree of lipid solubility and are cationic and ionized will penetrate the nerve membrane slowly and produce a slower onset of action.

The administration site also influences the onset of action. The onset of a nerve block is faster in an area with smaller diameters of

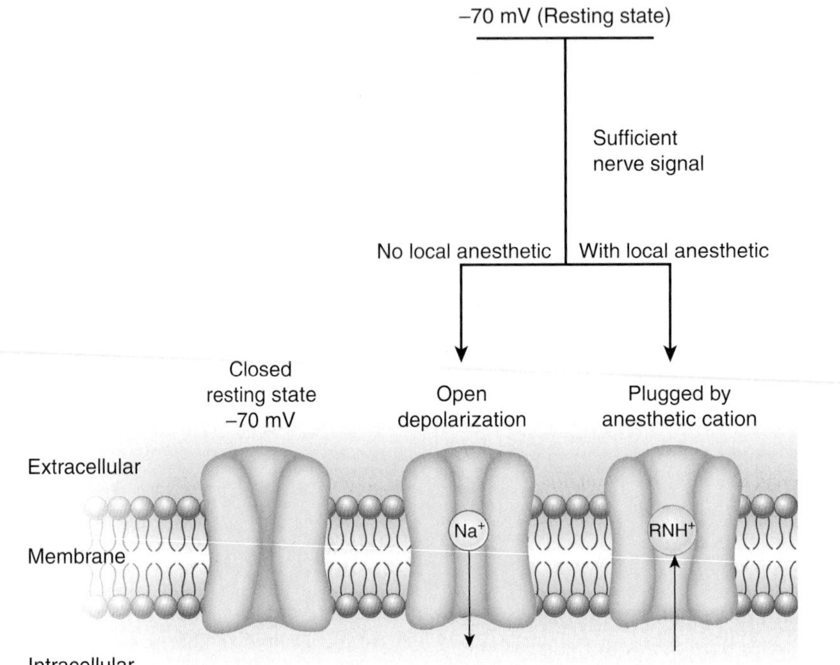

Fig. 3.8 Mode of action of local anesthetic agent. On the left is a closed channel, which remains closed to sodium ions in the resting state. The center channel is open (the usual configuration after a sufficient stimulus has been applied), allowing sodium (Na^+) ion influx through the nerve membrane. The right channel, although otherwise in the open configuration, has been closed by an anesthetic cation (RNH^+) that is bound to the receptor site in the channel.

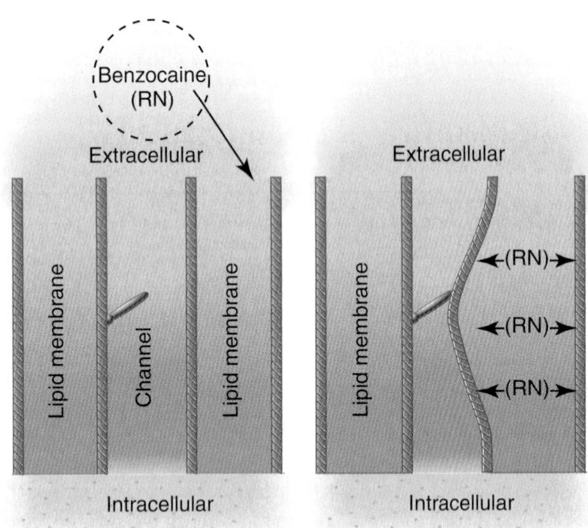

Fig. 3.9 Membrane expansion theory. Highly lipid-soluble anesthetics, such as benzocaine, insert themselves into the lipid bilayer of the cell membrane, expanding and narrowing the sodium channels preventing depolarization. (From Malamed SF: *Handbook of local anesthesia,* ed 7, St Louis, 2020, Elsevier.)

nerve trunks, and the onset is prolonged in areas with increased tissue or nerve sheath size.

Induction of Local Anesthetics

The process by which the local anesthetic moves from its extraneural site of deposition toward the nerve is called *diffusion* and is governed by the initial concentration of the anesthetic. The higher the concentration of the administered local anesthetic, the more readily the diffusion of its molecules through the nerve, producing a more rapid onset of action. As discussed in Chapter 2, the fasciculi in the mantle bundles are located near the outside of the nerve and innervate structures within close proximity, and fasciculi in the core bundles are located on the inside of the nerve and innervate structures at a distance. Using the IA nerve as an example, the mantle bundles innervate the molar area, and the core bundles innervate anterior teeth at the end of the nerve fiber[4] (Fig. 3.10). The location of the bundles in larger nerves has an effect on which bundles are affected by the local anesthetic first. Using the previous example, the local anesthetic, when administered, diffuses through the nerve to the mantle bundles (outer core), first providing concentrated anesthetic to the molar region and then diffusing to the

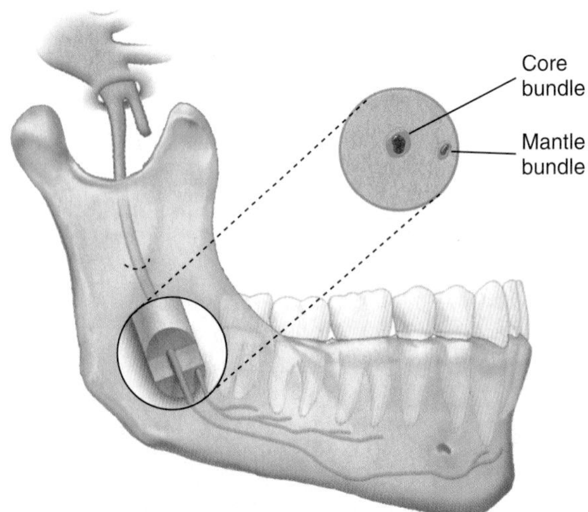

Fig. 3.10 The axons in the mantle bundle supply the molar teeth, and those in the core bundle supply the anterior teeth. The extraneural local anesthetic solution diffuses from the mantle to the core. (From Hargreaves KM, Berman LH: *Cohen's pathways of the pulp,* ed 11, St Louis, 2016, Elsevier.)

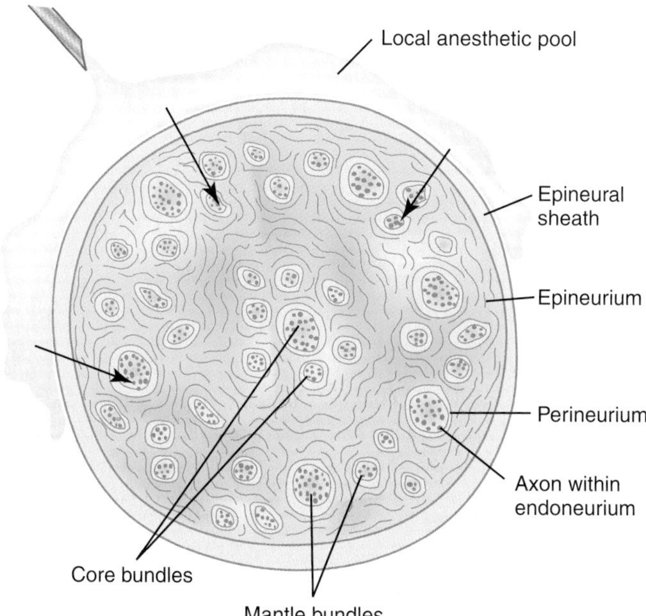

Fig. 3.11 The deposited local anesthetic solution near the nerve sheath must diffuse inward toward the core fibers, reaching the mantle fibers first.

core bundles (inner core), providing a more diluted anesthetic solution to the anterior mandibular teeth, including the lip and chin.[3,22] Because the mantle bundles are affected by the local anesthetic first, they are exposed to higher concentrations of the local anesthetic, causing a complete, rapid, and easy blockage of these fibers. The core bundles are located at a further distance inside the nerve; therefore they come in contact with a more diluted, lower concentration of local anesthetic[3] (Fig. 3.11). The anesthetic loses its concentration from tissue fluids, capillaries, and lymphatics at the site of administration and anatomic barriers of the nerve. This results in a slower onset of action in these fibers, and complete blockage is most likely never achieved.[3,4] Although the presence of anesthetic symptoms expressed by the patient is a good indication that successful anesthesia has been achieved, it is not an adequate indication of profound anesthesia. Areas of inadequate anesthesia may be a result of the anesthetic molecules not reaching the most inner core bundles.

Induction Time

Induction time is defined as the time interval between the initial deposition of the anesthetic solution at the nerve site and complete conduction blockade. Factors that control induction time of an anesthetic and its clinical actions are listed in Table 3.1.

Recovery From Local Anesthetic Block

Fasciculi in mantle bundles begin to lose anesthesia before the core bundles. As the local anesthetic begins diffusing out of the mantle bundles, the local anesthetic within the core bundles then diffuses into the mantle bundles. The core bundles will continue to slowly diffuse the anesthesia into the mantle bundles and the innermost core fibers will be the first nerves to completely lose anesthesia. The mantle bundles will retain the local anesthetic the longest and will be the last fibers to completely recover.[3] Using the IA nerve block as an example, anesthetic recovery will begin in the molar teeth, but as the anesthetic in the anterior teeth, chin, and lip (core bundles) begin to diffuse in the mantle bundles of the molar teeth, these structures will recover before the molar teeth. The molar teeth (mantle bundles) will completely recover last as the anesthetic solution diffuses out of the outermost fibers of the mantle bundles. Anesthetic recovery is a slower process than induction because the anesthetic binds to the receptor site in the Na^+ channel, releasing the anesthetic slowly into the systemic circulation. The degree of binding to the receptor site for each anesthetic determines the speed of recovery.

Reinjection of Local Anesthetic

When the procedure lasts longer than the duration of the anesthetic, a second injection may be required to finish the procedure. If the patient has pain, the nerve has returned to function and it is usually more difficult to achieve profound anesthesia again. Because emergence of local anesthetics begins in the mantle fibers, it is important to reinject the anesthetic before the mantle fibers have fully recovered. Partially recovered mantle fibers can achieve rapid onset of action after a new, high concentration of anesthetic is injected with a smaller volume than originally administered.[3] If the dental procedure lasts longer than the duration of the anesthetic and the mantle and core fibers have fully recovered, the reinjection of local anesthetic will be ineffective. A term used to describe this phenomenon is tachyphylaxis, which is described as an increased tolerance to a drug that is administered repeatedly.[3]

Duration of Anesthesia

The duration of local anesthetics is influenced by the following:

- *Protein binding:* Longer-acting local anesthetics such as bupivacaine are more firmly bound to the receptor sites than shorter-acting local anesthetics such as lidocaine. Increased protein binding allows the cations (RNH^+) to bind/cling more firmly so duration is increased.
- *Vascularity of the injection site:* Vascularity increases absorption of the anesthetic, allowing the drug to leave the injected area faster, decreasing potency and duration.
- *Presence or absence of a vasoconstrictor drug:* Added vasoconstrictors to a local anesthetic decrease the vasodilatory properties of local anesthetics by constricting the surrounding blood vessels at the site of administration, increasing the duration of the anesthetic.

Absorption of Local Anesthetics

The rate of systemic absorption of local anesthetics is dependent on the total dose and concentration of the drug administered, the route of administration, the vascularity of the tissue at the administration site, and the presence or absence of a vasoconstrictor in the anesthetic solution.

All local anesthetics are vasodilators and produce a pharmacologic effect on blood vessels, varying slightly from type to type.[3] The importance of these vasodilating properties is the increase in the rate of absorption of local anesthetics and the decrease in the rate of action. Higher blood levels of the drug increase the chance of the patient developing an overdose. The local anesthetic molecules diffuse out of the Na^+ channels and are carried into the bloodstream. To reduce the rate of absorption, vasoconstrictors are added to local anesthetics to decrease the vasodilating properties of the local anesthetic by constricting the blood vessels and reducing the blood supply to the area of injection (see Chapter 4). The vasoconstrictor will reduce rapid systemic absorption, which reduces systemic toxicity and increases the duration of the anesthetic. Of equal importance is the site where the anesthetic is injected. If the anesthetic is inadvertently injected intravascularly, it will be absorbed into the bloodstream rapidly, significantly increasing the possibility of an overdose.

Distribution of Local Anesthetics

After absorption of the local anesthetics into the bloodstream, local anesthetics are distributed throughout the body to all tissues. Highly vascular organs such as the brain, heart, liver, kidneys, and lungs have higher concentrations of anesthetics.[3] Local anesthetics easily cross the blood-brain barrier because nerves are predominantly susceptible to local anesthetics. The toxicity of local anesthetics is directly related to the amount of accumulation in the tissues.

Metabolism (Biotransformation) of Local Anesthetics

The intermediate chain of the local anesthetic molecule determines the classification of the drug as either an ester or an amide. It also determines the pattern of biotransformation.

The elimination half-life of a local anesthetic is the period of time it takes for 50% of the drug to be metabolized/removed from the body. The first half-life removes 50% of the anesthetic from the bloodstream, the second half-life removes another 25%, the third half-life removes another 12%, the next half-life removes another 6%, and so on until the drug is completely removed from the body.[23] For example, lidocaine has a half-life of 96 minutes, but by the time it gets through its last half-life, it takes approximately 10 hours for the drug to be completely removed from the body[6] (Table 3.3). The rate of absorption and the rate of elimination (half-life) of the local anesthetic from the blood and tissue influence the degree of toxicity. Also of important consideration are the drug-drug interactions with other medications that the patient may be taking that may compete with the metabolic process of the local anesthetic. This could increase the half-life of the local anesthetic and the possibility of an overdose (see Tables 3.3 and 3.4 and Chapter 7).

Ester Local Anesthetics

Esters are hydrolyzed in the plasma by the enzyme pseudocholinesterase and by liver esterases. Esters include benzocaine, tetracaine, and procaine. Benzocaine and tetracaine are commonly used in dentistry as topical anesthetics (see Chapter 6). Injectable esters are no longer manufactured in dental cartridges for use in dentistry because of their high potential for evoking allergic reactions. However, procaine is occasionally used in the medical profession and obtained in medical vials. Procaine is metabolized to para-aminobenzoic acid (PABA) and is the major metabolic by-product responsible for allergic reactions. Most patients are not allergic to the parent compound of ester drugs (e.g., procaine) but are allergic to the PABA metabolites. Approximately 1 in 2800 individuals has a hereditary condition known as *atypical pseudocholinesterase,* which causes the inability for these individuals to hydrolyze ester local anesthetics and other chemically related drugs. This condition causes higher anesthetic blood levels, increasing the risk for toxicity and therefore contraindicating the use of esters (see Chapter 7).[2]

TABLE 3.3 Half-Life Example for Lidocaine

Minutes	% Lidocaine Removed from Body
96	50
180	75
270	87
360	94
450	97
540	99
630	99.5

TABLE 3.4 Half-Life of Commonly Used Local Anesthetics

Drug	Half-Life Minutes	Half-Life Hours
Lidocaine	96	1.6
Mepivacaine	114	1.9
Prilocaine	96	1.6
Articaine	27[24*]	0.5
Bupivacaine	162	2.7

*Manufacturer product inserts list half-life of articaine at 43.8 minutes with 1:100,000 epinephrine and 44.4 minutes with 1:200,000 epinephrine.

Amide Local Anesthetics

Amides are primarily metabolized in the liver, and the process is much more complex than for esters. Amides include lidocaine, mepivacaine, prilocaine, articaine, and bupivacaine (see Chapter 5). Because the liver is the organ responsible for the entire metabolic process of most amides, the rate of biotransformation is slower in patients with significant liver dysfunction (e.g., cirrhosis) or patients with lower hepatic blood flow, causing an increased risk of systemic toxicity. Biotransformation for lidocaine, mepivacaine, and bupivacaine occurs completely in the liver. Prilocaine is metabolized in the liver and some also is metabolized in the lungs. Because prilocaine is metabolized in the lungs and in the liver, it is more rapidly biotransformed, and plasma levels decrease more quickly than with other anesthetics metabolized completely in the liver. Articaine is also an amide but contains a thiophene group/ester group. Only about 5% to 10% of articaine is biotransformed in the liver, with most of the drug being biotransformed by the enzyme plasma cholinesterase, the same route as esters. Amides that are primarily metabolized in the liver have a longer half-life, which increases the risk for systemic toxicity. Because articaine is metabolized by plasma cholinesterase, it has a very short half-life, approximately 27 minutes,[24]which decreases the risk for systemic toxicity.

Excretion of Local Anesthetics

The kidneys are the primary excretory organ for the metabolites of all local anesthetic agents. A small percentage is excreted unchanged in the urine. Esters are almost completely hydrolyzed in the blood and only small amounts are excreted unchanged in the urine. Amides are relatively resistant to hydrolysis, and therefore a greater percentage is excreted unchanged in the urine than that of an ester. With severe renal disease, such as end-stage renal disease, both the parent drug and the metabolites may accumulate in the kidneys, increasing the risk of systemic toxicity.

Systemic Effects of Local Anesthetics

Unlike most medications that must be absorbed by the bloodstream to produce the desired effect, local anesthetics are chemical agents that are deposited in the area of nerve conduction to block the action potential before they are absorbed through the bloodstream. Once absorbed into the circulatory system and before biotransformation, local anesthetics will affect the central nervous system (CNS) and the cardiovascular system (CVS). The higher the blood plasma level, the greater the effects on these systems. Adverse reactions and toxicity to local anesthetics are directly related to the following:

- *Nature of the drug.* Amount of vasodilation of the anesthetic and the inherent toxicity of each agent are contributory factors to toxicity.
- *Concentration of the drug and dose administered.* Higher concentrations and doses administered produce higher blood levels of a drug.
- *Route of administration.* Intravascular injections rapidly produce high blood levels of a drug. Topical anesthetics are administered in

high concentrations without vasoconstrictors and absorb quickly from the site of administration, increasing the possibility of toxicity.

- *Rate of injection.* Injections administered rapidly can increase the chance of toxicity because the tissue cannot accept the large, rapid volume of anesthetic.
- *Vascularity in the area of injection.* Vascularity in the area of the injection can be caused by a dental infection, inflammation as a response to an infection, or vasodilation from a local anesthetic agent without a vasoconstrictor. Vascularity from any of these factors causes an increase in the risk of systemic toxicity by allowing the local anesthetic drug to be rapidly absorbed into the circulation.
- *Age of the patient.* Children and older patients are more susceptible to total dose administered and adverse reactions because children's organs may not be fully developed to effectively metabolize the drug, whereas the older patient's organs may not be functioning properly to effectively metabolize the drug.
- *Weight of patient.* Variations in patient's weight affect blood levels of the drug. Maximum recommended doses must be calculated based on the patient's weight.
- *Patient's health.* Patients with systemic conditions that affect the biotransformation of local anesthetics should be given reduced doses to prevent toxicity.
- *The route and rate of metabolism and excretion of the drug.* Patients with liver dysfunction may be unable to metabolize the anesthetic and amides may accumulate in the liver; amides and both amide and ester metabolites may accumulate in the kidneys because of renal disease.[3,23]

Effect of Local Anesthetics on the Central Nervous System

Local anesthetics easily pass from the peripheral circulation into the CNS, which is especially sensitive to high blood levels of local anesthetics (more than any other system) because local anesthetics readily cross the blood-brain barrier. In general, the concentrations of local anesthetics required to elicit CNS effects are inversely proportional to their anesthetic potencies. Although CNS effects from a local anesthetic are rare, at high blood levels, the local anesthetic overdose manifests as CNS depression. At low blood levels, local anesthetics produce no significant effects on the CNS but may have some anticonvulsant properties.[3,4,25,26]

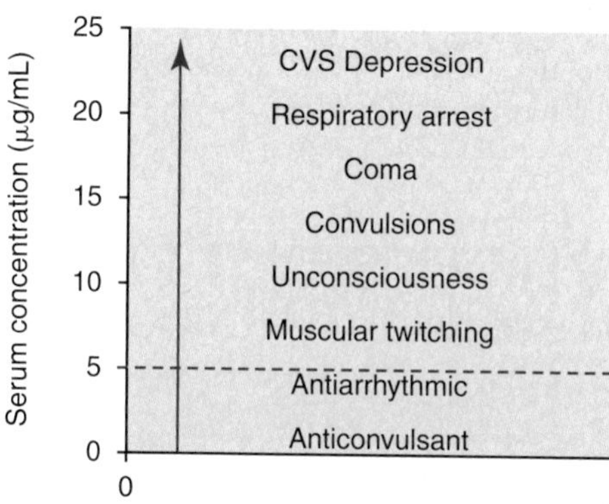

Fig. 3.12 Systemic influences of lidocaine. At low blood levels, local anesthetics have anticonvulsant properties. At much higher doses the effects on the central nervous system (CNS) is biphasic phase I, exhibiting initial excitatory signs progressing to phase II, the depressive phase, causing CNS depression, unconsciousness, and convulsions.

At much higher doses, the effects on the CNS are considered to be biphasic with phase I, exhibiting initial excitatory signs (e.g., muscle twitching, tremors) and progressing subsequently to phase II, the depressive phase that involves CNS depression, unconsciousness, convulsions, hypotension (because of the anesthetics varying degrees of vasodilation), and, eventually, respiratory arrest.[1-4,22,23,25] Fig. 3.12 demonstrates systemic influences of lidocaine, and Table 3.5 lists signs and symptoms of local anesthetic overdose on CNS. See Chapter 17 for more information on local anesthetic overdose.

Effect of Local Anesthetics on the Cardiovascular System

Local anesthetics can exert a variety of effects on the CVS. These effects are usually minimal. At mild overdose levels, the patient may exhibit a slight increase in blood pressure, heart rate, or respiration. Moderate overdose levels may occur with the administration of five cartridges of anesthetic. Similar to the CNS overdose symptoms, the CVS overdose symptoms are biphasic in nature and change from stimulation to a depression phase at the higher end of the overdose level, demonstrating signs of depression. Reduced heart rate, blood pressure, and respiration rate would be

TABLE 3.5 Signs and Symptoms of a Local Anesthetic Overdose on the Central Nervous System

Signs (Observable-Objective)	Symptoms (Subjectively Felt)
Low to moderate blood levels	Disorientation
• Circumoral and/or tongue numbness	Nervousness
• Metallic taste	Flushed skin color
• Excitatory-nervousness-talkativeness	Apprehension
• Slurred speech, general stutter	Twitching tremors
• Involuntary muscular twitching or shivering	Shivering
• General light-headedness, dizziness	Dizziness
• Tremor or twitching in muscles of face and distal extremities	Light-headedness
• Confusion, apprehension	Visual disturbances
• Sweating	Auditory disturbances
• Vomiting	Headache
• Elevated respiration	Tinnitus
• Elevated heart rate	Metallic taste
• Increased blood pressure	
Moderate to high blood levels	
• Convulsions, generally tonic-clonic	
• Respiratory depression (at high blood levels of drug)	
• Depressed blood pressure and heart rate	
• Central nervous system depression, coma, death	

observed. This decrease in myocardial contraction can lead to circulatory collapse and cardiac arrest[3,4,25,26] (Table 3.6 and Chapter 17).

The time lapse between the administration of the local anesthetic to the overdose reaction determines its severity. Symptoms that occur rapidly (within 5 minutes) are more likely to evolve into a more serious reaction. Delayed symptoms that occur after 5 minutes are usually easily resolved and do not develop into a serious reaction. In rare instances at extremely high levels, cardiac arrhythmia or hypotension and cardiovascular collapse occur (Table 3.7 and Chapter 17).

TABLE 3.6 Cardiovascular Effects of an Overdose*

Low to Moderate Overdose	Moderate to High Blood Levels
Elevated blood pressure	Cardiovascular depression (decreased blood pressure)
Elevated heart rate	Decreased excitability (decreased heart rate) Cardiac arrest

*All injectable and most topical local anesthetics are absorbed and carried to the cardiovascular system.

TABLE 3.7 Symptoms of Overdose on the Cardiovascular System

- Headache
- Lethargy
- Increased slurring of speech
- Increased disorientation
- Possible loss of consciousness

DENTAL HYGIENE CONSIDERATIONS

- High degree of hypersensitivity to ester local anesthetic metabolites (PABA) has been documented; consequently, injectable esters are no longer available for use in dentistry.
- Bupivacaine has the greatest degree of lipid solubility and is therefore the most potent local anesthetic.
- The higher the dissociation constant (pK_a) of an anesthetic, the slower the onset of action. Bupivacaine has the highest pK_a and the slowest onset of action. Topical benzocaine has the lowest pK_a and the quickest onset of action.
- Dental infections can impede the development of profound anesthesia because of the tissue acidity associated with these infections leaving fewer base molecules to penetrate the nerve.
- Anesthetic buffering provides the practitioner a way to neutralize the anesthetic prior to injection in vitro, and may improve anesthetic latency. In addition, it may provide more effective anesthesia in an area of dental infection.
- The degree of binding to the receptor site of each anesthetic determines the speed of recovery. Bupivacaine binds more firmly to the receptor site than shorter-acting local anesthetics.
- If more anesthetic is needed for a procedure, it is important to reinject the anesthetic before the mantle fibers have fully recovered. Partially recovered mantle fibers can achieve rapid onset of action with second dose at a smaller volume than initially administered.
- Tachyphylaxis is an increased tolerance to a drug that is administered repeatedly after the mantle and core bundles have fully recovered.
- Local anesthetics are vasodilators and increase the absorption of the drug by the blood.
- Vasoconstrictors are added to local anesthetics to counteract the vasodilatory properties of the anesthetic, increasing the duration and decreasing the risk of systemic toxicity.
- The rate of systemic absorption of local anesthetics is dependent on the total dose, concentration, route of administration, vascularity of tissue, and presence or absence of a vasoconstrictor.
- Intravascular injections significantly increase the possibility of an overdose.
- Before biotransformation, local anesthetics affect the central nervous system (CNS) and the cardiovascular system (CVS).
- Local anesthetics easily cross the blood-brain barrier.
- The degree of local anesthetic toxicity is dependent on the rate of absorption and elimination half-life. Articaine has a short half-life of approximately 27 minutes and has a low risk of systemic toxicity.
- Lidocaine, mepivacaine, and bupivacaine are biotransformed completely in the liver. Total dose for patients with liver dysfunction must be reduced.
- Prilocaine is biotransformed in the lungs and the liver. Total dose for patients with respiratory difficulties, such as asthma or chronic obstructive pulmonary disease (COPD), should be reduced.
- Articaine is biotransformed in the blood in the same manner as esters with only a slight amount (5%–10%) metabolized in the liver.

CASE STUDY 3.1 A Patient Experiences Difficulty With Reanesthetization

A patient is in the office for a 1-hour nonsurgical periodontal treatment of the mandibular left quadrant. The dental hygienist administers two cartridges of lidocaine 2% 1:100,000 epinephrine. The patient informs the dental hygienist that he feels very numb. The procedure is much more difficult than the dental hygienist expected, and the entire quadrant is not completed after the hour elapsed. The dental hygienist asks the patient if he is able to stay longer to complete the procedure because there is an opening in the schedule. After approximately a half hour into the continued treatment, the patient complains that he is feeling pain and asks for some more anesthetic. The dental hygienist administers another cartridge of anesthetic, but the patient does not get numb.

Critical Thinking Questions

- Why did the patient not get numb the second time the anesthetic was administered?
- What could the dental hygienist have done to prevent this from occurring?
- How should the dental hygienist handle this situation?

CHAPTER REVIEW QUESTIONS

1. Infection and inflammation causes the following effects when administering a local anesthetic:
   A. Increases the number of free base molecules
   B. Reduces the number of free base molecules
   C. Increases the duration of action of the local anesthetic
   D. Causes the inflamed tissue to have a high pH
2. All of the following are desirable properties of local anesthetics EXCEPT one. Which one is the EXCEPTION?
   A. Reversible
   B. Rapid onset
   C. Stability in solution
   D. Potent
   E. Slow biotransformation
3. Which characteristic enhances the effectiveness of local anesthetics?
   A. High lipid solubility
   B. High pK_a
   C. Low pH
   D. High concentration of cation molecules
4. Where is the action site for local anesthetics?
   A. The K^+ receptors in the K^+ channels
   B. All along the nerve membrane
   C. The structural proteins known as specific receptors in the K^+ channels
   D. The structural proteins known as specific receptors in the Na^+ channels
5. Which part of the chemical structure of a local anesthetic determines whether the local anesthetic agent is classified as an ester or an amide?
   A. Intermediate chain
   B. Aromatic ring
   C. Terminal amine
   D. Quaternary amine
6. Local anesthetics have their effect on myelinated nerves mostly in which way?
   A. All along the nerve membrane
   B. Mostly at the synapse
   C. Mostly at the cell bodies
   D. Mostly at the nodes of Ranvier
7. The quaternary form of the local anesthetic molecule:
   A. Is the ionized form in the cartridge and is responsible for binding to the receptor site
   B. Is the unionized form in the cartridge and is responsible for binding to the receptor site
   C. Is the ionized form of the molecule that penetrates the nerve membrane
   D. Is the unionized form of the molecule that penetrates the nerve membrane
8. Ester type local anesthetics are no longer manufactured in injectable form for dentistry because:
   A. Of their difficulty penetrating the nerve
   B. Of their high degree of hypersensitivity
   C. They decrease the potential for systemic overdose
   D. They have less vasodilatory properties
9. During manufacturing, local anesthetics are formulated as which of the following to render them water-soluble?
   A. Muriatic acid
   B. Sodium bisulfite
   C. Hydrochloride salt
   D. Sodium bicarbonate
10. Which of the following anesthetics will provide the most rapid onset based on its pK_a?
    A. Mepivacaine
    B. Lidocaine
    C. Bupivacaine
    D. Benzocaine
11. Which of the following local anesthetics is the most lipid-soluble?
    A. Mepivacaine
    B. Lidocaine
    C. Bupivacaine
    D. Prilocaine
12. The mantle bundles of the inferior alveolar nerve innervate which teeth?
    A. The molar area
    B. The anterior teeth
    C. The lingual tissue
    D. The buccal tissue of the three molar teeth
13. When the local anesthetic is administered, the solution reaches the core bundles first, and then diffuses to the mantle bundles.
    A. Both statements are correct.
    B. Both statements are NOT correct.
    C. The first statement is correct; the second statement is NOT correct.
    D. The first statement is NOT correct; the second statement is correct.
14. What is tachyphylaxis?
    A. A term used to describe the inability of the anesthetic to reach the nerve membrane because of anatomic barriers
    B. Reinjection of anesthetic before the mantle fibers have fully recovered
    C. Increased tolerance to a drug that is administered repeatedly
    D. A term used to describe only partial anesthesia
15. Recovery of local anesthetics after the inferior alveolar block begins in the posterior teeth, but as the anesthetic in the anterior teeth, chin, and lip (core bundles) begin to diffuse into the mantle region of the molar teeth, the anterior region will recover before the molar teeth.
    A. Both statements are correct.
    B. Both statements are NOT correct.
    C. The first statement is correct; the second statement is NOT correct.
    D. The first statement is NOT correct; the second statement is correct.
16. Which of the following are true regarding local anesthetics?
    1. They are potent vasodilators
    2. They exhibit anticonvulsant properties
    3. They cause hemostasis
    4. They cause hypotension
    5. They have a pH of 7.5

    A. 1, 4, 5
    B. 1, 2, 4
    C. 2, 3, 5
    D. 3, 4, 5
17. Which of the following is responsible for allergic reactions in ester anesthetics?
    A. The parent compound
    B. Para-amino benzoic acid
    C. Pseudocholinesterase
    D. Sodium bisulfite

18. Most amide local anesthetics are biotransformed in the:
A. Plasma
B. Lungs
C. Kidneys
D. Liver

19. Local anesthetic overdose has an effect on which system?
A. Central nervous system
B. Skeletal system
C. Lymphatic system
D. Respiratory system

20. The dissociation constant (pK_a) of an anesthetic predicts the proportion of the molecules that exist in the acid form verses the base form. The acid–base balance of the solution is manipulated by the manufacturer.
A. Both statements are correct.
B. Both statements are NOT correct.
C. The first statement is correct; the second statement is NOT correct.
D. The first statement is NOT correct; the second statement is correct.

REFERENCES

1. Becker D, Reed K. Essentials of local anesthetic pharmacology. *Anesth Program.* 2006;53:98–109.
2. Becker D, Reed K. Local anesthetics: review of pharmacological considerations. *Anesth Program.* 2012;59:90–102.
3. Malamed S. *Handbook of local anesthesia.* ed. 7. St Louis: Elsevier; 2020.
4. Jastak T, Yagiela J, Donaldson D. *Local anesthesia of the oral cavity.* St Louis: Saunders; 1995.
5. Fernandez C, Reader A, Beck M, Nusstein J. A prospective, randomized, double-blind comparison of bupivacaine and lidocaine for inferior alveolar nerve blocks. *J Endod.* 2005;31:499–503.
6. Reader A. Taking the pain out of restorative dentistry and endodontics: current thoughts and treatment options to help patients achieve profound anesthesia. Endodontics: Colleagues for Excellence Winter 2009. Chicago: American Association of Endodontists; 2009.
7. Lai TN, Lin CP, Kok SH, et al. Evaluation of mandibular block using a standardized method. *Oral Surg Oral Med Oral Pathol Oral Radiol Endod.* 2006;102:462–468.
8. Kanaa MD, Meechan JG, Corbert IP, Whitworth JM. Speed of injection influences efficacy of inferior alveolar nerve blocks: a double-blind randomized controlled trial in volunteers. *J Endod.* 2006;32:919–923.
9. Malamed SF, Faldel M. Buffered local anaesthetics: the importance of pH and CO2. *SAAD Dig.* 2013;29:9–17.
10. Malamed S. Buffering local anesthetics in dentistry. *The Pulse.* 2011;44(1):7–9.
11. Bowles WH, Frysh H, Emmons R. Clinical evaluation of buffered local anesthetic. *Gen Dent.* 1995;43(2):182.
12. Stewart JH, Cole GW, Klein JA. Neutralized lidocaine with epinephrine for local anesthesia. *J Dermatol Surg Oncol.* 1989;15(10):1081.
13. Catchlove RFH. The influence of CO_2 and pH on local anesthetic action. *J Pharmacol Exp Ther.* 1972;181(2):208.
14. Malamed SF, Tavana S, Falkel M. Faster onset and more comfortable injection with alkalinized 2% lidocaine with epinephrine 1:100,000. *Compend Contin Educ Dent.* 2013; 34 Spec No 1:10–20.
15. Davies JR. Buffering the pain of local anaesthetics: a systematic review. *Emerg. Med Australas.* 2003;15. 91-88.
16. Cepda MS, Tzortzopulou A, Thackrey M, et al. Adjusting the pH of lignocaine for reducing pain on injection. *Cochrane Database Syst Rev.* 2010;12:CD006581.
17. Primosch RE, Robinson L. Pain elicited during intraoral infiltration with buffered lidocaine. *Am J Dent.* 1996;9(1):5–10.
18. Whitcomb M, Drum M, Reader A, Nusstein M, Beck M. A prospective, randomized, double-blind study of the anesthetic efficacy of sodium bicarbonate buffered 2% lidocaine with 1:100,000 epinephrine in inferior alveolar nerve blocks. *Anesth Prog.* 2010;57, 59.
19. Scarfone RJ, Jasani M. Pain of local anesthetics: rate of administration and buffering. *Ann Emerg Med.* 1998;31:36–40.
20. Ackerman WE, Ware TR, Juneja M. The air-liquid interface and the pH and Pco_2 of alkalinized local anaesthetic solutions. *Can J Anaesth.* 1992;39(4):387.
21. de Jong RH. *Local anesthetics.* St Louis: Mosby; 1994.
22. Haveles B. *Applied pharmacology for the dental hygienist.* ed 8. St Louis: Elsevier; 2020.
23. Bahl R. Local anesthesia in dentistry. *Anesth Prog.* 2004;51:138–142.
24. Vice TB, Baars AM, van Oss GE, et al. High performance liquid chromatography and preliminary pharmacokinetics of articaine and its 2-carboxy metabolite in human serum and urine. *J Chromatogr.* 1988;424:240–444.
25. Finder RL, More PA. Adverse drug reactions to local anesthesia. *Dent Clin N Am.* 2002;46:447–457.
26. Patton K, Thibodeau G. *Anatomy and physiology.* ed 21. St Louis: Elsevier; 2019.

ADDITIONAL RESOURCES

Castro A, Merchut MP, Neafsey E, Wurster R. *Neuroscience: an outline approach.* St Louis: Mosby; 2002.

Haines D. *Fundamental neuroscience for basic and clinical applications.* ed 3. St Louis: Churchill Livingstone; 2006.

Liebgott B. *The anatomical basis of dentistry.* ed 4. St Louis: Mosby; 2018.

Nolte J. *Elsevier's integrated neuroscience.* St Louis: Mosby; 2007.

Rosenblatt MA, Abel M, Fischer GW, Itzkovich CJ, Eisenkraft JB. Successful use of a 20% lipid emulsion to resuscitate a patient after a presumed bupivacaine-related cardiac arrest. *Anesthesiology.* 2006;105:217–218.

Sisk A. Vasoconstrictors in local anesthesia for dentistry. *Anesth Prog.* 1992;39:187–193.

Tetzlaff JE. *Clinical pharmacology of local anesthetics.* Woburn, MA: Butterworth-Heinemann; 2000.

4

Pharmacology of Vasoconstrictors

Demetra Daskalos Logothetis, RDH, MS

LEARNING OBJECTIVES

1. Discuss the problems associated with the vasodilatory properties of local anesthetics.
2. Discuss the benefits of adding vasoconstrictors to local anesthetic solutions.
3. Name the two vasoconstrictors that are added to local anesthetics available in the United States.
4. Discuss the use of vasoconstrictors in dentistry.
5. Discuss epinephrine, including:
   - Mechanism of action
   - Epinephrine dilutions
   - Sodium bisulfite preservative
   - Actions of epinephrine on specific systems and tissue
   - Termination of action
   - Maximum recommended dose
6. Discuss levonordefrin, including:
   - Actions on specific systems and tissue
   - Levonordefrin dilution
   - Sodium bisulfite preservative
   - Termination of action
   - Maximum recommended dose
7. Discuss the effects, mechanisms of action, and uses of norepinephrine, phenylephrine, and felypressin.
8. Discuss the side effects and overdose of vasoconstrictors.

INTRODUCTION

Local anesthetics are vasodilators with the ester procaine having the greatest vasodilatory properties, compared with the amides mepivacaine and prilocaine that have the least. No matter how readily the anesthetic can penetrate the nerve and bind to the receptor sites, the local blood vessels in the area of injection will immediately begin to absorb the anesthetic by causing vasodilation of the blood vessels, leading to increased blood flow to the site of injection, causing:

- An increased rate of anesthetic absorption into the bloodstream by carrying the anesthetic away from the injection site.
- A decrease in the duration of the anesthetic's action by diffusing quickly from the site of administration.
- Higher blood levels of local anesthetics, increasing the risk of systemic toxicity.
- Increased bleeding in the area resulting from the increase in blood flow.[1]

Vasoconstrictors are combined with local anesthetics to counteract the vasodilating properties of local anesthetics. Simply stated, vasoconstrictor drugs work by contracting the smooth muscle in blood vessels, which causes the vessels to constrict. Vasoconstrictors are important additives to the local anesthetic solution because of their ability to constrict blood vessels, thus providing the following beneficial effects:

- A decrease in the blood flow by constricting the blood vessels in the area of anesthetic administration and the amount of anesthetic needed to produce profound anesthesia.
- An increased duration of the anesthetic's effect by localizing the high concentration of the drug in the area of injection, within the nerve, improving the success rate and intensity of the nerve block. Using lidocaine 2% as an example, the duration of pulpal anesthesia in a plain solution (without a vasoconstrictor) is approximately 5 to 10 minutes; the duration of action dramatically increases approximately six times when a vasoconstrictor is added to 60 minutes of pulpal anesthesia.
- Slowing absorption of local anesthetic into the cardiovascular system (CVS), resulting in lower drug levels in the blood, reducing the probability of systemic toxicity. The anesthetic metabolism is able to keep pace with drug absorption, providing hemostasis at the injection site, which is particularly useful in areas of heavy bleeding. Deep scaling procedures performed by the dental hygienist involve soft tissue manipulation, resulting in hemorrhage, especially with severely inflamed tissues. These procedures generally require the patient to be anesthetized, and vasoconstrictors added to the anesthetic solution counteract unwanted bleeding caused by local anesthetic drugs.

CHEMISTRY

There are two vasoconstrictors that are added to local anesthetic drugs available in the United States: epinephrine and levonordefrin. Epinephrine is the most commonly used vasoconstrictor in dental local anesthetics and is referred to as the benchmark. Vasoconstrictors used in dentistry are structurally identical with the natural, nonsteroid mediators of the sympathetic nervous system (see Chapter 2), epinephrine and norepinephrine, which are secreted by the adrenal medulla. Because these drugs mimic similar effects as those caused by stimulation of the adrenergic nerves, they are referred to as sympathomimetic or adrenergic drugs. The term catecholamine is also appropriate for these agents because they are naturally occurring catecholamines of the sympathetic nervous system and have a distinct structure of a benzene ring with two hydroxyl groups (Fig. 4.1). Epinephrine and norepinephrine are naturally occurring catecholamines of the sympathetic nervous system, and levonordefrin is a synthetic catecholamine. They increase heart rate, contract blood

	①	②
Epinephrine	H	CH_3
Levonordefrin	CH_3	H
Norepinephrine	H	H

Fig. 4.1 Structural formulas of sympathomimetic amines commonly used as vasoconstrictors in local anesthesia for dentistry. (From Jastak T, Yagiela J, Donaldson D: *Local anesthesia of the oral cavity,* St Louis, 1995, Saunders.)

vessels, dilate air passage, and participate in the "fight-or-flight" response of the sympathetic nervous system.

THE USE OF VASOCONSTRICTORS IN DENTISTRY

When a vasoconstrictor is not added to the local anesthetic solution, the drug is quickly removed from the injection site into the systemic circulation, increasing the possibility of systemic toxicity and decreasing the duration of action. As discussed previously, vasoconstrictors added to local anesthetic solutions have several potentially beneficial effects that counteract these undesirable properties of local anesthetics. However, epinephrine, which is the most widely used vasoconstrictor in dentistry, is not an ideal drug. Exogenous epinephrine is absorbed from the site of injection into the circulation just like local anesthetics, and measurable levels of epinephrine in the blood can affect the heart and blood vessels by causing the sympathomimetic fight-or-flight response of apprehension, increased heart rate, palpitations, and sweating.[1] This has caused continued debate regarding the harmful influences of vasoconstrictors in some situations.[1,2] The benefits of vasoconstrictor use should be carefully weighed against the risks for patients who are medically compromised by severe cardiovascular disease, high blood pressure, or hyperthyroidism. However, completely avoiding the use of vasoconstrictors in these patients can cause a lack of profound anesthesia, leading to pain during the dental procedure and subsequently stimulating a significant release of endogenous epinephrine from the adrenal gland. This endogenous release of epinephrine in response to inadequate anesthesia during the dental appointment can be much greater than the amount that reaches the circulation from an injection of anesthetic with a vasoconstrictor. Fig. 4.2 illustrates the blood levels of endogenous epinephrine during rest and during mild-to-severe stress. Blood levels of endogenous epinephrine release are higher than the maximum recommended dose of epinephrine, 0.04 mg per appointment, for a cardiovascularly compromised patient. (See Chapter 8 for dosing calculations of epinephrine.)

Another important consideration is the endogenous release of epinephrine by the adrenal gland for healthy patients experiencing anxiety and stress before and during the dental appointment. As shown in Fig. 4.2, endogenous release of epinephrine in minor-to-moderate stress is increased for particularly anxious patients. This can compound the adverse effects of exogenous administration of epinephrine via the anesthetic injection containing epinephrine (Fig. 4.3). Fortunately, the undesirable systemic effects of epinephrine are short-lived. The rapid inactivation of epinephrine by the reuptake of adrenergic nerves quickly reduces the vasoconstrictor's harmful effects. According to Sisk, when epinephrine is administered intravenously, it has a half-life of 1 to 3 minutes.[3]

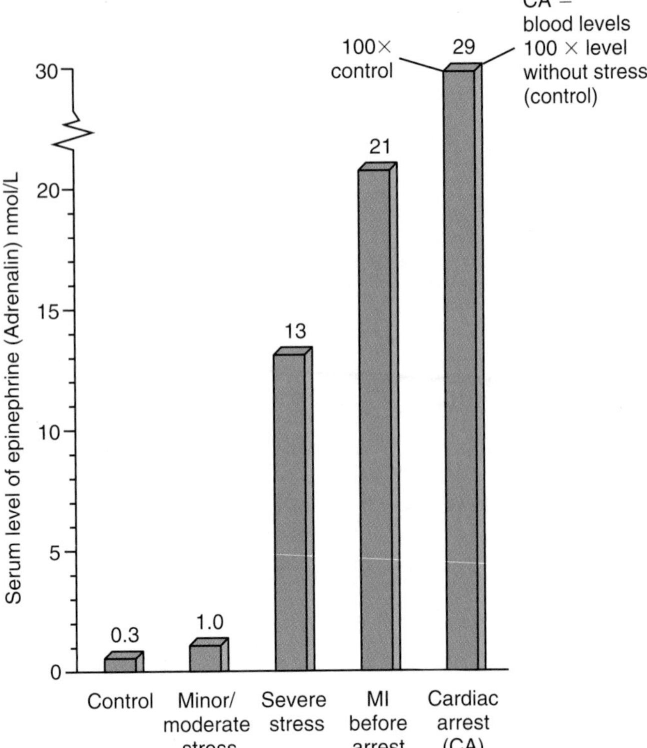

Fig. 4.2 Blood levels of endogenous epinephrine during rest; with minor, moderate, or severe stress; with myocardial infarction (MI); and with cardiac arrest (CA). (Modified from Haveles EB: *Applied pharmacology for the dental hygienist,* ed 8, St Louis, 2020, Elsevier.)

Patients with a recent myocardial infarction, coronary bypass surgery, or cerebrovascular accident within the past 6 months and those with uncontrolled hypertension, angina, arrhythmias, or hyperthyroidism should not be given an anesthetic with a vasoconstrictor until their medical condition is controlled.[4,5,6] Patients with a relative contraindication for vasoconstrictors can receive epinephrine-containing local anesthetic agents in the lowest possible dose, not to exceed the maximum recommended dose of 0.04 mg per appointment, using the best technique, which includes aspiration to reduce the risk of intravascular injection and injecting slowly to reduce the possibility of rapid systemic absorption. Depending on the severity of the condition, the clinician must determine whether a reduced amount of vasoconstrictor should be administered or whether no vasoconstrictor should be administered at all. In general, there are only a few absolute contraindications to the use of a vasoconstrictor, and in most situations limiting the amount of vasoconstrictor a patient can receive produces the benefits of vasoconstrictor use in local anesthetics without compromising the patient. Unless the vasoconstrictor is absolutely contraindicated, the inclusion of a vasoconstrictor should be considered routine. Absolute and relative contraindications to the use of vasoconstrictors are discussed in Chapter 7, and dosing information for vasoconstrictors is discussed in Chapter 8.

EPINEPHRINE (ADRENALIN)

As previously discussed, epinephrine is a naturally occurring catecholamine secreted by the adrenal medulla, consisting of approximately 80% of its secretions. It is also available as a synthetic catecholamine, which is identical in structure with the natural hormone epinephrine. Epinephrine is the most widely used vasoconstrictor in dentistry and

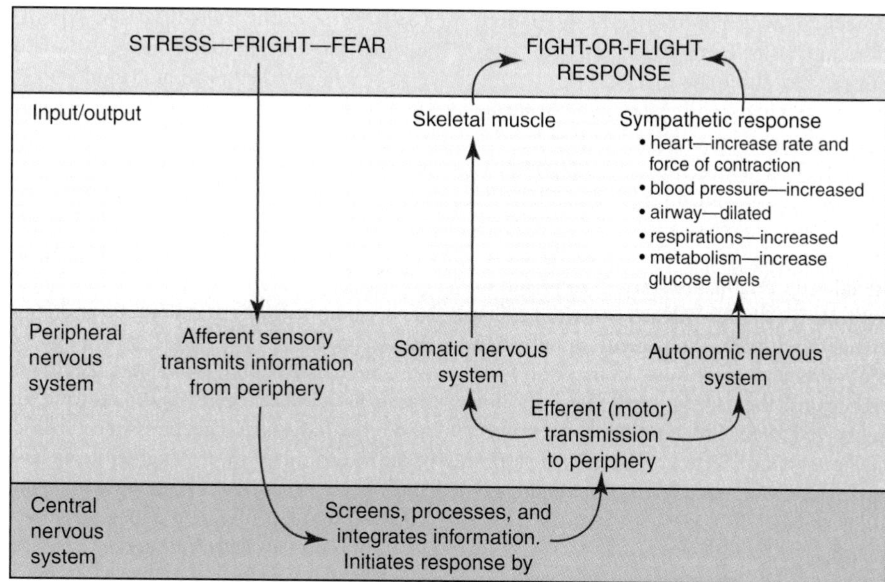

Fig. 4.3 Nervous system response during "fight-or-flight" or stress. (From McKenry L, Tessier E, Hogan M: *Mosby's pharmacology in nursing*, ed 22, St Louis, 2006, Mosby.)

TABLE 4.1 Epinephrine (Adrenalin) Dilutions and Uses in Dentistry

HO–(ring, HO)–$C(OH)(H)$–CH_2NHCH_3

Epinephrine

Concentration (Dilutions)	Anesthetic Preparations	Uses
1:1000	Epinephrine alone	Emergency treatment of anaphylaxis and acute asthma attacks
1:50,000	2% lidocaine	Most concentrated (least diluted) Provides greatest hemostasis Provides similar pain control as other anesthetic/vasoconstrictor preparations
1:100,000	2% lidocaine 4% articaine	Provides hemostasis but to a lesser degree than 1:50,000 dilution Provides similar pain control as other anesthetic/vasoconstrictor preparations Most commonly used dilution
1:200,000	4% articaine 4% prilocaine 0.5% bupivacaine	Least concentrated (most diluted) Provides hemostasis but to a lesser degree than 1:50,000 and 1:100,000 dilutions Provides similar pain control as other anesthetic/vasoconstrictor preparations Good alternative for patients with significant cardiovascular disease Good alternative for elderly patients sensitive to epinephrine

the most potent. Epinephrine is the standard by which all other vasoconstrictors are measured (Table 4.1).[1]

Mechanism of Action

Epinephrine and norepinephrine cause vasoconstriction by activating adrenergic receptors located in most tissues. According to Ahlquist,[2] these targeted receptor sites are divided into two major groups of adrenergic receptors, alpha (α) and beta (β), with several subtypes. Ahlquist recognized that α receptors have excitatory actions, and β receptors have inhibitory actions from catecholamines on smooth muscles. The excitatory action of α receptors by sympathomimetic drugs causes vasoconstriction of the smooth muscle in blood vessels. These α receptors have been further subcategorized into α_1 and α_2 depending on differences in their location and function, α_1 receptors are excitatory-postsynaptic and α_2 receptors are inhibitory-postsynaptic.[1,2,7] The inhibitory action of β receptors by sympathomimetic drugs causes smooth muscle relaxation (vasodilation and bronchodilation) and cardiac stimulation. The β receptors have also been further subcategorized into β_1 found in the heart (causing cardiac stimulation) and small intestines (causing lipolysis) and β_2 found in the bronchi, vascular beds, and uterus causing bronchodilation and vasodilation.[1,4,7]

Norepinephrine activates predominantly α receptors, and epinephrine activates both α and β receptors, causing vasoconstriction and vasodilation, respectively. α Receptors are less sensitive to epinephrine.[4] However, once the α receptor is stimulated by high levels of epinephrine, this activation will override the vasodilation caused by β

receptors and subsequently will cause vasoconstriction of the smooth muscle in peripheral arterioles and veins. This is the main reason sympathomimetic agents are added to local anesthetic solutions.

Stimulation of α receptors by adrenergic drugs such as epinephrine causes constriction of the smooth muscle in the blood vessels, also referred to as *vasoconstriction.* β_2 Receptor activation by epinephrine relaxes bronchial smooth muscles, causing the bronchi of the lungs to dilate. In addition, β_1 receptors have stimulatory effects that increase the rate and force of heart contractions. These stimulatory effects on β_1 receptors are undesirable side effects of incorporating sympathomimetic agents such as epinephrine into local anesthetic solutions. This is of particular concern in patients with preexisting cardiovascular and thyroid disease. The risks of adding the vasoconstrictor to the local anesthetic must be weighed against the benefits, and decreasing the amount of the drug administered should be considered (discussed next). Table 4.2 lists the major systemic effects of injected sympathomimetic agents involved in the cardiovascular and respiratory systems.

Epinephrine Dilutions

The concentration of vasoconstrictors in local anesthetic solutions is referred to as a ratio rather than a percentage as expressed by the local anesthetic drug. For example, a concentration of 1:100,000 means there is 1 g (or 1000 mg) of drug contained (dissolved/diluted) in a 100,000 mL solution, or 0.01 mg/mL. The most common dilutions of epinephrine combined with local anesthetics are 1:50,000 (0.02 mg/mL), 1:100,000 (0.01 mg/mL), and 1:200,000 (0.005 mg/mL). The 1:50,000 dilution is manufactured in combination with 2% lidocaine, the 1:100,000 dilution is manufactured in combination with 2% lidocaine and 4% articaine, and the 1:200,000 dilution is manufactured in combination with 4% prilocaine, 4% articaine, and 0.5% bupivacaine. Therefore in a typical dental anesthetic cartridge containing both a local anesthetic drug and vasoconstrictor, the label will identify both drugs (Fig. 4.4). Using prilocaine with epinephrine as an example, the cartridge may contain 4% prilocaine (referred to as a percentage) with 1:200,000 epinephrine (referred to as a ratio) (Fig. 4.4). Table 4.3 lists the vasoconstrictor dilutions combined with dental local anesthetics used in the United States and Canada.

The 1:50,000 dilution represents the highest concentration, and 1:200,000 dilution represents the lowest concentration and therefore produces fewer side effects.[1] Concentrations greater than 1:200,000 offer no advantage in prolonging the duration of anesthesia, reducing the plasma levels, or advancing pain control. Therefore because a 1:50,000 dilution offers no added benefits to most clinical situations and can produce more profound undesired sympathomimetic actions (fight or flight), there is questionable rationale for using a 1:50,000 dilution of epinephrine for pain control. However, higher concentrations of epinephrine, specifically the 1:50,000 dilution, are more effective for bleeding control (hemostasis). Local anesthetics with vasoconstrictors may be infiltrated for hemostasis even when pulpal anesthesia has been obtained. Therefore a 1:100,000 dilution of epinephrine for obtaining pulpal anesthesia may be used in combination with a relatively small infiltrated dose of 1:50,000 dilution of epinephrine into the papilla or gingival margin to decrease bleeding to less than half of that recorded from a similar volume of 1:100,000 (Fig. 4.5). This is particularly important for bleeding control during periodontal surgeries and for dental hygienists providing nonsurgical periodontal therapy.[8,9] (See Chapters 12 and 13.)

The selection of an appropriate vasoconstrictor dilution, if any, should be determined considering several factors such as the length of the dental procedure, the medical status of the patient, and the need for hemostasis.[1] As discussed earlier, the addition of a vasoconstrictor to an anesthetic such as lidocaine can dramatically increase the pulpal anesthesia and the clinical effectiveness of lidocaine. The medical status of the patient must be reviewed and considered when selecting a vasoconstrictor. In general, for patients with significant cardiovascular diseases ASA III and IV, patients with hyperthyroidism, patients with sulfite allergies, and patients taking certain medications, the severity of each of these conditions must be evaluated to determine the appropriateness of a selected vasoconstrictor.[5,6,10] The medical status of the patient in relationship to the use of vasoconstrictors will be covered thoroughly

TABLE 4.2 Systemic Effects of Adrenergic Amines on the Cardiovascular and Respiratory Systems

Cardiovascular System	Receptor Affected	Response
Heart rate	β_1, β_2	Increased (may be blocked or reversed by compensatory vagal reflex activity)
Contractile force	β_1, β_2	Increased
Coronary arterioles	α_1, α_2, β_2	Constriction/dilation (local regulatory processes largely govern blood flow)
Conduction velocity	β_1, β_2	Increased (may be blocked or reversed by compensatory vagal reflex activity)
Peripheral resistance	α_1, α_2, β_2	Increased/decreased
Respiratory System	**Receptor Affected**	**Response**
Bronchial smooth muscle	β_2	Relaxation
Bronchial glands	α_1, β_2	Decreased/increased
Pulmonary arterioles	α_1, β_2	Constriction/dilation

From Jastak JT, Yagiela JA, Donaldson D: *Local anesthesia of the oral cavity,* St Louis, 1995, Saunders.

TABLE 4.3 Vasoconstrictors Used in Dental Local Anesthetic Solutions

Generic Name	Proprietary Name	Dilutions
Epinephrine	Adrenalin	1:50,000 1:100,000 1:200,000
Levonordefrin	Neo-Cobefrin	1:20,000

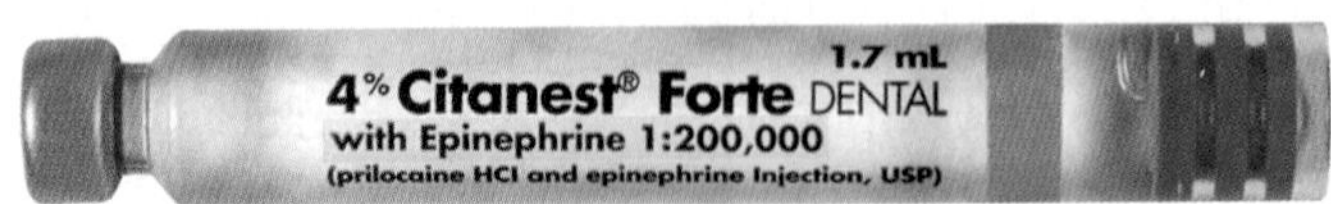

Fig. 4.4 Typical dental anesthetic cartridge containing both a local anesthetic drug (prilocaine) and vasoconstrictor (epinephrine). The label will identify both drugs and their concentrations.

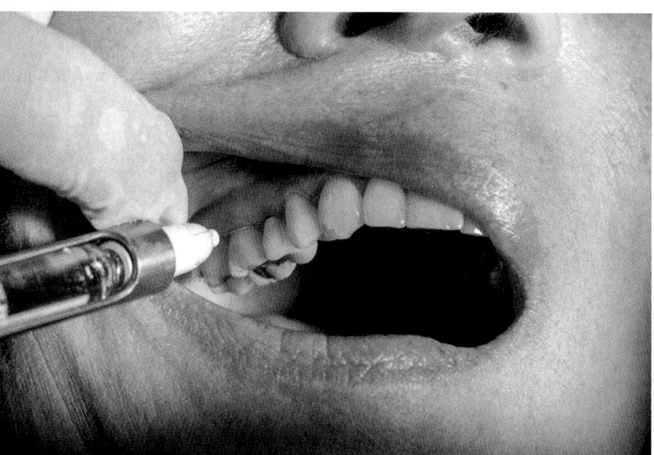

Fig. 4.5 Small amounts of lidocaine 1:50,000 epinephrine can be infiltrated into the papilla to decrease bleeding during nonsurgical periodontal therapy after pulpal anesthesia has been obtained using a lower concentration of epinephrine such as lidocaine 1:100,000 epinephrine.

in Chapter 7. Finally, the need for hemostasis should be considered. Epinephrine is effective in decreasing blood flow during surgical procedures and nonsurgical periodontal therapy. Because epinephrine possesses both α and β actions with α receptors being less sensitive to epinephrine than β receptors, higher doses of epinephrine are needed to produce the vasoconstriction action of α receptors. Although all epinephrine dilutions provide bleeding control, a 1:50,000 dilution (being double the concentration of 1:100,000 and four times the concentration of 1:200,000) provides the most rigorous bleeding control compared with the 1:100,000 and 1:200,000 dilutions. However, an important consideration is that as the tissue level of epinephrine begins to decline, it produces a rebound vasodilatory effect when the β_2 action begins to predominate. This vasodilatory action can potentially lead to postoperative bleeding approximately 6 hours after the procedure.[1]

Sodium Bisulfite Preservative

Synthetic epinephrine is not very stable and must include the addition of an acidic preservative to stabilize the solution to prevent oxidation of epinephrine. Because a local anesthetic is manufactured as an acid salt, the drug is highly soluble in water and acidic, with a pH of approximately 6.5. The addition of the preservative sodium bisulfite provides a shelf life of approximately 18 months because of its antioxidant properties.[1] However, there are disadvantages to the presence of this preservative. First, sodium bisulfite can further acidify the pH of the anesthetic solution to the range of 3.0 to 5.5, thus reducing the efficiency of the quaternary amine to dissociate (once injected) into the uncharged tertiary amine base necessary to penetrate the lipid-rich membrane of the nerve and slightly slowing the onset of action of the local anesthetic. This is of particular concern in an acidic tissue environment associated with an active infection (see Chapter 3). Second, according to the U.S. Food and Drug Administration (FDA), sulfites associated with vasoconstrictors may cause allergic-type reactions in certain susceptible persons, especially asthmatics. Patients who have a true allergy to sodium bisulfite should not receive an anesthetic/vasoconstrictor combination. However, for sulfite-containing epinephrine for injection for use in allergic emergency, the FDA states that "epinephrine is the preferred treatment for serious allergic or other emergency situations even though the product contains a sulfite that may in other products cause allergic-type reactions including anaphylactic symptoms or life-threatening or less severe asthmatic episodes in susceptible persons. The alternative to using epinephrine in a life-threatening situation may not be satisfactory. The presence of a sulfite(s) in the product should not deter administration of the drug for treatment of serious allergic or other emergency situations" *(CFR – Code of Federal Regulations Title 21)*. Cartridges that do not contain a vasoconstrictor, such as 3% mepivacaine and 4% prilocaine, do not contain sodium bisulfite and are therefore safe to be administered to patients with sulfite allergies. Because mepivacaine and prilocaine produce only minor vasodilation compared with other available anesthetics, they can still produce adequate pulpal anesthesia for short dental appointments when administering nerve blocks (see Chapter 5). People often confuse sulfites with sulfa medications; although both can cause allergic reactions in people, they are chemically unrelated.

Actions of Epinephrine on Specific Systems and Tissue

Mode of Action

Epinephrine exerts its action directly on the adrenergic receptors, including both α and β receptors, affecting β receptors predominantly.

Myocardium

The pharmacologic effect of epinephrine is essentially a result of its direct effect as an agonist on specific α and β receptors (β_1 and β_2). Epinephrine increases heart rate, stroke volume, and cardiac output by stimulating β_1 receptors.

Pacemaker Cells

Epinephrine stimulates β_1 receptors, increasing the incidence of dysrhythmias.

Coronary Arteries

Epinephrine increases coronary artery flow by dilating coronary arteries.

Blood Pressure

Small doses of epinephrine increase systolic pressure to a greater extent than the diastolic pressure (diastolic pressure may decrease). Higher doses of epinephrine increase diastolic pressure.

Cardiovascular System

The β_1 effects of epinephrine have direct stimulation on the CVS, which leads to an overall decrease in cardiac efficiency.

Vasculature

Epinephrine constricts the α receptors that are contained in the skin and mucous membranes. The effects of epinephrine on the blood vessels of the skeletal muscles, which contain both α and β_2 receptors, are dose dependent resulting from the predominance of β_2 receptors, which are more sensitive to epinephrine than α receptors. Therefore smaller doses are affected by β_2 actions and produce vasodilation, and larger doses are affected by α actions and produce vasoconstriction.

Metabolic System

Epinephrine inhibits insulin secretion, causing a rise in blood sugar and an increase in free fatty acids. This is of particular concern in brittle diabetics taking large doses of insulin, especially if, in addition, these individuals have cardiovascular disease. Inconsistent blood sugar levels, including severe hypoglycemia and hyperglycemia, may result. Well-controlled diabetics may receive epinephrine without precautions.[6]

Respiratory System

Epinephrine is a potent bronchial dilator resulting from the β_2 receptor effects. It is an invaluable drug for treating acute asthmatic attacks and anaphylactic reactions.[11,12]

Central Nervous System

In normal therapeutic doses, epinephrine does not stimulate the CNS. Overdose of epinephrine produces signs and symptoms of CNS stimulation, which may include anxiety, nausea, restlessness, weakness, tremor, headache, and hyperventilation.

Hemostasis

Epinephrine is added to local anesthetic solutions to provide hemostasis and is frequently used during surgical procedures. High doses stimulate α receptors, causing vasoconstriction, followed by β_2 vasodilation after 6 hours.[1,9]

Termination of Action

The absorption of epinephrine is retarded because of the drug's vasoconstricting properties. It may take several hours for absorption to be completed. The effects of epinephrine after inadvertent intravascular injection become apparent within 1 minute and, because of the body's efficiency at removing catecholamines, the effects of epinephrine in the blood last only 5 to 10 minutes. Once absorbed, the action of epinephrine is terminated primarily by the reuptake action of adrenergic nerves, and any epinephrine that escapes the reuptake action is inactivated rapidly in the blood by enzymes catechol-O-methyltransferase (COMT) and monoamine oxidase (MAO), both of which are present in the liver.[1,2] Only 1% of epinephrine is excreted unchanged in urine. Fig. 4.6 illustrates the distribution and fate of catecholamines injected into peripheral tissues.

Maximum Recommended Dose

The American Heart Association[13] and the New York Heart Association[14] indicate that the lowest possible effective dose should be used when administering local anesthetics with epinephrine to either healthy or medically compromised patients. Proper aspiration on several planes and slow injection should also be done when administering local anesthetics with epinephrine. The maximum recommended dose per visit of epinephrine for a healthy patient is 0.2 mg. The maximum recommended dose per visit of epinephrine for a cardiovascularly compromised patient or a patient needing treatment modifications (e.g., a patient taking a tricyclic antidepressant) is 0.04 mg. See Chapter 7 for medical history considerations when administering epinephrine. Maximum recommended doses for vasoconstrictors and local anesthetics, as well as calculation methods, are discussed in Chapter 8.

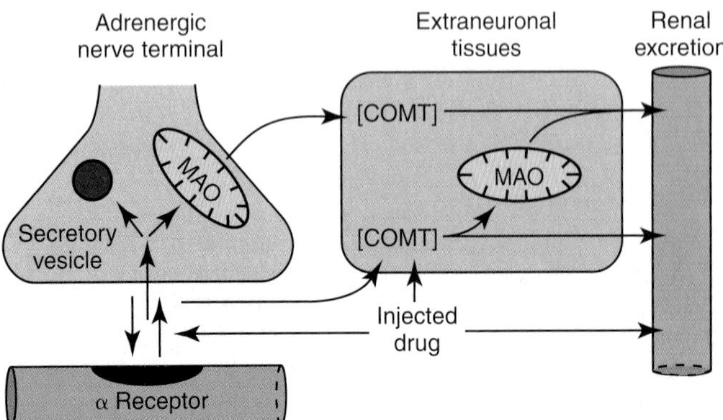

Fig. 4.6 The distribution and fate of catecholamines injected into peripheral tissue. *Dark arrows* indicate the predominant pathways for epinephrine and norepinephrine. *COMT,* Catechol-O-methyltransferase; *MAO,* monoamine oxidase. (From Jastak T, Yagiela J, Donaldson D: *Local anesthesia of the oral cavity,* St Louis, 1995, Saunders.)

LEVONORDEFRIN (NEO-COBEFRIN)

Levonordefrin is a synthetic vasoconstrictor that is approximately one-sixth (15%) as potent as epinephrine; it is manufactured in a higher concentration to achieve the same effects as epinephrine 1:100,000.[2] Levonordefrin is available in dentistry with only 2% mepivacaine in a 1:20,000 dilution, which is five times greater than epinephrine in a dilution of 1:100,000, but because it is one-sixth as potent as epinephrine, a 1:20,000 dilution of levonordefrin produces the same clinical effects as the epinephrine 1:100,000 dilution. Like epinephrine, levonordefrin contains the preservative sodium bisulfite to delay its deterioration (Table 4.4).

Actions of Levonordefrin on Specific Systems and Tissue

Mode of Action

Levonordefrin is a selective α_2 agonist (75%) and produces vasoconstriction in low systemic concentrations; it has much less β activity (only 25%) compared with epinephrine, which has 50% α and 50% β activity.[1]

Myocardium

The pharmacologic effect of levonordefrin on the myocardium is essentially the same as epinephrine by increasing cardiac output and heart rate, but to a lesser degree.

Pacemaker Cells

Levonordefrin acts the same as epinephrine by increasing dysrhythmias, but to a lesser degree.

Coronary Arteries

Levonordefrin increases coronary artery flow by dilating coronary arteries similar to epinephrine, but to a lesser degree.

Blood Pressure

Levonordefrin increases systolic pressure to a greater extent than the diastolic (diastolic pressure may decrease). Higher doses of levonordefrin increase diastolic pressure.

Cardiovascular System

Levonordefrin leads to a decrease in cardiac efficiency.

Vasculature

Effects on the vasculature are similar to epinephrine by providing α constriction of the skin and mucous membranes, but to a lesser degree.

Metabolic System

Levonordefrin inhibits insulin secretion, causing a rise in blood sugar and an increase in free fatty acids similar to epinephrine, but to a lesser degree.

TABLE 4.4 Levonordefrin (Neo-Cobefrin) Dilution and Uses in Dentistry

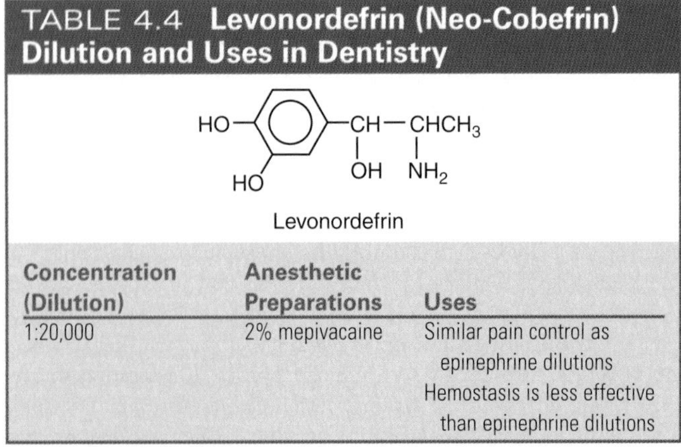

Concentration (Dilution)	Anesthetic Preparations	Uses
1:20,000	2% mepivacaine	Similar pain control as epinephrine dilutions Hemostasis is less effective than epinephrine dilutions

Respiratory System

Levonordefrin provides some bronchodilation but significantly less than epinephrine.

Central Nervous System

In normal therapeutic doses, levonordefrin does not stimulate the CNS. In an overdose, it is not a potent stimulant compared with epinephrine.

Hemostasis

Levonordefrin provides hemostasis but is significantly less effective than epinephrine.

Termination of Action

Levonordefrin is terminated by reuptake by adrenergic nerves, and escaped levonordefrin is inactivated by COMT. Levonordefrin is not terminated by MAO.[2]

Maximum Recommended Dose

The maximum recommended dose per visit of levonordefrin for a healthy patient is 1.0 mg. The maximum recommended dose per visit of levonordefrin for a cardiovascularly compromised patient or a patient needing treatment modifications is 0.2 mg. Some sources indicate that a cardiac dose is not necessary for levonordefrin and that for all patients the maximum dose is 1.0 mg or 11.1 cartridges.[1] This author and others recommend that the need for a cardiac dose of levonordefrin should be determined on an individual patient basis, utilizing physician consultations if necessary.[13,15,16] Levonordefrin should be avoided in patients taking tricyclic antidepressants to avoid hypertensive crises.[1,15] See Chapter 7 for medical history considerations when administering levonordefrin and Chapter 8 for maximum recommended dose and dosing methods.

OTHER VASOCONSTRICTORS

Norepinephrine (Levarterenol)

Norepinephrine is a naturally occurring catecholamine. Twenty percent of its production is from the adrenal medulla, but it is also available as a synthetic catecholamine. The usual dilution used in dentistry is 1:30,000. Norepinephrine has the same action as levonordefrin on α receptors. It almost exclusively activates α receptors (90%) and minimally activates β receptors (10%).[17] Because of this, norepinephrine produces intense peripheral vasoconstriction with a possible dramatic increase in blood pressure. Therefore its use in dentistry is *not recommended.* The intense vasoconstriction/hemostasis caused by norepinephrine is likely to produce tissue necrosis, especially on the palate (Fig. 4.7).

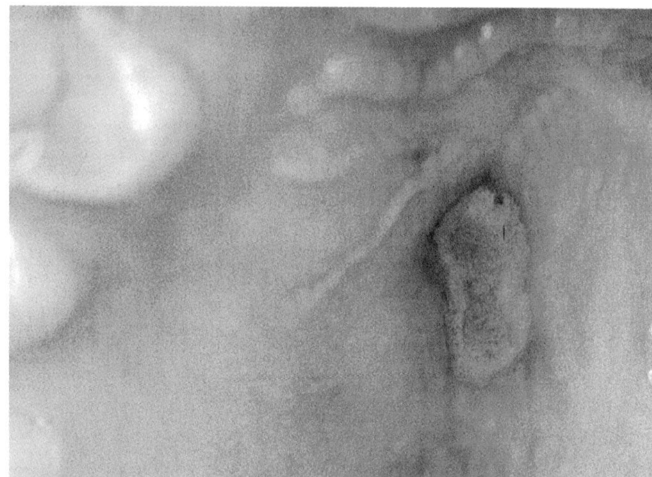

Fig. 4.7 Sterile abscess on the palate produced by excessive use of a vasoconstrictor. This is likely to be produced with epinephrine dilution of 1:50,000 or with norepinephrine. (From Malamed S: *Handbook of local anesthesia,* ed 7, St Louis, 2020, Elsevier.)

Phenylephrine (Neo-Synephrine)

Phenylephrine is a synthetic sympathomimetic amine that exerts its action predominantly on α receptors (95%), with very little β effects on the heart. It is a very weak vasoconstrictor (only 5%), is as potent as epinephrine, and is formulated at much higher concentrations than epinephrine (1:2500 dilution). It is not used in dentistry but is used in combination with local anesthetics for the management of hypotension and for nasal decongestants and ophthalmic solutions.[18]

Felypressin

Felypressin is a synthetic hormone analog of vasopressin.[1] It is a direct stimulator of vascular smooth muscles.[3] Felypressin causes few side effects because it has little or no direct effect on the myocardium or adrenergic nerve transmission. Therefore it may be safely administered to patients with uncontrolled hyperthyroidism or patients taking tricyclic antidepressants or MAO inhibitors. Felypressin is available in Great Britain and other countries usually in combination with 3% prilocaine. It is favorably compared with epinephrine in anesthesia for restorative dentistry.[1,9]

SIDE EFFECTS AND OVERDOSE OF VASOCONSTRICTORS

Overdose of vasoconstrictors from accidental intravenous injection or by administering more than the maximum recommended dose produces overstimulation of adrenergic receptors that can produce signs and symptoms normally observed from CNS stimulation. Table 4.5 lists the typical overdose responses to epinephrine.

With high plasma levels of epinephrine, dysrhythmias, ventricular fibrillation, dramatic increase in heart rate, and possible cardiac arrest are possible, more so in patients with increased susceptibility to the adverse cardiovascular effects of adrenergic drugs. Because the body is very efficient at removing vasoconstrictors, these adverse effects last only about 5 to 10 minutes. Even so, for patients with severe conditions such as unstable angina, recent myocardial infarction (within 6 months), recent coronary bypass surgery (within 6 months), uncontrolled hypertension, uncontrolled hyperthyroidism, uncontrolled dysrhythmias, or congestive heart failure, the risk of using a vasoconstrictor may outweigh the benefits.[1,5,6,15] The patient's physician should be consulted before using vasoconstrictors on these patients. These conditions, as well as drug interactions, are discussed in Chapter 7. For all patients, only the minimal effective dose should be administered, not to exceed the maximum recommended dose. (See Table 4.6 for recommended doses for vasoconstrictors.)

TABLE 4.5 Overdose Responses to Vasoconstrictors

Tension	Increased heart rate
Anxiety	Increased blood pressure
Apprehension	Throbbing headache
Nervousness	Hyperventilation
Tremors	

From Jastak T, Yagiela J, Donaldson D: *Local anesthesia of the oral cavity,* St Louis, 1995, Saunders.

TABLE 4.6 Recommended Maximum Dosages of Vasoconstrictors

Concentration (Dilution)	Maximum Recommended Dose (MRD) Per Appointment: Healthy Patient	Number of Cartridges: Healthy Patient (ASA I)	Maximum Recommended Dose (MRD) Per Appointment: Patient With Clinically Significant Cardiovascular Disease (ASA III or IV), Or Patients Needing Treatment Modifications	Number of Cartridges: Patient With Clinically Significant Cardiovascular Disease (ASA III or IV), Or Patients Needing Treatment Modifications
1:50,000 Epinephrine	0.2 mg	5.5	0.04 mg	1.1
1:100,000 Epinephrine	0.2 mg	11.1	0.04 mg	2.2
1:200,000 Epinephrine	0.2 mg	22.2	0.04 mg	4.4
1:20,000 Levonordefrin	1.0 mg*	11.1*	0.2 mg*	2.2*

Levonordefrin should be avoided in patients taking tricyclic antidepressants.[1,15]

*Data from other sources[1] indicate that for all patients, the maximum dose of levonordefrin should be 1.0 mg per appointment or 11.1 cartridges. This author and others recommend that the need for a cardiac dose of levonordefrin should be determined on an individual patient basis, utilizing physician consultations if necessary.[13,15,16]

DENTAL HYGIENE CONSIDERATIONS

- Vasoconstrictors are added to local anesthetics to counteract the vasodilating properties of the local anesthetic.
- Vasoconstrictors provide hemostasis, increase duration of action, decrease systemic toxicity, and decrease required dose of the local anesthetic drug.
- Vasoconstrictors are adrenergic drugs and stimulate the "fight-or-flight" response of the sympathetic nervous system and increase heart rate and blood pressure.
- Endogenous release of epinephrine associated with stress in an anxious patient may compound the adverse effects of exogenous administration of epinephrine. This is of even greater concern for patients who are cardiovascularly compromised.
- Patients with a recent myocardial infarction, coronary bypass surgery, or cerebrovascular accident within the past 6 months, and those with uncontrolled hypertension, angina, arrhythmias, and hyperthyroidism should not be given an anesthetic with a vasoconstrictor until their medical condition is under control.
- Mepivacaine 3% and prilocaine 4% plain have the lowest vasodilating properties of all the local anesthetic agents available in the United States and are good alternatives for patients who are unable to receive a local anesthetic with a vasoconstrictor.
- Prilocaine plain (block anesthesia) is the only intermediate-acting local anesthetic in dentistry without a vasoconstrictor.
- Epinephrine, once in the bloodstream, is rapidly inactivated predominantly by adrenergic nerves. Any epinephrine that escapes the reuptake action is inactivated rapidly in the blood by enzymes catechol-O-methyltransferase (COMT) and monoamine oxidase (MAO).
- Patients with relative contraindications to epinephrine can receive 0.04 mg of epinephrine per appointment.
- The maximum recommended dose per visit of epinephrine for a healthy patient is 0.2 mg. The maximum recommended dose per visit of epinephrine for a cardiovascularly compromised patient or a patient needing treatment modifications is 0.04 mg.
- More diluted formulations of epinephrine (1:200,000) are safer for patients who are cardiovascularly compromised or elderly patients sensitive to epinephrine.
- More concentrated formulations of epinephrine (1:50,000) provide the greatest bleeding control.
- As epinephrine begins to decline in the tissue, it produces rebound vasodilation and can potentially lead to postoperative bleeding.
- There is no difference in pain control between 1:50,000, 1:100,000, and 1:200,000 dilutions of epinephrine. Therefore since a 1:50,000 dilution can produce more profound undesired sympathomimetic actions (fight or flight), it should be reserved for bleeding control and not pain control.
- Sodium bisulfite is added to local anesthetic solutions that contain a vasoconstrictor to prevent the oxidation of the vasoconstrictor. Individuals who are allergic to sodium bisulfite should not receive an anesthetic containing a vasoconstrictor.
- The U.S. Food and Drug Administration (FDA) states that epinephrine is the preferred treatment for serious allergic or other emergency situations even though the patient may be allergic to sulfites.
- When sodium bisulfite is added to local anesthetic solutions that contain a vasoconstrictor, it decreases the pH of the local anesthetic even further, causing the solution to be even more acidic.
- Epinephrine in high doses (1:1000) is an invaluable drug for treating acute asthmatic attacks and anaphylactic reaction and should be in every dental emergency kit.
- Levonordefin is only formulated with 2% mepivacaine using a 1:20,000 dilution.
- Levonordefrin is only 15% as potent as epinephrine and therefore manufactured in a higher concentration. Levonordefrin has the same systemic actions as epinephrine but to a lesser degree.
- A 1:20,000 dilution of levonordefrin produces the same clinical effects as the epinephrine 1:100,000 dilution.
- Levonordefrin provides less hemostasis than epinephrine.
- The maximum recommended dose per visit of levonordefrin for a healthy patient is 1.0 mg. The maximum recommended dose per visit of levonordefrin for a cardiovascularly compromised patient or a patient needing treatment modifications is 0.2 mg.
- Levonordefrin should be avoided if patients are taking tricyclic antidepressants.

CASE STUDY 4.1 A Patient Requires Emergency Treatment for a Broken Tooth

A patient is in the office for emergency treatment of a broken tooth on #3. She is in severe pain, and, because of the severity of the breakage, the tooth cannot be saved. The dentist believes it will be an easy extraction, and therefore will extract the tooth using local anesthesia. The dentist asks the dental hygienist to administer the anesthesia. Upon review of the patient's medical history and consultation with the patient's physician, it is determined that the patient has uncontrolled hyperthyroidism.

Critical Thinking Question

Considering the patient's medical history, what type of anesthetic should be selected for the procedure and why?

CHAPTER REVIEW QUESTIONS

1. Once absorbed in the bloodstream, epinephrine is terminated primarily by:
   A. Hydrolysis by acetylcholinesterase
   B. Metabolism by monoamine oxidase (MAO)
   C. Metabolism by catecholamine-O-methyl transferase (COMT)
   D. Reuptake by adrenergic nerves
2. Which of the following is a sign of epinephrine toxicity?
   A. Fatigue
   B. Tachycardia
   C. Miosis
   D. Hypotension
   E. Sleepiness
3. What is the maximum recommended dose of epinephrine per appointment for a patient with significant cardiovascular disease?
   A. 0.02 mg
   B. 0.04 mg
   C. 0.2 mg
   D. 0.4 mg
   E. 2.0 mg
4. Epinephrine should be avoided in patients with:
   A. Untreated hyperthyroidism
   B. Hypotension
   C. Controlled diabetes
   D. Myocardial infarction or stroke within the prior 6 months
   E. A and D
   F. C and D
5. What is epinephrine used for?
   A. Seizures
   B. Angina pectoris
   C. Anaphylactic reactions
   D. Syncope
   E. Gout
6. An effect of epinephrine used in dentistry is to:
   A. Increase vasoconstriction and slow bleeding
   B. Decrease duration of anesthetic
   C. Calm down a nervous patient
   D. Increase dissociation of cation
7. Which of the following is a systemic effect of vasoconstrictors used with local anesthetics?
   A. Increased diastolic blood pressure
   B. Decreased systolic blood pressure
   C. Increased systolic blood pressure
   D. Decreased heart rate
   E. A and C
8. Vasoconstrictors are added to local anesthetics for what reason(s)?
   A. Reduce bleeding
   B. Counteract the vasodilatory effects of local anesthetics
   C. Decrease possibility of an anesthetic overdose
   D. A and B above
   E. B and C above
   F. A, B, C above
9. Which of the following is the preservative added to local anesthetic solutions containing epinephrine to prevent its oxidation?
   A. Sodium bisulfite
   B. Sodium chloride
   C. Sodium bicarbonate
   D. None of the above
10. There is no difference in pain control when using a 1:50,000, 1:100,000, or 1:200,000 dilution of epinephrine. A 1:200,000 dilution of epinephrine offers the most rigorous bleeding control.
    A. Both statements are correct.
    B. Both statements are NOT correct.
    C. The first statement is correct; the second statement is NOT correct.
    D. The first statement is NOT correct; the second statement is correct.
11. Epinephrine causes direct stimulation of which of the following adrenergic receptors resulting in cardiac stimulation?
    A. α
    B. β_1
    C. β_2
    D. None of the above; epinephrine does not stimulate the cardiovascular system.
12. Which of the following vasoconstrictors can safely be administered to a patient with uncontrolled hyperthyroidism?
    A. Norepinephrine
    B. Phenylephrine
    C. Felypressin
    D. Levonordefrin
13. The half-life of epinephrine is approximately:
    A. 1 to 3 minutes
    B. 5 to 7 minutes
    C. 10 to 3 minutes
    D. 15 to 20 minutes
14. What is a 1:1000 dilution of epinephrine used for?
    A. Increase hemostasis
    B. Increase duration of anesthetic
    C. Treatment of anaphylaxis
    D. Prevent systemic overdose
15. Levonordefrin is added to which of the following local anesthetics?
    A. 2% lidocaine
    B. 2% mepivacaine
    C. 3% mepivacaine
    D. 4% prilocaine
16. Vasoconstrictor drugs are known as all of the following EXCEPT one. Which one is the EXCEPTION?
    A. Sympathomimetic amines
    B. Catecholamines
    C. Adrenergic drugs
    D. Vasodilators
17. Epinephrine and norepinephrine are endogenous hormones excreted by:
    A. Adrenal gland
    B. Pituitary gland
    C. Parotid gland
    D. Pancreas
18. Which adrenergic receptor causes epinephrine to have inhibitory actions that cause vasodilation and bronchodilation?
    A. α_1
    B. β_1
    C. β_2
    D. α_2
19. Which of the following concentrations of epinephrine is the most diluted?
    A. 1:50,000
    B. 1:100,000
    C. 1:200,000
    D. 1:1000
20. Signs and symptoms of a vasoconstrictor overdose manifest as:
    A. Central nervous system depression
    B. Central nervous system stimulation
    C. Cardiovascular depression
    D. Respiratory depression

REFERENCES

1. Malamed S. *Handbook of local anesthesia.* ed 7. St Louis: Elsevier; 2020.
2. Ahlquist RP. A study of adrenotropic receptors. *Am J Physiol.* 1948;153:586–600.
3. Sisk A. Vasoconstrictors in local anesthesia for dentistry. *Anesth Prog.* 1992;39:187–193.
4. Yagiela JA. Epinephrine and the compromised heart. *Orofac Pain Manage.* 1991;1:5–8.
5. Goulet JP, Perusse R, Turotte JY. Contraindications to vasoconstrictors in dentistry. Part I. Cardiovascular diseases. *Oral Surg Oral Med Oral Pathol.* 1992;74:579–686.
6. Goulet JP, Perusse R, Turotte JY. Contraindications to vasoconstrictors in dentistry. Part II. Hyperthyroidism, diabetes, sulfite sensitivity, cortico-dependent asthma, and pheochromocytoma. *Oral Surg Oral Med Oral Pathol.* 1992;74:587–691.
7. Haveles EB. *Applied pharmacology for the dental hygienist.* ed 8. St. Louis: Elsevier; 2020.
8. Bowen DM, Pieren JA. *Darby and Walsh dental hygiene: theory and practice.* ed 5. St. Louis: Elsevier; 2020.
9. Jastak T, Yagiela J, Donaldson D. *Local anesthesia of the oral cavity.* St Louis: Saunders; 1995.
10. Goulet JP, Perusse R, Turotte JY. Contraindications to vasoconstrictors in dentistry. Part III. Pharmacologic interactions. *Oral Surg Oral Med Oral Pathol.* 1992;74:592–697.
11. Epinephrine drug monograph. ClinicalKey. http://www.clinicalkey.com.
12. Shah R, Saltoun CA. Chapter 14: acute severe asthma (status asthmaticus). *Allergy Asthma Proc.* 2012;33(suppl 1):S47–S50.
13. Management of dental problems in patients with cardiovascular disease: report of a working conference jointly sponsored by the American Dental Association and American Heart Association. *J Am Dent Assoc.* 1964;68:333–342.
14. Use of epinephrine in connection with procaine in dental procedures: report of the Special Committee of the New York Heart Association, Inc., on the use of epinephrine in connection with procaine in dental procedures. *J Am Dent Assoc.* 1955;50:108.
15. Little JW, Falace DA, Miller CS, Rhodus NL. *Dental management of the medically compromised patient.* ed 9. St Louis: Elsevier; 2018.
16. Paarmann C. Decision making and local anesthesia. *Dimens Dent Hyg.* 2008;6(10):24.
17. Norepinephrine drug monograph. ClinicalKey. http://www.clinicalkey.com.
18. Phenylephrine drug monograph. ClinicalKey. http://www.clinicalkey.com.

ADDITIONAL RESOURCES

Bahl R. Local anesthesia in dentistry. *Anesth Prog.* 2004;51:138–142.

Becker D, Reed K. Essentials of local anesthetic pharmacology. *Anesth Prog.* 2006;53:98–109.

Berecek KH, Brody MJ. Evidence for a neurotransmitter role for epinephrine derived from the adrenal medulla. *Am J Physiol.* 1982;242:H593–H601.

Finder RL, More PA. Adverse drug reactions to local anesthesia. *Dent Clin N Am.* 2002;46:447–457.

Hargreaves KM, Berman LH. *Cohen's pathways of the pulp.* ed 11. St Louis: Elsevier; 2016.

Malamed SF, Sykes P, Kubota Y, et al. Local anesthesia: a review. *Anesth Pain Control Dent.* 1992;1:11–24.

Stiell IG, Hebert PC, Weitzman BN, et al. High-dose epinephrine in adult cardiac arrest. *N Engl J Med.* 1992;327(15):1045–1050.

Yagiela JA. Adverse drug interactions in dental practice: interactions associated with vasoconstrictors. Part V of a series. *J Am Dent Assoc.* 1999;130:701–709.

5

Local Anesthetic Agents

Demetra Daskalos Logothetis, RDH, MS

LEARNING OBJECTIVES

1. List and describe the composition of local anesthetic agents.
2. Define ester and amide local anesthetics.
3. List and discuss amide local anesthetics using their generic and proprietary names.
4. Discuss the selection considerations when choosing a local anesthetic.
5. Describe the factors that determine the duration of a local anesthetic.
6. Discuss posttreatment pain control in relation to local anesthetics.
7. Differentiate between a relative and an absolute contraindication.
8. Summarize allergies that affect local anesthetic selection.
9. Stress why hemostasis control is needed.
10. Discuss the properties, helpful tips for anesthetic selection, precautions, and maximum recommended dose for the following amide local anesthetics:
    - Lidocaine
    - Mepivacaine
    - Prilocaine
    - Articaine
    - Bupivacaine
11. Discuss procaine and other ester local anesthetics.

COMPOSITION OF LOCAL ANESTHETIC AGENTS

Local anesthetics used in dentistry are manufactured in single-use cartridges. Local anesthetic cartridges are designed to contain 2.0 mL of solution. However, when the silicone rubber stopper is added to the cartridge, it is capable of containing only 1.8 mL of solution. Although most local anesthetic cartridges contain 1.8 mL of solution, not all are labeled as such. Some manufacturers label and market their anesthetics as containing 1.7 mL of solution (Box 5.1). Local anesthetics are formulated as 2% agents (36 mg per cartridge), 3% agents (54 mg per cartridge), 4% agents (72 mg per cartridge), and 0.5% agents (9 mg per cartridge). See Chapter 8 for dosing facts and calculations. In addition to the local anesthetic drug, the dental cartridge may contain several other ingredients, such as the following:

- *Vasoconstrictor:* As discussed in Chapter 4, there are two vasoconstrictors currently added to local anesthetic agents in the United States: epinephrine and levonordefrin. Epinephrine is available in 1:50,000, 1:100,000, and 1:200,000 dilutions, and levonordefrin is available in a 1:20,000 dilution and with only 2% mepivacaine. All local anesthetics are vasodilators, and vasoconstrictors are added to local anesthetic agents to delay the absorption of local anesthetics, which reduces the potential for systemic toxicity and prolongs the duration of action. Because vasoconstrictors counteract the vasodilatory properties of local anesthetics, they are also beneficial for providing hemostasis.
- *Vasoconstrictor preservative:* Sodium bisulfite, metabisulfite, or acetone sodium bisulfite is only added to local anesthetic agents that contain vasoconstrictors.[1] Because vasoconstrictors are unstable and have a short shelf life, sodium bisulfite is added to delay the deterioration of the vasoconstrictor. Sodium bisulfite is manufactured as an acid salt, rendering it soluble in water and decreasing the pH of the agent, making it significantly more acidic than the same solution without a vasoconstrictor. As discussed in Chapter 3, local anesthetic agents that are more acidic have a greater quantity of charged cation molecules (RNH^+) than the uncharged base (anion) molecules (RH). This slows the efficiency of the local anesthetic agent to diffuse into the axoplasm, delaying the onset of action.
- *Sodium hydroxide:* Sodium hydroxide is a buffer that alkalinizes, or adjusts, the pH of the solution between 6 and 7.[2]
- *Sodium chloride:* Sodium chloride is a buffer, which when added to a local anesthetic creates an injectable isotonic solution.

Methylparaben is a bacteriostatic agent and preservative that was added to local anesthetic agents without vasoconstrictors before 1984 to prevent bacterial growth. Allergic reactions developed from repeated exposures to parabens led to the removal of this agent from dental anesthetic solutions. Dental patients who developed allergic reactions from local anesthetics containing methylparaben in the past may indicate on their medical history that they are allergic to local anesthetics. If this occurs, further dialogue is necessary to determine when the allergic reaction occurred. If the reaction occurred before 1984, it could indicate an allergy to methylparaben. Currently, no dental local anesthetic cartridges contain methylparaben.

SELECTION OF LOCAL ANESTHETIC AGENTS

There are two main classifications of local anesthetic agents: esters and amides. Esters are metabolized in the plasma by plasma cholinesterase, and most amides are metabolized in the liver, the exception being articaine, which is predominantly metabolized in the blood similar to esters. Because there is a greater propensity of patients who are hypersensitive to injectable esters, all injectable local anesthetics manufactured for dentistry today are in the amide group. As discussed in Chapter 3, the intermediate hydrocarbon chain of the anesthetic molecule determines whether the anesthetic is classified as an ester or an amide. There are five generic classifications of amide local anesthetics

BOX 5.1 Cartridge Variations of Anesthetic Volumes

Local anesthetic glass cartridges are designed to contain 2.0 mL of solution; however, when the silicone rubber stopper is added to the cartridge, it can only contain a maximum of 1.8 mL of solution. There has been some confusion among dentists, hygienists, dental students, and dental hygiene students regarding the manufacturer labeling changes of local anesthetic volumes. Currently, some manufacturer product inserts and anesthetic labels identify the cartridge as containing 1.7 mL of solution instead of the traditional labeling of 1.8 mL of solution. This change in the labeling of some cartridges of local anesthetics came about when articaine was undergoing the U.S. Food and Drug Administration (FDA) approval in the late 1990s. The FDA asked the manufacturer of articaine if it could guarantee that every cartridge contained 1.8 mL of solution. Because local anesthetic cartridges are filled by a machine and slight variations will occur between cartridges, and the average dental cartridge in the United States contains 1.76 mL of solution, the manufacturer cannot guarantee that all cartridges contain 1.8 mL of solution. However, the manufacturer can guarantee that every cartridge contains a minimum of 1.7 mL of solution, and therefore are labeled as such. More manufacturers are likely to market and label their anesthetic in this manner. So, how does this affect drug calculations? Because there will be only a slight variation of +/− 0.1 between cartridges, this should not alter the calculation formula of anesthetics labeled as 1.7 mL and will provide a margin of safety if 1.8 mL of solution is actually in the cartridge. Therefore the use of 1.8 mL will continue to be the recommended volume of solution in one cartridge when determining maximum recommended doses (see Chapter 8 for dosing calculations). However, to add to this confusion, some regional dental hygiene local anesthesia board examinations require licensure candidates to calculate doses based on 1.7 mL of solution rather than the recommended 1.8 mL, whereas other testing organizations require calculations based upon 1.8 mL. Licensure candidates must be prepared to alter the calculation formulas with the specified amount of solution identified on the examination. Appendix 8.2 will provide drug calculation information based on 1.7 mL of solution to assist licensure candidates who are taking such examinations.

available in North America for use in dentistry. Table 5.1 lists some generic and proprietary names. These amide local anesthetic formulations come in various concentrations, with or without vasoconstrictors. The formulations are as follows:

- *Lidocaine:* 2% 1:50,000 epinephrine; 2% 1:100,000 epinephrine
- *Mepivacaine:* 3% plain; 2% 1:20,000 levonordefrin
- *Prilocaine:* 4% plain; 4% 1:200,000 epinephrine
- *Articaine:* 4% 1:100,000 epinephrine; 4% 1:200,000 epinephrine
- *Bupivacaine:* 0.5% 1:200,000 epinephrine

The selection of a local anesthetic agent should be determined by the dental hygienist on a patient-by-patient basis, taking into consideration the efficacy, safety, individual patient assessment, consultations, and dental or dental hygiene care plan. Most dental hygiene care requiring the use of local anesthetics is typically nonsurgical periodontal treatment. However, dental practices in some states hire dental hygienists whose main responsibility in the practice is to administer local anesthetics for many of the procedures performed by the dentist. A dental hygienist may also be asked to administer the anesthesia for the dentist on a case-by-case basis. It is therefore essential for the dental hygienist to fully understand the need for pain control in all dental situations. The following are important considerations in determining the appropriate local anesthetic selection:

- The duration of pain control based upon the length of the procedure
- The need for posttreatment pain control

TABLE 5.1 Amide Local Anesthetics

Generic Name	Proprietary Name
Lidocaine	Xylocaine, Lignospan, Octocaine
Mepivacaine	Carbocaine, Arestocaine, Isocaine, Polocaine, Scandonest
Prilocaine	Citanest, Citanest Forte
Articaine	Septocaine, Zorcaine, Articadent
Bupivacaine	Marcaine, Vivacaine

- The patient's health assessment and current patient medications
- A local anesthetic, sodium bisulfite, or metabisulfite allergy
- The need for hemostasis

Duration of Action and Operative Pain Control

As discussed in Chapter 3, there are several physical properties that determine the local anesthetic's onset and duration of action. Table 5.2 lists the properties for the local anesthetic agents that are currently available. The drug's pK_a determines the anesthetic's distribution of cations and anions. The lower the pK_a, the more anions are present in base form for better penetration through the lipid-rich nerve, which provides a more rapid onset of action. The protein-binding capacity and the lipid solubility of the anesthetic are related to its duration of action. The lipid solubility also determines the anesthetic's potency. Bupivacaine has the highest percentage of protein binding and is the most lipid-soluble of all the local anesthetics; it therefore has the longest duration and is the most potent. However, bupivacaine has the highest pK_a and therefore the slowest onset of action. The vasodilating properties of anesthetics also play a significant role in both the potency and duration of action. Mepivacaine and prilocaine have the least vasodilating effects, allowing the anesthetic to remain in the area of disposition longer, especially after a nerve block[3,4] (Table 5.3). For this reason, both anesthetics are quite effective without a vasoconstrictor, and both are good alternatives when a vasoconstrictor is contraindicated.

The duration of local anesthetic agents is divided into three main categories, which are influenced by the presence or absence of a vasoconstrictor:

1. Short-acting anesthetics provide pulpal anesthesia of approximately 30 minutes and do not contain a vasoconstrictor. These include:
   - 3% Mepivacaine: 20 minutes (supraperiosteal) and 40 minutes (block)
   - 4% Prilocaine: 10 - 15 minutes (supraperiosteal)
2. Intermediate-acting anesthetics provide pulpal anesthesia of approximately 60 minutes and contain a vasoconstrictor, except for 4% prilocaine when administered as a nerve block. These include:
   - 2% Lidocaine; 1:50,000 epinephrine
   - 2% Lidocaine; 1:100,000 epinephrine
   - 2% Mepivacaine; 1:20,000 levonordefrin
   - 4% Prilocaine (intermediate only when administering a nerve block, may provide 60 minutes of pulpal anesthesia)
   - 4% Prilocaine; 1:200,000 epinephrine (categorized as intermediate but provides slightly longer duration of 60-90 minutes)
   - 4% Articaine; 1:100,000 epinephrine (categorized as intermediate but provides slightly longer duration of 60-75 minutes)
   - 4% Articaine; 1:200,000 epinephrine
3. Long-acting anesthetics provide pulpal anesthesia of approximately 90 minutes or more and contain a vasoconstrictor. Bupivacaine is the only long-acting anesthetic available in the United States.
   - 0.5% Bupivacaine; 1:200,000 epinephrine

TABLE 5.2 Physical Properties of Local Anesthetics

Local Anesthetic	PK$_a$*	Onset of Action (Min)	Vasodilating†	T½‡ (Min)	Lipid Solubility§	Protein Binding‖ (5%)
Lidocaine	7.7	3–5	1	96	2.9	65
Mepivacaine	7.6 (Plain and w/VC)	3–5	0.8	114¶	0.8	75
Prilocaine	7.7 (Plain) 7.9 (w/VC)	3–5	0.5	96	0.9	55
Articaine	7.8	Supraperiosteal 1–2 Block 2–2.5	1¶	Approx. 27**	1.5	54
Bupivacaine	8.1	Up to 6–10	2.5	162	27.5	95

*pK$_a$, Dissociation constant; rate of onset.
†Vasodilating; lidocaine (as the benchmark) given value of 1.
‡Half-life (minutes).
§Lipid solubility oil/water solubility; intrinsic potency, increased penetrability.
‖Protein binding duration of action.
¶Estimated.
**Vice TB, Baars AM, van Oss GE, et al: High performance liquid chromatography and preliminary pharmacokinetics of articaine and its 2-carboxy metabolite in human serum and urine, *J Chromatogr* 424:240–444, 1988. Manufacturer product inserts list half-life of articaine at 43.8 minutes with 1:100,000 epinephrine, and 44.4 minutes with 1:200,000 epinephrine.
Modified from Haveles EB: *Applied pharmacology for the dental hygienist,* ed 8, St Louis, 2020, Mosby.

TABLE 5.3 Duration of Pulpal Anesthesia of Local Anesthetics Without Vasoconstrictors by Injection Type

Local Anesthetic	Supraperiosteal (Duration in Minutes)	Nerve Block (Duration in Minutes)
3% Mepivacaine	20	40
4% Prilocaine	10–15	40–60

Table 5.4 lists the local anesthetics by their duration of action categorized by short, intermediate, and long-acting, and both pulpal and soft tissue anesthesia. Fig. 5.1 illustrates the duration of action for soft tissue anesthesia after the administration of a nerve block, and Fig. 5.2 illustrates the duration of action for pulpal anesthesia after the administration of a nerve block.

Duration of anesthesia varies among patients depending on individual response to anesthetic, accuracy of anesthetic administration, vascularity of tissue, variation of anatomic structure, and injection technique:

- *Individual response to anesthetic.* In general, individuals respond as expected to the onset and duration of action as listed in Table 5.4. However, some individuals are less or more sensitive to the administered anesthetic and expected duration is either decreased or increased accordingly. There are three types of individual responses to the administration of local anesthetics: *normal responders, hyperresponders,* and *hyporesponders.*[4] These categories are used to determine the duration of action of a local anesthetic. Using lidocaine 2% 1:100,000 epinephrine as an example, approximately 70% of patients would fall in the normal responder category, representing a typical duration of 60 minutes of pulpal anesthesia. Hyperresponders represent approximately 15% of individuals who overly respond to local anesthetics and may have pulpal anesthesia of approximately 70 to 80 minutes or longer. Hyporesponders represent the final 15% of individuals who under respond to local anesthetics and may have pulpal anesthesia of approximately 45 minutes or less. Individual patient responses should be anticipated from time to time. Once it is determined that a patient does not respond to the anesthetic drug as expected, a notation should be made in the patient's chart to signal the practitioner of the variation in the patient's response to the anesthetic and to document any modifications that were made to achieve appropriate duration of anesthesia (Box 5.2).
- *Accuracy of anesthetic administration.* Accuracy of anesthetic administration is most difficult when administering a **nerve block**, an injection of local anesthetic in the vicinity of a nerve trunk to anesthetize the nerve's area of innervations, such as with the inferior alveolar (IA) block; it is least difficult when administering a **supraperiosteal injection**, an injection that anesthetizes a small area by depositing anesthetic near the terminal nerve endings. To successfully achieve profound anesthesia of the IA block, the anesthetic agent should be deposited as close to the nerve trunk as possible. Because of the depth of penetration required for an IA block, it is necessary to advance the needle through significant soft tissue, allowing a greater possibility for needle deflection, which can influence the accuracy of the injection.
- *Vascularity of tissue.* In healthy tissue, the onset of action and the duration of the anesthetic are more predictable. However, inflamed tissue has increased vascularity resulting from infection, slowing the onset of action and decreasing the duration because of rapid absorption (see Chapter 3).
- *Variation of anatomic structure.* Anatomic variations are difficult to predict and often decrease the duration of local anesthetic action. Decreased anesthetic duration and effectiveness in the maxillae may be caused by the following:[5]
  - Density of bone. The density of the alveolar bone of the maxillae is typically less than the alveolar bone of the mandible, providing easy anesthetic diffusion and increased duration of pain control. Extra dense bone in this area decreases the success and duration of pain control.
  - Flaring of palatal roots of maxillary molars may affect the anesthetic's action.
  - A lower than normal zygomatic arch, commonly seen in children, may prevent or decrease the duration of the anesthetic's action in the maxillary molars.

TABLE 5.4 Categories of Duration of Action of Local Anesthetic Agents (Plain and With a Vasoconstrictor) Available in the United States

GENERAL CATEGORIES		
Short Duration (Pulpal = Approximately 30 Min)	**Intermediate Duration (Pulpal Approximately 60 Min)**	**Long Duration (Pulpal >90 Min)**
	Lidocaine 2% 1:50,000 or 1:100,000 epinephrine	Bupivacaine 0.5% 1:200,000 epinephrine
Mepivacaine 3% plain (supraperiosteal/nerve block)[†]	Mepivacaine 2% 1:20,000 levonordefrin	
Prilocaine 4% plain (supraperiosteal)[‡]	Prilocaine plain (nerve block)[‡]	
	Prilocaine 4% 1:200,000 epinephrine[§]	
	Articaine 4% 1:100,000 epinephrine[§]	
	Articaine 4% 1:200,000 epinephrine	

PULPAL AND SOFT TISSUE ANESTHESIA		
Local Anesthetics	**Pulpal (Min)**	**Soft Tissue (Min)**
Lidocaine 2% 1:50,000 or 1:100,000 epinephrine	60	180–300
Mepivacaine 3% plain (supraperiosteal/block)[†]	20 (supraperiosteal) 40 (nerve block)	120–180
Mepivacaine 2% 1:20,000 levonordefrin	60	180–300
Prilocaine 4% plain (supraperiosteal/block)[‡]	10–15 (supraperiosteal) 40–60 (nerve block)	90–120 (supraperiosteal) 120–240 (nerve block)
Prilocaine 4% 1:200,000 epinephrine[§]	60–90	180–480
Articaine 4% 1:100,000 epinephrine[§]	60–75	180–360
Articaine 4% 1:200,000 epinephrine	45–60	120–300
Bupivacaine 0.5% 1:200,000 epinephrine	90–180	240–540 (reports up to 720)

[†]Mepivacaine plain is a short-acting anesthetic when administered by supraperiosteal or nerve blocks, but the duration is increased with a nerve block.
[‡]Prilocaine plain administered as a supraperiosteal is a short-acting anesthetic. When administered as a nerve block, it increases its duration to an intermediate action.
[§]4% Prilocaine 1:200,000 and 4% articaine 1:100,000 are categorized as intermediate durations but provide a slightly longer duration than the other intermediate drugs, extending the duration to 60 to 90 minutes for prilocaine and 60 to 75 minutes for articaine.

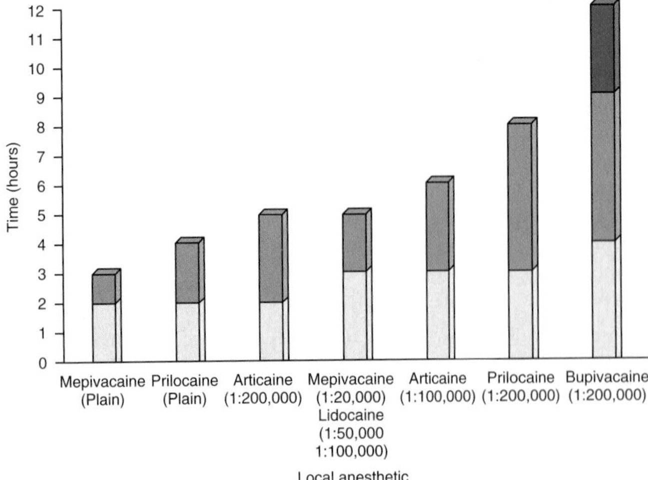

Fig. 5.1 Duration of anesthesia in soft tissue after a nerve block. Color shading differences demonstrate the range.

Decreased anesthetic duration and effectiveness in the mandible may include the following[5]:

- The height of the mandibular foramen
- Width of the mandible
- Width and length of the ramus
- Volume of musculature and adipose tissue
- Injection technique. Soft tissue and pulpal anesthesia is increased when a nerve block, rather than a supraperiosteal, is administered.

Posttreatment Pain Control

For effective pain management, the selection of an appropriate anesthetic agent for a dental procedure should take into consideration posttreatment pain control. For half mouth (two quadrants) nonsurgical periodontal therapy, profound anesthesia and a longer appointment time may be necessary. Although nonsurgical periodontal therapy usually does not require posttreatment pain control, long-duration agents may be needed on occasion for some individuals if posttreatment discomfort is anticipated.[5] Most dental procedures performed by the dentist and dental hygienist fall within the intermediate range of pain control. Examples of procedures that may require postoperative pain control may include, but are not limited to, extractions (impacted third molars) and periodontal surgeries. If the dental hygienist is administering anesthesia for a nondental hygiene procedure, consultation with the dentist before selecting the local anesthetic is appropriate. Anesthetics that provide longer posttreatment durations of pulpal and soft tissue anesthesia are 0.5% bupivacaine 1:200,000 epinephrine (long acting), and 4% prilocaine 1:200,000 epinephrine (which can provide intermediate to long pain control; see

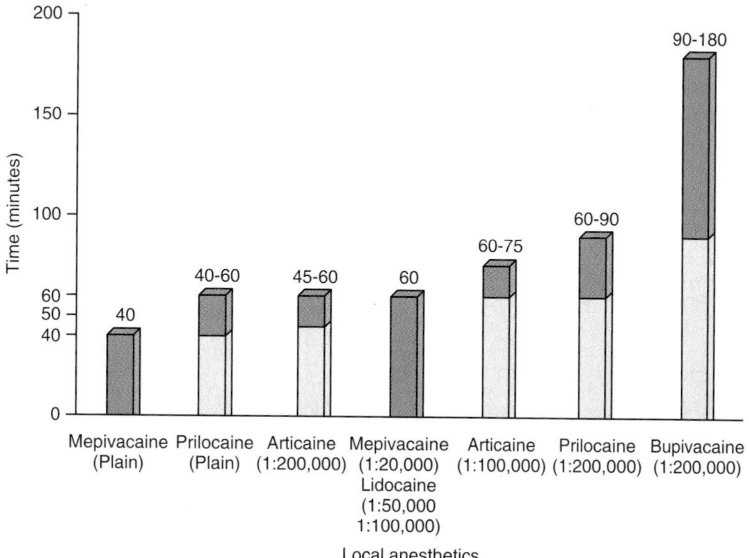

Fig. 5.2 Duration of pulpal anesthesia after a nerve block. Color shading differences demonstrate the range.

BOX 5.2 Treatment Notes for a Periodontally Involved Patient Seeing the Dental Hygienist for Nonsurgical Periodontal Therapy Using Local Anesthesia

4/30/21

Medical history reviewed, no significant findings. Patient consented to treatment with local anesthesia. Nonsurgical periodontal therapy of the mandibular right quadrant: 36 mg of 2% lidocaine 1:100,000 epinephrine (0.018 mg) was administered for the IA, B blocks. No reaction to the anesthesia. Post-operative instructions were provided. Patient was still profoundly numb after the 60-minute appointment. At next visit, ask patient how long the duration of anesthesia lasted and adjust anesthetic accordingly for hyperresponder.

D Logothetis

B, Buccal; *IA*, inferior alveolar.

Table 5.4). Longer-acting local anesthetic agents should be avoided for children and individuals with special needs to prevent the possibility of self-mutilation by accidentally biting or chewing on the lip or tongue (see Chapters 14 and 16).

Patient Health Assessment and Current Patient Medications

Local anesthetics used in dentistry today are reliable and, when administered correctly, produce effective pain control with little toxicity.[6] However, certain medical conditions, such as cardiovascular disease, hepatic disease, hyperthyroidism, brittle diabetes, allergies, and drug interactions (e.g., tricyclic antidepressants, cimetidine, nonselective beta blockers), may influence the type and volume of anesthetic or vasoconstrictor that the patient may safely receive. The patient's medical history must be thoroughly evaluated and discussed at each dental appointment to determine whether a relative or absolute contraindication exists for the local anesthetic agent or vasoconstrictor. A **relative contraindication** means that the administration of the offending drug may be used judiciously, and an **absolute contraindication** means the offending drug should not be administered to the individual under any circumstances. Once the dental hygienist determines whether any contraindications exist using consultations as needed, the **maximum recommended dose** (MRD) for the individual patient can be determined. The MRD is the maximum quantity of drug a patient can safely tolerate during an appointment based on their physical status. Chapter 7 discusses in detail the relative and absolute contraindications to local anesthetic agents and vasoconstrictors based on the patient's physical status and current medications. Chapter 8 discusses the calculation of MRDs.

Local Anesthetic, Sodium Bisulfite, and Metabisulfite Allergy

The addition of the sodium bisulfite preservative may cause allergic reactions in individuals who are sensitive to sulfites, including respiratory reactions in asthmatics (predominantly steroid-dependent asthmatics). It has been reported that 5 to 10% of the asthmatic population are allergic to bisulfites. Asthmatic patients who receive a local anesthetic with vasoconstrictor should be observed for signs and symptoms of an asthmatic attack.[1,7,8] Sulfites are one of the top food allergens. Sulfites are used in wine to prevent fermentation and oxidation and are often used as a preservative in dried fruits and dried potato products. Individuals who are allergic to such foods or other sulfite-containing products should not be given an anesthetic with a vasoconstrictor. Bisulfite allergies typically manifest as a severe respiratory allergy, commonly bronchospasm. Amide local anesthetic allergies are essentially free of this risk.[4] A documented drug allergy would indicate the need for an alternative drug selection and may represent an *absolute contraindication* to the offending drug. Sulfite sensitivities have been well documented[1,4,9,10] and may rule out anesthetic formulations that contain vasoconstrictors. Table 5.5 summarizes allergies that affect local anesthetic selection, and see Chapter 17 for more information on local anesthetic allergic reactions.

Need for Hemostasis

When vasoconstrictors are added to local anesthetic agents, there is no difference in pain control associated with the various vasoconstrictor

TABLE 5.5 Allergies That Affect the Selection of Local Anesthetic Agents or Vasoconstrictors

Reported Allergy	Type of Contraindication	Drugs to Avoid	Potential Problem(s)	Alternative Drug
Local anesthetic allergy, documented	Absolute	All local anesthetics in same chemical class (esters vs amides)	Allergic response, mild (e.g., dermatitis, bronchospasm) to life-threatening reactions	Local anesthetics in different chemical class (esters vs amides)
Sodium bisulfate or metabisulfite	Absolute	Local anesthetics containing a vasoconstrictor	Severe bronchospasm, usually in asthmatics	Local anesthetic without vasoconstrictor

From Bowen DM, Pieren JA: *Darby and Walsh dental hygiene: theory and practice,* ed 5, St Louis, 2020, Elsevier.

dilutions. However, when hemostasis control is needed, adrenergic vasoconstrictors offer considerable value to the selection of an anesthetic, and the concentration of the vasoconstrictor is a significant factor in the amount of bleeding control they provide.[4,6] All local anesthetics containing a vasoconstrictor offer some degree of hemostasis. As discussed in Chapter 4, because epinephrine possesses both α and β actions, with α receptors being less sensitive to epinephrine than β receptors, higher doses of epinephrine are needed to produce the vasoconstriction action of α receptors. Therefore a 1:50,000 dilution provides the greatest hemostasis properties compared with the 1:100,000 and 1:200,000 dilutions. For nonsurgical periodontal therapy, a 1:100,000 epinephrine dilution will provide adequate hemostasis. In patients with heavy bleeding, the dental hygienist may consider using a 1:100,000 epinephrine dilution for pain control, and use small amounts of a 1:50,000 epinephrine dilution to infiltrate into papilla for bleeding control in the direct area of instrumentation (see Chapters 12 and 13). Levonordefrin is a selective α_2 agonist (75%) and produces vasoconstriction in low systemic concentrations. Although levonordefrin has significant effects on α receptors, it does not provide the same powerful vasoconstriction of the peripheral vasculature as epinephrine. Therefore epinephrine provides better bleeding control than levonordefrin.

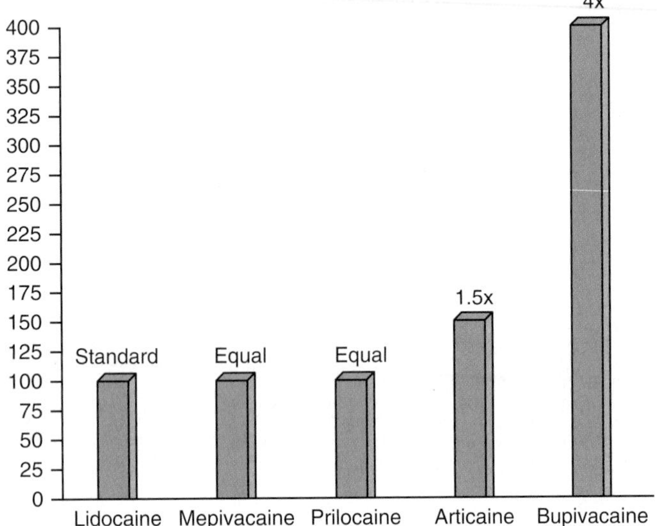

Fig. 5.3 Relative potency values for amide local anesthetics compared with lidocaine. Using lidocaine as the benchmark with the reference value of 100% for the comparison. This figure demonstrates that mepivacaine and prilocaine are equal to lidocaine in potency. Articaine is 1.5 times more potent than lidocaine, and bupivacaine is four times more potent.

AMIDE LOCAL ANESTHETICS

Lidocaine

Lidocaine was the first amide local anesthetic suitable for nerve blocks in dentistry and because of its reliability is currently the most commonly used local anesthetic solution in dentistry in the United States. It has become the standard with which other local anesthetics are compared. Pharmacologically, lidocaine is a xylidine derivative. It is approximately two times more potent than the ester procaine and when injected intraorally produces greater depth of anesthesia.[6]

Because lidocaine is a potent vasodilator, it only offers pulpal anesthesia of 5 to 10 minutes and, therefore, is rarely used in dentistry without a vasoconstrictor. However, when the commonly used formulation of 1:100,000 epinephrine is used, it provides profound pulpal anesthesia of approximately 60 minutes and soft tissue anesthesia of up to 5 hours with low risk of systemic toxicity and no documented allergic reactions.[6] The 1:50,000 formulation provides no further duration and depth of pulpal anesthesia than the 1:100,000 formulation and increases the risk of adverse cardiovascular reactions. Elderly patients are more likely to be hyperresponders to vasoconstrictors, and in these individuals the 1:100,000 formulation should be used.[4,11] However, the 1:50,000 formulation does provide greater vasoconstriction, offering better hemostasis than the 1:100,000 formulation, and therefore should be reserved for procedures that require bleeding control with only small volumes infiltrated directly into the areas needing hemostasis (see Chapter 4).

Lidocaine is equal in potency to mepivacaine and prilocaine. It is two-thirds as potent as articaine and one-fourth as potent as bupivacaine (Fig. 5.3). Lidocaine is similar in toxicity to articaine. It is slightly more toxic than mepivacaine (approximately 25% more) and prilocaine (approximately 40% more). It is far less toxic than bupivacaine, specifically only one-fourth as toxic (Fig. 5.4).

Lidocaine has anticonvulsant properties and may be used to terminate or decrease the duration of grand mal and petit mal seizures. These anticonvulsant properties occur at blood levels below that which lidocaine produces seizure activity in an overdose. Lidocaine decreases the excitability of neurons due to its depressant actions on the central nervous system (CNS), thus raising seizure thresholds.[4] In addition, patients may experience initial sedative effects from lidocaine compared with other local anesthetic agents. During toxic overdose reactions from local anesthetics, initial CNS stimulation is followed by CNS depression (Fig. 5.5). With lidocaine, the stimulation phase may be nonexistent or brief, displaying signs and symptoms of initial CNS depression rather than CNS stimulation[2] (see Fig. 5.5).

Lidocaine is also an effective topical anesthetic and is currently the only topical amide anesthetic on the market (see Chapter 6). Lidocaine is metabolized in the liver through a complex pattern that uses several hepatic enzymes, and less than 10% of lidocaine is excreted unchanged by the kidneys.[4] Individuals with significant hepatic disease can receive lidocaine but at a reduced dose (see Chapters 7 and 8).

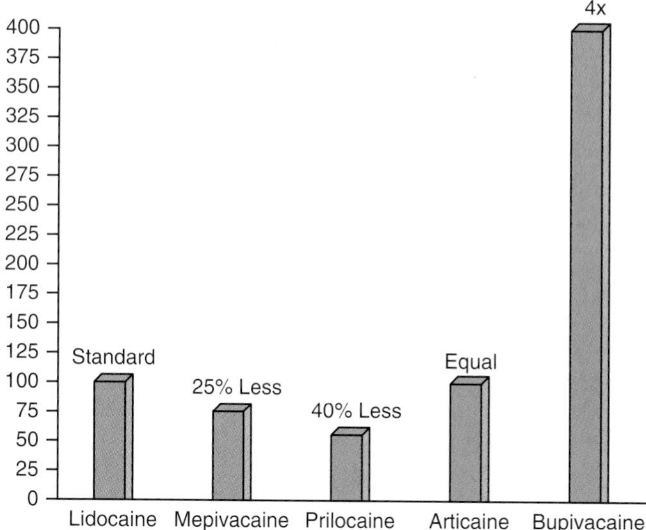

Fig. 5.4 Relative toxicity values for amide local anesthetics compared with lidocaine. Using lidocaine as the benchmark with the reference value of 100% for the comparison, this figure demonstrates that articaine is equal in toxicity to lidocaine, mepivacaine is 25% less toxic than lidocaine, and prilocaine is 40% less toxic than lidocaine. Bupivacaine is the most toxic and is four times more toxic than lidocaine.

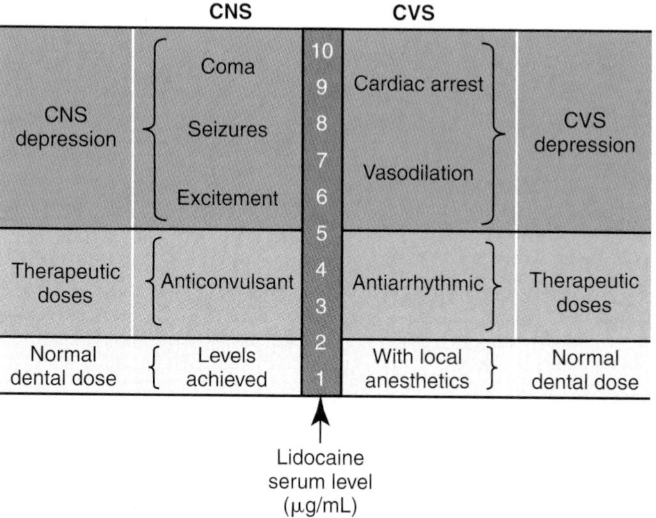

Fig. 5.5 Relationship among levels of local anesthesia in serum and the pharmacologic and adverse effects. *CNS,* Central nervous system; *CVS,* cardiovascular system. (From Haveles EB: *Applied pharmacology for the dental hygienist,* ed 8, St Louis, 2020, Elsevier.)

Lidocaine is available in two different formulations: 2% 1:50,000 epinephrine and 2% 1:100,000 epinephrine. Table 5.6 lists the main properties of lidocaine, and Tables 5.7 and 5.8 give helpful tips for anesthetic selection and precautions for lidocaine formulations (also see Chapter 7 for specific guidelines related to the precautions for local anesthetics and vasoconstrictors).

The MRD for lidocaine is 3.2 mg/lb or 7.0 mg/kg, and the absolute U.S. Food and Drug Administration (FDA) MRD is 500 mg (see Table 5.9 for lidocaine MRDs and Chapter 8 for calculation guidelines).

Mepivacaine

Pharmacologically like lidocaine, mepivacaine is a xylidine derivative. Mepivacaine is similar to lidocaine in its onset of action, duration, potency, toxicity, and no reported allergic reactions. Mepivacaine is available in two different formulations: 3% mepivacaine plain and 2% mepivacaine 1:20,000 levonordefrin. Because mepivacaine produces less vasodilation than lidocaine, it is an effective anesthetic without a vasoconstrictor and is supplied in this manner only in the 3% formulation. It can be used for short appointments providing pulpal anesthesia of approximately 20 minutes via supraperiosteal injections, and 40 minutes via nerve blocks, and 2 to 3 hours of soft tissue anesthesia when profound pulpal anesthesia is not necessary. It is therefore a good alternative if the use of a vasoconstrictor is contraindicated. However, caution should be taken to avoid systemic toxicity related to using plain anesthetics, especially in children (see Chapter 14). Two percent mepivacaine is the only anesthetic that is formulated with levonordefrin as its vasoconstrictor in the United States, and it provides equivalent depth and duration of pulpal (60 minutes) and soft tissue (3–5 hours) anesthesia as lidocaine with epinephrine. Levonordefrin, however, does not provide the same intensity of hemostasis as epinephrine. Similar to lidocaine, mepivacaine also has anticonvulsant properties.

Mepivacaine is equal in potency to lidocaine and prilocaine, and it is two-thirds as potent as articaine and one-fourth as potent as bupivacaine (see Fig. 5.3). Mepivacaine is similar in toxicity to lidocaine and articaine (about equal or slightly less [25%]). It is more toxic than prilocaine (approximately 25% more). It is far less toxic than bupivacaine, specifically only one-fourth as toxic (see Fig. 5.4). Unlike lidocaine, the signs and symptoms of an overdose to mepivacaine follow the more typical pattern of CNS stimulation followed by CNS depression.

Mepivacaine is not effective as a topical anesthetic. Like lidocaine, mepivacaine is metabolized in the liver using several hepatic enzymes with variable excretion of unchanged mepivacaine from zero to 16% by the kidneys. Individuals with significant hepatic disease can receive mepivacaine but at a reduced dose (see Chapters 7 and 8). Table 5.10 describes the main properties of mepivacaine, and Tables 5.11 and 5.12 give helpful tips for anesthetic selection and precautions for mepivacaine formulations (also see Chapter 7 for specific guidelines related to the precautions for local anesthetics and vasoconstrictors).

The MRD for mepivacaine is 3.0 mg/lb or 6.6 mg/kg, and the absolute FDA MRD is 400 mg (see Table 5.13 for mepivacaine MRDs and Chapter 8 for calculation guidelines).

Prilocaine

Pharmacologically, prilocaine is similar to both lidocaine and mepivacaine. Chemically, prilocaine is a secondary amino derivative of toluidine, and lidocaine and mepivacaine are xylidine derivatives.

Prilocaine is equal in potency to lidocaine and mepivacaine and two-thirds as potent as articaine and one-fourth as potent as bupivacaine (see Fig. 5.3). Prilocaine is much less toxic (approximately half) than lidocaine and articaine and slightly less toxic than mepivacaine. It is much less toxic than bupivacaine, approximately one-fifth as toxic (see Fig. 5.4). It is the least toxic anesthetic currently available because it has a significantly larger volume of distribution and greater clearance rate, which permits its safe formulation as a 4% solution. It minimally affects the CNS and cardiovascular system (CVS). Compared with lidocaine with a similar intravenous (IV) dose, CNS toxicity after the administration of prilocaine is shorter and less severe.[4]

Like mepivacaine, prilocaine produces very little vasodilation and is an effective plain anesthetic. In fact, when 4% prilocaine is administered as a nerve block, it increases its duration from short- to intermediate-action, providing pulpal anesthesia for approximately 40 to 60 minutes and soft tissue anesthesia for approximately 2 to 4 hours[4] (see Table 5.4).

TABLE 5.6 Lidocaine

Chemical formula 2-(diethylamino)-2′,6′–acetoxylidide hydrochloride	
Proprietary names	Xylocaine, Lignospan, Octocaine
Formulations in dentistry	2% lidocaine 1:50,000 epinephrine 2% lidocaine 1:100,000 epinephrine
Vasoactivity	Significantly less vasodilatory properties compared with procaine Causes more vasodilation than mepivacaine and prilocaine
Duration of action (see Tables 5.3 and 5.4)	Pulpal duration: Intermediate 60 min Soft tissue duration 180–300 min
Potency	Equal potency to mepivacaine and prilocaine 2/3 as potent as articaine 1/4 as potent as bupivacaine
Toxicity	Similar toxicity to articaine, slightly more toxic than mepivacaine (approximately 25% more) 40% more toxic than prilocaine 1/4 as toxic as bupivacaine
Metabolism	Liver
Excretion	Kidneys, less than 10% excreted unchanged
pK_a	7.7
pH	3.3–4.4
Onset of action	3–5 min
Half-life	Approximately 96 min (1.6 hours)
Dosage	7.0 mg/kg 3.2 mg/lb
Maximum recommended dose	500 mg
Pregnancy/Lactation	Generally safe during pregnancy; safe during lactation (use with caution)

Structure: 2,6-dimethylphenyl ring (CH_3, CH_3) –NH-CO-CH_2-N(C_2H_5)(C_2H_5)

From Jastak T, Yagiela J, Donaldson D: *Local anesthesia of the oral cavity,* St Louis, 1995, Saunders; Malamed S: *Handbook of local anesthesia,* ed 7, St Louis, 2020, Elsevier; Product monographs.

Prilocaine is especially effective when slightly longer duration of action is needed than that of mepivacaine and lidocaine. Prilocaine plain has a slightly longer duration than mepivacaine plain, and prilocaine with 1:200,000 epinephrine has a slightly longer duration than lidocaine 1:100,000 epinephrine. Prilocaine 1:200,000 is also useful when a lower concentration of epinephrine is needed for patients with cardiovascular disease (such as ASA III) who are epinephrine-sensitive. The epinephrine dilution of 1:200,000 is half the potency of the 1:100,000 dilution; therefore patients with cardiovascular disease can receive twice as many cartridges (4.4) of prilocaine with epinephrine as they can cartridges (2.2) of lidocaine 1:100,000 epinephrine.

Prilocaine is metabolized more easily by the liver than lidocaine and mepivacaine. Because, as discussed previously, prilocaine is a toluidine derivative, it has a greater clearance rate than xylidine-based anesthetics and leaves the circulation faster than its delivery to the liver via the bloodstream. Therefore, although the liver plays a major role in the metabolism of prilocaine, it is predicted that some of the drug is already metabolized by alternate sites in the lungs and kidneys before it reaches the liver.[6,12,13] Prilocaine is a secondary amine differing significantly from lidocaine and mepivacaine, causing the drug to be metabolized by hepatic amidases directly into orthotoluidine and *N*-propylalanine with the major end-product being carbon dioxide. The primary limiting factor for clinical use of prilocaine is methemoglobinemia, which is a side effect caused by the metabolite orthotoluidine. Methemoglobinemia is characterized by the presence of a higher than normal level of methemoglobin in the blood that does not bind to oxygen. In large doses of prilocaine (more than the MRD), clinical cyanosis of the lips and mucous membranes can be observed. This is a relative contraindication to the use of prilocaine, and minimal doses should be administered to patients with idiopathic or congenital methemoglobinemia or receiving treatment with methemoglobin-inducing agents, anemia, hemoglobinopathies (sickle cell anemia), or cardiac or respiratory failure evidenced by hypoxia because methemoglobin levels are increased, decreasing oxygen-carrying capacity.[4,14-16] Moreover, prilocaine is relatively contraindicated in patients receiving acetaminophen or phenacetin, both of which produce elevations in methemoglobin levels (see Chapter 7 for more information).[4]

Topical uses of prilocaine can be found in combination with lidocaine in products such as Oraqix (Dentsply Pharmaceutical) and EMLA (AstraZeneca; see Chapter 6). Table 5.14 lists the main properties of prilocaine, and Tables 5.15 and 5.16 give helpful tips for anesthetic selection and precautions for prilocaine formulations (also see Chapter 7 for specific guidelines related to the precautions for local anesthetics and vasoconstrictors).

TABLE 5.7

Lidocaine 2% 1:50,000 Epinephrine

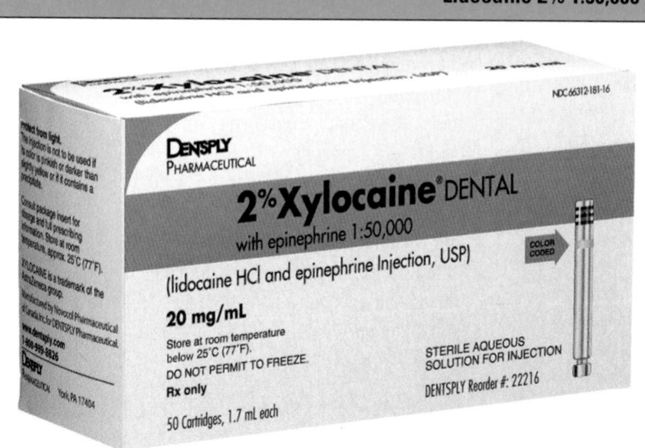

Helpful Tips for Anesthetic Selection

- Intermediate duration
- Low risk of systemic toxicity
- Best choice for bleeding control
- Highest concentration of epinephrine
- No difference in duration or depth of anesthesia compared with the 1:100,000 or 1:200,000 formulations of anesthetics, therefore, should be reserved only for patients requiring hemostasis (recommended to infiltrate small amount directly into areas requiring hemostasis)
- Not recommended for patients with significant cardiovascular disease or patients needing treatment modifications due to epinephrine interactions and elderly patients sensitive to epinephrine

Precautions Associated with the Vasoconstrictor*

- Patients with significant cardiovascular disease or elderly patients sensitive to epinephrine
- Patients taking nonselective beta blockers
- Patients taking central nervous system stimulants
- Patients allergic to sodium bisulfite
- Steroid-dependent asthmatics
- Patients taking tricyclic antidepressants
- Patients taking phenothiazides
- Patients taking digitalis glycosides
- Patients taking large doses of thyroid hormones
- Cocaine and methamphetamine abusers
- Patients with brittle diabetes
- Patients with hyperthyroidism
- Patients with hypertension
- Patients with sickle cell anemia
- Patients with recent myocardial infarction
- Patients with recent cerebrovascular accident
- Patients with recent coronary bypass surgery
- Patients with angina

Precautions Associated with the Local Anesthetic*

- Hepatic disease
- Patients taking cimetidine
- Patients taking beta blockers
- Patients taking central nervous system depressants
- Severe renal dysfunction
- Risk of malignant hyperthermia with large doses

*See Chapter 7 for detailed explanations of local anesthetic and vasoconstrictor precautions.
Images courtesy Dentsply Pharmaceutical, York, PA.

The FDA MRD for prilocaine is 3.6 mg/lb or 8.0 mg/kg, and the absolute MRD is 600 mg (see Table 5.17 for prilocaine MRDs and Chapter 8 for calculation guidelines).

Articaine

Articaine (Septocaine) 1:100,000 epinephrine was approved for use in the United States in 2000. It is 1.5 times as potent as lidocaine, mepivacaine, and prilocaine, and 3 times less potent than bupivacaine. Articaine is similar in toxicity to lidocaine. It is slightly more toxic than mepivacaine (approximately 25% more) and prilocaine (approximately 40% more). It is far less toxic than bupivacaine, specifically only one-fourth as toxic (see Figs. 5.3 and 5.4). In August 2006, 4% articaine 1:200,000 epinephrine was approved. Studies have shown that the duration and pulpal effectiveness is comparable to the 1:100,000 formulation. However, this formulation of articaine provides another alternative for patients with significant cardiovascular disease and for patients who are taking medications that enhance the systemic effect of epinephrine. Both formulations provide intermediate duration of action of approximately 60 to 75 minutes of pulpal anesthesia and 3 to 6 hours of soft tissue anesthesia (see Table 5.4).

Pharmacologically, articaine is derived from thiophene, which makes it different from other amide anesthetics and allows better lipid

TABLE 5.8

Lidocaine 2% 1:100,000 Epinephrine	
	Helpful Tips for Anesthetic Selection • Most commonly used local anesthetic • Intermediate duration • Low risk of systemic toxicity • Effective bleeding control but less than 1:50,000 formulation • Generally safe during pregnancy • Can be used for significant cardiovascular disease, or patients needing treatment modifications at decreased dose of 0.04 mg per appointment (2.2 cartridges) • Contains half as much epinephrine compared with the 1:50,000 dilution
	Precautions Associated with Vasoconstrictor* • Patients with significant cardiovascular disease • Patients taking nonselective beta blockers • Patients taking central nervous system stimulants • Patients allergic to sodium bisulfite • Steroid-dependent asthmatics • Patients taking tricyclic antidepressants • Patients taking phenothiazides • Patients taking digitalis glycosides • Patients taking large doses of thyroid hormones • Cocaine and methamphetamine abusers • Patients with brittle diabetes • Patients with hyperthyroidism • Patients with hypertension • Patients with sickle cell anemia • Patients with recent myocardial infarction • Patients with recent cerebrovascular accident • Patients with recent coronary bypass surgery • Patients with angina **Precautions Associated with Local Anesthetic*** • Hepatic disease • Patients taking cimetidine • Patients taking beta blockers • Patients taking central nervous system depressants • Severe renal dysfunction • Risk of malignant hyperthermia with large doses

*See Chapter 7 for detailed explanations of local anesthetic and vasoconstrictor precautions.
Images courtesy Dentsply Pharmaceutical, York, PA.

solubility, which permits better diffusion through tissue and enhanced ability to cross lipid membranes. Another basic property of articaine that differs from the other amides is that it contains an extra ester linkage. This causes articaine to be hydrolyzed quickly by plasma esterase as well as enzymes in the liver. Approximately 90% to 95% of articaine is metabolized in the blood and only 5% to 10% is metabolized in the liver. This feature is clearly demonstrated when the half-life of articaine is compared with that of lidocaine. The elimination half-life for lidocaine is approximately 96 minutes; for articaine, it is approximately 27 minutes according to Vice et al.[17] However, manufacturer product inserts list the half-life of articaine at 43.8 minutes with 1:100,000 epinephrine and 44.4 minutes with 1:200,000 epinephrine. Articaine has an advantage over the other local anesthetics for patients with significant hepatic disease because it predominantly avoids liver metabolic pathways. Amides that are primarily metabolized in the liver have a longer half-life, increasing the risk for systemic toxicity. Articaine's major metabolite is articainic acid. It is inactive as a local anesthetic, and systemic toxicity has not been observed.[7] This finding is important because an active metabolite may affect toxicity and may exert undesirable side effects. In comparison, lidocaine has active metabolites. Because of articaine's rapid metabolism and its inactive metabolites, it may be a safer drug to readminister later during a dental visit if more anesthetic is necessary. In addition, because articaine possesses both ester and amide characteristics and is metabolized in the

TABLE 5.9

Lidocaine Maximum Recommended Doses Healthy Patient (Based on 1.8 mL of Solution)					
2% 1:50,000 Epinephrine			2% 1:100,000 Epinephrine		
Maximum milligrams and cartridges based upon body weight 2% solution = 36 mg/cartridge 7 mg/kg 3.2 mg/lb Absolute maximum recommended dose = 500 mg					
Weight kg	**Maximum mg (7 mg/kg)**	**Maximum Cartridges**	**Weight lb**	**Maximum mg (3.2 mg/lb)**	**Maximum** Cartridges
10	70	1.9	30	96	2.6
20	140	3.8	50	160	4.4
28	196	5.4	62	198	5.5
30	210	5.8	70	224	6.2
40	280	7.7	90	288	8.0
50	350	9.7	110	352	9.7
56	392	10.8	125	400	11.1
60	420	11.6	130	416	11.5
65	455	12.6	140	448	12.4
70	490	13.6	150	480	13.3
80	560 (500 max)	15.5 (13.8 max)	170	544 (500 max)	15.1 (13.8 max)
90	630 (500 max)	17.5 (13.8 max)	190	608 (500 max)	16.8 (13.8 max)
100	700 (500 max)	19.4 (13.8 max)	210	672 (500 max)	18.6 (13.8 max)
Green-shaded area: Absolute maximum dose for 2% lidocaine 1:50,000 is 5.5 cartridges.					
Red-shaded area: Absolute maximum dose for 2% lidocaine 1:100,000 is 11.1 cartridges. (Vasoconstrictor will be the limiting drug for a healthy patient weighing greater than 56 kg or 125 lbs)					
Shaded area: Over maximum recommended dose because the vasoconstrictor is the limiting drug					

See Chapter 8 for information on anesthetic and vasoconstrictor doses and calculations.

TABLE 5.10 Mepivacaine

Chemical formula 1-methyl-2′,6′–pipecoloxylidide hydrochloride		
Proprietary names	Carbocaine, Arestocaine, Isocaine, Polocaine, Scandonest	
Formulations in dentistry	3% mepivacaine plain 2% mepivacaine 1:20,000 levonordefrin	
Vasoactivity	Weak vasodilator	
Duration of action: 3% mepivacaine (see Tables 5.3 and 5.4)	Pulpal duration: Short	20 min supraperiosteal 40 min block
	Soft tissue duration	120–180 min
Duration of action: 2% mepivacaine 1:20,000 levonordefrin (see Tables 5.3 and 5.4)	Pulpal duration: Intermediate Soft tissue duration: with levonordefrin	60 min 180–300 min
Potency	Equal potency to lidocaine and prilocaine 2/3 as potent as articaine 1/4 as potent as bupivacaine	

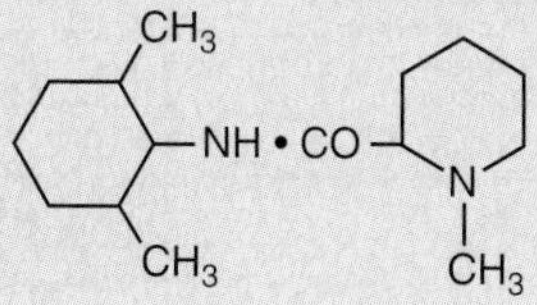

(Continued)

TABLE 5.10 Mepivacaine (*Cont.*)

Toxicity	Slightly less toxic than lidocaine and articaine (approximately 25% less) Approximately 25% more toxic than prilocaine 1/4 as toxic as bupivacaine	
Metabolism	Liver	
Excretion	Kidneys, up to 16% excreted unchanged	
pK_a	7.6	
pH	Plain	5.5–6.0
	Vasoconstrictor added	3.0–4.0
Onset of action	3–5 min	
Half-life	Approximately 114 min (1.9 hours)	
Dosage	6.6 mg/kg 3.0 mg/lb	
Maximum recommended dose	400 mg	
Pregnancy/Lactation	Use with caution during pregnancy; enters breast milk (use with caution)	

From Jastak T, Yagiela J, Donaldson D: *Local anesthesia of the oral cavity,* St Louis, 1995, Saunders; Malamed S: *Handbook of local anesthesia,* ed. 7, St Louis, 2020, Elsevier; Product monographs.

TABLE 5.11

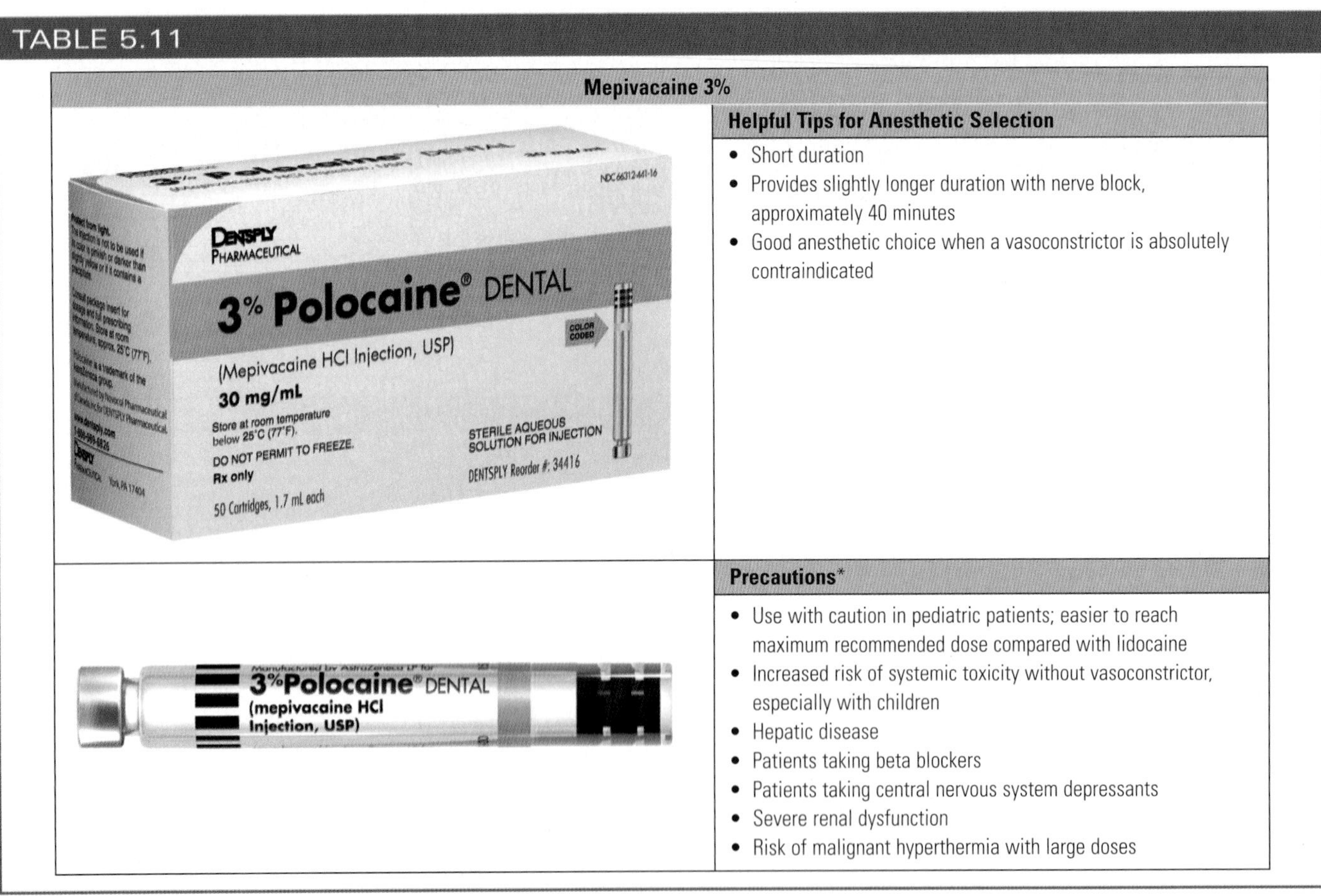

Mepivacaine 3%	
	Helpful Tips for Anesthetic Selection
	• Short duration • Provides slightly longer duration with nerve block, approximately 40 minutes • Good anesthetic choice when a vasoconstrictor is absolutely contraindicated
	Precautions*
	• Use with caution in pediatric patients; easier to reach maximum recommended dose compared with lidocaine • Increased risk of systemic toxicity without vasoconstrictor, especially with children • Hepatic disease • Patients taking beta blockers • Patients taking central nervous system depressants • Severe renal dysfunction • Risk of malignant hyperthermia with large doses

*See Chapter 7 for detailed explanations of local anesthetic precautions.
Images courtesy Dentsply Pharmaceutical, York, PA.

TABLE 5.12

Mepivacaine 2% 1:20,000 Levonordefrin

Helpful Tips for Anesthetic Selection

- Intermediate duration
- Low risk of systemic toxicity
- Provides bleeding control but not as effective as epinephrine dilutions
- Epinephrine is preferred over levonordefrin when hemostasis is needed
- Can be used for significant cardiovascular disease, or patients needing treatment modifications at decreased dose of 0.2 mg per appointment (2.2 cartridges)
- Therapeutically indistinguishable from epinephrine 1:100,000 except for bleeding control
- Dosage calculation for levonordefrin is identical to the 1:100,000 epinephrine dilution

Precautions Associated with Vasoconstrictor*

- Patients with significant cardiovascular disease
- Patients taking nonselective beta blockers
- Patients taking central nervous system stimulants
- Patients allergic to sodium bisulfite
- Steroid-dependent asthmatics
- Avoid using on patients taking tricyclic antidepressants
- Patients taking phenothiazides
- Patients taking digitalis glycosides
- Patients taking large doses of thyroid hormones
- Cocaine and methamphetamine abusers
- Patients with brittle diabetes
- Patients with hyperthyroidism
- Patients with hypertension
- Patients with sickle cell anemia
- Patients with recent myocardial infarction
- Patients with recent cerebrovascular accident
- Patients with recent coronary bypass surgery
- Patients with angina

Precautions Associated with Local Anesthetic*

- Hepatic disease
- Patients taking beta blockers
- Patients taking central nervous system depressants
- Severe renal dysfunction
- Risk of malignant hyperthermia with large doses

*See Chapter 7 for detailed explanations of local anesthetic and vasoconstrictor precautions.
Images courtesy Carestream Health, Inc., Rochester, NY.

plasma and the liver, it can be administered safely to a patient with atypical plasma cholinesterase, a genetic deficiency in the enzyme serum cholinesterase that is responsible for the biotransformation of esters (see Chapter 7).[18] Only about 2% of articaine is excreted unchanged by the kidneys. Although articaine has an ester linkage, it is not linked to higher rates of allergy like the ester anesthetic agents that metabolize to para-aminobenzoic acid (PABA), the agent responsible for anesthetic allergic reactions. Therefore articaine has the same allergy profile as the other amide agents. Like prilocaine, articaine has been reported during regional anesthesia purposes to cause methemoglobinemia if administered IV in very high doses. However, there have been no reported cases of this at the recommended dose used in dentistry.[4]

Articaine contains a thiophene ring instead of benzene as lidocaine does. This gives the molecule better diffusion properties than lidocaine.[19] Some dentists who use articaine claim that they seldom miss an IA block and that buccal supraperiosteal injections in the maxillary arch were often enough before an extraction of a molar. In addition, some studies have demonstrated that after a supraperiosteal injection of articaine in the mandible of adult patients is significantly more successful than lidocaine because of articaine's bone penetration properties.[20,21]

TABLE 5.13

Mepivacaine Maximum Recommended Doses Healthy Patient (Based on 1.8 mL of Solution)					
Maximum milligrams and cartridges based upon body weight 2% solution = 36 mg/cartridge 3% solution = 54 mg/cartridge 6.6 mg/kg 3.0 mg/lb Absolute maximum recommended dose = 400 mg					
2% 1:20,000 Levonordefrin					
Weight kg	**Maximum mg (6.6 mg/kg)**	**Maximum Cartridges**	**Weight lb (3.0 mg/lb)**	**Maximum mg**	**Maximum Cartridges**
10	66	1.8	30	90	2.5
20	132	3.6	50	150	4.1
30	198	5.5	70	210	5.8
40	264	7.3	90	270	7.5
50	330	9.1	110	330	9.1
60	396	11.0	133	396	11.0
65	429 (400 max)	11.9 (11.1 max)	140	420 (400 max)	11.6 (11.1 max)
70	462 (400 max)	12.8 (11.1 max)	150	450 (400 max)	12.5 (11.1 max)
80	528 (400 max)	14.6 (11.1 max)	170	510 (400 max)	14.1 (11.1 max)
90	594 (400 max)	16.5 (11.1 max)	190	570 (400 max)	15.8 (11.1 max)
100	660 (400 max)	18.3 (11.1 max)	210	630 (400 max)	17.5 (11.1 max)
Shaded Areas: Above absolute maximum dose of 400 mg and 11.1 cartridges					
3% Plain					
Weight kg	**Maximum mg (6.6 mg/kg)**	**Maximum Cartridges**	**Weight lb (3.0 mg/lb)**	**Maximum mg**	**Maximum Cartridges**
10	66	1.2	30	90	1.6
20	132	2.4	50	150	2.7
30	198	3.6	70	210	3.8
40	264	4.8	90	270	5.0
50	330	6.1	110	330	6.1
60	396	7.3	133	399	7.3
65	429 (400 max)	7.9 (7.4 max)	140	420 (400 max)	7.7 (7.4 max)
70	462 (400 max)	8.5 (7.4 max)	150	450 (400 max)	8.3 (7.4 max)
80	528 (400 max)	9.7 (7.4 max)	170	510 (400 max)	9.4 (7.4 max)
90	594 (400 max)	11.0 (7.4 max)	190	570 (400 max)	10.5 (7.4 max)
100	660 (400 max)	12.2 (7.4 max)	210	630 (400 max)	11.6 (7.4 max)
Shaded Areas: Above absolute maximum dose of 400 mg and 7.4 cartridges					

See Chapter 8 for information on anesthetic and vasoconstrictor doses and calculations.

TABLE 5.14 **Prilocaine**

Chemical formula 2-(propylamino)-*o*-propionotoluidine hydrochloride

CH_3-(benzene ring)-NH • CO • CH(CH_3) • N(C_3H_7)(H)

Proprietary names	Citanest, Citanest Forte	
Formulations in dentistry	4% plain 4% Prilocaine 1:200,000 epinephrine	
Vasoactivity	Produces slight vasodilation	
Duration of action: 4% prilocaine plain (see Tables 5.3 and 5.4)	Pulpal duration: plain (supraperiosteal)	10–15 min
	Pulpal duration: intermediate plain (block)	45–60 min
	Soft tissue duration: plain (supraperiosteal)	90–120 min
	Soft tissue duration: plain (block)	120–240 min

TABLE 5.14 **Prilocaine (*Cont.*)**		
Duration of action: 4% prilocaine 1:200,000 (see Tables 5.3 and 5.4)	Pulpal duration: intermediate	60–90 min
	Soft tissue duration	180–480 min
Potency	Equal potency to mepivacaine and lidocaine 2/3 as potent as articaine	
	1/4 as potent as bupivacaine	
Toxicity	40% less toxic than lidocaine and articaine	
	1/5 as toxic as bupivacaine	
Metabolism	Simpler hepatic metabolism than lidocaine and mepivacaine by hepatic amidases directly into orthotoluidine and *N*-propylalanine	
	Primarily the liver, but it is predicted that the drug is also metabolized by the lungs before it reaches the liver	
Excretion	Kidneys, small fraction unchanged in urine	
pK_a	7.7 plain	
	7.9 with vasoconstrictor	
pH	Plain	6.0–6.5
	Vasoconstrictor added	3.0–4.0
Onset of action	3–5 min	
Half-life	Approximately 96 minutes (1.6 hours)	
Dosage	8.0 mg/kg	
	3.6 mg/lb	
Maximum recommended dose	600 mg	
Pregnancy/Lactation	Generally safe during pregnancy; unknown safety during lactation	

From Jastak T, Yagiela J, Donaldson D: *Local anesthesia of the oral cavity,* St Louis, 1995, Saunders; Malamed S: *Handbook of local anesthesia,* ed 7, St Louis, 2020, Elsevier; Product monographs.

TABLE 5.15

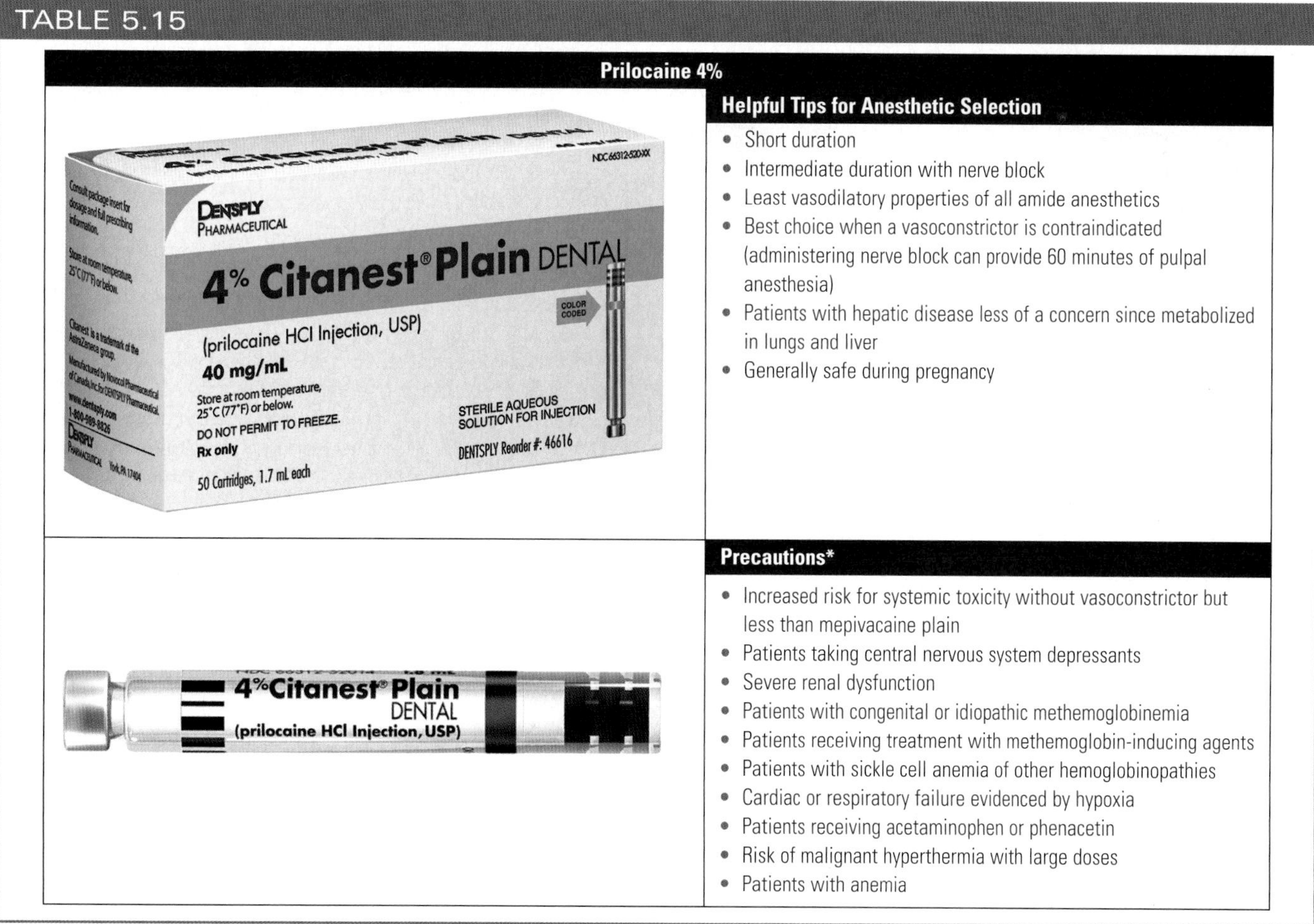

Prilocaine 4%

Helpful Tips for Anesthetic Selection

- Short duration
- Intermediate duration with nerve block
- Least vasodilatory properties of all amide anesthetics
- Best choice when a vasoconstrictor is contraindicated (administering nerve block can provide 60 minutes of pulpal anesthesia)
- Patients with hepatic disease less of a concern since metabolized in lungs and liver
- Generally safe during pregnancy

Precautions*

- Increased risk for systemic toxicity without vasoconstrictor but less than mepivacaine plain
- Patients taking central nervous system depressants
- Severe renal dysfunction
- Patients with congenital or idiopathic methemoglobinemia
- Patients receiving treatment with methemoglobin-inducing agents
- Patients with sickle cell anemia of other hemoglobinopathies
- Cardiac or respiratory failure evidenced by hypoxia
- Patients receiving acetaminophen or phenacetin
- Risk of malignant hyperthermia with large doses
- Patients with anemia

*See Chapter 7 for detailed explanations of local anesthetic precautions.
Images courtesy Dentsply Pharmaceutical, York, PA.

TABLE 5.16

Prilocaine 4% 1:200,000 Epinephrine	
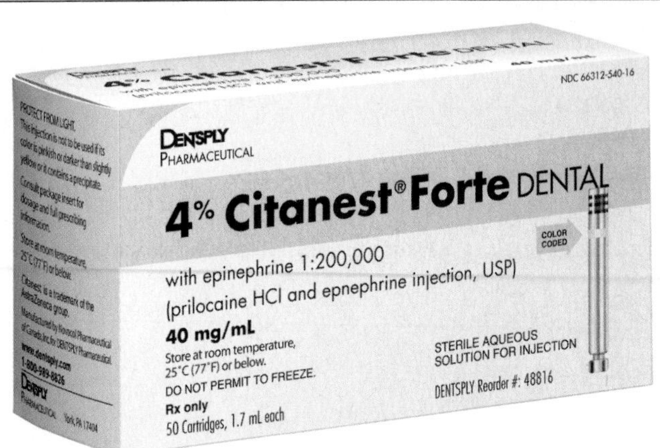	**Helpful Tips for Anesthetic Selection** • Intermediate duration, slightly longer than lidocaine and mepivacaine with vasoconstrictors • Low risk of systemic toxicity • Least toxic of all amide local anesthetics • Effective bleeding control but less than epinephrine 1:50,000 and 1:100,000 dilutions • Generally safe during pregnancy • Best choice for patients with significant cardiovascular disease or patients needing treatment modifications due to epinephrine interactions at decreased dose of 0.04 mg per appointment (4.4 cartridges) • Good choice for elderly patients hyper-sensitive to epinephrine • Patients with hepatic disease less of a concern since metabolized in lungs and liver • Contains half as much epinephrine compared with 1:100,000 dilution
	Precautions Associated with Vasoconstrictor* • Patients with significant cardiovascular disease • Patients taking central nervous system stimulants • Patients allergic to sodium bisulfite • Steroid-dependent asthmatics • Patients taking tricyclic antidepressants • Patients taking phenothiazides • Patients taking digitalis glycosides • Patients taking large doses of thyroid hormones • Cocaine and methamphetamine abusers • Patients with brittle diabetes • Patients with hyperthyroidism • Patients with hypertension • Patients with sickle cell anemia • Patients with recent myocardial infarction • Patients with recent cerebrovascular accident • Patients with recent coronary bypass surgery • Patients with angina
	Precautions Associated with Local Anesthetic* • Patients with anemia • Patients with cardiac or respiratory failure evidenced by hypoxia • Patients taking central nervous system depressants • Patients with congenital or idiopathic methemoglobinemia • Patients receiving treatment with methemoglobin-inducing agents • Patients with sickle cell anemia of other hemoglobinopathies • Cardiac or respiratory failure evidenced by hypoxia • Patients receiving acetaminophen or phenacetin • Risk of malignant hyperthermia with large doses

*See Chapter 7 for detailed explanations of local anesthetic and vasoconstrictor precautions.
Images courtesy Dentsply Pharmaceutical, York, PA.

TABLE 5.17

Prilocaine Maximum Recommended Doses Healthy Patient (Based on 1.8 mL of Solution)					
4% Plain			**4% 1:200,000 Epinephrine**		
Maximum milligrams and cartridges based upon body weight 4% solution = 72 mg/cartridge 8.0 mg/kg 3.6 mg/lb Absolute maximum recommended dose = 600 mg Limiting drug "anesthetic"					
Weight kg	**Maximum mg (8.0 mg/kg)**	**Maximum Cartridges**	**Weight lb**	**Maximum mg (3.6 mg/lb)**	**Maximum Cartridges**
10	80	1.1	30	108	1.5
20	160	2.2	50	180	2.5
30	240	3.3	70	252	3.5
40	320	4.4	90	324	4.5
50	400	5.5	110	396	5.5
60	480	6.6	130	468	6.5
65	520	7.2	140	504	7.0
70	560	7.7	150	540	7.5
75	600	8.3	166	598	8.3
80	640 (600 max)	8.8 (8.3 max)	170	612 (600 max)	8.5 (8.3 max)
90	720 (600 max)	10.0 (8.3 max)	190	684 (600 max)	9.5 (8.3 max)
100	800 (600 max)	11.1 (8.3 max)	210	756 (600 max)	10.5 (8.3 max)
Shaded Areas: Above absolute maximum dose of 600 mg and 8.3 cartridges. (Anesthetic will be the limiting drug for a healthy patient.)					

See Chapter 8 for information on anesthetic and vasoconstrictor doses and calculations.

Since the FDA approval of articaine in 2000, there has been intense discussion regarding the frequent (many anecdotal) reports of paresthesia. Paresthesia can be defined as persistent anesthesia beyond the expected duration or altered sensation, such as tingling or itching, beyond a normal level. Articaine is delivered as a 4% agent, whereas lidocaine is delivered as a 2% agent. One possible disadvantage of the higher concentration of the local anesthetic agent is that it has been determined that local anesthetic-induced nerve injury is concentration dependent, with injuries increasing as concentration increases.[4,22-25] Some authors[19,22] have made recommendations to avoid using articaine for IA blocks because of the potential for paresthesia. However, this is still controversial.[26,27] Paresthesia has also been reported with 4% prilocaine. It is essential that the dental hygienist remains abreast of the current research of all anesthetics and only administers a drug if the benefits outweigh the risks. Paresthesia and articaine will be discussed in detail in Chapter 16.

Table 5.18 describes the main properties of articaine, and Tables 5.19 and 5.20 describe helpful tips for anesthetic selection and precautions for articaine formulations (also see Chapter 7 for specific guidelines related to the precautions for local anesthetics and vasoconstrictors).

The MRD for articaine is 3.2 mg/lb or 7.0 mg/kg. There is no MRD listed for articaine (see Table 5.21 for articaine MRDs and Chapter 8 for calculation guidelines). For pediatric patients under the age of 4, the safety and efficacy of articaine have not been established (see Chapter 14).

Bupivacaine

Bupivacaine is the most potent and toxic of all amide anesthetics. It is four times more potent than lidocaine, mepivacaine, and prilocaine and three times more potent than articaine. It is four times more toxic than lidocaine, mepivacaine, and articaine and six times more toxic than prilocaine[4] (see Figs. 5.3 and 5.4). Pharmacologically, bupivacaine is structurally similar to mepivacaine, except the butyl group in

TABLE 5.18 **Articaine**

Chemical formula 3-N-Propylamino-proprionylamino-2-carbomethoxy-4-methylthiophene hydrochloride	
S, $COOCH_3$ • HCl H_3C $NHCOCHNHCH_2CH_2CH_3$ CH_3	
Proprietary names	Septocaine, Zorcaine, Articadent
Formulations in dentistry	4% Articaine 1:100,000 epinephrine 4% Articaine 1:200,000 epinephrine

(Continued)

TABLE 5.18 (*Cont.*)		
Vasoactivity	Equal to lidocaine	
Duration of action (see Tables 5.3 and 5.4)	Pulpal duration: intermediate	60–75 min (1:100,000)
		45–60 min (1:200,000)
	Soft tissue duration:	180–360 min (1:100,000)
		120–300 min (1:200,000)
Potency	1.5 times more potent than lidocaine, mepivacaine, and prilocaine 1/3 as potent as bupivacaine	
Toxicity	Similar to lidocaine and slightly more than mepivacaine (approximately 25% more) 40% more toxic than prilocaine 1/4 as toxic as bupivacaine	
Metabolism	95% in plasma and 5% in liver—amide anesthetic that also contains ester component	
Excretion	Kidneys, less than 10% excreted unchanged	
pK_a	7.8	
pH	1:100,000 epinephrine	4.0–5.5
	1:200,000 epinephrine	4.0–5.5
Onset of action	Supraperiosteal (1:100,000)	1–2 min
	Block	2–2.5 min
	Supraperiosteal (1:200,000)	1–2 min
	Block	2–3 min
Half-life	Approximately 27 min*	
Dosage	7.0 mg/kg 3.2 mg/lb	
Maximum recommended dose	No FDA absolute maximum recommended dose	
Pregnancy/Lactation	Use with caution during pregnancy; unknown safety during lactation	

FDA, U.S. Food and Drug Administration.
*Vice TB, Baars AM, van Oss GE, et al: High performance liquid chromatography and preliminary pharmacokinetics of articaine and its 2-carboxy metabolite in human serum and urine, *J Chromatogr* 424:240–444, 1988. Manufacturer product inserts list half-life of articaine at 43.8 minutes with 1:100,000 epinephrine and 44.4 minutes with 1:200,000 epinephrine.
From Jastak T, Yagiela J, Donaldson D: *Local anesthesia of the oral cavity,* St Louis, 1995, Saunders; Malamed S: *Handbook of local anesthesia,* ed 7, St Louis, 2020, Elsevier; Product monographs.

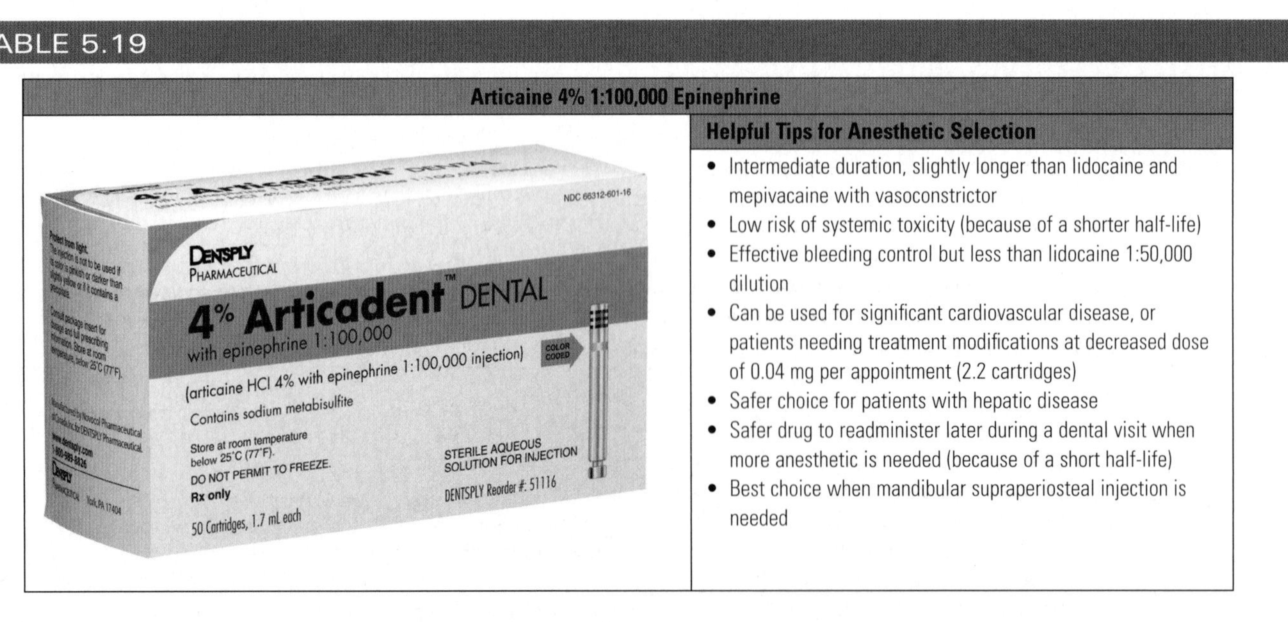

TABLE 5.19

Articaine 4% 1:100,000 Epinephrine	
	Helpful Tips for Anesthetic Selection
	• Intermediate duration, slightly longer than lidocaine and mepivacaine with vasoconstrictor • Low risk of systemic toxicity (because of a shorter half-life) • Effective bleeding control but less than lidocaine 1:50,000 dilution • Can be used for significant cardiovascular disease, or patients needing treatment modifications at decreased dose of 0.04 mg per appointment (2.2 cartridges) • Safer choice for patients with hepatic disease • Safer drug to readminister later during a dental visit when more anesthetic is needed (because of a short half-life) • Best choice when mandibular supraperiosteal injection is needed

TABLE 5.19 (*Cont.*)

Precautions Associated with Vasoconstrictor*

- Patients with significant cardiovascular disease
- Patients taking central nervous system stimulants
- Patients allergic to sodium bisulfite
- Steroid-dependent asthmatics
- Patients taking tricyclic antidepressants
- Patients taking phenothiazides
- Patients taking digitalis glycosides
- Patients taking large doses of thyroid hormones
- Cocaine and methamphetamine abusers
- Patients with brittle diabetes
- Patients with hyperthyroidism
- Patients with hypertension
- Patients with sickle cell anemia
- Patients with recent myocardial infarction
- Patients with recent cerebrovascular accident
- Patients with recent coronary bypass surgery
- Patients with angina

Precautions Associated with Anesthetic*

- Patients with myasthenia gravis
- Patients taking central nervous system depressants
- Patients with congenital or idiopathic methemoglobinemia
- Patients receiving treatment with methemoglobin-inducing agents
- Risk of malignant hyperthermia with large doses

*See Chapter 7 for detailed explanations of local anesthetic and vasoconstrictor precautions.
Images courtesy Dentsply Pharmaceutical, York, PA.

TABLE 5.20

Articaine 4% 1:200,000 Epinephrine

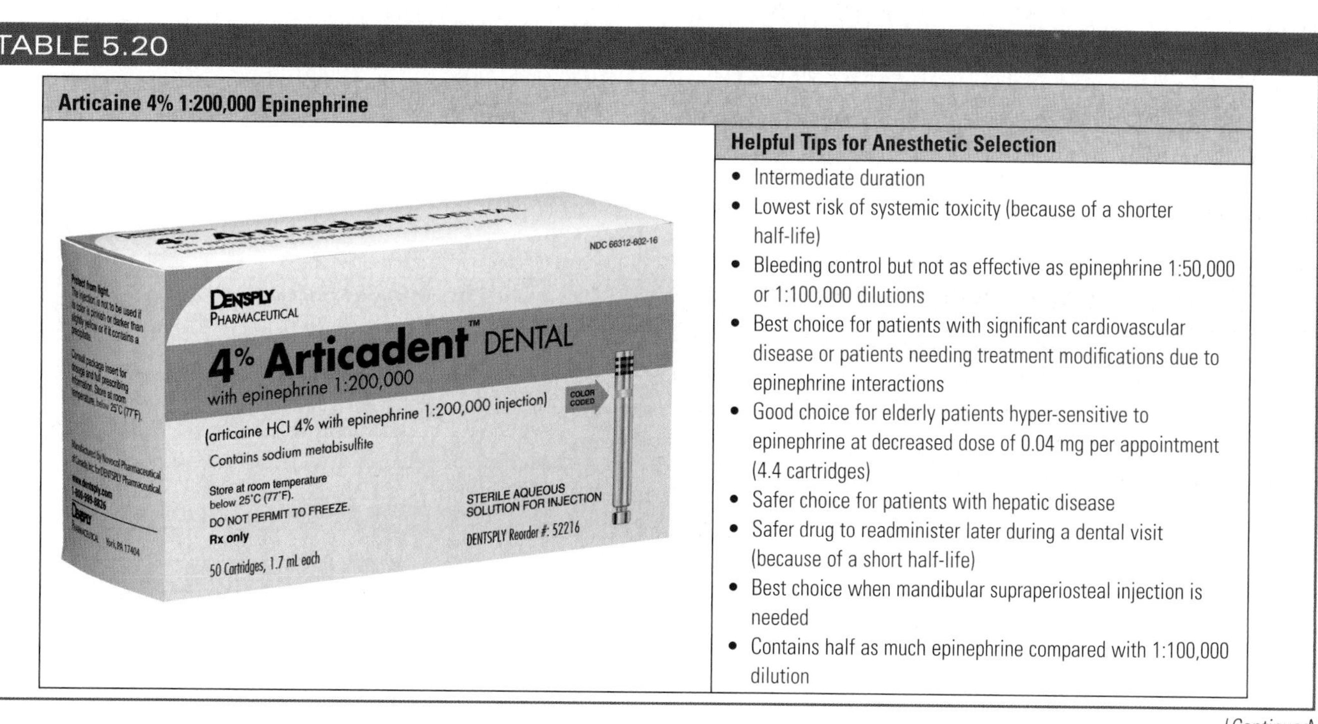

Helpful Tips for Anesthetic Selection

- Intermediate duration
- Lowest risk of systemic toxicity (because of a shorter half-life)
- Bleeding control but not as effective as epinephrine 1:50,000 or 1:100,000 dilutions
- Best choice for patients with significant cardiovascular disease or patients needing treatment modifications due to epinephrine interactions
- Good choice for elderly patients hyper-sensitive to epinephrine at decreased dose of 0.04 mg per appointment (4.4 cartridges)
- Safer choice for patients with hepatic disease
- Safer drug to readminister later during a dental visit (because of a short half-life)
- Best choice when mandibular supraperiosteal injection is needed
- Contains half as much epinephrine compared with 1:100,000 dilution

(*Continued*)

TABLE 5.20 (Cont.)

Precautions Associated with the Vasoconstrictor*

- Patients with significant cardiovascular disease
- Patients taking central nervous system depressants
- Patients allergic to sodium bisulfite
- Steroid-dependent asthmatics
- Patients taking tricyclic antidepressants
- Patients taking phenothiazines
- Patients taking digitalis glycosides
- Patients taking large doses of thyroid hormones
- Cocaine and methamphetamine abusers
- Patients with brittle diabetes
- Patients with hyperthyroidism
- Patients with hypertension
- Patients with sickle cell anemia
- Patients with recent myocardial infarction
- Patients with recent cerebrovascular accident
- Patients with recent coronary bypass surgery
- Patients with angina

Precautions Associated with the Anesthetic*

- Patients with myasthenia gravis
- Patients taking central nervous system depressants
- Patients with congenital or idiopathic methemoglobinemia
- Patients receiving treatment with methemoglobin-inducing agents
- Risk of malignant hyperthermia with large doses

*See Chapter 7 for detailed explanations of local anesthetic and vasoconstrictor precautions.
Images courtesy Dentsply Pharmaceutical, York, PA.

TABLE 5.21

Articaine Maximum Recommended Doses Healthy Patient (Based on 1.8 mL of Solution)					
4% 1:100,000 Epinephrine			**4% 1:200,000 Epinephrine**		
Maximum milligrams and cartridges based upon body weight 4% solution = 72 mg/cartridge 7 mg/kg 3.2 mg/lb Absolute maximum recommended dose = No FDA approved maximum recommended dose					
Weight kg	**Maximum mg (7 mg/kg)**	**Maximum Cartridges**	**Weight lb**	**Maximum mg (3.2 mg/lb)**	**Maximum Cartridges**
10	70	0.97	30	96	1.3
20	140	1.9	50	160	2.2
30	210	2.9	70	224	3.1
40	280	3.8	90	288	4.0
50	350	4.8	110	352	4.8
60	420	5.8	130	416	5.7
65	455	6.3	140	448	6.2
70	490	6.8	150	480	6.6
80	560	7.7	170	544	7.5
90	630	8.7	190	608	8.4
100	700	9.7	210	672	9.3
104	728	10.1	230	736	10.2
113	791	10.9	250	800	11.1
Vasoconstrictor will be the limiting drug for a healthy patient weighing greater than 250 pounds.					

FDA, U.S. Food and Drug Administration.
See Chapter 8 for information on anesthetic and vasoconstrictor doses and calculations.

TABLE 5.22 Bupivacaine

Chemical formula I-Butyl-1′,6′–pipecoloxylidide hydrochloride		
Proprietary names	Marcaine, Vivacaine	
Formulations in dentistry	0.5% 1:200,000 epinephrine	
Vasoactivity	Greater than lidocaine, mepivacaine, prilocaine, and articaine but less than procaine	
Duration of action (see Tables 5.3 and 5.4)	Pulpal duration: long with epinephrine	90–180 min
	Soft tissue duration:	240–540 min (reports up to 720 min)
Potency	Four times more potent than lidocaine, mepivacaine, and prilocaine	
	Three times more potent than articaine	
Toxicity	Four times more toxic than lidocaine, articaine, and mepivacaine	
	Six times more toxic than prilocaine	
Metabolism	Liver	
Excretion	Kidneys, 16% excreted unchanged	
pK_a	8.1	
pH	Vasoconstrictor added	3.0–4.5
Onset of action	6–10 min	
Half-life	162 min (2.7 h)	
Dosage	2.0 mg/kg (No FDA weight-based recommendations; values based on Canadian weight-based recommendations)	
	0.9 mg/lb (No FDA weight-based recommendations; values based on Canadian weight-based recommendations)	
Maximum recommended dose	90 mg (No FDA weight-based recommendations; values based on Canadian weight-based recommendations)	
Pregnancy/Lactation	Use with caution during pregnancy; unknown safety during lactation	

From Jastak T, Yagiela J, Donaldson D: *Local anesthesia of the oral cavity*, St Louis, 1995, Saunders; Malamed S: *Handbook of local anesthesia*, ed 7, St Louis, 2020, Elsevier; Product monographs.

bupivacaine is exchanged for the methyl group in mepivacaine. This substitution allows for a fourfold increase in potency, allows for toxicity, and provides bupivacaine with a major advantage of increased duration of action compared with other amides.[4,6] Bupivacaine is the only anesthetic that provides a long duration of action, and does so despite its intense vasodilating properties, second only to procaine and significantly more than lidocaine, and it is therefore only formulated with 1:200,000 epinephrine. Bupivacaine is highly lipid soluble and binds powerfully to protein receptor sites in the sodium channels. It provides approximately 1.5 to 3 hours of pulpal anesthesia and 4 to 9 hours of soft tissue anesthesia. Because of its long duration, bupivacaine may not be clinically practical for many dental procedures, including nonsurgical periodontal therapy. In an overdose, bupivacaine has equal effects on the CNS and CVS. Bupivacaine's long half-life (2.7 hours) further increases the risk for systemic toxicity.

The use of bupivacaine is indicated when long pulpal anesthesia is needed (greater than 1.5 hours) and/or postoperative pain control is expected to be needed (e.g., periodontal surgery, endodontics, oral surgery). In many situations, it may be prudent to administer after long procedures have been completed and immediately before the patient's discharge from the office. This provides the benefit of extended pain control, allowing time for oral pain medications to take effect. In addition, it is a good alternative when profound anesthesia has been difficult to attain with other anesthetic formulations. With the highest pK_a of the amide anesthetics, bupivacaine has a slightly slower onset of action, but the duration of anesthesia is almost twice that of lidocaine. Bupivacaine is not recommended for use on patients who are prone to self-mutilation (patients with special needs and young children). It is metabolized by liver enzymes in the same manner as lidocaine and mepivacaine, and up to 16% is excreted unchanged by the kidneys. Individuals with significant hepatic disease can receive bupivacaine but at a reduced dose (see Chapters 7 and 8). Table 5.22 lists the main properties of bupivacaine, and Table 5.23 gives helpful tips for anesthetic selection and precautions for bupivacaine (also see Chapter 7 for specific guidelines related to the precautions for local anesthetics and vasoconstrictors).

The FDA MRD for bupivacaine is 0.9 mg/lb or 2.0 mg/kg (based on Canadian weight-based recommendations; there are no FDA weight-based recommendations), and the absolute MRD is 90 mg (see Table 5.24 for bupivacaine MRDs and Chapter 8 for calculation guidelines).

ESTER LOCAL ANESTHETIC

Because of the high degree of hypersensitivity to injectable esters, all injectable local anesthetics manufactured for dentistry (in single-use dental cartridges) today are in the amide group. Injectable ester anesthetics are no longer used in dentistry, therefore only procaine is discussed here because it is still available for use in medicine. Table 5.25 lists the ester local anesthetics of PABA and benzoic acid.

TABLE 5.23

Bupivacaine 0.5% 1:200,000 Epinephrine

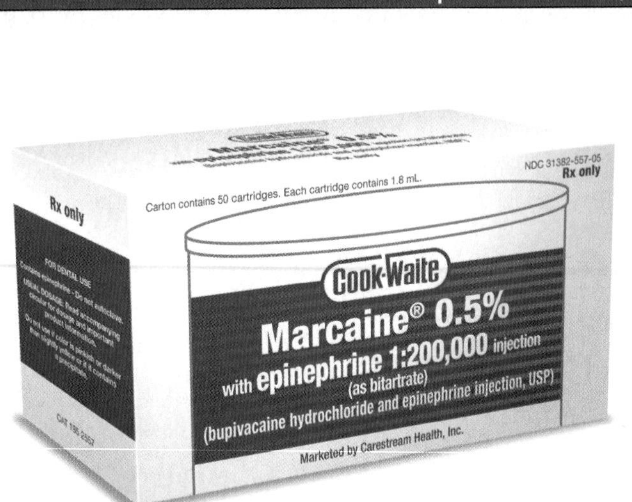

Helpful Tips for Anesthetic Selection

- Long duration
- Greater risk of systemic toxicity because of a longer half-life
- Bleeding control but not as effective as epinephrine 1:50,000 or 1:100,000 formulations
- Can be used for significant cardiovascular disease at decreased dose of 0.04 mg per appointment (4.4 cartridges)
- Safer choice for patients with significant cardiovascular disease or patients needing treatment modifications because of epinephrine interactions if long duration is needed
- Good choice for elderly patients hypersensitive to epinephrine if long duration is needed
- Best choice for long extensive dental procedures and surgical procedures
- Best choice for postoperative pain control
- Infrequently used for routine restorative dentistry and nonsurgical periodontal therapy
- Good alternative when profound anesthesia is difficult to attain with other anesthetic formulations

Precautions Associated with Vasoconstrictor*

- Patients with significant cardiovascular disease
- Patients taking nonselective beta blockers
- Patients taking central nervous system stimulants
- Patients allergic to sodium bisulfite
- Steroid-dependent asthmatics
- Patients taking tricyclic antidepressants
- Patients taking phenothiazines
- Patients taking digitalis glycosides
- Patients taking large doses of thyroid hormones
- Cocaine and methamphetamine abusers
- Patients with brittle diabetes
- Patients with hyperthyroidism
- Patients with hypertension
- Patients with sickle cell anemia
- Patients with recent myocardial infarction
- Patients with recent cerebrovascular accident
- Patients with recent coronary bypass surgery
- Patients with angina

Precautions Associated with the Local Anesthetic*

- Hepatic disease
- Patients taking beta blockers
- Patients taking central nervous system depressants
- Severe renal dysfunction
- Patients prone to self-mutilation (patients with special needs and young children)
- Risk of malignant hyperthermia with large doses

*See Chapter 7 for detailed explanations of local anesthetic and vasoconstrictor precautions.
Images courtesy Carestream Health, Inc., Rochester, NY.

TABLE 5.24

Bupivacaine Maximum Recommended Doses Healthy Patient (Based on 1.8 mL of Solution)					
0.5% 1:200,000 Epinephrine					
Maximum milligrams and cartridges based upon body weight 0.5% solution = 9 mg/cartridge 2 mg/kg mg (No FDA weight-based recommendations; values based on Canadian weight-based recommendations) 0.9 mg/lb mg (No FDA weight-based recommendations; values based on Canadian weight-based recommendations) Absolute maximum recommended dose = 90 mg (No FDA weight-based recommendations; values based on Canadian weight-based recommendations) Limiting drug "anesthetic"					
Weight kg	**Maximum mg (2.0 mg/kg)**	**Maximum Cartridges**	**Weight lb (0.9 mg/lb)**	**Maximum mg**	**Maximum Cartridges**
10	20	2.2	30	27	3.0
20	40	4.4	50	45	5.0
30	60	6.6	70	63	7.0
40	80	8.8	90	81	9.0
50	100 (90 max)	11.1 (10.0 max)	110	99 (90 max)	11.0 (10.0 max)
60	120 (90 max)	13.3 (10.0 max)	130	117 (90 max)	13.0 (10.0 max)
65	130 (90 max)	14.4 (10.0 max)	140	126 (90 max)	14.0 (10.0 max)
70	140 (90 max)	15.5 (10.0 max)	150	135 (90 max)	15.0 (10.0 max)
80	160 (90 max)	17.7 (10.0 max)	170	153 (90 max)	17.0 (10.0 max)
90	180 (90 max)	20.0 (10.0 max)	190	171 (90 max)	19.0 (10.0 max)
100	200 (90 max)	22.2 (10.0 max)	210	189 (90 max)	21.0 (10.0 max)
Shaded Areas: Above absolute maximum dose of 90 mg and 10.0 cartridges. Local anesthetic is the limiting drug.					

FDA, U.S. Food and Drug Administration.
See Chapter 8 for information on anesthetic and vasoconstrictor doses and calculations.

TABLE 5.25 **Ester Local Anesthetics**

Esters of Para-Aminobenzoic Acid	Esters of Benzoic Acid
Procaine (Novocaine 2%)	Butacaine Piperocaine
Propoxycaine (0.4%): used in combination with procaine until its removal from the U.S. market in January 1996	Benzocaine (Ethyl amino benzoate)
Ravocaine = procaine 2% propoxycaine 0.4% and Levophed 1:30,000 or Neo-Cobefrin 1:20,000	Cocaine
Chloroprocaine	Hexylcaine
	Piperocaine
	Tetracaine

Procaine

Although injectable esters are not available for use in dentistry, procaine is still available in multidose vials and is used as an antiarrhythmic. Formulations include 2% procaine plain, 4% procaine plain, 2% procaine with 1:100,000 epinephrine, and 4% procaine with 1:100,000 epinephrine. Procaine is significantly less potent and toxic compared with all other amide local anesthetics. Procaine (Novocaine) was the first injectable local anesthetic and was used routinely in dentistry until amide local anesthetics became available. Procaine produces the greatest vasodilating properties of all local anesthetics and provides no pulpal anesthesia.[4] Procaine's high degree of allergic reactions and its vasodilating properties made it less desirable, and its use was discontinued. Procaine is metabolized via plasma cholinesterase to PABA, which is the major metabolic by-product responsible for allergic reactions.

DENTAL HYGIENE CONSIDERATIONS

- Local anesthetic cartridges containing a vasoconstrictor contain the preservative sodium bisulfite, which may cause allergic reactions including respiratory reactions in asthmatics (predominantly steroid-dependent asthmatics).
- Methylparaben is a bacteriostatic agent/preservative added to local anesthetic cartridges before 1984 and is known to cause allergic reactions. Currently no anesthetic cartridges contain methylparaben.
- Ester anesthetics are no longer manufactured for use in dentistry.
- The selection of the local anesthetic drug should be determined by the dental hygienist on an individual patient basis, taking into consideration the efficacy, safety, individual patient assessment, and dental or dental hygiene care plan.
- Intermediate action anesthetics are most commonly used for regular restorative dentistry and nonsurgical periodontal therapy.
- Lidocaine is the standard by which all other local anesthetics are compared.
- Lidocaine is the most commonly used anesthetic in dentistry in the United States; it provides profound anesthetic without extensive duration.
- There is no difference in pain control between a 1:50,000, 1:100,000, and 1:200,000 formulation of epinephrine.
- Lidocaine 1:50,000 epinephrine should be reserved for hemostasis by infiltrating small amounts into the papilla for bleeding control in the direct area of instrumentation.
- 2% mepivacaine is formulated only with 1:20,000 levonordefrin.
- Mepivacaine and prilocaine have the least vasodilating properties and are effective when a vasoconstrictor is contraindicated. Prilocaine plain may have intermediate duration when administered as a nerve block.
- Lidocaine, mepivacaine, and bupivacaine are metabolized in the liver by amidases. These anesthetics should be administered in lower doses to a patient with significant hepatic disease.
- Prilocaine is metabolized in the liver and additionally by the lungs and kidneys as alternative sites.
- Because of prilocaine's metabolite orthotoluidine, when administered in high doses, some individuals may develop methemoglobinemia by reducing the blood's oxygen-carrying capacity. This is a relative contraindication for at-risk patients.
- Prilocaine is the least toxic of the local anesthetics.
- Articaine is the only amide anesthetic that has an ester component attached to the aromatic ring structure. It is metabolized primarily in the plasma by plasma cholinesterase, and therefore it has the shortest half-life.
- Articaine can be safely administered to a patient with atypical plasma cholinesterase.
- Bupivacaine is the only long-acting local anesthetic available in the United States.
- Anesthetics that provide longer posttreatment durations of pulpal and soft tissue anesthesia are 0.5% bupivacaine 1:200,000 (long acting over 90 minutes) and 4% prilocaine 1:200,000 (intermediate to long acting 60 – 90 minutes).

CASE STUDY 5.1 The Patient Is Nervous About her Extraction

A patient is in your office for an impacted third molar extraction of tooth #1. The dentist asks the dental hygienist to administer the local anesthesia. The patient's blood pressure is 110/85 mm Hg and her weight is 102 lb. She has a history of atypical plasma cholinesterase, and she is very nervous about her dental appointment.

Critical Thinking Questions

- What are the medical considerations when choosing a local anesthetic?
- Choose and justify an appropriate local anesthetic for this patient.

CHAPTER REVIEW QUESTIONS

1. What is the most important advantage of amide over ester local anesthetics?
   A. Quicker onset
   B. Longer duration
   C. Less allergenicity
   D. Cheaper cost
2. Which local anesthetic is the longest acting?
   A. 2% Mepivacaine 1:20,000
   B. 4% Prilocaine
   C. 0.5% Bupivacaine 1:200,000
   D. 4% Prilocaine 1:200,000
   E. 4% Articaine 1:100,000
3. Which local anesthetic has the least vasodilatory effect when used without epinephrine?
   A. Mepivacaine
   B. Lidocaine
   C. Cocaine
   D. Procaine
4. Which local anesthetic has the greatest vasodilatory effect when used without epinephrine?
   A. Mepivacaine
   B. Lidocaine
   C. Articaine
   D. Procaine
5. One cartridge of anesthetic contains how much solution?
   A. 1.8 mL
   B. 1.8 g
   C. 1.8 mg
   D. 1.8 L
6. Important factors to consider when selecting a local anesthetic include all of the following EXCEPT one. Which one is the EXCEPTION?
   A. Duration of pain control
   B. An absolute or relative contraindication to the local anesthetic
   C. Requirement for hemostasis
   D. Vitamin intake
7. All of the following statements are correct, EXCEPT one. Which one is the EXCEPTION?
   A. Injectable esters are not commercially available for use in dentistry.
   B. Procaine is an ester.
   C. Topical benzocaine is an amide.
   D. Prilocaine is an amide.
8. Which of the following local anesthetics is metabolized in the plasma and liver?
   A. Lidocaine
   B. Bupivacaine
   C. Prilocaine
   D. Articaine

9. Which of the following is an advantage of having a local anesthetic metabolized in the plasma and liver?
   A. Increased duration of action of drug
   B. Shorter half-life of drug
   C. Decreased vasoactivity of drug
   D. Easy excretion of metabolites
10. Which of the following local anesthetics is metabolized in the lungs and liver?
   A. Mepivacaine
   B. Bupivacaine
   C. Prilocaine
   D. Articaine
11. Methylparaben is a:
   A. Local anesthetic preservative that prevents oxidation of epinephrine
   B. Bacteriostatic agent that is no longer added to dental cartridges because of high incidence of allergic reactions
   C. Buffer that alkalinizes the anesthetic solution
   D. Buffer that creates an isotonic solution
12. How is 3% mepivacaine formulated?
   A. 3% plain
   B. 3% 1:20,000 levonordefrin
   C. 3% 1:100,000 epinephrine
   D. 3% 1:200,000 epinephrine
13. Which of the following is a concern when selecting bupivacaine?
   A. Patient self-mutilation
   B. Decreased risk of toxicity
   C. Concentration of anesthetic
   D. Ease of biotransformation
14. Which of the following local anesthetics is the BEST option for readministration of anesthetic to provide a lessened likelihood of blood concentration build-up?
   A. Lidocaine
   B. Mepivacaine
   C. Prilocaine
   D. Articaine
   E. Bupivacaine
15. The lower the pK_a of a drug, the more anions are present, which decreases the onset of action. The higher the pKa of a drug, the more cations are present, which increases the onset of action.
   A. Both statements are correct.
   B. Both statements are NOT correct.
   C. The first statement is correct; the second statement is NOT correct.
   D. The first statement is NOT correct; the second statement is correct.
16. Which of the following is NOT a factor in the duration of a local anesthetic?
   A. Individual response to anesthetic
   B. Anatomic structure
   C. Patient health assessment
   D. Injection technique
17. Which of the following local anesthetics used without a vasoconstrictor provides intermediate duration of action when administering a block?
   A. Lidocaine
   B. Mepivacaine
   C. Prilocaine
   D. Bupivacaine
18. Which of the following is the BEST reason for choosing a local anesthetic that provides a long duration?
   A. Need for postoperative pain control
   B. Medical status of patient
   C. Dense bone in the area of administration
   D. Infection in the area
19. When is lidocaine 1:50,000 epinephrine most effective?
   A. When postoperative pain control is needed
   B. When hemostasis is needed
   C. When treating a patient with cardiovascular disease
   D. When more profound pain control is needed
20. Where is procaine metabolized?
   A. Liver
   B. Lungs
   C. Plasma
   D. Plasma and liver

REFERENCES

1. Stevenson DD, Simon RA. Sensitivity to ingested metabisulfites in asthmatic subjects. *J Allergy Clin Immunol.* 1981;68:26–32.
2. Haveles EB. *Applied pharmacology for the dental hygienist.* ed 8. St Louis: Elsevier; 2020.
3. Bahl R. Local anesthesia in dentistry. *Anesth Prog.* 2004;51:138–142.
4. Malamed S. *Handbook of local anesthesia.* ed 7. St Louis: Elsevier; 2020.
5. Bowen DM, Pieren JA. *Darby and Walsh dental hygiene: theory and practice.* ed 5. St Louis: Elsevier; 2020.
6. Jastak T, Yagiela J, Donaldson D. *Local anesthesia of the oral cavity.* St Louis: Saunders; 1995.
7. Stevenson DD, Simon RA. Sulfites and asthma. *J Allergy Clin Immunol.* 1984;74:469–472.
8. Matheson DA, Stevenson DD, Simon RA. Precipitating factors in asthma. Aspirin, sulfites, and other drugs and chemicals. *Chest.* 1985;87(1 Suppl): 50S–54S.
9. Sher TH, Schwartz HJ. Bisulfite sensitivity manifesting an allergic reaction to aerosol therapy. *Ann Allergy.* 1985;54:224–226.
10. Borghesan F, Basso D, Chieco Bianchi F, et al. Allergy to wine. *Allergy.* 2004;59:1135–1136.
11. Young ER, Mason DR, Saso MA, et al. Some clinical properties of Octocaine 200 (2 percent lidocaine with epinephrine 1:200,000). *J Can Dent Assoc.* 1989;55:987–991.
12. Akerman B, Astrom A, Ross S, Telc A. Studies on the absorption, distribution and metabolism of labeled prilocaine and lidocaine in some animal species. *Acta Pharmacol Toxicol (Copenh).* 1966;24:389–403.
13. Geddes IC. The metabolism of prilocaine (Citanest), established by means of C-14 and H3 isotopes. *Anesth Analg (Paris).* 1966;24:213–224.
14. Gutenberg LL, Chen JW, Trapp L. Methemoglobin levels in generally anesthetized pediatric patients receiving prilocaine verses lidocaine. *Anesth Prog.* 2013;60:99–108.
15. Trapp L, Will J. Acquired methemoglobinemia revisited. *Dent Clin N Amer.* 2010;54:665–675.
16. Doko Y, Iranami H, Fujii K, Yamazaki A, Shimogai M, Hatano Y. Severe methemoglobinemia after dental anesthesia: a warning about propitocaine-induced methemoglobinemia in neonates. *J Anesth.* 2010;24:935–937.
17. Vice TB, Baars AM, van Oss GE, et al. High performance liquid chromatography and preliminary pharmacokinetics of articaine and its 2-carboxy metabolite in human serum and urine. *J Chromatogr.* 1988;424:240–444.
18. Malamed S. *Medical emergencies in the dental office.* ed 7. St Louis: Elsevier; 2015.
19. Isen DA. Articaine: pharmacology and clinical use of a recently approved local anesthetic. *Dent Today.* 2000;19:72–77.

20. Kanaa MD, Whitworth JM, Corbett IP, Meechan JG. Articaine and lidocaine mandibular buccal infiltration anesthesia: a prospective randomized double-blind cross-over study. *J Endod.* 2006;32(4):296–298.
21. Robertson D, Nusstein J, Reader A, Beck M, McCartney M. The anesthetic efficacy of articaine in buccal infiltration of mandibular posterior teeth. *J Am Dent Assoc.* 2007;138(8):1104–1112.
22. Oertel R, Rahn R, Kirch W. Clinical pharmacokinetics of articaine. *Clin Pharmacokinet.* 1997;33:417–425.
23. Oertel R, Richter K. Plasma protein binding of the local anaesthetic drug articaine and its metabolite articainic acid. *Pharmazie.* 1998;53:646–647.
24. Haas DA, Lennon D. A 21-year retrospective study of reports of paresthesia following local anesthetic administration. *J Can Dent Assoc.* 1995;61:319–330.
25. Dower JS. A review of paresthesia. *Dent Today.* 2003;22:64–69.
26. Malamed SF. Local anesthetics: dentistry's most important drugs-clinical update 2006. *J Calif Dent Assoc.* 2006;34(12):971–976.
27. Malamed SF. Articaine versus lidocaine: the author responds (comment on Dower JS Jr. Articaine vs lidocaine). *J Calif Dent Assoc.* 2007;35(4):240, 242, 244.

ADDITIONAL RESOURCES

Bartlett SZ. Clinical observation on the effect of injections of local anaesthetics preceded by aspiration. *Oral Surg.* 1972;33:520–525.

Becker D, Reed K. Essentials of local anesthetic pharmacology. American Dental Society of Anesthesiology. *Anesth Program.* 2006;53:98–109.

Buckley JA, Ciancio SG, McMullen JA. Efficacy of epinephrine concentration in local anesthesia during periodontal surgery. *J Periodontol.* 1984;55: 653–657.

De Jong RH. *Local anesthetics.* St Louis: Mosby; 1994.

Finder RL, More PA. Adverse drug reactions to local anesthesia. *Dent Clin N Am.* 2002;46:447–457.

Haas DA, Harper DG, Saso MA, Young ER. Comparison of articaine and prilocaine anesthesia by infiltration in maxillary and mandibular arches. *Anesth Prog.* 1990;37:230–237.

Hargreaves KM, Berman LH. *Cohen's pathways of the pulp.* ed 11. St Louis: Elsevier; 2016.

Isen DA. Articaine: Pharmacology and clinical use of a recently approved local anesthetic. *Dent Today.* 2000;19:72–77.

Jakobs W. Local anaesthesia and vasoconstrictive additional components. *Newslett Int Fed Dent Anesthesiol Soc.* 1989;2:1–3.

Jakobs W, Ladwig B, Cichon P, Oertel R, Kirch W. Serum levels of articaine 2% and 4% in children. *Anesth Prog.* 1995;42:113–115.

Malamed SF, Gagnon S, Leblanc D. A comparison between articaine HCL and lidocaine HCL in pediatric dental patients. *Am Acad Ped Dent.* 2000;22: 307–311.

Malamed SF, Gagnon S, Leblanc D. Efficacy of articaine: a new amide local anesthetic. *J Am Dent Assoc.* 2000;131:635–642.

Malamed SF, Gagnon S, Leblanc D. Articaine hydrochloride: a study of the safety of a new amide local anesthetic. *J Am Dent Assoc.* 2001;132:177–184.

Oertel R, Ebert U, Rahn R, Kirch W. The effect of age on the pharmacokinetics of the local anesthetic drug articaine. *Regional Anesth Pain Med.* 1999;24: 524–528.

Sisk A. Vasoconstrictors in local anesthesia for dentistry. *Anesth Prog.* 1992;39: 187–193.

Van der Meer AD, Burm AG, Stienstra R, van Kleef JW, Vletter AA, Olieman W. Pharmacokinetics of prilocaine after intravenous administration in volunteers: enantioselectivity. *Anesthesiology.* 1999;90(4):988–992.

APPENDIX 5.1: Summary of Amide Local Anesthetic Agents and Vasoconstrictors

Generic Name	Lidocaine		Mepivacaine		Prilocaine		Articaine		Bupivacaine
Available formulations	2% 1:50,000 Epinephrine Green	2% 1:100,000 Epinephrine Red	3% Plain Tan	2% 1:20,000 Levonordefrin Brown	4% Plain Black	4% 1:200,000 Epinephrine Yellow	4% 1:100,000 Epinephrine Gold	4% 1:200,000 Epinephrine Silver	0.5% 1:200,000 Epinephrine Blue
ADA color coding band									
pKa	7.7	7.7	7.6	7.6	7.7	7.9	7.8	7.8	8.1
Onset of action (in minutes)	3–5	3–5	3–5	3–5	3–5	3.5	1–2 (S) 2.0–2.5 (B)	1–2 (S) 2–3 (B)	6–10
pH	3.3–4.4	3.3–4.4	5.5–6.0	3.0–4.0	6.0–6.5	3.0–4.0	4.0–5.5	4.0–5.5	3.0–4.5
Duration category	Intermediate	Intermediate	Short	Intermediate	Short (S) Intermediate (B)	Intermediate	Intermediate	Intermediate	Long
Duration pulpal (in minutes)	60	60	20 (S) 40 (B)	60	10–15 (S) 40–60 (B)	60–90§	60–75§	45–60	90–180
Duration soft tissue (in minutes)	180–300	180–300	120–180	180–300	90–120 (S) 120–240 (B)	180–480	180–360	120–300	240–540 (Reports up to 720)
Half-life (in minutes)	96	96	114	114	96	96	Approx. 27*	Approx. 27*	162
MRD (mg/lb)	3.2	3.2	3.0	3.0	3.6	3.6	3.2	3.2	0.9†
MRD (mg/kg)	7.0	7.0	6.6	6.6	8.0	8.0	7.0	7.0	2.0†
MRD Absolute mg	500	500	400	400	600	600	None listed	None Listed	90
Relative potency (reference value = Lidocaine @100%)	100%	100%	100%	100%	100%	100%	150%	150%	400%
Relative toxicity (reference value = Lidocaine @100%)	100%	100%	75%	75%	60%	60%	100%	100%	Less than 400%

ADA, American Dental Association; *MRD,* maximum recommended dose; *S,* Supraperiosteal; *B,* block.

*Vice TB, Baars AM, van Oss GE, et al: High performance liquid chromatography and preliminary pharmacokinetics of articaine and its 2-carboxy metabolite in human serum and urine, *J Chromatogr* 424:240–444, 1988. Manufacturer product inserts list half-life of articaine at 43.8 minutes with 1:100,000 epinephrine and 44.4 minutes with 1:200,000 epinephrine.

§4% Prilocaine 1:200,000 and 4% articaine 1:100,000 are categorized as intermediate durations but provide a slightly longer duration than the other intermediate drugs, extending the duration to 60 to 90 minutes for prilocaine and 60 to 75 minutes for articaine.

†Canadian recommendations; no U.S. recommendations available.

6

Topical Anesthetic Agents

Diana Burnham Aboytes, RDH, MS

LEARNING OBJECTIVES

1. Discuss the purpose of topical anesthetics.
2. Identify ideal properties of topical anesthetics and discuss their mechanism of action.
3. List common forms of topical anesthetics and describe the methods for delivery of topical anesthetic drugs.
4. Identify and describe the common topical anesthetic agents used in dentistry, including classification, available concentrations, onset of action, duration, considerations, and maximum recommended dosages.
5. Identify and describe topical anesthetic drug combinations used in dentistry.
6. Discuss special considerations when dealing with topical anesthetics in dentistry, including recognizing signs and symptoms of adverse reactions to topical anesthetics.

INTRODUCTION

An important component of the local anesthesia armamentarium is topical anesthetic. **Topical** implies that the anesthetic will be applied to a body surface such as the skin or mucous membrane. In dentistry, topical anesthetics are used routinely to provide pain management before conventional local anesthetic injections. They contribute by minimizing the pain associated with needle insertion. Topical anesthetics are also frequently used for the treatment of minor injuries of the gingiva and oral mucosa, to increase comfort during minor dental and dental hygiene procedures, and to reduce the patient's gag reflex while taking radiographs and impressions.

There are limitations to topical anesthetics, and they should not be used as a substitute for local anesthesia. Topical anesthetics do not provide pulpal anesthesia and will not be effective if root sensitivity is a concern.

Some topical anesthetic agents are available over the counter to the public and can be purchased at local food and drug stores. People use them to ease pain caused by braces, aphthous ulcers (canker sores), dentures, or toothaches.

Whether being applied professionally or in the comfort of your home (Tables 6.1 and 6.2), an intraoral topical anesthetic should ideally be nonallergenic and produce no damage to the tissue to which it is applied. It should consist of a pain-free application, have an acceptable taste, and be able to remain at the site of application. Also, it must produce reliable, effective anesthesia with a sufficient duration and not induce systemic toxicity (Box 6.1).

MECHANISM OF ACTION OF TOPICAL ANESTHETICS

The mechanism of action of topical anesthetics is similar to that of their injectable counterparts. Topical anesthetics, however, have a higher concentration and do not contain a vasoconstrictor in order to diffuse through the mucous membrane. The permeability of sodium ions to the nerve cell is decreased, resulting in decreased depolarization and an increased excitability threshold. Topical anesthesia, unlike a local infiltration, supraperiosteal, or nerve block, only blocks free nerve endings closest to the mucosal surface where it is applied. (Fig. 6.1)

TOPICAL ANESTHETIC FORMS AND METHODS OF DELIVERY

Topical anesthetic agents are available in a variety of commercial forms, including gels, ointments, sprays (both metered and unmetered), creams, liquids, and lozenges. The type of preparation can affect the efficacy. Depending on the form used, effective concentrations range from 0.2% to 20%.[1,2] Delivery methods include the use of cotton-tip applicators, sprays, brushes, patches, blunted cannulas and/or syringes, and single-dose applicator swabs (Fig. 6.2).

When professionals apply topical anesthetics, each form and method of delivery is considered on an individual patient basis. Medical and dental histories should always be reviewed before the anesthetic is applied, and manufacturer's directions should be followed.

To provide pain management before the administration of conventional local anesthetic injections, topical gels or ointments are applied with a cotton-tip applicator (see Procedure 6.1). The site of penetration should first be dried using a 2 × 2 gauze square to increase visibility and accurate placement of the topical anesthetic (Fig. 6.3). Only a small amount of gel or ointment on the applicator tip is necessary to achieve the desired result (Fig. 6.4). Student dental hygienists and even experienced clinicians often apply excessive amounts of topical anesthesia, leading to an unnecessary effect on surrounding tissue. This excess mixes with the saliva and may anesthetize unwanted areas such as the tongue, soft palate, or pharynx. The topical agent should remain at the site of penetration for 1 to 2 minutes (depending on the concentration of the topical anesthetic) to ensure effectiveness (Fig. 6.5). If these steps are followed, anesthesia should be achieved to a depth of approximately 2 mm to 3 mm into the tissue. This helps provide comfort during the initial penetration of the needle.

Topical anesthetics in liquid form are also used in dentistry. Liquids provide anesthesia to a wide area. They are especially useful when trying to decrease a patient's gag reflex, thereby making placement of

TABLE 6.1 Common Topical Agents Administered Professionally

Product Name	Gel	Spray	Liquid	Ointment	Patch	Lozenge	Cream	Single Unit Dose	Active Ingredient
Anacaine				X					Benzocaine 10%
BeeGentle	X								Benzocaine 20%
Benzo-Jel	X								Benzocaine 20%
CaineTips								X	Benzocaine 20%
Cetacaine	X	X	X						Benzocaine 14%, butamben 2%, tetracaine hydrochloride 2%
ComfortCaine	X								Benzocaine 20%
Cora-Caine				X					Benzocaine 16%
Gingicaine	X		X						Benzocaine 18%
HurriCaine	X	X	X					X	Benzocaine 20%
HurriPak			X						Benzocaine 20%
Kolorz	X								Benzocaine 20%
Lidocaine				X					Lidocaine 5%
Lollicaine								X	Benzocaine 20%
ProJel-20	X								Benzocaine 20%
One Touch Advanced	X								Benzocaine 14%, butamben 2%, tetracaine hydrochloride 2%
Oraqix	X								Lidocaine 2.5% and prilocaine 2.5%
Topex	X	X	X						Benzocaine 20%
Topex HandiCaine Stix								X	Benzocaine 20%
Topicale	X			X	X				Benzocaine regular 18%, extra strength 20%
Ultracare	X								Benzocaine 20%
Xylonor	X	X							Lidocaine 15%

impression materials or radiograph film more comfortable and tolerable. The use of a liquid for a more site-specific procedure requires an applicator. Cetacaine (Cetylite, Pennsauken, NJ), which is available only by prescription, is administered either by a cotton pellet or via blunted cannula to deliver the anesthetic subgingivally (Fig. 6.6). Another liquid, HurriPak (Beutlich Pharmaceuticals) is designed primarily for the use of subgingival placement by using irrigation syringes with plastic tips (Fig. 6.7). These are indicated when attempting to increase comfort during prophylaxis or nonsurgical periodontal therapy procedures.

Gels, ointments, and liquids often come in multidose containers, but some products are packaged in single unit-dose applications. Lollicaine (Centrix), HandiCaine Stix (Topex Sultan Healthcare), and CaineTips (J Morita) are some of the products available through dental suppliers. These single unit–dose applications can also be found in over-the-counter products such as Orajel medicated tooth swabs (Fig. 6.8). Individual packaging is less messy, helps prevent possible cross-contamination, and allows monitoring of the dose.

Sprays are also used to deliver topical anesthesia. Unmetered sprays are not recommended because they do not allow control of the amount of anesthetic dispensed, nor are they easily contained at a specific site. However, the use of a metered spray with a disposable nozzle enables control over the amount of agent being dispensed, thus decreasing the risk for systemic toxicity (Fig. 6.9). Both the Institute of Safe Medication Practices (ISMP) and the U.S. Food and Drug Administration (FDA) have released advisory statements informing the public of the association between benzocaine and methemoglobinemia, wherein methemoglobin builds up in the blood, hindering the effective transport of oxygen to body tissues (see Chapter 7).

BOX 6.1 Ideal Properties of an Intraoral Topical Anesthetic

- Nonallergenic
- Produce no local damage to tissue
- Allow pain-free application
- Have an acceptable taste
- Remain at the site of application
- Produce reliable anesthesia
- Produce sufficient duration of anesthesia
- Produce no systemic toxicity

From Meechan JG: Intra-oral topical anesthetics: a review, *J Dent* 28:3–14, 2000.

TABLE 6.2 Common Over-the-Counter Topical Anesthetic Agents Self-Administered by Patients

Product Name	Gel	Spray	Liquid	Ointment	Patch	Lozenge	Cream	Single Unit Dose	Active Ingredient
Anbesol	X		X						Benzocaine: Jr 10%, max strength 20%
BiZets						X			Benzocaine 15 mg
Cepacol		X				X			Benzocaine-spray 5% Lozenges 7.5 mg to 15 mg
Chloraseptic						X			Benzocaine 6 mg
Dentapaine	X								Benzocaine 20%
HDA Toothache	X								Benzocaine 6.5%
Kank-A	X		X			X			Benzocaine-gel and liquid 20%, bead 3 mg
Orabase									Benzocaine 20% comes in a paste
Orajel Adult	X						X	X	Benzocaine-regular 10%, ultra and denture 15%, medicated swab 20%, PM max strength 20%
Ora-Film									Benzocaine 10% comes in a thin film strip
Red Cross Canker				X					Benzocaine 20%
Sucrets						X			Dyclonine hydrochloride Children 1.2 mg, max strength 3 mg
Tanac			X						Benzocaine 10%
Thorets						X			Benzocaine 10 mg
Zilactin-B	X								Benzocaine 10%, max strength 20%

A newer product, Kovanaze, delivers dental anesthetic by way of nasal spray. The 3% tetracaine hydrochloride with 0.05% oxymetazoline HCl combination is administered via the nasal mucosa and diffuses into the maxillary superior dental plexus. It provides anesthesia to both hard and soft tissues of teeth #A through #J or #4 through #13. A product that provides anesthesia without a needle offers great promise for the dental profession by giving options to patients who avoid or put off treatment because of the fear associated with the needle injection in this area.

Nerve block
Supraperiosteal injection
Infiltration
Topical

Fig. 6.1 Shows comparison of how topical anesthesia reaches only the free nerve endings nearest the mucosal surface compared with infiltrations, supraperiosteal injections, or nerve blocks.

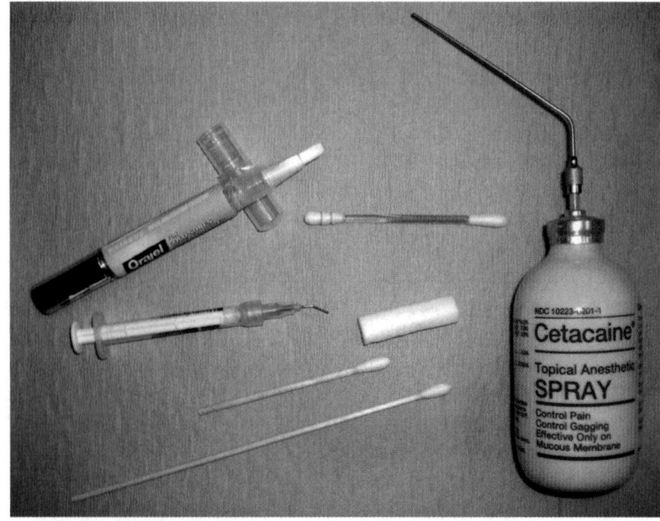

Fig. 6.2 Methods used to deliver topical anesthetics.

PROCEDURE 6.1 Basic Topical Anesthesia Technique Used Prior to Local Anesthesia Injection

Step 1 Review medical and dental history.

Step 2 Set up armamentarium.

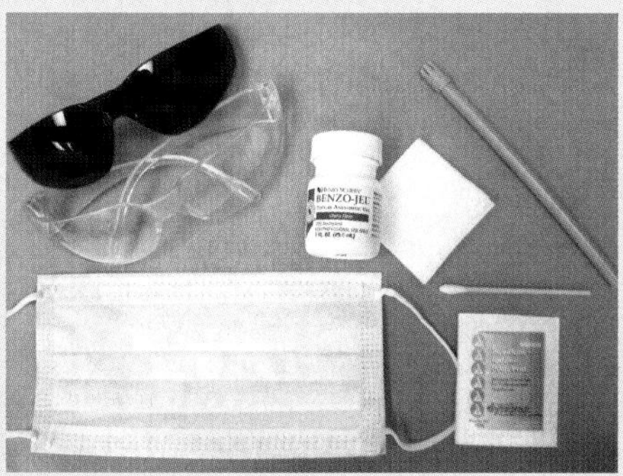

2 × 2 gauze
Cotton-tip applicator
Saliva ejector
Topical anesthetic
Topical antiseptic (optional)
Personal protective equipment (PPE) and patient safety eyewear

Step 3 Have on all PPE and make sure patient is wearing protective eyewear.

Step 4 Place patient in supine position.

Step 5 Prepare cotton-tip applicator with proper amount of topical anesthetic.

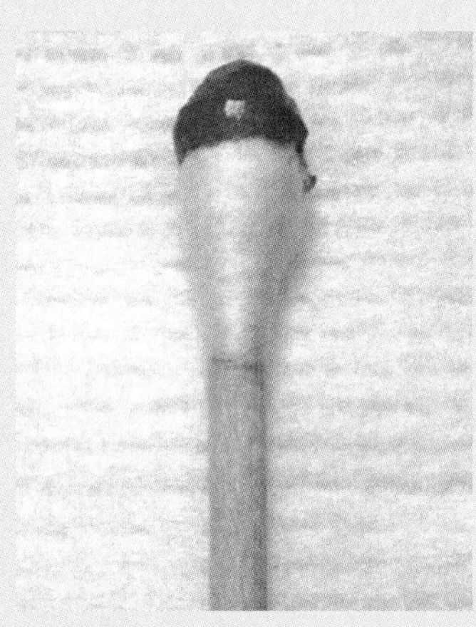

Remember: Only a small amount is necessary to achieve the desired results.

Step 6 Perform intraoral inspection of the areas where topical anesthesia is to be placed. Assess area for abrasions, lacerations, or any trauma that would affect absorption and increase risk for toxicity.

Step 7 Identify landmarks. Using 2 × 2 gauze, gently wipe the area dry, removing any debris from the area.

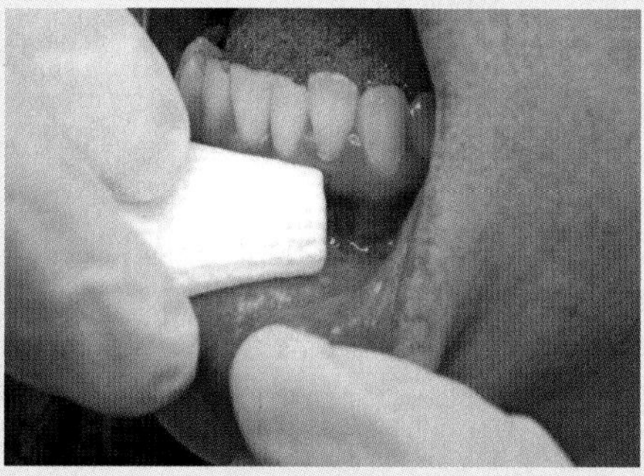

Step 8 (Optional) Wipe area using a topical antiseptic such as Betadine (povidone-iodine). This step helps decrease the risk for infection but is considered optional.

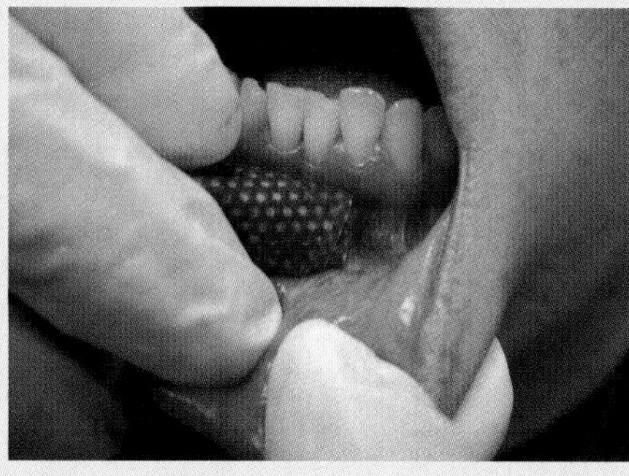

Step 9 Place topical anesthesia at site of penetration. Leave in place for 1–2 minutes to ensure effectiveness.

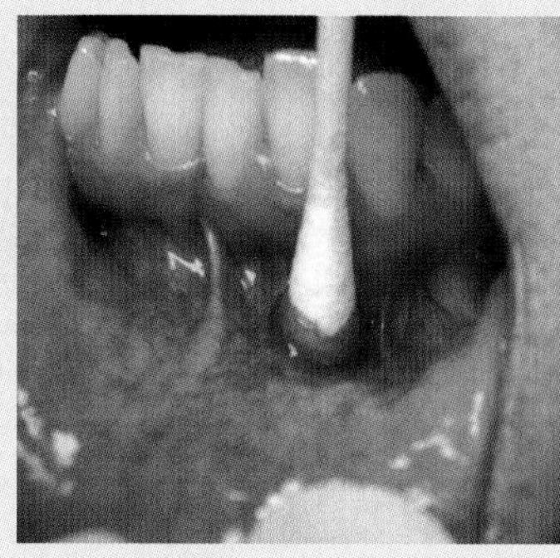

Step 10 Remove cotton-tip applicator, provide suction as necessary, and continue with the injection.

Patch delivery of a topical anesthetic is advantageous because the patch can be placed directly on the delivery site, and then it adheres to the tissue. Transdermal patches are used regularly in medicine on intact skin to administer certain medications or to provide local dermal analgesia. For example, Synera (ZARS Pharma, Salt Lake City, Utah) is an FDA-approved peel-and-stick topical anesthetic patch that numbs intact skin before minor needle procedures and superficial dermatologic procedures.[3] Lidoderm (Endo Pharmaceuticals, Chadds Ford, PA) is also an FDA-approved adhesive patch that provides pain relief from postherpetic neuralgia, commonly

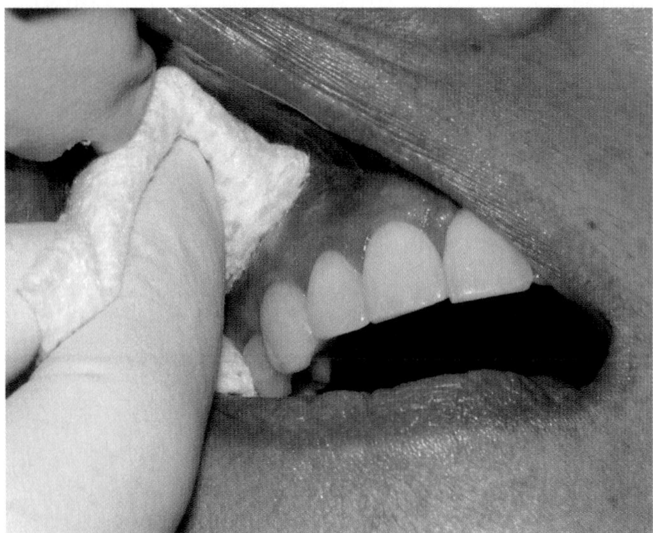

Fig. 6.3 A 2 × 2 gauze square is used to gently wipe and dry tissue at the site of needle penetration.

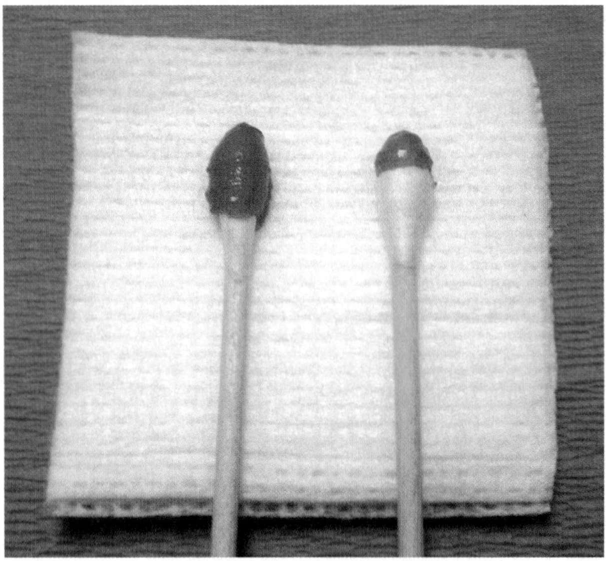

Fig. 6.4 Cotton-tip applicator on left shows excessive amount of topical anesthesia. Cotton-tip applicator on the right shows correct amount of topical anesthesia to be applied at each penetration site.

called after-shingles pain.[4] These patches are not used intraorally, however.

Patches available for intraoral topical anesthesia are limited. Noven Pharmaceuticals introduced the first FDA-approved transoral anesthetic patch, DentiPatch, in 1996, but the manufacturer has since discontinued the product. Currently the only patch available for intraoral use is Topicale GelPatch (Premier Dental Co.) (Fig. 6.10).

Regardless of the form and method of delivery, there is more than one option for delivering topical anesthetics to dental patients. Furthermore, dental hygienists must be aware that patients often self-medicate using these same drugs in over-the-counter formulations and should query their patients before administering any anesthetic agents.

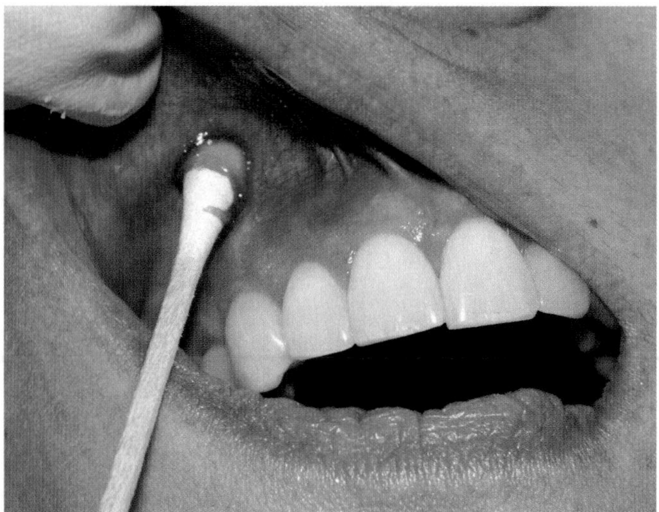

Fig. 6.5 Topical anesthetic placed at the site of needle penetration for 1 to 2 minutes.

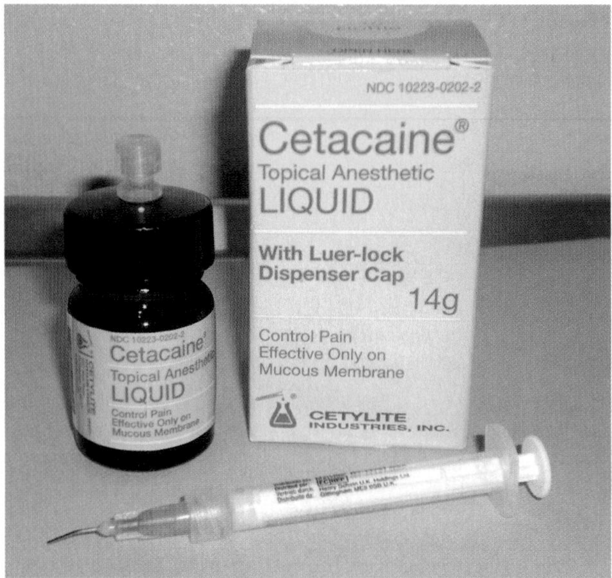

Fig. 6.6 Cetacaine liquid with syringe applicator.

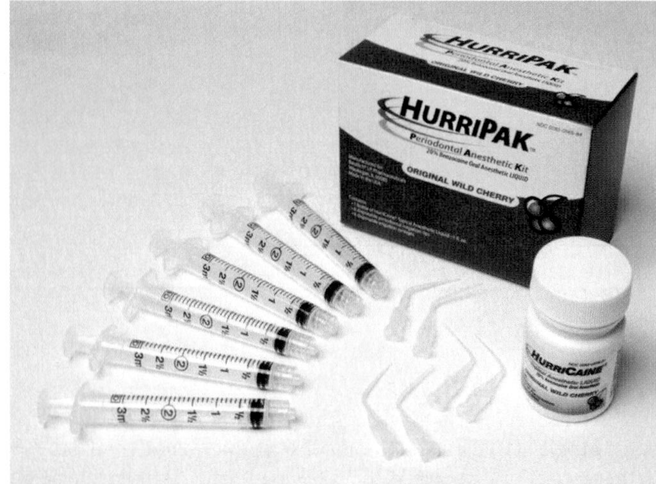

Fig. 6.7 HurriPak liquid topical anesthesia with plastic irrigation syringes and tips.

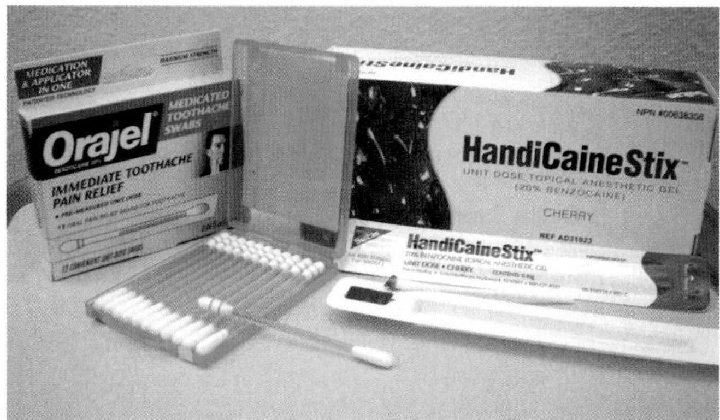

Fig. 6.8 Single unit–dose applicator.

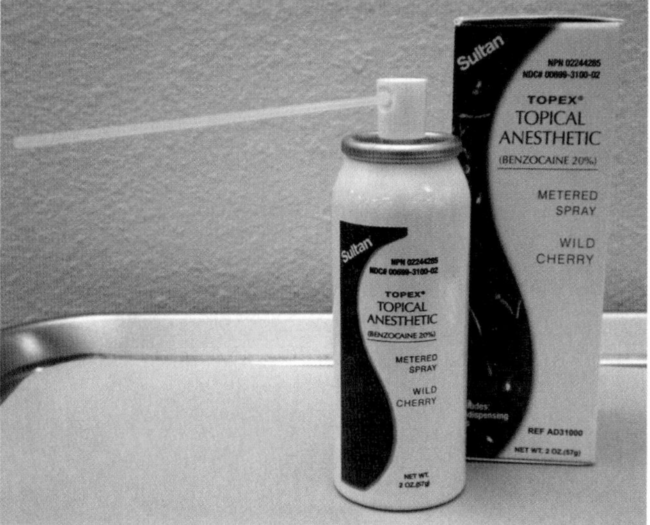

Fig. 6.9 Metered spray with disposable nozzle.

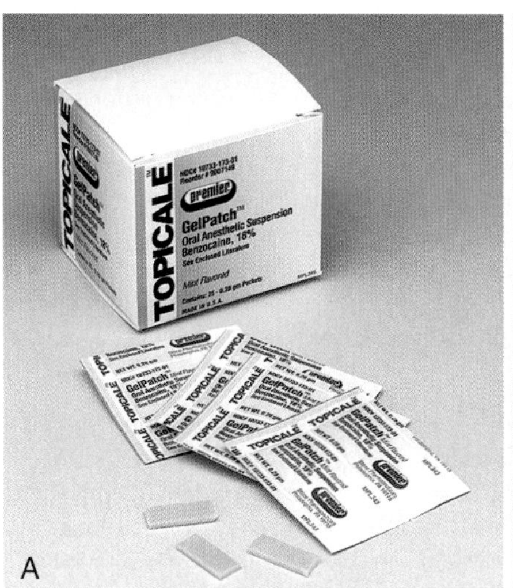

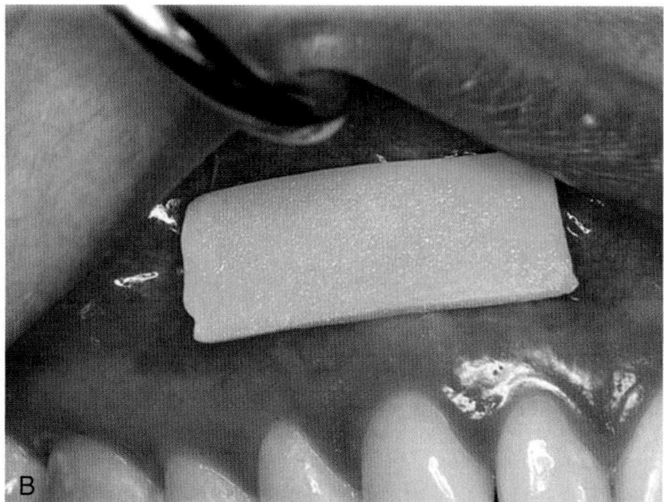

Fig. 6.10 (A) Transoral adhesive Topicale GelPatch. (B) Adhesive GelPatch placed intraorally.

COMMON TOPICAL AGENTS USED IN DENTISTRY

Benzocaine

Benzocaine is one of the more common and widely used topical anesthetics. It is available in gel, cream, ointment, lozenge, liquid solution, spray, and patch (Fig. 6.11). It exists almost entirely in its base form, making absorption into the circulation slow and therefore having a very low potential for systemic toxicity in healthy individuals.

- **Classification:** Benzocaine is an ester.
- **Available concentration:** The most commonly used concentration in dentistry is 20%, although it is available in concentrations ranging from 6% to 20%.
- **Onset of action:** The onset is rapid, or as early as 30 seconds, and it has its peak effect at 2 minutes.
- **Duration:** 5 to 15 minutes.
- **Maximum recommended dose:** There are no published maximum dosage recommendations.[5]
- **Metabolism/excretion:** Benzocaine is metabolized via hydrolysis in the plasma and to a lesser extent in the liver by cholinesterase. Excretion occurs primarily through the kidneys with only a small portion remaining unchanged in the urine.
- **Pregnancy/lactation:** Animal studies have shown a risk, but controlled human studies have not been conducted, or studies are not available in humans or animals. It is given only after risks to the fetus are considered. Use with caution with lactation.

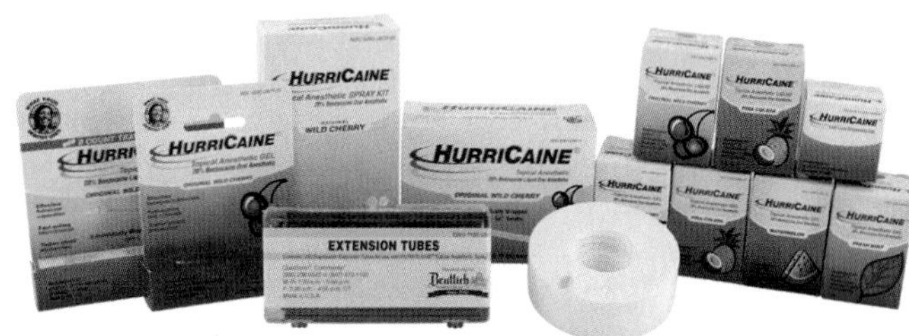

Fig. 6.11 Varieties of products used professionally that contain benzocaine.

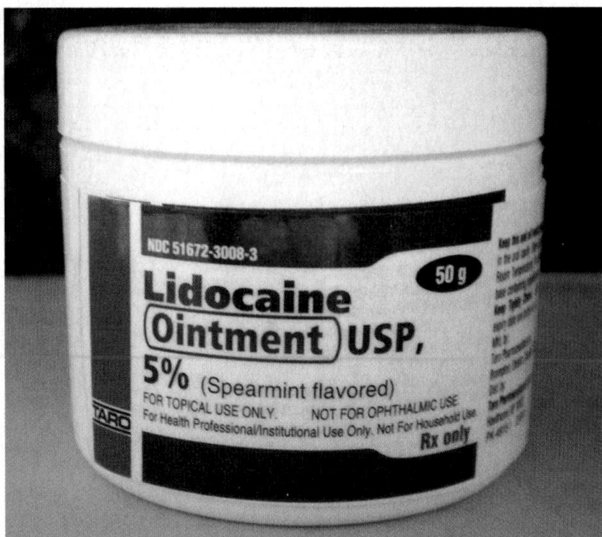

Fig. 6.12 Lidocaine products.

- **Special considerations:** Methemoglobinemia has been reported after topical anesthetic use of benzocaine, particularly with higher concentrations of 14% to 20% spray applications applied to the mouth and mucous membrane. Always apply as directed. Benzocaine should not be used on children younger than 2 years of age.

Lidocaine

Lidocaine is a good alternative if a patient has sensitivity to esters. The most common topical preparation is an ointment (Fig. 6.12), but it can be found as a patch, as a spray, and in a solution. It is available in two forms, as a base or a hydrochloride salt. The base form is poorly soluble in water and has poor penetration and absorption abilities. The hydrochloride salt form, on the other hand, is water soluble and can easily penetrate and be absorbed in the tissues, significantly increasing the risk of toxicity. The base form is preferred for application to mucous membranes and for covering large areas.

- **Classification:** Lidocaine is an amide.
- **Available concentration:** The most common is in 2% or 5% preparations.
- **Onset of action:** The onset is between 2 and 10 minutes.
- **Duration:** This depends on method of application but is approximately 15 to 45 minutes.
- **Maximum recommended dose:** 200 mg (300 mg manufacturer recommendation).
- **Metabolism/excretion:** It is metabolized in the liver and excreted via the kidney with less than 10% remaining unchanged.
- **Pregnancy/lactation:** Animal reproduction studies have not indicated fetal risk, and human studies have not been conducted, or animal studies have shown a risk, but controlled human studies have not.
- **Special considerations:** Always follow the manufacturer's application directions and ask questions of the physician staff if necessary.

Dyclonine Hydrochloride

Dyclonine hydrochloride has a unique classification in that it is neither an ester nor an amide agent, but rather it is a ketone. This unique property is beneficial for patients with sensitivities to traditional topical anesthetics. As a topical anesthetic, dyclonine hydrochloride is available by prescription, and to patients it is available over the counter in Sucrets lozenges (Fig. 6.13).

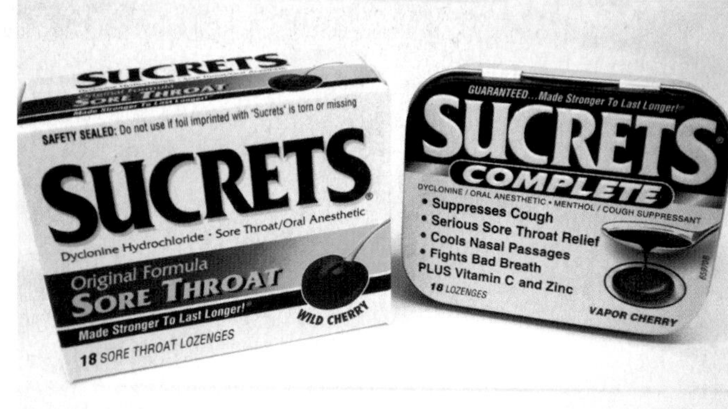

Fig. 6.13 Over-the-counter products containing dyclonine hydrochloride.

- **Classification:** Dyclonine hydrochloride is a ketone.
- **Available concentration:** It is formulated for use in dentistry as a 0.5% or 1% solution.
- **Onset of action:** The onset is slow; it may take up to 10 minutes to become effective.
- **Duration:** The average duration is 30 minutes; however, effects may last up to 1 hour.
- **Maximum recommended dose:** 200 mg (40 mL of 0.5% solution or 20 mL of a 1% solution).
- **Metabolism/excretion:** No information is available on the metabolism and excretion of dyclonine hydrochloride.
- **Pregnancy/lactation:** Animal studies have shown a risk, but controlled human studies have not been conducted, or studies are not available in humans or animals. It is given only after risks to the fetus are considered. Use with caution during lactation.

Tetracaine Hydrochloride

Tetracaine hydrochloride is considered the most potent of the topical anesthetics. It is not made available for injection and with topical preparations is typically combined with other drugs.

- **Classification:** Tetracaine hydrochloride is an ester.
- **Available concentration:** 2% in topical preparations.
- **Onset of action:** The onset is slow; peak effects may take up to 20 minutes.
- **Duration:** Approximately 45 minutes.
- **Maximum recommended dose:** 20 mg for topical administration; 1 mL of a 2% solution.
- **Metabolism/excretion:** It is metabolized by plasma pseudocholinesterase and excreted in the kidneys.
- **Pregnancy/lactation:** Animal studies have shown a risk, but controlled human studies have not been conducted, or studies are not available in humans or animals. It is given only after risks to the fetus are considered. Use with caution during lactation.
- **Special considerations:** It is highly soluble in lipids, making absorption into local tissues very rapid.

COMBINATIONS OF TOPICAL DRUGS

Topical anesthetic agents are also mixed and used in combinations to increase the anesthetic effect.

Compounded Topical Agents

There are instances when individual topical anesthetics agents may not be enough to meet the patient's needs. Dental providers may opt for a compounded topical anesthetic, which is a custom formulation that combines individual agents to create a new tailored product. There are a variety of formulations that can be developed, each available by prescription, but lidocaine, prilocaine, and tetracaine are among the most commonly combined anesthetics. Additionally, unlike traditional topical anesthetic agents, which do not contain a vasoconstrictor, compounded agents can have a vasoconstrictor such as phenylephrine added to most formulations.

A few examples of topical anesthetic compounds include the following:

- Lidocaine 10%, prilocaine 10% and tetracaine 4%
  - Referred to as Profound, Tricaine Blue, or DepBlu
- Lidocaine 3%, prilocaine 10%, tetracaine 12.5%, and 3% phenylephrine
  - Referred to as the Baddest Topical in Town (BTT)
- Lidocaine 20%, tetracaine 4%, and phenylephrine 2%
  - Referred to as TAC 20 Alternate

Individual medications used for compounding have approval from the FDA. However, when these are combined, the quality, safety, or effectiveness of these newly compounded topical anesthetics have not been evaluated by the FDA and thus do not have FDA approval.

Compounded topical anesthetics have the ability to penetrate deeper into the tissue, providing more comfort to complete a variety of soft tissue surgical procedures, such as a frenectomy and gingivectomy, and during nonsurgical periodontal therapies. Studies have shown that when administered in the periodontal pocket, compounded topical anesthetics can travel through the periodontal ligament and down to the apices, resulting in anesthesia of the tooth's pulp. This could be particularly beneficial for dental hygienists when performing nonsurgical periodontal therapy of a localized area.

Benzocaine, Butamben, and Tetracaine

One topical anesthetic combination commonly used in the dental office is Cetacaine (Cetylite Industries). It contains the triple-action formula of benzocaine, butamben, and tetracaine hydrochloride. The benzocaine provides a quick onset while the properties of tetracaine allow deeper penetration of the agent, thus contributing to an increase in the duration of action. It is available by prescription only in spray, liquid, and gel forms (Fig. 6.14).

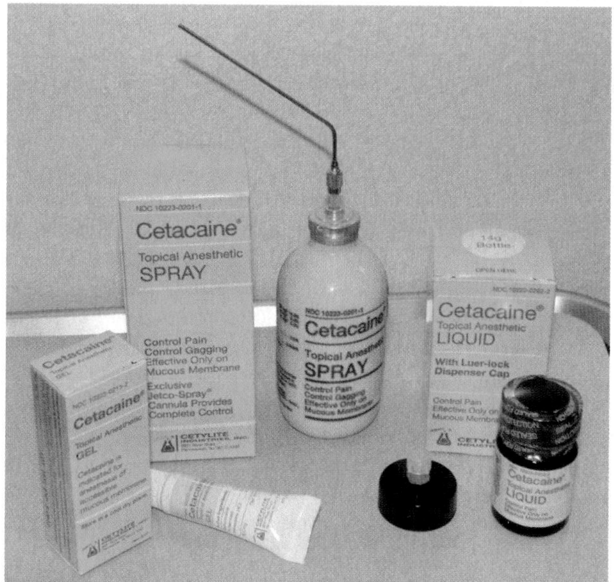

Fig. 6.14 Benzocaine, butamben, and tetracaine products available. Cetacaine (Cetylite Industries).

- **Classification:** Benzocaine, butamben, and tetracaine hydrochloride are all esters.
- **Available concentration:** Triple-active formula of benzocaine 14%, butamben 2%, and tetracaine hydrochloride 2%.
- **Onset of action:** The onset is rapid, or approximately 30 seconds.
- **Duration:** Typically 30 to 60 minutes.
- **Maximum recommended dose:** 200 mg, which is equivalent to 1 spray or ¼ to ½ pearl.
- **Metabolism/excretion:** Hydrolysis via cholinesterase.
- **Pregnancy/lactation:** Animal studies have shown a risk, but controlled human studies have not been conducted, or studies are not available in humans or animals. It is given only after risks to the fetus are considered. Use with caution during lactation.
- **Special considerations:** Tetracaine is highly lipid-soluble, making absorption into local tissues very rapid. It is not suitable for injection.[6]

Eutectic Mixtures

A eutectic mixture is a mixture of two or more elements that, when combined, have a lower melting temperature than the individual components. This increases the concentration and enhances the drug's properties, resulting in a faster, deeper-penetrating, longer-acting agent.

EMLA: 2.5% Lidocaine/2.5% Prilocaine Cream

The first major breakthrough for surface anesthesia on intact skin was a 2.5% lidocaine and 2.5% prilocaine oil-in-water emulsion referred to as an EMLA (eutectic mixture of local anesthetic). EMLA is available commercially as a cream or disc and often requires an occlusive dressing to allow the release of the drug into the epidermal and dermal layers. This FDA-approved combination of lidocaine/prilocaine has been well recognized in the medical community and has been used to provide efficacious topical anesthesia for a variety of medical procedures, such as venipuncture, circumcision, and minor gynecologic procedures.[7,8] When used as directed, the risk of systemic toxicity remains low; however, if not used as prescribed, the systemic absorption of lidocaine and prilocaine can also become a side effect of the desired effect because the amount of drug absorbed depends on the surface area and the duration of the application. Although EMLA is FDA approved, the FDA released a public health advisory in 2007 expressing concerns and warning the public of potential danger associated with the use of the topical anesthetic drug (Box 6.2).

The first documented use of lidocaine/prilocaine in the oral cavity was done in 1985 by Holst and Evers.[9] Since then, many more studies have been conducted that show great promise for the use of EMLA intraorally.[10–15]

Oraqix: 2.5% Lidocaine/2.5% Prilocaine Gel

Though studies do exist on the effectiveness of EMLA cream used intraorally, EMLA cream is not approved by the FDA for intraoral use. However, there is a prescription eutectic mixture available for use in the oral cavity that consists of a 2.5% lidocaine and 2.5% prilocaine gel called Oraqix (Dentsply Sirona, Charlotte, NC). Oraqix is a microemulsion in which the oil phase is a eutectic mixture in a ratio of 1:1 weight. Oraqix can only be administered by means of a special applicator and does not work with standard dental syringes (Fig. 6.15). Although Oraqix remains in liquid form at room temperature in the cartridge, it begins to thicken into a gel upon application into the periodontal pocket and reaching body temperature.

BOX 6.2 U.S. Food and Drug Administration Releases Public Health Advisory to Consumers

Even though topical anesthetics are generally regarded as safe, if used improperly they can produce adverse reactions ranging in severity from mild to life threatening or fatal. In 2007 the U.S. Food and Drug Administration (FDA) released a public health advisory alerting consumers of this potential risk by informing the public of two instances in which women, aged 22 and 25 years old, subsequently died from the toxic effects of the topical anesthetic drug. To lessen the pain of laser hair removal, both women were instructed to apply topical anesthetics to their legs and then wrap their legs in plastic wrap to increase the cream's numbing effect. Both women suffered seizures, fell into comas, and eventually died of the toxic effect of the anesthetic drugs. In 2009 the FDA released the public health advisory again to remind the public of their concerns.

Full version of the public health advisory may be obtained at the FDA website: https://www.fda.gov/Drugs/DrugSafety/PostmarketDrugSafetyInformationforPatientsandProviders.

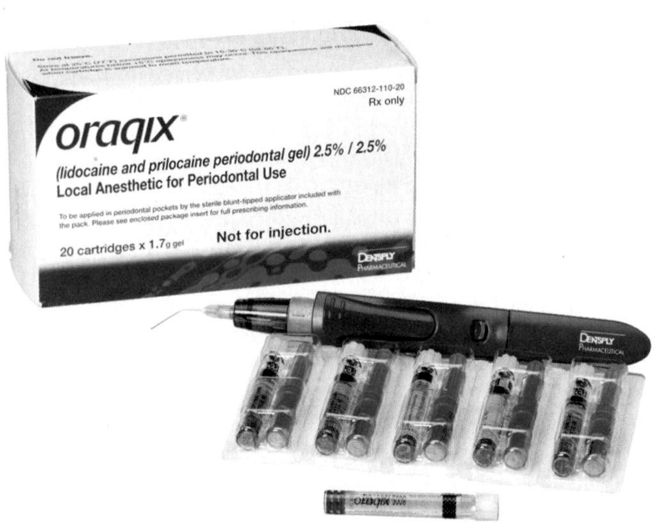

Fig. 6.15 Oraqix delivery system applicator.

Even though pulpal anesthesia is not achieved, Oraqix is indicated to provide comfort to the gingival tissues during prophylaxis, periodontal assessment, and nonsurgical periodontal therapy. Assembly of the dispenser is quick and easy, making it available for use within seconds (Procedure 6.2).

- **Classification:** Lidocaine and prilocaine are amides.
- **Available concentration:** 5% periodontal gel (2.5% lidocaine and 2.5% prilocaine).
- **Onset of action:** The onset occurs by 30 seconds. Longer wait time does not enhance the anesthetic effect.
- **Duration:** Approximately 20 minutes (average, 14–31 minutes).
- **Maximum recommended dose:** Five cartridges at one treatment session.
- **Metabolism/excretion:** It is mainly metabolized in the liver.
- **Pregnancy/lactation:** Animal reproduction studies have not indicated fetal risk, and human studies have not been conducted, or animal studies have shown a risk, but controlled human studies have not. (Previous FDA Category B.)
- **Special considerations:** Do not inject. (Source: Oraqix prescribing information, DentsplySirona Charlotte, NC, https://www.dentsply-sirona.com.)

SPECIAL CONSIDERATIONS

The concentration of topical anesthetic agents is higher than that of their injectable counterparts. This is necessary to facilitate diffusion of the agent through the mucous membranes. In addition, topical anesthetics do not contain a vasoconstrictor. With these higher concentrations and the lack of vasoconstriction abilities, the risk of local and systemic absorption increases, thus increasing the risk of toxicity (see Chapter 4).

High plasma concentrations of topical anesthetics can produce adverse effects and results when patients are exposed to excessive amounts of the drugs. Children, the elderly, and medically compromised individuals are more susceptible to the adverse reactions of topical anesthetics. Methemoglobinemia, a rare but serious condition, can occur, resulting in a decrease in the amount of oxygen being carried through the bloodstream. Signs and symptoms of methemoglobinemia include pale, gray, or blue-colored skin, lips, and/or nailbeds; fatigue; shortness of breath; headache; and lightheadedness. These signs and symptoms can occur within minutes to hours after topical benzocaine administration. Most of the cases reported are in children under 2 years of age, prompting the FDA to release a safety announcement in 2011 regarding over-the-counter benzocaine teething preparations and, more recently, another in 2014 regarding prescription viscous lidocaine use for soothing gums in children (Box 6.3). Adult patients with breathing problems such as asthma, emphysema, and chronic obstructive lung disease (COPD), those with heart disease, and smokers are also at a greater risk for complications related to methemoglobinemia.

Possible localized adverse effects include irritation, stinging or burning at the site of application, sloughing, tissue discoloration, and temporary alteration in taste perception. The most prominent of the systemic effects of topical anesthetics are in the central nervous system and cardiovascular system. Excitatory effects of the central nervous system are often displayed at the initial signs and symptoms of overdose. Some of these signs and symptoms include dizziness, visual disturbances, tinnitus, disorientation, unusual nervousness or apprehension, and localized involuntary muscular activity. The excitatory manifestations may be very brief or not occur at all, in which case the first manifestation would be a depressant response, such as slurred speech, drowsiness, and respiratory impairment. Toxic overdoses result in seizures, unconsciousness, and respiratory arrest. In the cardiovascular system, patients may experience bradycardia and hypotension, leading to rare cases of cardiac arrest (see Chapter 17).

Allergic reactions associated with topical anesthetics are rare. Benzocaine and tetracaine are both esters, which increases the potential for an allergic reaction; however the risks are still low. Anaphylaxis is very rare with topical anesthetics. Any reaction would likely be delayed and not present itself until after the patient has left the dental office. Those mild allergic reactions can include swelling, raised welts on the skin, itching, or burning. Some allergic reactions occur up to 2 days after the anesthetic is given.

Although these adverse reactions are rare, the potential does exist. It is important to take all precautions necessary to minimize or avoid or prevent them (Box 6.4).

PROCEDURE 6.2 **Preparing the Dispenser for the Administration of Oraqix**

Step 1 Parts of the applicator include the body (*right*) and the tip (*left*). The blunt-tip applicator and cartridge of Oraqix come packaged together in a blister pack.

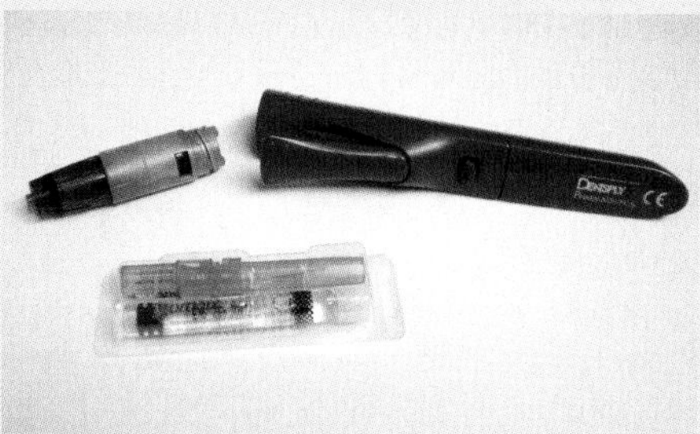

Step 2 Remove blunt-tip applicator and cartridge of Oraqix from the blister pack.

Step 3 Twist to break the seal of blunt-tip applicator cap and attach it into the tip of the Oraqix dispenser. Twist to lock in place.

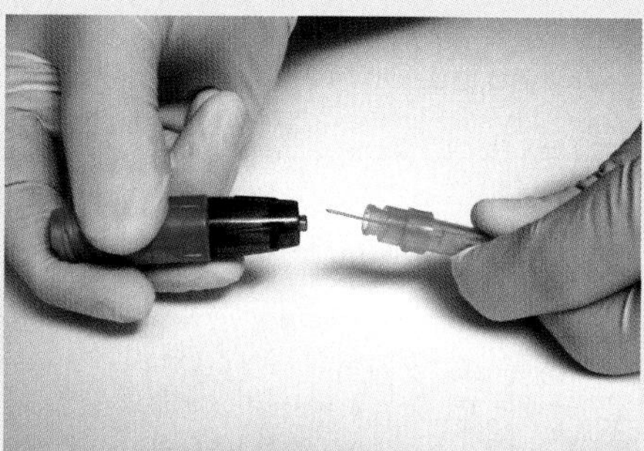

Step 4 With thumb, press the mechanism-reset button down toward the back end of the body.

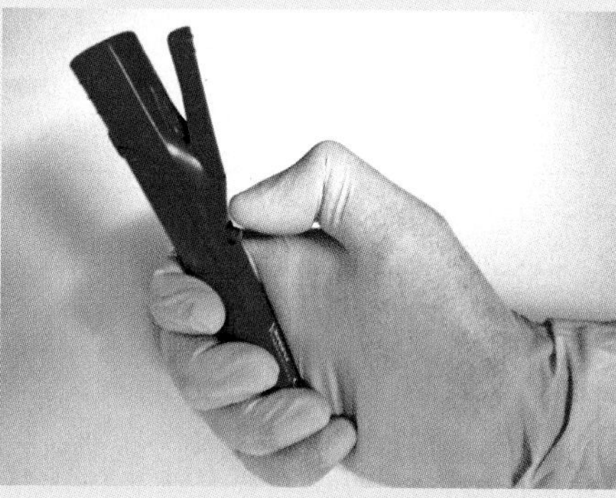

Step 5 Load the Oraqix cartridge into the body of the dispenser. The side with the rubber stopper should be placed into the body of the dispenser.

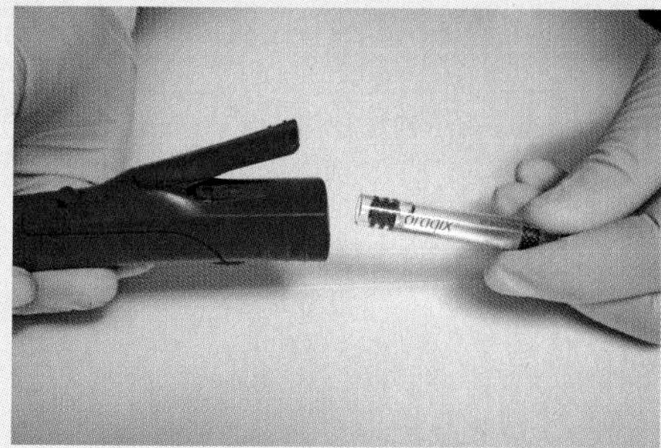

Step 6 Join together the tip and the body of the dispenser. Twist and lock in place.

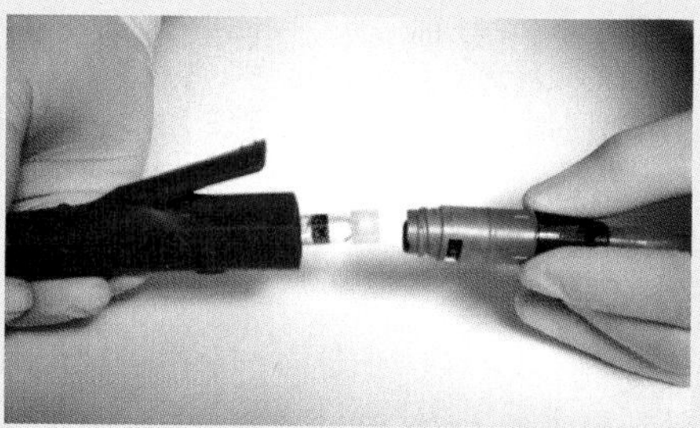

Step 7 Remove applicator cap. Use the cap to bend the applicator tip. Use a double-bend technique if a bend greater than 45 degrees is desired.

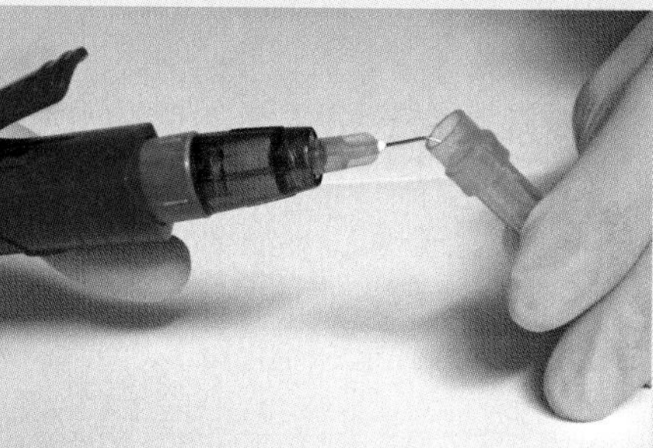

Step 8 Using a modified pen grasp, begin dispensing Oraqix by pressing down on the paddle.

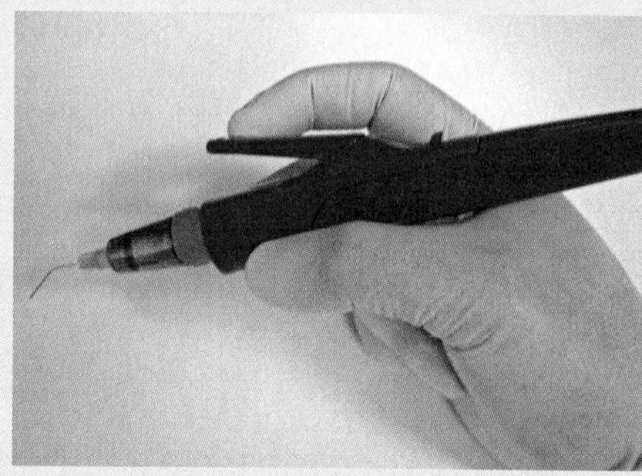

Step 9 Apply Oraqix in two steps: (A) first to the gingival margin around the selected teeth and (B) then after 30 seconds, to the base of the periodontal pockets. Wait 30 seconds to begin procedure.

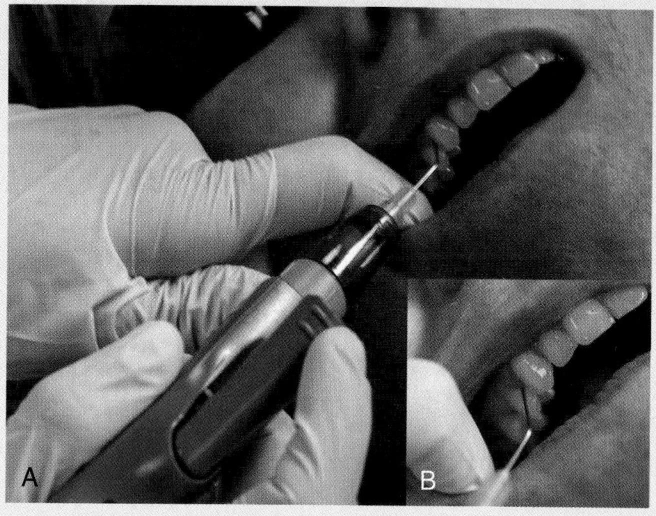

Adapted and summarized from https://www.dentsplysirona.com. Full detailed dispenser directions available at https://www.dentsplysirona.com/content/dam/dentsply/pim/manufacturer/Preventive/Anesthesia/Non_Injectable_Anesthesia/Oraqix_lidocaine_and_prilocaine_periodontal_gel/PHA_66400/OraqixDispenser-DFU_PI_Art4.pdf.

BOX 6.3 U.S. Food and Drug Administration Safety Announcements Regarding the Use of Teething Agents in Children

In 2018, the U.S. Food and Drug Administration (FDA) released a safety announcement recommending that people discontinue the use of over-the-counter benzocaine gels and liquids in children under the age of 2 years old. The FDA stated that the risks associated with benzocaine-induced methemoglobinemia in this population are greater than the benefits when used to treat sore gums from teething. Manufacturers have been urged to cease marketing of these over-the-counter products for infants and children less than 2 years and to add a warning to the label regarding methemoglobinemia. The FDA encourages parents/caregivers to follow the recommendations of the American Academy of Pediatrics for pain associated with teething and simply rub or massage a child's gums and/or give the child a chilled (not frozen) teething ring. This recommendation comes after years of concerns that prompted two previously released safety statements 2014 and 2011.

The full version can be accessed at FDA website using the following links:
https://www.fda.gov/drugs/drug-safety-and-availability/risk-serious-and-potentially-fatal-blood-disorder-prompts-fda-action-oral-over-counter-benzocaine
https://www.fda.gov/Drugs/DrugSafety/ucm402240.htm
https://www.fda.gov/Drugs/DrugSafety/ucm250024.htm

BOX 6.4 How to Avoid Toxic Reactions From Topical Anesthesia

1. Know the relative *toxicity* of the drug being used.
2. Know the *concentration* of the drug being used.
3. Use the *smallest* volume.
4. Use the *lowest* concentration.
5. Use the *least toxic* drug to satisfy clinical requirements.
6. Limit the *area of application* (avoid sprays).

From Haveles EB: *Applied pharmacology for the dental hygienist*, ed 8, St Louis, 2020, Mosby.

DENTAL HYGIENE CONSIDERATIONS

- Topical anesthesia is an important component of the local anesthesia armamentarium and is used routinely in dentistry to provide pain control before conventional local anesthetic injections.
- Topical anesthesia comes in a variety of preparations including gels, ointments, creams, liquids, sprays, and lozenges.
- Topical anesthesia is available as a prescription or over the counter with concentrations ranging from 0.2% to 20%.
- Be aware that products available over the counter can have concentrations just as high as those used professionally in the dental office.
- Only a minimal amount of topical anesthesia is needed to obtain the desired effect. Placing the topical anesthesia at a site for 1–2 minutes will provide anesthesia 2–3 mm into the tissue or mucosa.
- Even though adverse and allergic reactions are rarely noted with use of topical anesthetics, a thorough review of the patient's medical history is always necessary before their application.
- With the many varieties of topical anesthesia available, it is important to select a product that is safe and will provide the most benefit for the patient.

CASE STUDY 6.1 A Patient Who Is Fearful of Needles

Age: 69 years
Blood pressure: 140/90

A patient presents to your office to begin treatment. Upon reviewing her medical history, you discover she has a complex medical history. You determine that her American Society of Anesthesiologists (ASA) physical status is a class III, but there are no immediate contraindications for treatment today.

She is to have four quadrants of nonsurgical periodontal therapy to remove moderate subgingival and supragingival calculus and to treat her severe inflammation. She expresses to you a great fear of needles. She asks if you can use "the gel on a cotton swab" like her sister had done at her office in Colorado. You agree and begin applying 20% benzocaine gel on the upper right quadrant. Partially through the procedure she winces and asks you to add more because she is still having some discomfort. You add more benzocaine and continue to work quadrant by quadrant. As you begin the final quadrant, you notice that the patient is becoming restless and appears strangely apprehensive. She tells you she hears ringing in her ears and you notice that her left cheek begins to twitch. You ask how she is feeling, and she responds, "I feel very sleepy." Her speech is noticeably slurred. You immediately stop and assess the patient more thoroughly.

Critical Thinking Questions

- What should you suspect is happening with the patient as you are beginning the final quadrant?
- If no anesthesia was injected, how could this happen?
- What are some other treatment options that should have been offered to this patient?

CHAPTER REVIEW QUESTIONS

1. Which of the following topical anesthetics is classified as an amide?
   A. Benzocaine
   B. Lidocaine
   C. Tetracaine
   D. Dyclonine

2. Benzocaine is available in all of the following preparations EXCEPT one. Which one is the EXCEPTION?
   A. Cream
   B. Gel
   C. Spray
   D. Patch
   E. Injectable

3. All of the following statements are true EXCEPT one. Which one is the EXCEPTION?
   A. Allergic reactions associated with topical anesthetics are rare.
   B. Topical anesthetics are made available over the counter.
   C. The more topical placed at the site of needle penetration, the better.
   D. Tetracaine hydrochloride is considered the most potent of the topical anesthetics.
4. Which of the following topical anesthetics is generally safe during pregnancy?
   A. Tetracaine hydrochloride
   B. Benzocaine
   C. Lidocaine
   D. Dyclonine hydrochloride
5. Which of the following would be an indication for use of a topical anesthetic?
   A. To minimize patients' gag reflexes
   B. To numb patients' tongue so they will stop talking so much
   C. To achieve pulpal anesthesia
   D. To achieve anesthesia of the bone
6. All of the following are true regarding maximum recommended doses for topical anesthesia EXCEPT one. Which one is the EXCEPTION?
   A. It is difficult to monitor exact doses being administered.
   B. Patches are a good way to monitor doses.
   C. Maximum recommended dose does not exist for all topical anesthetics.
   D. Exact doses can be measured using a cotton-tip applicator.
7. Concentrations available in over-the-counter products can be as high as those administered professionally in the dental office.
   A. True
   B. False
8. All of the following topical anesthetics require a prescription EXCEPT one. Which one is the EXCEPTION?
   A. EMLA
   B. Cetacaine
   C. Oraqix
   D. Benzocaine
9. All of the following are considered ideal properties of a topical anesthetic EXCEPT one. Which one is the EXCEPTION?
   A. It should produce no damage to the tissue.
   B. It should have an acceptable taste.
   C. It should not induce systemic toxicity.
   D. It should be allergenic.
10. Which method of delivery is recommended to decrease the risk of methemoglobinemia?
    A. Unmetered spray
    B. Metered spray
    C. Unmetered spray with disposable nozzle
    D. Metered spray with disposable nozzle
11. Topical anesthetics generally penetrate _____ into the tissue.
    A. 1 to 2 mm
    B. 2 to 3 mm
    C. 3 to 4 mm
    D. 5 to 6 mm
12. Which of the following local anesthetic agents is found in Oraqix?
    A. Mepivacaine
    B. Prilocaine
    C. Procaine
    D. Benzocaine
    E. Articaine
13. The concentrations of topical anesthetics are greater than those of their injectable counterparts. Topical anesthetics do not contain vasoconstrictors.
    A. Both statements are correct.
    B. Both statements are NOT correct.
    C. The first statement is correct; the second statement is NOT correct.
    D. The first statement is NOT correct; the second statement is correct.
14. All of the following describes advantages of single unit–dose applications of topical anesthetics EXCEPT one. Which one is the EXCEPTION?
    A. It prevents cross-contamination.
    B. Doses administered can be monitored.
    C. It is less messy.
    D. It requires less administration time.
15. EMLA is approved by the U.S. Food and Drug Administration for use on which of the following areas?
    A. Intact skin
    B. Mucous membranes
    C. Hard palate
    D. Soft palate
16. Pulpal anesthesia can be achieved using 2.5% lidocaine and 2.5% prilocaine gel mixture.
    A. True
    B. False
17. Which of the following topical anesthetic agents is considered a ketone?
    A. Benzocaine
    B. Dyclonine hydrochloride
    C. Lidocaine
    D. A and B
18. If plasma concentrations in the body become too high, the most prominent systemic effect will occur in which of the following systems?
    A. Respiratory system
    B. Cardiovascular system
    C. Central nervous system
    D. B and C
19. Allergic reactions associated with topical anesthetics are rare. It is not necessary to review a patient's medical history before applying a topical anesthetic agent.
    A. Both statements are correct.
    B. Both statements are NOT correct.
    C. The first statement is correct; the second statement is NOT correct.
    D. The first statement is NOT correct; the second statement is correct.
20. All of the following are possible localized adverse reactions associated with topical anesthesia EXCEPT one. Which one is the EXCEPTION?
    A. Burning or stinging
    B. Sloughing
    C. Tissue discoloration
    D. Increased heart rate

REFERENCES

1. Malamed S. *Handbook of local anesthesia.* ed 7. St Louis: Elsevier; 2020.
2. Yagiela JA. Injectable and topical local anesthetics. *American Dental Association guide to dental therapeutics.* Chicago: Donnelley & Sons; 2000:1–16.
3. SYNERA: complete prescribing information. Salt Lake City: ZARS Pharma; 2018. https://www.synera.com.
4. LIDODERM: *Complete Prescribing Information.* Chadds Ford: Endo Pharmaceuticals; 2018. https://www.endo.com/endopharma/our-products.
5. Yagiela JA. Injectable and topical local anesthetics. In: Ciancio SG, ed. *American Dental Association guide to dental therapeutics.* ed 3. ADA Publishing: Chicago; 2003.
6. Cetacaine product information available from Cetylite Industries, Pennsauken, NJ; 2017. https://www.cetylite.com/dental/topical-anesthetics.
7. Zilbert A. Topical anesthesia for minor gynecological procedures: a review. *Obstet Gynecol Surv.* 2002;57:171–177.
8. Mansell-Gregory M, Romanowski B. Randomised double trial of EMLA for the control of pain related to cryotherapy in the treatment of genital HPV lesions. *Sex Transm Infect.* 1998;74(4):274–275.
9. Holst A, Evers H. Experimental studies of new topical anaesthetics on the oral mucosa. *Swed Dent J.* 1985;9:185–191.
10. Daneshkazemi A, Abrisham SM, Daneshkazemi P, Davoudi A. The efficacy of eutectic mixture of local anesthetics as a topical anesthetic agent used for dental procedures: a brief review. *Anesth Essays Res.* 2016;10(3):383–387.
11. Nayak R, Sudah P. Evaluation of three topical anaesthetic agents against pain: a clinical study. *Ind J Dent Res.* 2006;17(4):155–160.
12. Abu M, Anderson L. Comparison of topical anesthetics (EMLA/Oraqix vs. benzocaine) on pain experienced during palatal needle injection. *Oral Surg Oral Med Oral Path Oral Radiol Endod.* 2007;103:16–20.
13. Meechan JG. The use of EMLA for an intraoral soft tissue biopsy in a needle phobic: a case report. *Anesth Prog.* 2001;48:32–42.
14. Vickers ER, Punnia-Moorthy A. A clinical evaluation of three topical anaesthetic agents. *Aust Dent J.* 1992;37:266–270.
15. Svensson P, Petersen JK. Anesthetic effect of EMLA occluded with Orahesive oral bandages on oral mucosa. A placebo-controlled study. *Anesth Progr.* 1992;39:79–82.

ADDITIONAL RESOURCES

Haveles EB. *Applied pharmacology for the dental hygienist.* ed 8. St Louis: Elsevier; 2020.

Kundu S, Achar S. Principles of office anesthesia: part II. Topical anesthesia. *Am Fam Physician.* 2002;66(1):99–102.

Meechan JG. Effective topical anesthetic agents and techniques. *Dent Clin North Am.* 2002;46:759–766.

Meechan JG. Intra-oral topical anaesthetics: a review. *J Dent.* 2000;28:3–14.

Mosby's dental drug reference. ed 11. St Louis: Mosby; 2013.

Oraqix. Product information available from DentsplySirona, Charlotte, NC. https://www.dentsplysirona.com.

Overman P. Controlling the pain. *Dimens Dent Hyg.* 2004;2(11):10–14.

Tetzlaff JE. *Clinical pharmacology of local anesthetics.* Woburn, MA: Butterworth-Heinemann; 2020.

Yagiela JA. Safely easing the pain for your patients. *Dimens Dent Hyg.* 2005;3(5):20.

Yagiela JA. *Pharmacology and therapeutics for dentistry.* ed 6. St Louis: Mosby; 2010.

PART 3

Patient Assessment

CHAPTER 7 Preanesthetic Assessment, 94

APPENDIX 7.1 Sample Medical History Form in English/Spanish, 111

CHAPTER 8 Determining Drug Doses, 114

APPENDIX 8.1 Summary of Local Anesthetic Agents and Vasoconstrictors, 126

APPENDIX 8.2 Comparison of Previous and Current Maximum Recommended Doses of Anesthetic Drugs per Appointment for Healthy Patients, 127

APPENDIX 8.3 Dosing Information for Regional Local Anesthesia Board Examinations Requiring Calculations Based on 1.7 mL of Solution, 128

7

Preanesthetic Assessment

Demetra Daskalos Logothetis, RDH, MS

LEARNING OBJECTIVES

1. Discuss the importance of obtaining a patient's medical history, dental history, and dialogue history.
2. Discuss the role of emotional status, blood pressure, pulse, respiration, and weight in selection/utilization of local anesthetics.
3. Describe dental fear and how dental professionals deal with patient fears through psychological, physical, and chemical parameters.
4. Determine the relative risk presented by a patient prior to administering local anesthesia by interpretation of the health history.
5. Differentiate between relative and absolute contraindications.
6. Describe the drug-to-drug interactions that may occur between the vasoconstrictor and other drugs.
7. Describe vasoconstrictor and systemic disease interactions and summarize vasoconstrictor contraindications.
8. List the concerns for patients with cardiovascular disease, hyperthyroidism, asthma, sickle cell anemia, and allergies when selecting local anesthetics and scheduling treatment.
9. Summarize the ester derivative local anesthetic interactions.
10. Discuss the importance of amide local anesthetic drug–drug interactions.
11. List the concerns about other amide local anesthetic interactions for patients with malignant hyperthermia, methemoglobinemia, liver disease, kidney disease, pregnancy, and bleeding disorders.

INTRODUCTION

To meet the human need for safety, a thorough medical history evaluation using appropriate dental and medical consultations of the patient's current health status is an essential requirement before providing dental hygiene care. The administration of local anesthetic and vasoconstricting agents provides an additional rationale for a thorough health history and health status review. This chapter will focus on further evaluating the patient's medical and psychological status to determine the appropriateness of administering local anesthetic and vasoconstrictor agents. This important preanesthetic information will assist the dental hygienist in choosing the appropriate technique, agent, and dosage to prevent or minimize local anesthetic complications or emergencies.[1] Most healthy patients can tolerate the standard recommended doses of local anesthetics without any adverse reactions. Other patients, including medically compromised patients, may also safely receive local anesthetics if all precautions are recognized and appropriate drug modifications are rendered. These modifications to treatment are categorized into relative contraindications and absolute contraindications (see Contraindications to Local Anesthetics).

All drugs exert their actions on multiple body systems; local anesthetics and vasoconstrictors are no exception. Local anesthetics exert their actions by depressing excitable membranes of the central nervous system (CNS) and cardiovascular system (CVS). These actions are dependent on the amount of local anesthetic agent in the systemic circulation and are influenced by the administration technique (aspirating to prevent intravenous [IV] injection) and successful ability of the body to metabolize the drug in the liver (for most amides) and the plasma (for esters and articaine), as well as the ability of the kidneys to excrete any unmetabolized drug.[2] Other commonly observed responses that result from the administration of local anesthetics are due to psychological responses and include the commonly observed reactions of syncope, or hyperventilation, and other less common reactions such as tonic-clonic convulsions, bronchospasm, and angina pectoris.[2]

The dental hygienist must evaluate, through the health history, the patient's physical and psychological ability to tolerate the administration of a local anesthetic or vasoconstrictor, a history of anesthetic hypersensitivity, and current medications that may have an interaction with the anesthetic drug being administered. This preanesthetic evaluation should be determined using a team approach of consultation with the dentist, patient's physician, and any specialists involved in the patient's medical care. For dental hygienists working in alternative settings such as nursing homes, hospitals, public health programs, collaborative dental hygiene practices, or other settings without the physical presence of a dentist, it is of the utmost importance to use a multidisciplinary approach to patient evaluation. The collection of preanesthetic data guides the dental hygienist in determining the following:

- Appropriateness of administering a local anesthetic or vasoconstrictor
- Need for a medical consultation
- Need for modification of the dental hygiene care plan
- Type of anesthetic most appropriate for the patient's treatment
- Contraindications to any of the medications to be employed

The preanesthetic evaluation should include a complete medical/dental history, a dialogue history, and a physical and psychological examination.

MEDICAL, DENTAL, AND DIALOGUE HISTORY

The most common and efficient method of obtaining a medical/dental history in the dental office is by a printed questionnaire filled out by the patient followed by a dialogue history, allowing the dental hygienist to follow up on questions to gain further information. The health history questionnaire constitutes a legal document. In the case of a minor, this form must be completed by the parent or legal guardian. These medical history forms should be updated at each patient visit. Information gleaned from the patient's medical history should include data regarding current and past medical and dental conditions; current and past medications including over-the-counter drugs, herbs, and supplements; any adverse reactions to medications including local anesthetic agents; and any problems with past dental experiences.

Medications currently being taken by the patient are in their system when a local anesthetic is administered. This is referred to as concomitant: two or more drugs given at the same time or in the same day.[3] Concomitant drug administration can alter the efficiency and safety of the local anesthetic by decreasing the efficiency of its metabolism and excretion. This may affect the type of anesthetic selected and its safe dosage level. The dental hygienist should use a current *Physicians' Desk Reference (PDR)* or other drug references to research all drugs the patient is currently taking and determine the safest anesthetic drug selection and the safest dosage a patient can tolerate.

The dialogue history is invaluable in gaining more information regarding the patient's medical status, as well as determining the patient's personal fears associated with local anesthetic administration. In addition, the dialogue history provides an opportunity for the dental hygienist to assess the patient's individual response to local anesthetic agents categorized as *normal responders, hyperresponders,* or *hyporesponders.* (See Chapter 5.)

Many medical history forms are available, including one from the American Dental Association (https://www.ada.org). The content details of most medical history forms are essentially similar and should be modified to meet the specific needs of individual dental practices. Appendix 7.1 is an example of a medical history form in English and in Spanish. Other multilingual medical history forms are available at https://www.metdental.com. Table 7.1 explains each medical history question and its implications on the administration of local anesthesia.

TABLE 7.1 Medical History Questions Explained

Medical History Question	Local Anesthetic Implications
Are you in good health?	Treatment modifications may be considered for patients who reveal a significant disability or medical or psychological condition. Significant medical conditions or medications the patient is taking may contraindicate or limit the use of a local anesthetic or vasoconstrictor. Patients with special needs and children should not receive bupivacaine because of the possibility of self-mutilation.
Are you currently under the care of a physician?	Dental hygiene care modifications should be considered for a patient with a medically compromising condition. Determine whether the patient is taking any medications to manage the problem. Significant medical conditions or medications the patient is taking may contraindicate or limit the use of a local anesthetic or vasoconstrictor. Medical consultation with the patient's general physician or specialist may be indicated before anesthetic selection and treatment.
Has there been any change in your general health within the past year?	A recent change may indicate needed treatment modifications that may influence anesthetic selection.
Have you had any serious illness or operation or been hospitalized in the past 5 years?	Identify local anesthesia precautions that may be needed if there is a prior history of serious illness. Dental hygiene treatment and the use of local anesthetics with vasoconstrictors may need to be postponed if the patient has had surgery within 6 months. Existing or chronic medical conditions may indicate the need for modifications in care. Stress reduction protocols implemented for patients with medical conditions that could be exacerbated by stress/anxiety from the administration of local anesthetics and dental hygiene care.
Have you had any problems with or during dental treatment?	Complications often are a source of patient dissatisfaction and fear; if possible, avoid repeating the complication. Stress reduction for the anxious patient. Selection of local anesthetic of adequate duration for effective postoperative pain control.
Are you allergic or had any reaction to any medications (including local anesthetics)?	ADRs are common. Most ADRs are labeled by patients as an allergic reaction and, on occasion, by the health care provider. However, despite the frequency of reported allergic reactions, true documented allergic drug reactions to local anesthetics are rare and essentially nonexistent. Patients may report an allergy to "epinephrine" or "adrenaline." Most of these reports are simply an exaggerated "fight-or-flight" response to the release of endogenous catecholamines from the act of receiving the local anesthetic injection. (See Chapter 4.) Evaluate further to determine whether a true allergy exists. (See Chapter 17.) Patient should be referred to an allergist if there is still concern regarding a local anesthetic allergy or if, after questioning the patient, the dental hygienist is unsure if the patient has a true allergy to local anesthetics. If the patient has a true allergy to sulfites, vasoconstrictors should be avoided.
Do you have any other allergies, such as metals, latex, food, or pollen?	Patient has an increased risk for a latex allergy from the rubber stopper and diaphragm of the glass cartridge. However, no documented allergies to latex from the anesthetic cartridge have been reported. Patients who have many allergies to foods, metals, or pollen may be more susceptible to allergic reactions to sulfites or ester topical anesthetics. Food allergies are seen in 8% of children and 5% of adults.[9] The presence of an allergy alone represents an ASA class II risk.[9]

(Continued)

TABLE 7.1 Medical History Questions Explained (*Cont.*)

Medical History Question	Local Anesthetic Implications
Do you have any artificial heart valves or shunts?	The primary concern is to determine whether antibiotic prophylaxis is required. Consultation with the patient's physician (e.g., the cardiologist) is appropriate prior to treatment. The administration of local anesthetics does not require antibiotic prophylaxis, except for the PDL injection. However, nonsurgical periodontal treatment performed by the dental hygienist requires antibiotic prophylaxis for the susceptible patient. Nature of dental treatment will dictate the need for antibiotic prophylaxis. Clinicians should remain current in the American Dental Association, American Academy of Orthopaedic Surgeons, and the American Heart Association premedication guidelines. Patients with prosthetic heart valves usually represent an ASA class II or III risk.[9]
Do you have cardiovascular disease, such as heart trouble, heart attack, angina, high blood pressure, or hardening of the arteries?	**Heart attack (myocardial infarction):** Delay treatment for 6 months, as these patients are considered an ASA IV risk; after 6 months, patients are considered to be an ASA III risk unless there is little or no residual damage to the myocardium, then the patient is considered an ASA class II risk: Decrease the amount of epinephrine to 0.04 mg per appointment and levonordefrin to 0.2 mg per appointment. (See dosage guidelines for vasoconstrictors in Chapter 8.)
	Heart failure: Assess degree of heart failure (weakness of the "pump"). Specific treatment modifications are warranted for patients with CHF or dyspnea (labored breathing) at rest. Presence of dyspnea at rest represents an ASA IV risk. The clinician should assess the need for supplemental O_2 during treatment. Effective pain control for heart failure patients who are ASA II and ASA III is essential to prevent increase in cardiac workload; therefore local anesthetics with vasoconstrictors are indicated to provide adequate pain control duration using the cardiac dose. (See dosage guidelines for vasoconstrictors in Chapter 8.)
	Angina: Angina is the sensation of pain that is an aching, heavy, squeezing pressure in the chest brought on by exertion and alleviated by rest, resulting from temporary ischemia of the myocardium. Unstable angina: ASA IV, increased risk of severe angina attack. Dental hygiene treatment should be postponed until condition is under control. Absolute contraindication to vasoconstrictors until condition is under control. Stable angina: ASA III—adequate pain control will decrease the risk of angina attack caused by apprehension and nervousness. Vasoconstrictors can be administered, but at a decreased dose of 0.04 mg per appointment for epinephrine and 0.2 mg for levonordefrin.
	High blood pressure: Elevated BP is common in the dental environment and caused by the added stress associated with a visit to the dental office. It is important to determine whether the patient is taking medications to control high BP and any possible interactions to drugs that might be used during the dental procedure. Uncontrolled high blood pressure: Dental hygiene treatment should be postponed until blood pressure is under control; absolute contraindication to vasoconstrictors until blood pressure is under control. Controlled blood pressure with beta blockers: This indicates a relative contraindication to vasoconstrictors and to amide local anesthetics metabolized in the liver. Monitor BP after initial local anesthetic injection and posttreatment for signs of increased BP.
Have you ever had a stroke?	CVA "stroke": This is caused by sudden interruption of oxygenated blood to the brain. Focal necrosis of the brain tissue occurs from ischemia. Delay treatment for 6 months as the patient is an ASA class IV risk. After 6 months the patient is an ASA class III risk, and effective pain control is essential with local anesthesia and vasoconstrictors. Decrease the amount of vasoconstrictors to 0.04 mg per appointment for epinephrine and 0.2 mg for levonordefrin. Avoid intravascular injections of vasoconstrictors.
Have you taken cortisone in the past 2 years?	Identify patients at risk for adrenal insufficiency. Use a stress reduction protocol and consider nitrous oxide or IV sedation to further reduce stress.
Were you born with any heart problems?	Usually patients can safely receive dental care with the use of local anesthetics and vasoconstrictors. Medical consultation as needed.
Do you have sinus trouble, asthma, hay fever, or skin rashes?	**Asthma:** This is chronic inflammatory disease of the airways resulting in episodes of dyspnea, coughing, and wheezing commonly precipitated by stress. Well-controlled asthmatic patients represent an ASA II risk, and well-controlled but stress-induced asthmatic patients represent an ASA III risk. Adequate pain control is essential to not precipitate attack. Stress reduction protocol. Sodium bisulfite preservative for vasoconstrictors may cause respiratory reactions in asthmatics (predominantly steroid-dependent asthmatics). (See Chapter 4).
Do you have fainting spells, seizures, epilepsy, or convulsions?	**Vasodepressor Syncope:** Vasodepressor syncope is the most common medical emergency in the dental office and more likely to occur during the administration of local anesthesia, resulting from anxiety during injection. Prior recognition of dental anxiety and using a stress reduction protocol can result in prevention of the syncopal episode.

TABLE 7.1 Medical History Questions Explained (*Cont.*)

Medical History Question	Local Anesthetic Implications
	Epilepsy: Adequate pain control is important to not precipitate seizures in epileptic patients. Local anesthetics are sensitive to CNS depressants; avoid higher doses of local anesthetic drugs when a patient is taking anticonvulsants such as phenytoin (Dilantin). Stress reduction protocol. Epileptic patients with well-controlled seizures (occur infrequently) are ASA class II risk; those with more frequent episodes of seizures are ASA class III or IV risk. Local anesthetic overdose symptoms manifest as tonic-clonic seizure activity (see Chapter 17).
Do you have diabetes?	Epinephrine is associated with the inhibition of peripheral glucose uptake by the tissues and opposes the action of insulin. Concentrations of epinephrine used in dentistry do not significantly raise the glucose blood levels. **Uncontrolled "brittle" diabetes** (ASA class IV): Dental hygiene treatment should be postponed until condition is under control. Use epinephrine with caution. **Controlled diabetes:** Blood glucose levels should be evaluated before dental hygiene treatment. Morning appointments after a meal. Vasoconstrictors can be administered.
Do you have hepatitis, yellow jaundice, cirrhosis, or liver disease?	Decreased liver function increases the half-life of the amides metabolized in the liver, increasing risk of overdose. Limit the dose of amides metabolized in the liver. Articaine may be a safer choice because it is predominantly metabolized in the blood.
Do you have AIDS or HIV infection?	Universal precautions should be used on all patients. Proper care and handling of the local anesthetic handpiece and disposal of contaminated needles in all situations should be implemented to avoid accidental needlestick injury. Follow postexposure protocols (Chapter 18).
Do you have thyroid problems (goiter)?	Hyperthyroid patients have an increased sensitivity to epinephrine. **Uncontrolled hyperthyroidism:** Postpone dental hygiene treatment until condition is under control. Absolute contraindication to vasoconstrictors. **Controlled hyperthyroidism:** Vasoconstrictors can be administered but use minimal effective dose not to exceed 0.04 mg per appointment for epinephrine and 0.2 mg per appointment for levonordefrin. **Pheochromocytoma** (catecholamine-producing tumor): Postpone dental hygiene treatment until condition is under control. Absolute contraindication to vasoconstrictors.
Do you have respiratory problems, emphysema, or bronchitis?	Emphysema is a form of COPD. Supplemental O_2 is recommended for patients with emphysema. Prilocaine is metabolized in the lungs and liver; limit the dose. Stress reduction protocol.
Have you ever had a joint replacement?	The administration of local anesthetics does not require antibiotic prophylaxis, except for the PDL injection. However, nonsurgical periodontal treatment performed by the dental hygienist may require antibiotic prophylaxis. Clinicians should remain current in the American Dental Association and the American Academy of Orthopaedic Surgeons premedication guidelines to determine the need for antibiotic prophylaxis.
Have you ever had kidney trouble or dialysis treatment?	Usual doses do not pose an increased risk. Significant renal disease: medical consultation needed. Limiting the amount of anesthetic is recommended depending on severity.
Do you have anemia or blood disorders?	Avoid block injections for clotting disorders. **Methemoglobinemia:** Substitute other amides for prilocaine and topical lidocaine for topical benzocaine or use minimal effective dose of prilocaine. **Atypical plasma cholinesterase**: Substitute ester topical anesthetics with lidocaine. **Sickle cell anemia:** A hereditary blood disorder characterized by an abnormality in the oxygen-carrying hemoglobin molecule in red blood cells. For routine dental care, appointments should be short (to reduce stress). Physician consultation is recommended to determine cardiac status. No dental treatment or local anesthesia should be administered during a crisis. The use of local anesthesia is acceptable. However, congenital or idiopathic methemoglobinemia represents a relative contraindication to prilocaine. The inclusion of small amounts of epinephrine should be limited to treatment where profound anesthesia is warranted and to obtain hemostasis.[4]
Have you been diagnosed with alcoholism?	Decreased liver function increases the half-life of the amides metabolized in the liver, increasing risk of overdose. Limit the dose of amides metabolized in the liver. Articaine may be a safer choice because it is predominantly metabolized in the blood.
Do you use recreational drugs?	Vasoconstrictors administered the same day that a patient has used cocaine or methamphetamine can be life-threatening.

(*Continued*)

TABLE 7.1 Medical History Questions Explained (*Cont.*)

Medical History Question	Local Anesthetic Implications
Are you pregnant or nursing a baby?	Elective dental hygiene care with anesthesia can be safely administered in any trimester, in consultation with the patient's physician. Conservative approach: Avoid elective treatment with anesthesia until the second trimester. Choose a safe local anesthetic. Choose a safe anesthetic for lactation.
Are you taking any medications, including any nonprescription medications or natural supplements?	Decrease amount of amide local anesthetic for patients taking cimetidine, beta blockers, and CNS depressants. No topical esters for patients taking sulfonamides and cholinesterase inhibitors. Decrease the amount of epinephrine per appointment for patients taking tricyclic antidepressants, beta blockers, phenothiazides, large doses of thyroid hormones. Use epinephrine in consultation with patient's physician for patients taking digitalis glycosides. Avoid levonordefrin for patients taking tricyclic antidepressants.

AIDS, Acquired immune deficiency syndrome; *ADRs,* adverse drug reactions; *ASA,* American Society of Anesthesiologists; *BP,* blood pressure; *CHF,* congestive heart failure; *CNS,* central nervous system; *COPD,* chronic obstructive pulmonary disease; *CVA,* cerebrovascular accident; *HIV,* human immunodeficiency virus; *IV,* intravenous; *PDL,* periodontal ligament.

PHYSICAL EXAMINATION

Visual Examination

A simple visual examination can provide valuable information regarding the patient's general health and well-being. For instance, observing the patient's posture, body movements, speech patterns, and skin can help identify the anxious patient, which is an important consideration when administering local anesthetics.

Vital Signs

Preanesthetic vital signs are important to provide the dental hygienist with baseline values as comparison standards in the event that an emergency situation should occur. Another benefit to obtaining vital signs is to identify diagnosed or undiagnosed conditions that may require modifications to treatment, drug selection, and dosage. Vital signs should be recorded on the patient's permanent record at each visit requiring anesthetic administration.

Blood Pressure

The administration of a local anesthetic agent will further elevate the existing blood pressure of patients, and to a greater extent in the anxious patient.[2] Obtaining a preanesthetic blood pressure provides valuable baseline information. Many local anesthetic emergencies alter a patient's blood pressure, and preanesthetic numbers are critical in assessing the severity of the emergency. Furthermore, the use of a vasoconstrictor may need to be limited or avoided in the presence of hypertension. See Table 7.2 for adult blood pressure guidelines for dental management of the hypertensive patient. An accurate blood pressure recording is essential. See Fig. 7.1 for guidelines for proper blood pressure cuff size and Box 7.1 for common errors in blood pressure assessment.

TABLE 7.2 Adult Blood Pressure Guidelines Used in the Dental Hygiene Process of Care

Blood Pressure (mm Hg)	ASA Physical Status Classification	Dental and Dental Hygiene Therapy Consideration and Interventions Recommended
<120 systolic and <80 diastolic (normal)	I	No unusual precautions related to patient management based on blood pressure readings. Recheck at next continuing care appointment.
120–129 systolic and/or 80–89 diastolic	I	Routine dental treatment is permitted.
130–139 systolic and/or 80–89 diastolic	I	Routine dental treatment is permitted. Assess risk factors and refer for consultation with physician of record.
≥140 systolic and/or ≥90 diastolic	II	Routine dental hygiene treatment is permitted. Refer for consultation with the physician of record.
160–180 systolic and/or 100– < 110 diastolic	III	Recheck blood pressure in 5 minutes; if still elevated, seek medical consultation before dental or dental hygiene appointment. Initiate stress-reduction protocols, such as administration of nitrous oxide–oxygen analgesia.
>180 systolic and/or >120 diastolic	IV	Recheck blood pressure in 5 minutes; discontinue appointment; immediate medical consultation if still elevated. Postpone all dental or dental hygiene therapy until the elevated BP is corrected Refer to hospital if immediate dental therapy is indicated.

ASA, American Society of Anesthesiologists; *BP,* blood pressure; *IV,* intravenous.
Modified from Bowen DM, Pieren JA: *Darby and Walsh dental hygiene: theory and practice,* ed 5, St Louis, 2020, Elsevier.

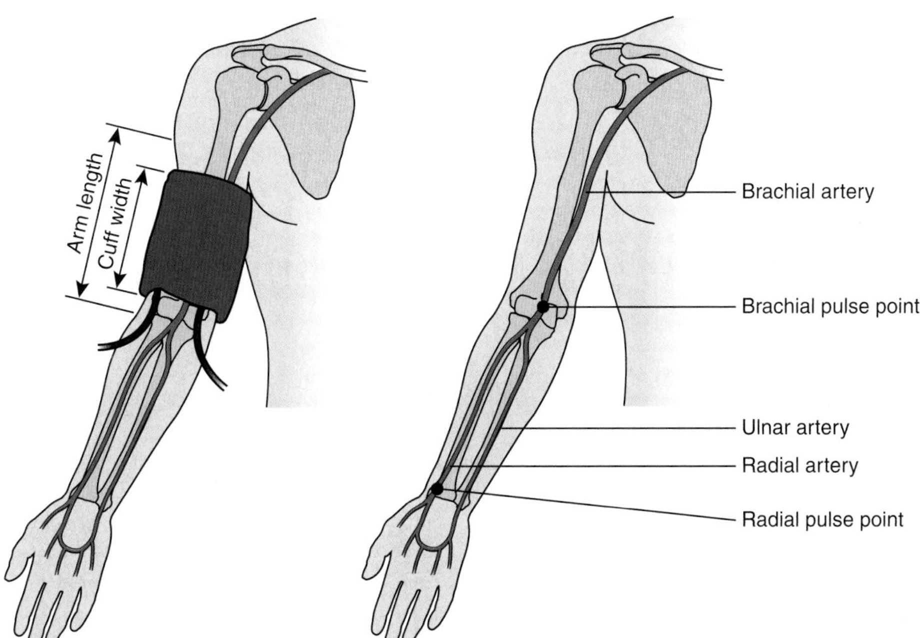

Fig. 7.1 Proper placement of blood pressure cuff. Guidelines for cuff size: Cuff width = 20% more than upper arm diameter or 40% of circumference and two-thirds of arm length. (From Bowen DM, Pieren JA: *Darby and Walsh dental hygiene: theory and practice,* ed 5, St Louis, 2020, Elsevier.)

BOX 7.1 Common Errors in Blood Pressure Detection

False high readings	Bladder or cuff too small, too narrow, or too short Cuff wrapped too loosely or unevenly Deflating cuff too slowly (false high diastolic reading) Arm is below heart level Arm is not supported Cuff is inflated too slowly Repeating assessments too quickly (false high systolic) Bladder not fully deflated before beginning measurement Legs are crossed Patient is not resting quietly for 3–5 minutes before assessment
False low readings	Failure to identify the auscultatory gap Bladder or cuff too wide Arm is above heart level Stethoscope is pressed too firmly (produces a false low systolic) Stethoscope pressed too firmly (false low diastolic) Inflation level is inadequate (produces false low systolic)

Modified from Bowen DM, Pieren JA: *Darby and Walsh dental hygiene: theory and practice,* ed 5, St Louis, 2020, Elsevier.

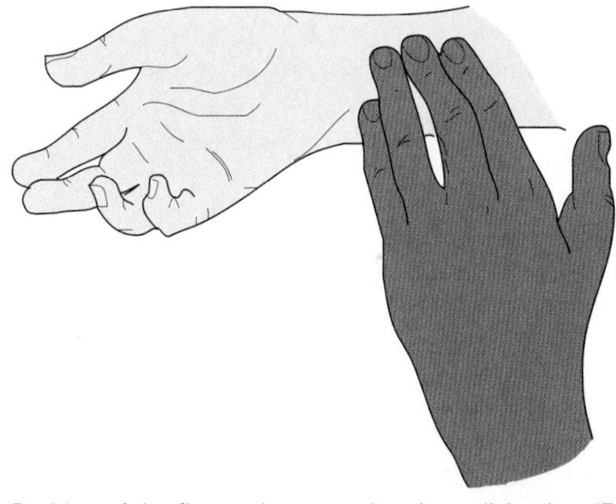

Fig. 7.2 Position of the fingers in measuring the radial pulse. (From Potter PA, Perry AG, Stockert PA, et al: *Fundamentals of nursing,* ed 9, St Louis, 2017, Elsevier.)

Pulse

The most common procedure for assessing the pulse rate is to palpate the radial artery on the thumb side of the wrist for 1 minute (Fig. 7.2). Tachycardia (>100 beats per minute) is an abnormally elevated heart rate and may be a sign of a cardiovascular disease or influenced by stress and anxiety. Bradycardia (<60 beats per minute) is a slow heart rate.[4] Table 7.3 lists the acceptable ranges of heart (pulse) rate, and Table 7.4 discusses the factors that influence heart (pulse) rate. Local anesthetics containing epinephrine are contraindicated in patients with uncontrolled cardiac dysrhythmias.

TABLE 7.3 Acceptable Ranges of Heart (Pulse) Rate

Age	Heart Rate (Beats per Minute)
Toddler	90–140
Preschooler	80–110
School-age child	75–100
Adolescent	60–90
Adult	60–100

(Modified from Potter PA, Perry AG, Stockert PA, et al: *Fundamentals of nursing,* ed 9, St Louis, 2017, Elsevier.)

Respiration

Respiration can be evaluated before or after the pulse rate is assessed while the dental hygienist's fingers are in the pulse monitoring position. The rate and depth of the respiration is observed by the rise and fall of

TABLE 7.4 Factors That Influence Heart (Pulse) Rate

Factor	Increased Pulse Rate	Decreased Pulse Rate
Exercise	Short-term exercise	Heart conditioned by long-term exercise, resulting in lower resting pulse and quicker return to resting level after exercise
Temperature	Fever and heat	Hypothermia
Emotions	Sympathetic stimulation increased by acute pain and anxiety, affecting heart rate; effect of chronic pain on heart rate varies	Parasympathetic stimulation increased by unrelieved severe pain affecting heart rate, relaxation
Medications	Positive chronotropic drugs (e.g., epinephrine)	Negative chronotropic drugs (e.g., digitalis, beta and calcium blockers)
Hemorrhage	Sympathetic stimulation increased by loss of blood	
Postural changes	Standing or sitting	Lying down
Pulmonary conditions	Diseases causing poor oxygenation such as asthma, COPD	

COPD, Chronic obstructive pulmonary disease.
(Modified from Potter PA, Perry AG, Stockert PA, et al: *Fundamentals of nursing,* ed 9, St Louis, 2017, Elsevier.)

TABLE 7.5 Acceptable Ranges of Respiratory Rate According to Age

Age	Rate (Breaths per Minute)
Toddler (2 years)	25–32
Child	20–30
Adolescent	16–20
Adult	12–20

(Modified from Potter PA, Perry AG, Stockert PA, et al: *Fundamentals of nursing,* ed 9, St Louis, 2017, Elsevier.)

the resting patient's chest. Hyperventilation (breathing that is deeper and more rapid than normal) is a common occurrence in apprehensive patients, especially before the administration of a local anesthetic injection. (See Table 7.5 for acceptable ranges of respiratory rate, and see Chapter 17 for signs, symptoms, and treatment of hyperventilation.)

Weight

The weight of a patient is used before the administration of a local anesthetic to determine the patient's maximum recommended dose (MRD). Consideration should be given to lowering the MRD for children with excess weight. In this situation, the MRD may allow a greater volume of anesthetic to be administered based upon the child's weight, but their immature liver may not be able to readily biotransform the anesthetic, putting the child at risk for an overdose. (See Chapters 8 and Chapter 14.)

PSYCHOLOGICAL EXAMINATION

Dental phobia is any objectively unfounded fear or morbid dread of dental treatment. Dental phobia is a real affliction that affects many individuals, usually caused by a traumatic, difficult, and/or painful dental experience (Box 7.2).

The evaluation of a patient's attitude and psychological fears is an important component to the preanesthetic assessment. The typical medical history form should include a few questions regarding the patient's past dental history and any previous trouble associated with the treatment. Further dialogue should be conducted by the dental hygienist to recognize possible stresses and anxiety that can exacerbate medical problems such as angina, asthma, hyperventilation, seizures, or vasodepressor syncope.[1,2,4] Anxiety and fear can be recognized by increases in vital signs and visual observation of the patient's body movements, skin color (paleness), cold sweats, posture, trembling, and verbal communication (Box 7.3).

BOX 7.2 Common Origins of Dental Fear

- Previously painful or negative dental experiences including careless comments made by dental professionals
- Severe discomfort with feeling helpless or out of control in the oral health care setting
- Embarrassment caused by dental neglect and fear of ridicule or belittlement
- Scary stories of negative dental experiences learned vicariously from family and friends
- Negative portrayals of dentists in movies, on television, or in printed materials
- A sense of depersonalization in the oral health care setting, intensified by the use of masks, gloves, and shields
- Fear of pain
- Fear of injections
- Fear the injection will not work
- Feelings of helplessness and loss of control
- Loss of personal space (i.e., physical closeness of practitioner to the patient's face)
- A general fear of the unknown
- A previous bad experience that unknowingly has become associated with dentistry

From Bowen DM, Pieren JA: *Darby and Walsh dental hygiene: theory and practice,* ed 5, St Louis, 2020, Elsevier.

BOX 7.3 Clinical Signs of Moderate Anxiety

- Unnaturally stiff posture
- Nervous play
- White-knuckle syndrome
- Perspiration on forehead and hands
- Overwillingness to cooperate with clinician
- Nervous conversation
- Quick answers

From Bowen DM, Pieren JA: *Darby and Walsh dental hygiene: theory and practice,* ed 5, St Louis, 2020, Elsevier.

The body's response to fear provokes the stress response referred to as *fight or flight.* These symptoms include a state of alarm and adrenaline production causing an increase in heart rate and blood pressure, as well as irritability, muscular tension, and the inability to concentrate (Box 7.4). These symptoms can be further intensified by the

BOX 7.4 Effects of Stress on the Body

- Dilated pupils
- Decreased salivation (tight, dry throat)
- Chest pain
- High blood pressure
- Shortness of breath
- Increased heart rate
- Increased blood cholesterol and blood glucose
- Gastrointestinal disturbances
- Headache
- Back and neck aches
- Clenched jaws
- Grinding of teeth (bruxism)
- Indigestion
- Increased perspiration (e.g., sweaty hands, visible perspiration beads above upper lip)
- Insomnia
- Increase or decrease in weight
- Hives
- Dry mouth (xerostomia)
- Irritation of gastrointestinal tract lining (e.g., stomach ulcers)
- Decreased immune response

From Bowen DM, Pieren JA: *Darby and Walsh dental hygiene: theory and practice*, ed 5, St Louis, 2020, Elsevier.

BOX 7.5 Stress Reduction Protocol

- Recognize the patient's level of anxiety (be a good observer)
- Open communication about fears or concerns
- Complete medical consultation before care, as needed
- Preoperative sedation: short-acting benzodiazepine (e.g., triazolam 0.125–0.25 mg) 1 hour before the appointment and possibly the night before the day of the appointment, as needed
- Short appointments (preferably morning)
- Minimize the patient's waiting time
- Monitor and record preoperative vital signs and postoperative vital signs
- Consider psychosedation during therapy (see Chapter 15)
- Select an anesthetic agent with appropriate posttreatment pain control
- Administer adequate pain control during therapy
- Follow up with postoperative pain and anxiety control
- Telephone the highly anxious or fearful patient later the same day that treatment was delivered

administration of exogenous epinephrine (see Chapter 4). Fear and apprehension also lower the patient's pain reaction threshold, and even minor, nonpainful procedures may be perceived as painful (see Chapter 1). A stress reduction protocol is essential for the apprehensive patient and should start before the dental appointment and continue through the postoperative period if necessary[2] (Box 7.5).

Adequate Pain Control and Fear of the Needle

Adequate pain control is essential to provide thorough nonsurgical periodontal therapy and is best accomplished by the administration of local anesthetics. The apprehensive patient who fears the dental needle may resist the administration of local anesthetics for nonsurgical periodontal therapy. The dental hygienist should explain the advantages of profound anesthesia during these procedures and that care will be taken to reduce the discomfort of the injection (Box 7.6). (See Chapter 11 for basic injection techniques.)

BOX 7.6 Benefits of Adequate Pain Control and Nonsurgical Periodontal Therapy

- Dental hygienist can provide more thorough treatment on a relaxed patient
- The periodontal therapy will be less traumatic for the patient
- The less traumatic the experience, the more likely the patient will return to complete treatment
- Without adequate pain control, sedation and stress reduction are impossible to achieve

Selection of Local Anesthetic for the Anxious Patient

To reduce stress and anxiety during nonsurgical periodontal therapy, it is critical that adequate pain control be obtained. The potentially adverse actions of the released catecholamines on cardiovascular function in the patient with clinically significant heart or blood vessel disease warrant the inclusion of vasoconstrictors in the local anesthetic solution. Without adequate control of pain, sedation and stress reduction are impossible to achieve. Therefore the anesthetic must outlast the dental treatment, and the inclusion of a vasoconstrictor is the best way to ensure this occurrence. In most situations, cardiovascularly involved patients may receive vasoconstrictors in limited doses. This is referred to as the cardiac dose, or a safe dose of vasoconstricting drugs that can be administered to a patient with significant cardiovascular disease. It limits the amount of epinephrine to 0.04 mg per appointment and 0.2 mg per appointment for levonordefrin. If the dental hygienist selects a vasoconstrictor dilution of 1:200,000, the patient can safely receive 4.4 cartridges of anesthetic with epinephrine, which should be adequate for most nonsurgical periodontal procedures. A 1:100,000 dilution can be safely administered, but this patient should only receive 2.2 cartridges of anesthetic with epinephrine. (See Chapter 8 for dosage calculations.)

RISK ASSESSMENT

Once a thorough medical history, expanded by dialogue of relevant issues with the patient, and vital signs have been obtained, the data must be evaluated to determine whether a patient can physiologically and psychologically safely undergo dental treatment and receive local anesthetics. Based on this information, modifications to dental treatment or selection of an anesthetic may be required. The American Society of Anesthesiologists has developed a system to express the anxiety and medical risk of a patient receiving dental care regardless of the type of procedure or anesthesia used (Table 7.6). As the classification level increases, the risk for dental care increases as well.[4] Another helpful tool for determining the at-risk patient is evaluating the ABCs of risk assessment (Table 7.7).[4]

CONTRAINDICATIONS TO LOCAL ANESTHESIA

Local anesthetic agents and vasoconstrictors are relatively safe drugs when administered using the appropriate standard of delivery (see Chapter 11). However, certain medical conditions and drug interactions may necessitate limiting or avoiding their use. Modifications to the selection of a local anesthetic agent and the dental hygiene care plan are determined when the patient's assessment has been thoroughly reviewed and standard procedures are contraindicated. Contraindications to local anesthetics and vasoconstrictors are divided into two categories:

Absolute contraindication. The administration of the offending drug increases the possibility of a life-threatening situation and should not be administered to the individual under any circumstances.

TABLE 7.6 ASA Physical Status Classification System

Classification	Description of Classification
ASA class I	A normal, healthy patient
ASA class II	A patient with a mild systemic disease, but this does not interfere with daily activity (e.g., healthy patient [ASA class I] with extreme anxiety and fear toward dentistry, adult patient with systolic BP between 140 and 159 mm Hg and/or diastolic BP between 90 and 94 mm Hg, healthy pregnant patient, patient who has well-controlled type 2 diabetes or controlled epileptic and/or well-controlled asthma, patient with a history of hyperthyroid or hypothyroid conditions who is under care and presently in a euthyroid condition)
ASA class III	A patient with moderate to severe systemic disease that limits activity but is not incapacitating but may affect daily activity (e.g., patient with well-controlled type 1 diabetes, patient with symptomatic hyperthyroid or hypothyroid disease, patient stable angina, patient with exercise-induced asthma, patient with postmyocardial infarction or cerebrovascular accident more than 6 months before treatment, patient with uncontrolled dysrhythmias, patient with severe COPD)
ASA class IV	A patient with an incapacitating systemic disease that is a constant threat to life (e.g., patient with a myocardial infarction within past 6 months or cerebrovascular accident within 6 months, patient with uncontrolled epilepsy or uncontrolled diabetes, patient with BP greater than 200 and/or a diastolic BP or 115 mm Hg or higher, patient with severe heart failure, patient with severe COPD, patient with uncontrolled epilepsy)
ASA class V	A moribund patient not expected to survive 24 hours with or without an operation
ASA class VI	A declared brain-dead patient whose organs are being removed for donor purposes

ASA, American Society of Anesthesiologists; *BP,* blood pressure; *COPD,* chronic obstructive pulmonary disease.
Modified from Little JW, Falace DA, Miller CS, Rhodus NL: *Dental management of the medically compromised patient,* ed 9, St Louis, 2018, Elsevier.

Relative contraindication. The administration of the offending drug is preferably avoided because of the increased possibility of an adverse reaction to the drug. However, if an acceptable alternative drug is not available, the drug may be used judiciously (i.e., administration of a minimal effective dose).

VASOCONSTRICTOR DRUG–DRUG INTERACTIONS

Epinephrine and other vasoconstrictors may produce drug-to-drug interactions with prescribed medications the patient may be taking (see Table 7.8 for a complete list of vasoconstrictor modifications and Table 7.9 for vasoconstrictor absolute contraindications). The dental hygienist should administer vasoconstrictors with great caution or eliminate them entirely when the patient is taking the drugs described in the following paragraphs. The dental hygienist should consult the patient's physician if uncertain that a vasoconstrictor can be safely administered.

TABLE 7.7 ABCs of Risk Assessment

	Possible Issues
A:	
*A*ntibiotics	Antibiotic requirement (prophylactic or therapeutic)
*A*nalgesics	Is the patient taking aspirin or other NSAIDs that may increase bleeding? Will analgesics be needed after the procedure?
*A*nesthesia	Any potential problems associated with local anesthetics or vasoconstrictors
*A*nxiety	Patient requirement for sedation
*A*llergy	Possible allergy to prescribed drug or anesthetic
B:	
*B*leeding	Possibility of abnormal hemostasis
*B*reathing	Does the patient have any difficulty breathing, or is the breathing abnormally fast or slow?
*B*lood pressure	Is the blood pressure well controlled, or is it likely to increase or decrease during dental treatment?
C:	
*C*hair position	Patient's tolerance to supine positioning
D:	
*D*rugs	Interactions, adverse effects, side effects, allergies
*D*evices	Prosthetic valves, prosthetic joints, stents, pacemakers, A-V fistulas that may require consideration
E:	
*E*quipment	Potential problems or concerns associated with x-rays, ultrasonic scaler, oxygen supply
*E*mergencies	Potential for occurrence
F:	
*F*ollow-up	Is any follow-up care indicated? Should the patient be contacted at home to assess her or his response to treatment?

NSAIDs, Nonsteroidal antiinflammatory drugs.
Modified from Little J, Falace D, Miller C, Rhodus N: *Dental management of the medically compromised patient,* ed 9, St Louis, 2018, Elsevier.

Tricyclic Antidepressants

Tricyclic antidepressants are commonly prescribed for the management of severe depression, and when used in combination with exogenously administered vasoconstrictors, the patient's cardiovascular actions are enhanced.[4] An exaggerated increase in the pressor (increase in blood pressure) effects is likely to occur after the administration of local anesthetics with vasoconstrictors in patients taking tricyclic antidepressants.[4] The pressor effects of epinephrine are potentiated twofold, and the enhancement with levonordefrin and norepinephrine is fivefold to tenfold. If the patient also has arrhythmias, the situation is of even greater concern.[4] For dental treatment, levonordefrin and norepinephrine should be avoided, and epinephrine should be administered at the lowest effective dose similar to that recommended for a cardiovascularly involved patient (0.04 mg per appointment for epinephrine). See Box 7.7 for commonly prescribed tricyclic antidepressants.

Nonselective Beta Blockers

Nonselective beta blockers are antihypertensive drugs used to lower systolic and diastolic blood pressure. However, when used with exogenously administrated vasoconstrictors, especially epinephrine, the combined effect leads to blockade of beta-adrenergic receptors in the skeletal muscles and may cause hypertension and reflex bradycardia.

TABLE 7.8 **Drug–Drug Interactions That Affect the Use of Vasoconstrictors**

Medication	Type of Contraindication	Significance	Vasoconstrictor Dose/Drug Modification
Patients taking tricyclic antidepressants	Relative	Increases effects of vasoconstrictor; both epinephrine and levonordefrin may cause acute hypertension and cardiac dysrhythmia but levonordefrin to a greater degree	Avoid levonordefrin; limit epinephrine to cardiac dose of 0.04 mg per appointment; do not use 1:50,000 epinephrine
Patients taking nonselective beta blockers (propranolol, nadolol)	Relative	Increased hypertension resulting in rebound bradycardia; potential cardiac arrest	If vasoconstriction is necessary, limit vasoconstrictor to cardiac dose; 0.04 mg per appointment for epinephrine; 0.2 mg per appointment for levonordefrin; do not use 1:50,000 epinephrine
Phenothiazides Promethazine (Phenergan): chlorpromazine (Thorazine): Mellaril (Thioridazine)	Relative	May reverse the pressor effect of vasoconstrictors resulting in an increased risk of hypotension, and they have been noted to antagonize the peripheral vasoconstrictive effects of epinephrine	Limit vasoconstrictor to cardiac dose; 0.04 mg per appointment for epinephrine; 0.2 mg per appointment for levonordefrin; do not use 1:50,000 epinephrine
Digitalis glycosides (digoxin, digitoxin)	Relative	Epinephrine increases the potential for cardiac arrhythmias	Use epinephrine in consultation with patient's physician
Levodopa, thyroid hormones (levothyroxine, liothyronine)	Relative	Large doses beyond replacement doses may risk cardiac toxicity	Use vasoconstrictor with caution
Catecholamine-*O*-methyltransferase inhibitors (tolcapone, entacapone)	Relative	May enhance systemic actions of vasoconstrictors	Use vasoconstrictor with caution
CNS stimulants (amphetamine, methylphenidate); ergot derivatives (dihydroergotamine, methysergide)	Relative	Effects of stimulant or vasoconstrictor may occur	Use vasoconstrictor with caution

ASA, American Society of Anesthesiologists; *CNS,* central nervous system.

TABLE 7.9 **Absolute Contraindications: Do Not Use Vasoconstrictors**

Health Condition	Type of Contraindication	Significance
Recent myocardial infarction within 6 months	Absolute	Increases cardiovascular effects to dangerous levels; ASA IV until recuperation Avoid all dental care until condition is under control
Recent coronary bypass surgery within 6 months	Absolute	Increases cardiovascular effects to dangerous levels; ASA IV until recuperation Avoid all dental care until condition is under control
Uncontrolled high blood pressure	Absolute	Increases blood pressure to dangerous levels Avoid all dental care until condition is under control
Uncontrolled angina	Absolute	Increases risk of severe angina attack Avoid all dental care until condition is under control
Uncontrolled arrhythmias	Absolute	Increases cardiovascular effects to dangerous levels Avoid all dental care until condition is under control
Sulfite allergies	Absolute	Avoid vasoconstrictors in true allergic reaction
Pheochromocytoma: catecholamine-producing tumors	Absolute	Tumor of the adrenal gland, causes adrenal insufficiency Avoid all dental care until condition is under control
Uncontrolled hyperthyroidism	Absolute	Risk of thyroid crisis, thyroid storm Avoid all dental care until condition is under control
Cocaine or methamphetamine abusers	Absolute	Potentiates the adrenergic effects on the heart with the potential for a heart attack Avoid use of vasoconstrictors until cocaine has been withheld for at least 24 hours

ASA, American Society of Anesthesiologists.

The antihypertensives listed in Box 7.8 may potentiate the action of epinephrine and other adrenergic amines. The basis for concern with the use of nonselective beta-adrenergic blocking agents is that muscle vasculature mediated by β_2 receptors is inhibited by these drugs, and injection of epinephrine, and levonordefrin, may result in uncompensated peripheral vasoconstriction because of unopposed stimulation of α_1 receptors. The vasoconstrictive effect could potentially cause a significant elevation in blood pressure and a compensatory bradycardia.[5,6]

BOX 7.7 Commonly Prescribed Tricyclic Antidepressants

- Amitriptyline (Elavil)
- Amoxapine (Asendin)
- Clomipramine (Anafranil)
- Desipramine (Norpramin, Pertofrane)
- Doxepin (Sinequan, Adapin)
- Nortriptyline (Aventyl, Pamelor)
- Imipramine (Tofranil)
- Protriptyline (Vivactil)
- Trimipramine (Surmontil)

BOX 7.8 Commonly Prescribed Nonselective Beta Blockers

- Propranolol (Inderal, Betachron)
- Metoprolol (Lopressor)
- Timolol (Blocadren)
- Nadolol (Corgard)
- Pindolol (Visken)
- Betaxolol (Kerlone)
- Acebutolol (Sectral)
- Esmolol (Brevibloc)
- Bisoprolol (Zebeta)
- Sotalol (Betapace)
- Carteolol (Cartrol)

Several cases of this interaction have been reported in the literature, but it appears to be dose-dependent.[7,8] If vasoconstriction is needed, use with caution, limiting their use to the lowest effective dose (not to exceed 0.04 mg per appointment for epinephrine and 0.2 mg per appointment for levonordefrin). If vasoconstrictors are administered, preanesthetic and postanesthetic vital signs should be monitored and documented. In addition, the patient should be monitored throughout treatment for symptoms of altered (increased) blood pressure.

Cardiac Drugs

Digitalis glycosides (digoxin, digitoxin) are used for the treatment of congestive heart failure. The combination of digitalis glycosides and epinephrine increases the potential for cardiac arrhythmias. Avoid use of epinephrine or use in consultation with the patient's physician.[4]

Phenothiazides

Phenothiazides are prescribed for the management of serious psychotic disorders. The drug interaction between epinephrine and phenothiazides occurs because phenothiazides are alpha blockers that antagonize the beta effects of epinephrine. When this occurs, the beta (vasodilatory) effects of epinephrine predominate. Phenothiazides such as promethazine (Phenergan), thioridazine (Mellaril), and chlorpromazine (Thorazine) may reverse the pressor effect of vasoconstrictors, resulting in an increased risk of hypotension. Phenothiazides have been noted to antagonize the peripheral vasoconstrictive effects of epinephrine. The minimal effective dose of epinephrine should be administered, similar to that recommended for a cardiovascularly involved patient (0.04 mg per appointment).

Illegal (Recreational) Drugs (Cocaine, Methamphetamine)

Cocaine is a local anesthetic drug that significantly stimulates the CNS and CVS. Cocaine stimulates the release of norepinephrine and inhibits the adrenergic nerve reuptake, causing tachycardia, severe hypertension, and arrhythmias.[4] Methamphetamine affects the neurotransmitter epinephrine by either increasing its release or stopping its metabolic breakdown and reuptake, resulting in a hypertensive crisis. The clinician should be on the alert for signs and symptoms that may indicate substance abuse. Vasoconstrictors should **not** be administered to a patient who is suspected of using cocaine or methamphetamine within 24 hours of dental treatment; it may lead to a hypertensive crisis, stroke, or myocardial infarction.

VASOCONSTRICTORS AND SYSTEMIC DISEASE INTERACTIONS

Few health conditions absolutely contraindicate the administration of vasoconstrictors, and in these situations, patients are not usually seen for elective dental procedures such as nonsurgical periodontal therapy until the systemic disease is under control. The dental hygienist must carefully weigh the benefits of the administration of vasoconstrictors with the risks involved to determine whether a vasoconstrictor should be administered. Table 7.9 summarizes the vasoconstrictor absolute contraindications, and Table 7.10 summarizes the vasoconstrictor relative contraindications.

Cardiovascular Disease

Stress provoked by dental procedures is likely to increase blood pressure, pulse, and possibly respiration (hyperventilation) in many patients. Patients with cardiovascular disease are more susceptible than healthy patients to these responses, producing further adverse effects on their already compromised system. Therefore authorities[2–4,9,10] recommend small amounts (cardiac dose) of epinephrine; 0.04 mg per appointment (2.2 cartridges containing 1:100,000 dilution) compared with a maximum of 0.2 mg in a healthy adult (approximately 13.8 cartridges of lidocaine with epinephrine) to be administered to cardiovascular patients in category ASA III for most dental procedures, including nonsurgical periodontal therapy. Most postmyocardial infarction (MI) patients are considered to be an ASA III risk 6 or more months after the episode. Profound local anesthesia is indicated to minimize release of endogenous epinephrine in response to pain. Adequate aspiration is critical to prevent intravascular injection. The use of concentrated vasoconstrictors 1:50,000 epinephrine for bleeding control is contraindicated.

Patients with significant cardiovascular disease (ASA IV) should not receive elective dental procedures or vasoconstrictors until their disease is controlled. The following are absolute contraindications to the use of vasoconstrictors (see Table 7.9):

- Blood pressure greater than 180/110 mm Hg
- Treatment within 6 months after a heart attack or stroke
- Severe cardiovascular disease
- Daily episodes of angina pectoris or unstable (preinfarction) angina
- Cardiac dysrhythmias despite appropriate therapy
- Treatment within 6 months of coronary artery bypass surgery

Hyperthyroidism

Hyperthyroidism is a condition that occurs because of excessive production of thyroid hormone by the thyroid gland. Patients with hyperthyroidism are sensitive to catecholamines, which may precipitate an exaggerated response to vasoconstrictors, resulting in cardiac stimulation and risk of developing thyrotoxicosis, more commonly known as *thyroid storm*. Uncontrolled hyperthyroidism is an absolute contraindication to vasoconstrictors because of the possibility of causing a thyroid crisis. Patients should not receive elective dental care or vasoconstrictors until the situation is controlled, and then only the minimal effective

TABLE 7.10 **Health Conditions That Require Modifications to the Amount of Vasoconstrictor Administered**

Health Condition	Type of Contraindication	Reason for Modification	Vasoconstrictor Dose/Drug Modification
Cardiovascular disease	Relative	Vasoconstrictors will enhance the cardiovascular effects; ASA III patients are treatable with appropriate drug modifications	Limit vasoconstrictor to cardiac dose; 0.04 mg per appointment for epinephrine; 0.2 mg per appointment for levonordefrin; do not use 1:50,000 epinephrine
Diabetes	Relative	Vasoconstrictors directly oppose effect of insulin, possible changes in blood levels of glucose; amounts used in dentistry are generally safe and do not significantly raise blood sugar levels	Use with caution. Limit the dose of vasoconstrictor for patients with uncontrolled "brittle" diabetes
Controlled hyperthyroidism	Relative	Sensitivity to vasoconstrictors increasing their effect	Surgically corrected or medication controlled respond normally to vasoconstrictors
Sickle cell anemia	Relative	No dental treatment during a crisis; vasoconstrictors will increase stress	Routine dental care appointments should be short. Use of local anesthesia is acceptable. The inclusion of small amounts of epinephrine (1:200,000) should be limited to treatment where profound anesthesia is warranted and to obtain hemostasis

ASA, American Society of Anesthesiologists.

dose should be administered, not to exceed 0.04 mg per appointment for epinephrine and 0.2 mg per appointment for levonordefrin.

Asthma

Asthma is a chronic inflammatory disease of the airways resulting in episodes of dyspnea, coughing, and wheezing commonly precipitated by stress. Asthma may be induced by anxiety related to the administration of local anesthetics, so stress reduction is paramount. The addition of sodium bisulfite, or metabisulfite, to prevent the oxidation of vasoconstrictors may cause respiratory reactions in asthmatics (predominantly steroid-dependent asthmatics). It has been reported that 5 to 10% of the asthmatic population are allergic to bisulfites. Asthmatic patients who receive a local anesthetic with a vasoconstrictor should be observed for signs and symptoms of an asthmatic attack. Bisulfite allergies typically manifest as a severe respiratory allergy, commonly bronchospasm.[10–15]

Sickle Cell Anemia

Sickle cell anemia is a hereditary blood disorder characterized by an abnormality in the oxygen-carrying hemoglobin molecule in red blood cells. This leads to a propensity for the cells to assume an abnormal, rigid, sickle-like shape under certain circumstances. Sickle cell disease is associated with a number of acute and chronic health problems, such as severe infections, attacks of severe pain ("sickle cell crisis"), stroke, and there is an increased risk of death. For routine dental care, appointments should be short (to reduce stress). The use of local anesthesia is acceptable (avoid prilocaine). Physician consultation is recommended to determine cardiac status. No dental treatment or local anesthesia should be administered during a crisis. The inclusion of small amounts of epinephrine in the local anesthetic is controversial; however, the benefits probably outweigh the risks and should be limited to treatment where profound anesthesia is warranted and to obtain hemostasis.[4,16]

ALLERGIES

Amino esters are derivatives of para-aminobenzoic acid (PABA), which have been associated with acute allergic reactions. Amino amides are not associated with PABA and do not produce allergic reactions with the same frequency.

Since the removal of methylparaben, a local anesthetic preservative (structurally similar to PABA) from local anesthetic solutions, the possibility of an amide local anesthetic allergic reaction is extremely rare and essentially nonexistent.[4,9] Moreover, there are no confirmed cases of a true allergy to a pure amide anesthetic. However, patients often claim they are allergic to local anesthetics. These patients must be further questioned to rule out the possibility of misinformation or misdiagnosis. Also, patients who may have experienced rapid adrenergic symptoms from the vasoconstrictor or experienced a local anesthetic overdose may confuse these symptoms with an allergic reaction. A well-documented allergic reaction to a local anesthetic represents an absolute contraindication to that class of drugs, and an unrelated drug should be selected. A patient who has an allergic reaction to one agent is likely to experience hypersensitivity to another agent in the same group. Cross-hypersensitivity between esters and amides is unlikely.

As discussed in Chapter 4, local anesthetics with adrenergic vasoconstrictors contain the antioxidant sodium bisulfite, or metabisulfite. Documented allergic reactions have been reported to these agents.[10-15] Patients who have demonstrated a true allergy to sulfites should not receive a local anesthetic agent containing vasoconstrictors (an absolute contraindication). Table 7.11 summarizes allergies that affect the selection of local anesthetic agents.

ESTER DERIVATIVE LOCAL ANESTHETIC INTERACTIONS

Injectable esters are no longer available for use in dentistry because of their well-documented risk of allergic reactions. However, because topical ester anesthetics continue to be administered in dentistry, these drug–drug interactions will be discussed.

Sulfonamides

Procaine and tetracaine undergo hydrolysis to PABA, a major metabolic by-product. Sulfonamides competitively inhibit PABA in microorganisms. PABA derivatives, therefore, may antagonize the antibacterial activity of sulfonamides, rendering them ineffective. Because the use of ester injectable local anesthetics is no longer available in dentistry, this

TABLE 7.11 Allergies That Affect the Selection of Local Anesthetic Agents or Vasoconstrictors

Reported Allergy	Type of Contraindication	Drugs to Avoid	Potential Problem(s)	Alternative Drug
Local anesthetic allergy, documented	Absolute	All local anesthetics in same chemical class (esters vs amides)	Allergic response, mild (e.g., dermatitis, bronchospasm) to life-threatening reactions	Local anesthetics in different chemical class (esters vs amides)
Sodium bisulfite or metabisulfite	Absolute	Local anesthetic containing a vasoconstrictor	Allergic reaction, severe bronchospasm, usually in asthmatics	Local anesthetic without vasoconstrictor

Modified from Bowen DM, Pieren JA: *Darby and Walsh dental hygiene: theory and practice,* ed 5, St Louis, 2020, Elsevier.

TABLE 7.12 Drug–Drug Interactions That Affect the Use of Local Anesthetics

Medication	Type of Contraindication	Significance	Local Anesthetic Dose/ Drug Modification
CNS depressants (e.g., alcohol, antidepressants, antihistamines, benzodiazepines, antipsychotics, muscle relaxants, opioids or opioid derivatives, antianxiety drugs, phenothiazines, and barbiturates)	Relative	May increase the risk of a local anesthetic overdose; could potentiate drowsiness. Barbiturates induce hepatic microsomal enzymes that could alter the rate of amide-type local anesthetic metabolism	Use amides in lower doses
Patients taking H_2-receptor blocker cimetidine (Tagamet), Zantac (ranitidine) on a regular basis	Relative	Drug reduces capacity of liver to metabolize lidocaine	Reduce dose of lidocaine; greater clinical significance in patients with CHF (ASA III or greater)
Patients taking beta blockers, predominantly Inderal (propranolol)	Relative	Inhibits metabolism of amides by decreasing hepatic blood flow, increasing risk of toxic overdose	Reduce dosage of amides metabolized in the liver

ASA, American Society of Anesthesiologists; *CHF,* congestive heart failure; *CNS,* central nervous system.

is unlikely to occur. However, ester topical anesthetics should not be given to a patient taking sulfonamides. Instead use lidocaine.

Atypical Plasma Cholinesterase

Ester anesthetics are metabolized in the plasma by cholinesterase enzymes. Some individuals, approximately one in every 2820, demonstrate an atypical form of plasma pseudocholinesterase.[4] This is an uncommon autosomal recessive genetic trait that impairs the patient's ability to effectively metabolize ester-type injectable and topical anesthetics.[9] Amide local anesthetics can be safely administered to these patients.

AMIDE LOCAL ANESTHETIC DRUG–DRUG INTERACTIONS

Only a few amide local anesthetic interactions occur with prescribed drugs. These typically manifest by delaying the metabolism of the local anesthetic agent. The importance of each interaction is summarized in Table 7.12.

Histamine H_2 Receptor Blockers

Amide local anesthetics that are primarily metabolized in the liver have a potential for drug interactions with other drugs that influence hepatic metabolism. Tagamet (cimetidine) decreases hepatic blood flow and inhibits hepatic metabolism of amides, particularly lidocaine, by competing for binding to hepatic oxidative enzymes, and therefore increases the half-life of the amide anesthetic, augmenting the risk for toxic overdose. Caution should be used when administering large doses of lidocaine. The interaction between lidocaine and cimetidine is of greater concern in patients with a history of congestive heart failure (ASA III or greater) because of the decrease in blood delivered to the liver; an increase in blood delivered to the brain increases the risk of an anesthetic overdose.[2]

Beta Blockers

Beta adrenergic blocking drugs, such as propranolol and metoprolol, share the same effect as cimetidine on amide biotransformation, particularly lidocaine. Beta blockers inhibit metabolism of amides by decreasing hepatic blood flow and interfere with the delivery of amide to the liver for biotransformation.[9] An increasing risk for toxic overdose is possible. Caution should be used when administering large doses of lidocaine. Not all antihypertensives behave in this manner. Dental hygienists should use a current *PDR* for specific drug interactions.

MEDICAL CONDITIONS THAT AFFECT THE USE OF AMIDE LOCAL ANESTHETICS

See Table 7.13 for a summary of medical conditions and affect the use of amide local anesthetics, and recommended dose or drug modifications.

Malignant Hyperthermia

Malignant hyperthermia is an inherited syndrome triggered by exposure to certain drugs used for general anesthesia and the neuromuscular blocking agent succinylcholine. It is a rare occurrence affecting approximately 1:15,000 children and 1:50,000 adults.[9] It can produce drastic uncontrolled skeletal muscle oxidative metabolism, which overwhelms the body's capacity to supply oxygen, remove carbon dioxide, and regulate body temperature, eventually leading to circulatory collapse and death if not treated quickly.

TABLE 7.13 Medical Conditions That Affect the Use of Local Anesthetics

Health Condition	Type of Contraindication	Reason for Modification	Local Anesthetic Dose/Drug Modification
Significant liver disease	Relative	Amides primarily metabolized in the liver increase possibility of toxic overdose	Reduce dosage of amides metabolized in the liver. Articaine is preferred
Renal dysfunction	Relative	Slight risk of toxicity with severe renal dysfunction	Use local anesthetics but use judiciously
Malignant hyperthermia	Relative	Life-threatening syndrome caused by general anesthetics	Medical consultation is recommended; use amides but reduce dosage
Methemoglobinemia	Relative	Potential for clinical cyanosis	Use amides but avoid prilocaine or topical benzocaine
Atypical plasma cholinesterase	Relative	Inability of esters to be metabolized in the plasma by cholinesterase enzymes	Should not be given ester derivative anesthetics
Pregnancy	Relative	Anesthetics are not teratogenic and pose little danger to the fetus	For the most conservative approach, use lidocaine or prilocaine anesthetics only after first trimester

The trait may never be identified in many individuals and may occur only after several episodes of anesthetic administration. Symptoms are characterized by a high fever, tachycardia, cardiac dysrhythmias, and cyanosis. Complications may be life threatening and are associated with the administration of general anesthesia.[4,9]

Although general anesthetics are known to trigger the episode, the ability for amide local anesthetics to act in the same manner is controversial. It is therefore recommended that a medical consultation be conducted before treating these patients, and when treating these patients, one should follow the guidelines from the Malignant Hyperthermia Association of the United States (MHAUS).[9,10,17–21]

Methemoglobinemia

Prilocaine (and possibly topical benzocaine) administered in high doses may produce methemoglobinemia, a rare hereditary condition characterized by the inability of the blood to bind to oxygen. Prilocaine is metabolized to *orthotoluidine* and is characterized by the presence of higher than normal levels of methemoglobin in the blood that is unable to bind and transport oxygen. Moreover, it impairs the ability of unaffected oxyhemoglobin to release its oxygen to the tissues. Clinical cyanosis of the lips and mucous membranes may be observed.[22–24]

Prilocaine is relatively contraindicated in patients with idiopathic or congenital methemoglobinemia or receiving treatment with methemoglobin-inducing agents, sickle cell anemia, anemia, or cardiac or respiratory failure evidenced by hypoxia because methemoglobin levels are increased, decreasing oxygen-carrying capacity. Moreover, prilocaine is relatively contraindicated in patients receiving acetaminophen or phenacetin, both of which produce elevations in methemoglobin levels. Lower the dose of prilocaine using the minimum effective dose or substitute with other amide anesthetics as an alternative anesthetic and topical lidocaine for benzocaine.[25–27]

Liver Disease

Biotransformation of amide local anesthetics is more complex than that of the esters. Virtually the entire metabolic process of lidocaine, mepivacaine, and bupivacaine occurs in the liver. The rate of biotransformation of these amide anesthetics is dependent on the liver function and hepatic perfusion. Therefore patients with lower than normal hepatic blood flow, hypotension, congestive heart failure, or significant liver disease (ASA III) such as cirrhosis and hepatitis B may be unable to adequately biotransform the amides that are primarily metabolized in the liver, causing an interruption in the process. Interruption of the biotransformation of amides could lead to systemic toxicity. Liver disease represents a relative contraindication to amides, and the minimal effective dose should be administered. Because articaine is primarily metabolized in the plasma, this anesthetic may provide a better choice over lidocaine, mepivacaine, and bupivacaine in some situations.

Kidney Disease

Only a small percentage of unmetabolized local anesthetics are excreted in the urine, and usual doses of anesthetics do not pose any additional risk. Toxic serum levels of anesthetic could develop in patients with significant renal dysfunction, but this occurrence is rare.

Pregnancy

Local anesthetics administered during pregnancy are not teratogenic and pose little danger to the fetus. Pregnancy is represented as a temporary contraindication relative to elective dental hygiene care, with the administration of local anesthetics.[4,9] Pregnant women can receive elective dental hygiene care with anesthesia in any trimester, in consultation with the patient's physician.[4,28] Lidocaine and prilocaine administered with epinephrine are generally considered safe for use during pregnancy. Lidocaine is the preferred drug of choice during pregnancy because of its low risk for both the mother and developing fetus, and it is not associated with methemoglobinemia (as is prilocaine). Articaine, bupivacaine, and mepivacaine are typically safe, although they should be used with caution. Topical lidocaine is considered safe during pregnancy. Topical benzocaine might be acceptable but should be used with caution.[4,28] Because of adverse effects associated with high levels of local anesthetics, it is important not to exceed the manufacturer's maximum recommended dose. The conservative approach when administering local anesthetics to a pregnant patient is to wait until the second trimester and to choose topical and injectable lidocaine.

Bleeding Disorders

A patient with a blood clotting disorder should be assessed for the potential to develop excessive bleeding as a result of puncturing a blood vessel. Local anesthetic injection techniques that pose a greater risk of positive aspirations are the posterior superior alveolar (PSA) block, inferior alveolar (IA) block, mental/incisive (M/I) block, and infraorbital (IO) block and should be avoided in favor of supraperiosteal and periodontal ligament injections or other techniques that do not pose a threat of excessive bleeding.

DENTAL HYGIENE CONSIDERATIONS

- The dental hygienist must evaluate, through a comprehensive medical history, the patient's physical ability to tolerate the administration of a local anesthetic or vasoconstrictor.
- The dental hygienist must evaluate medications that the patient is taking for the possibility of any local anesthetic/vasoconstrictor drug–drug interactions.
- The evaluation of the patient's attitude and psychological fears are important components to the preanesthetic assessment. Fear and anxiety provoke the "fight-or-flight" response.
- Medical consultation with the patient's physician or specialist should be completed as necessary before the administration of the local anesthetic agent.
- Maximum recommended doses for the selected local anesthetic drug must be calculated before administration of the agent. These doses are dependent on the patient's medical condition(s).
- Stress reduction protocols must be implemented for patients with medical conditions that could be exacerbated by stress and anxiety.
- True allergic reactions to a pure amide local anesthetic agent are extremely rare. If an allergic reaction exists, it will most likely be the result of the vasoconstrictor preservative, sodium bisulfite.
- Many patients confuse signs and symptoms of an anesthetic or vasoconstrictor overdose with an allergic reaction. Dialogue with the patient is invaluable in gaining more information regarding the patient's medical status.
- Treatment should be delayed if the patient has had a heart attack or stroke within 6 months of treatment.
- Decreased liver function increases the half-life of the amides metabolized in the liver, increasing the risk for overdose.
- Vasoconstrictors administered the same day a patient has used cocaine or methamphetamines can be life threatening.
- Preanesthetic baseline vital signs are essential to provide a standard of comparison in an emergency.
- The proper duration of anesthetic for treatment and postoperative pain control is important to reduce patient stress and anxiety. Patients who feel pain during the procedure or on the way home could have potentially adverse reactions to endogenous release of catecholamines.
- An absolute contraindication means that the drug should not be administered under any circumstances.
- A relative contraindication means that the drug can be administered but precautions should be taken, and the drug should be used judiciously.
- The dental hygienist should be familiar with all absolute and relative contraindications to local anesthetic and vasoconstrictor drugs. These contraindications should be reviewed periodically during practice.
- Nerve blocks (posterior superior alveolar [PSA], infraorbital [IO], inferior alveolar [IA], mental/incisive [M/I]) should be avoided in patients with bleeding disorders. Supraperiosteal and periodontal ligament (PDL) injections are less likely to produce a hematoma and excessive bleeding.

CASE STUDY 7.1 Local Anesthesia Medical History Considerations

A patient comes to your office for nonsurgical periodontal therapy of the mandibular right quadrant. He is very sensitive and local anesthesia will be needed. His blood pressure is 150/100 mm Hg and his weight is 180 lb. He has a history of chronic asthma and is taking Tagamet for an ulcer. Everything else is within normal limits (WNL).

Critical Thinking Questions

- What are the medical considerations when choosing a local anesthetic?
- Choose an appropriate local anesthetic for this patient.
- What treatment modifications should be made for this patient, if any?
- Are any dosage modifications indicated for the drug selected?

CASE STUDY 7.2 Local Anesthesia Medical History Considerations

A patient is in your office for nonsurgical periodontal therapy. Her blood pressure is 135/90 mm Hg and her weight is 128 lb. She has a history of malignant hyperthermia, and she is taking Elavil. Everything else is within normal limits (WNL).

Critical Thinking Questions

- What are the medical considerations when choosing a local anesthetic?
- Choose an appropriate local anesthetic for this patient.
- What treatment modifications should be made for this patient, if any?
- Are any dosage modifications indicated for the drug selected?

CASE STUDY 7.3 Local Anesthesia Medical History Considerations

A patient is in your office for nonsurgical periodontal therapy. She is very sensitive and local anesthesia will be needed. Her blood pressure is 130/85 mm Hg and her weight is 150 lb. The patient has diabetes, which is controlled. She has a history of hypertension and is taking Inderal.

Critical Thinking Questions

- What are the medical considerations when choosing a local anesthetic?
- Choose an appropriate local anesthetic for this patient.
- What treatment modifications should be made for this patient, if any?
- Are any dosage modifications indicated for the drug selected?

CHAPTER REVIEW QUESTIONS

1. Which drug is most likely to exhibit a drug interaction with epinephrine?
   A. Sulfonamides
   B. Monoamine oxidase inhibitors
   C. Tricyclic antidepressants
   D. Serotonin specific reuptake inhibitors
   E. Acetaminophen
2. Before injecting a patient with a local anesthetic with or without a vasoconstrictor, the dental hygienist should perform all of the following EXCEPT one. Which one is the EXCEPTION?
   A. Review the patient's health history
   B. Take the patient's blood pressure
   C. Determine whether the patient has a history of allergies
   D. Determine whether any contraindications exist to the selected anesthetic
   E. Administer nitrous oxide
3. Patients with bleeding disorders will most likely be susceptible to:
   A. Technique of anesthetic administration
   B. Vasoconstrictors
   C. Ester anesthetics
   D. Amide anesthetics
4. After the administration of a local anesthetic with a vasoconstrictor, the patient experiences mild itching and a slight rash. This is most likely caused by:
   A. The amide anesthetic
   B. Methylparaben
   C. Sodium bisulfite
   D. The epinephrine
5. Patients with an artificial heart valve need premedication before a local anesthetic injection.
   A. True
   B. False
6. Which of the following is an absolute contraindication to the use of vasoconstrictors?
   A. Blood pressure 175/95 mm Hg
   B. Heart attack 5 months ago
   C. Use of tricyclic antidepressants
   D. Controlled diabetes
7. Which of the following drugs is the best choice to administer when a patient has a history of hepatitis B?
   A. Mepivacaine
   B. Lidocaine
   C. Bupivacaine
   D. Articaine
8. Which of the following anesthetics should be avoided if a patient has methemoglobinemia?
   A. Bupivacaine
   B. Prilocaine
   C. Lidocaine
   D. Procaine
9. Which local anesthetic is considered the safest choice to be administered during pregnancy?
   A. Lidocaine
   B. Bupivacaine
   C. Articaine
   D. Mepivacaine
10. It is recommended to monitor a patient's blood pressure throughout treatment for symptoms of altered (increased) blood pressure when a patient is taking which of the following medications?
    A. Phenothiazines
    B. Monoamine oxidase inhibitors
    C. Nonselective beta blockers
    D. Insulin
    E. Barbiturates
11. When a patient is taking a tricyclic antidepressant and is also given levonordefrin, blood pressure enhancement is fivefold greater than with levonordefrin alone.
    A. True
    B. False
12. Select the local anesthetic that is most likely to inhibit the antibacterial activity of sulfonamides.
    A. Lidocaine
    B. Prilocaine
    C. Articaine
    D. Procaine
    E. Bupivacaine
13. Patients with atypical plasma cholinesterase should not receive which classification of drugs?
    A. All amides
    B. All esters
    C. Vasoconstrictors
    D. Sulfonamides
14. Methemoglobinemia is caused by the metabolite:
    A. Orthotoluidine
    B. Benzene
    C. Para-amino benzoic acid
    D. Xylidine
15. Which of the following treatment modifications are important for patients with alcoholism?
    A. Avoid amide local anesthetics
    B. Administer the minimal effective dose of articaine
    C. Administer the minimal effective dose of lidocaine, mepivacaine, or bupivacaine
    D. No treatment modifications are necessary for all amides
    E. Administer the minimal effective dose of epinephrine
16. Patients taking Elavil should:
    A. Not receive amide local anesthetics
    B. Receive amide local anesthetic when administered in the minimal effective dose
    C. Not receive ester local anesthetics
    D. Receive lowest effective dose of epinephrine similar to that recommended for a cardiovascularly involved patient
17. ASA II describes a patient:
    A. With a mild systemic disease that does not interfere with daily activity
    B. With a mild systemic disease that interferes with daily activity
    C. With a moderate to severe systemic disease that limits activity but is not incapacitating
    D. Who is healthy
18. Which of the following can cause a false high blood pressure reading?
    A. Blood pressure cuff is too narrow
    B. Bladder or cuff is too wide
    C. Cuff is deflated too quickly
    D. Arm is above heart level

19. Which of the following is a relative contraindication to the use of an amide local anesthetic?
    A. Patient is taking tricyclic antidepressants
    B. Patient is taking Tagamet
    C. Patient is taking monoamine oxidase inhibitors
    D. Patient has diabetes and is taking antidiabetic medication

20. A patient is considered to have tachycardia if beats per minute are greater than 80.
    A. True
    B. False

REFERENCES

1. Bowen DM, Pieren JA. *Darby and Walsh dental hygiene: theory and practice.* ed 5. St. Louis: Elsevier; 2020.
2. Malamed S. *Medical emergencies in the dental office.* ed 7. St Louis: Elsevier; 2015.
3. Haveles EB. *Applied pharmacology for the dental hygienist.* ed 8. St Louis: Elsevier; 2020.
4. Little JW, Falace DA, Miller CS, Rhodus NL. *Dental management of the medically compromised patient.* ed 9. St Louis: Elsevier; 2018.
5. Houben H, Thien T, van 't Laar A. Effect of low-dose epinephrine infusion on hemodynamics after selective and nonselective beta-blockade in hypertension. *Clin Pharmacol Ther.* 1982;31:685–690.
6. Reeves RA, Boer WH, DeLeve L, Leenen FH. Nonselective beta-blockade enhances pressor responsiveness to epinephrine, norepinephrine, and angiotensin II in normal man. *Clin Pharmacol Ther.* 1984;35:461–466.
7. Kram J, Bourne HR, Melmon KL, Maibach H. Propranolol (letter). *Ann Intern Med.* 1974;80:282.
8. Mito RS, Yagiela JA. Hypertensive response to levonordefrin in a patient receiving propranolol: report of case. *J Am Dent Assoc.* 1988;116:55–57.
9. Malamed S. *Handbook of local anesthesia.* ed 7. St Louis: Elsevier; 2020.
10. Jastak T, Yagiela J, Donaldson D. *Local anesthesia of the oral cavity.* St Louis: Saunders; 1995.
11. Schwartz HJ. Sensitivity to ingested metabisulfites; variation in the clinical presentation. *J Allergy Clin Immunol.* 1983;71:487.
12. Simon RA, Green L, Stevenson DD. The incidence of ingested metabisulfite sensitivity in an asthmatic population. *J Allergy Clin Immunol.* 1982;69:118.
13. Stevenson DD, Simon RA. Sulfites and asthma. *J Allergy Clin Immunol.* 1984;74:469–472.
14. Matheson DA, Stevenson DD, Simon RA. Precipitating factors in asthma. Aspirin, sulfites, and other drugs and chemicals. *Clin Transl Allergy.* 2015;5:34.
15. Sher TH, Schwartz HJ. Bisulfite sensitivity manifesting an allergic reaction to aerosol therapy. *Ann Allergy.* 1985;54:224–226.
16. Lockhart PB. *Dental care of the medically complex patient.* ed 5. St Louis: Wright Elsevier; 2004.
17. Becker D, Reed K. Essentials of local anesthetic pharmacology. American Dental Society of Anesthesiology. *Anesthesia Program.* 2006;53.
18. De Jong RH. *Local anesthetics.* St Louis: Mosby; 1994.
19. Bahl R. Local anesthesia in dentistry. *Anesth Prog.* 2004;51:138–142.
20. Finder RL, More PA. Adverse drug reactions to local anesthesia. *Dent Clin N Am.* 2002;46:447–457.
21. Litman R, Rosenberg H. Malignant hyperthermia: update on susceptibility testing. *JAMA.* 2005;293(23):2918–2924.
22. Gutenberg LL, Chen JW, Trapp L. Methemoglobin levels in generally anesthetized pediatric patients receiving prilocaine versus lidocaine. *Anesth Prog.* 2013;60:99–108.
23. Trapp L, Will J. Acquired methemoglobinemia revisited. *Dent Clin N Amer.* 2010;54:665–675.
24. Doko Y, Iranami H, Fujii K, Yamazaki A, Shimogai M, Hatano Y. Severe methemoglobinemia after dental anesthesia: a warning about propitocaine-induced methemoglobinemia in neonates. *J Anesth.* 2010;24:935–937.
25. Prilocaine-induced methemoglobinemia—Wisconsin, 1993. *Morb Mortal Wkly Rep.* 1994:43:555–657.
26. Bellamy MC, Hopkins PM, Halsall PJ, et al. A study into the incidence of methemoglobinemia after 'three-in-one' block with prilocaine. *Anaesthesia.* 1992;47:1084–1085.
27. Daly DJ, Davenport J, Newland MC. Methemoglobinemia following the use of prilocaine. *Br J Anaesth.* 1964;36:737–739.
28. Donaldson M, Goodchild JH. Pregnancy, breast-feeding and drugs used in dentistry. *J Am Dent Assoc.* 2012;143(8):858–864.

ADDITIONAL RESOURCES

Adams V, Marley J, McCarroll C. Prilocaine induced methaemoglobinaemia in a medically compromised patient. Was this an inevitable consequence of the dose administered? *Br Dent J.* 2007;203(10):585–587.

Bartlett SZ. Clinical observation on the effect of injections of local anesthetics preceded by aspiration. *Oral Surg.* 1972;33:520–525.

Buckley JA, Ciancio SG, McMullen JA. Efficacy of epinephrine concentration in local anesthesia during periodontal surgery. *J Periodontol.* 1984;55:653–657.

Isen DA. Articaine: pharmacology and clinical use of a recently approved local anesthetic. *Dent Today.* 2000;19:72–77.

Jacobs W. Local anaesthesia and vasoconstrictive additional components. *Newslett Int Fed Dent Anesthesiol Soc.* 1989;2:1–3.

Jacobs W, Ladwig B, Cichon P, Oertel R, Kirch W. Serum levels of articaine 2% and 4% in children. *Anesth Prog.* 1995;42:113–115.

Oertel R, Ebert U, Rahn R, Kirch W. The effect of age on the pharmacokinetics of the local anesthetic drug articaine. *Regional Anesth Pain Med.* 1999;24:524–528.

Sisk A. Vasoconstrictors in local anesthesia for dentistry. *Anesth Prog.* 1992;39:187–193.

van der Meer AD, Burm AG, Stienstra R, van Kleef JW, Vletter AA, Olieman W. Pharmacokinetics of prilocaine after intravenous administration in volunteers: enantioselectivity. *Anesthesiology.* 1999;90(4):988–992.

APPENDIX 7.1: SAMPLE MEDICAL HISTORY FORM IN ENGLISH/SPANISH

MEDICAL ALERT **Sample Medical History Form in English/Spanish**

Date/Fecha

Name/Nombre

Last Apellido	**First** Nombre	**Initial** Inicial	**Soc. Sec. #** Num. de Seguro Social	**Home Phone** Teléfono	**Business Phone** Teléfono del Trabajo

Address Dirección	**City** Ciudad	**State** Estado	**Zip code** Código Postal	**Occupation** Ocupación	**Employer** Empleador

Birthdate Fecha de Nacimiento	**Sex** Sexo	**Height** Estatura	**Weight** Peso	**Marital Status** Estado Civil	Dr. **Previous Dentist's Name** Nombre de su Dentista	**Previous Dentist's Phone** Núm. Telefónico de su Dentista

Dr. **Physician's Name** Nombre de su Doctor	**Phone #** Número deTeléfono	**Person to contact in case of emergency** Persona a llamar en caso de emergencia	**Phone #** Num. Telefónico

For the following questions, check yes or no, whichever applies. Your answers will be considered confidential. Please note that during each of your visits you will be asked questions about your responses to this questionnaire and there may be additional questions concerning your health.
Para las siguentes preguntas, marque si o no para la respuesta que mejor aplique. Sus respuestas serán consideradas confidenciales. Por favor note que durante su visita inicial será cuestionado sobre sus respuestas a ésta forma y posiblemente habrá preguntas adicionales relacionadas con su salud.

Yes SI	**No** No	**Check each item.** Marque cada pregunta	**Provider's comments** Comentarios del Proveedor
		Are you in good health? ¿Está en buena salud?	
		Are you currently under the care of a physician? If not, when was your last visit? ¿Está bajo cuidado médico?	
		Has there been any change in your general health within the past year? ¿Hubo algún cambio en su salud durante el año pasado?	
		Have you had any serious illness operation, or been hospitalized? ¿Ha tenido una enfermedad seria, operación o ha sido hospitalizado?	
		Have you had any problems with or during dental treatment? ¿Ha tenido algún problema durante un tratamiento dental?	
		Are you allergic to or had reactions to any medications including local anesthetics? If yes, please list. ¿Sufre de alergias o ha tenido alguna reacción alérgica a alguna medicina, incluyendo la anestesia local?	
		Do you have any other allergies (metals, latex, food, pollen, etc.)?	
		Please check below if you have or had any of the following diseases or problems. *Por favor marque en las lineas debajo si padece o ha padecido de alguna enfermadad o problema mencionado.*	
		Artificial heart valves or shunts Válvulas cardiacas dañadas, válvulas cardiacas artificiales, marca pasos, soplo de corazón o fiebre reumática	
		Cardiovascular disease (heart trouble, heart attack, angina, high blood pressure, hardening of the arteries, stroke, etc.) Enfermedad cardiovascular como problemas del corazón, ataque cardiaco, angina de pecho, alta presión, endurecimiento de las arterias, infarto, etc.	
		Have you taken Cortisone in the last two years?	

Yes SI	No No	Check each item. Marque cada pregunta	Provider's comments Comentarios del Proveedor
		Were you born with any heart problems? ¿Nacío con algún problema cardiaco (del corazón)?	
		Sinus trouble Problemas de sinusitis	
		Asthma, hayfever, or skin rashes Asma o catarro asmático	
		Fainting spells, seizures, epilepsy or convulsions Desmayos, convulsiones o ataques epilépticos	
		Persistent diarrhea, weight loss, or vomiting Diarrea persistente, pérdida de peso o vómitos	
		Diabetes (sugar problems) Diabetis (azúcar alta en la sangre)	
		Hepatitis, yellow jaundice, cirrhosis, or liver disease Hepatitis, itericia, cirrosis u alguna otra enfermedad hepática(del higado)	
		AIDS or HIV infection SIDA (Sindrome de Immunodeficiencia Adquirida) or VIH (Virus de Immunodeficiencia Humana)	
		Thyroid problems (goiter) Problemas con las glándulas tiroides	
		Respiratory problems, emphysema, bronchitis, black lung, etc. Problemas respiratorios, enfisema, bronquitis, etc.	
		Arthritis or painful swollen joints Artritis o inflamación en las coyonturas	
		Have you ever had a joint replacement? Utiliza prótesis (ex: coyonturas, válvulas, aparatos auditivos, implantes, etc.) además de la dentadura	
		Kidney trouble or dialysis treatment Algún problema con los riñones o le han hecho diálisis	
		Tuberculosis or positive TB skin test Tuberculosis o ha salido positivo en un examen de tuberculosis	
		Anemia or blood disorders Anemia o alguna otra enfermedad sanguinea (de la sangre)	
		Gonorrhea, syphilis, herpes, or other similar diseases Gonorrea, sífilis, herpes u otra enfermedad parecida	
		Problems with mental health or nerves Trastornos mentales o nerviosos	
		Cancer Cáncer	
		Stomach ulcer, hyperacidity, or other GI problems Úlceras estomacales, acidez u otros problemas gastrointestinales	
		Do you use tobacco or snuff products? ¿Fuma o mastica tabaco?	
		Have you been diagnosed with alcoholism? ¿Ha sido diagnosticado(a) con alcoholismo o esta recuperandose del mismo?	
		Do you have vision or hearing problems? Problemas visuales o auditivos	
		Do you use recreational drugs? ¿Usa drogas recreativas?	
		Are you pregnant or nursing a baby? ¿Está embarazada o amamantando?	

Are you taking any medicine(s), including any non-prescription medicine or natural remedies? If yes, please list below in left column.
¿Está tomando algún medicamento, incluyendo medicinas sin receta médica o suplementos naturales? (ejemplo; pastillas anticonceptivas, calcio, ginseng ajo etc.)

Medication Name:	Condition Used For:	Dental Implications: (Provider Comments)	Resource: (Provider Comments)

I certify that I have read and understand the above questionnaire, and have answered the questions willingly, truthfully, and to the best of my ability.
Yo certifico que he leído y comprendido este cuestionario y que mi condición médica puede afectar mi salud y tratamiento dental. He respondido a las preguntas voluntariamente, con sinceridad y a lo mejor de mi abilidad.

______________________________ ______________

Signature of Patient or Legal Guardian **Date**
Firma del Paciente o Tutor Legal Fecha

______________________________ ______________

Signature of Dental Provider **Date**
Firma del Dentista o Profesorado Fecha

Vital signs: Blood Pressure __________ **Pulse** __________ **Respiration** __________

From the University of New Mexico, Division of Dental Hygiene

8

Determining Drug Doses

Demetra Daskalos Logothetis, RDH, MS

LEARNING OBJECTIVES

1. Define maximum recommended dose (MRD) for a local anesthetic and discuss factors involved.
2. Name the steps to calculate MRDs for local anesthetics and perform calculations as needed.
3. Discuss why some cartridges are labeled 1.7 mL and others are labeled 1.8 mL and how it affects the drug calculation.
4. Calculate the following:
   - Maximum number of cartridges based on MRD
   - Milligrams of anesthetic administered
   - Additional dosages of the same drug
   - Additional dosages of different drugs
5. Discuss the factors involved in calculating MRDs for vasoconstrictors for medically compromised and elderly patients and perform calculations as needed.
6. Discuss the issues to take into consideration when giving a local anesthetic to children and perform pediatric dosage calculations as needed.
7. Name the two potentially limiting drugs in the local anesthetic solution when administering local anesthetics with vasoconstrictors.
8. Discuss vasoconstrictor dilutions and the MRD for vasoconstrictor drugs.
9. Name the steps to calculate vasoconstrictor drug doses and perform calculations as needed.
10. Calculate milligrams of vasoconstrictor administered and additional doses of the same vasoconstrictor.
11. Determine the limiting drug when a local anesthetic agent and a vasoconstrictor are combined in an anesthetic cartridge.

INTRODUCTION

All drugs, if administered in excess, can produce an overdose reaction. To increase the safety of the patient during the administration of local anesthetics and vasoconstrictors, the dental hygienist must always administer the smallest clinically effective dose. This is especially critical when administering anesthetics and vasoconstrictors to the medically compromised patient, children, and the elderly. Each cartridge of solution may contain either one drug (the anesthetic) or two drugs (the anesthetic and vasoconstrictor, including a preservative for the vasoconstrictor). The maximum recommended dose (MRD) of the solution that contains both the anesthetic and vasoconstrictor is dependent on which of the two drugs reaches its MRD first. The drug that limits the total amount of volume delivered is referred to as the limiting drug (see Box 8.1).

All drugs have maximum dose levels, including local anesthetics and vasoconstrictors, which are determined by the manufacturer based on results from animal and human studies. These doses can be found in the product inserts. The maximum doses determined by the manufacturer have been approved by the U.S. Food and Drug Administration (FDA). The dental hygienist must determine the maximum dose of injectable local anesthetic based on the treatment to be delivered and the health status of the patient. The information presented in this chapter assists the dental hygienist in determining the appropriate dosage to be administered.

MAXIMUM RECOMMENDED DOSES OF LOCAL ANESTHETIC DRUGS

The MRD for a local anesthetic is defined as the highest amount of an anesthetic drug that can be safely administered without complication to a patient while maintaining its efficacy. MRDs should also be adjusted to consider the patient's overall health and any mitigating medical factors that could hamper the patient's recovery. These amounts are determined based on maximum dosage for each appointment. The dosage calculation is based on the patient's weight and is calculated based on milligrams per pound (mg/lb) or milligrams per kilogram (mg/kg). These values were modified from the first edition of this text (2012), which were more conservative and did not always follow the manufacturer recommended doses. This edition, as in the second edition, will follow the FDA-approved MRDs (Table 8.1 and Appendix 8.1). In most cases these values are significantly higher than previously listed recommendations. The dental hygienist can continue to use the conservative dosages as they offer an additional level of safety while maintaining efficacy and patient comfort and do not exceed the FDA-approved MRDs (see Appendix 8.2). Fortunately, maximum doses are unlikely to be reached for most dental hygiene procedures. If the dental hygiene care plan involves nonsurgical periodontal therapy (NSPT) for a quadrant, the administration of one to two cartridges often suffices. There is seldom a need to administer more than four cartridges during an appointment involving dental hygiene care. Table 8.1[1,2] provides the FDA-approved MRDs per appointment for each local anesthetic. Note that even though most individuals will respond predictably to an anesthetic agent, there is still a wide range of patient responses to blood levels of local anesthetics. Hyporesponders to elevated local anesthetic blood levels will not experience any adverse reactions until the blood levels are well above the MRDs. In contrast, hyperresponders may show adverse reactions at blood levels that are considerably lower than the doses normally necessary to exhibit such reactions. To maintain safety during the administration of local anesthetics to all patients, the clinician cannot assume

BOX 8.1 Limiting Drug

The limiting drug of the anesthetic solution is determined when an anesthetic drug and a vasoconstrictor drug are combined into one cartridge. The limiting drug is the drug (local anesthetic or vasoconstrictor) that reaches its maximum recommended dose (MRD) first based upon the patient's medical status. For example, using 2% lidocaine 1:100,000 epinephrine, to determine the limiting drug for a 150-lb healthy patient using the U.S. Food and Drug Administration (FDA)-approved MRD in milligrams/pounds, the calculation below demonstrates that the limiting drug will be the vasoconstrictor and not the anesthetic drug, lidocaine.

Begin by calculating the number of maximum cartridges for both drugs:

For the local anesthetic (lidocaine) calculation

2% = 20 mg/mL x 1.8 mL = 36 mg (in one cartridge of lidocaine)

150 x 3.2 mg/lb = 480 mg MRD

480 mg ÷ 36 mg = 13.3 cartridges maximum

For the vasoconstrictor (epinephrine) calculation

1:100,000 = 1 mg/100 mL = 0.01 mg/1 mL x 1.8 mL = 0.018 mg (in one cartridge of 1:100,000 epinephrine dilution)

0.2 mg (MRD of vasoconstrictor for healthy patient) ÷ 0.018 mg = 11.1 cartridges maximum

Because 11.1 cartridges of epinephrine is lower than 13.3 cartridges of lidocaine, epinephrine is the limiting drug in this example.

that administering the all-patient MRD means that the individual is safe. Therefore the clinician should always administer the smallest clinically effective dose to all patients.

Calculation of Maximum Recommended Dose for Local Anesthetic Drugs

All MRDs per appointment are calculated first based on milligrams (see Box 8.2 for dosing facts). Information needed to complete the MRD calculation includes:

1. The patient's weight
2. The drug concentration expressed as a percentage: 0.5%, 2%, 3%, or 4%
3. The amount of local anesthetic in a standard cartridge (1.8 mL for US cartridges)
4. The MRD for the selected anesthetic based upon milligrams per pound or milligrams per kilogram (see Table 8.1)

For clinical practicality, this amount can then be converted to maximum number of cartridges per appointment and maximum number of milliliters per appointment. The following are steps for calculating MRDs (see Table 8.2 for summary of steps).

Step 1: Obtain Necessary Patient Information

The dental hygienist must first obtain the necessary patient information before beginning the drug calculation. The selection of the anesthetic drug that will be administered will be determined by the treatment to be rendered and the patient's medical history (see Chapter 7). Once the drug is determined, the dental hygienist must obtain the patient's weight to determine the local anesthetic calculation.

Step 2: Calculate Milligrams of Selected Anesthetic Drug in One Cartridge

The number of milligrams of anesthetic drug in one cartridge is determined by the percentage of local anesthetic drug per milliliter of solution. Most standard local anesthetic cartridges are designed to contain 1.8 mL of solution; some manufacturers label their cartridges as containing a minimum of 1.7 mL of solution (Box 8.3).

TABLE 8.1 FDA Maximum Recommended Doses of Local Anesthetic Agents per Appointment for Healthy Patients*

Anesthetic	mg/lb	mg/kg	Maximum Milligrams per Appointment
Lidocaine	3.2	7.0	500 mg
Mepivacaine	3.0	6.6	400 mg
Prilocaine	3.6	8.0	600 mg
Articaine	3.2	7.0	None listed
Bupivacaine	0.9**	2.0**	90 mg

FDA, U.S. Food and Drug Administration.

*Maximum recommended dose (MRD) listed for the local anesthetic drug is determined for the anesthetic drug only, not the vasoconstrictor; dosages must be reduced for children, the elderly, and medically compromised patients.

**Canadian recommendations; no US recommendations available.

BOX 8.2 Dosing Facts for Local Anesthetic Agents

Converting Pounds to Kilograms: 1 kilogram (kg) = 2.2 pounds (lb)

lb to kg = lb ÷ 2.2 = kg

kg to lb = kg x 2.2 = lb

Cartridge Facts

1 cartridge = 1.8 mL of solution

Some cartridges are marketed as a minimum of 1.7 mL of solution. In these cases, 1.8 mL will be used in all calculation formulas.

1 cc = 1 mL

1.8 cc = 1.8 mL

1 g = 1000 mg

Local Anesthetic Concentrations

2% solution = 2 g/100 mL, so 2% = 2000 mg/100 mL or 20 mg/1 mL

3% solution = 3 g/100 mL, so 3% = 3000 mg/100 mL or 30 mg/1 mL

4% solution = 4 g/100 mL, so 4% = 4000 mg/100 mL or 40 mg/1 mL

0.5% solution = 0.5 g/100 mL, so 0.5% = 500 mg/100 mL or 5 mg/1 mL

Maximum recommended dose calculation for the local anesthetic agent is weight dependent.

Vasoconstrictor Concentrations

1:20,000 dilution = 1 g/20,000 mL = 1000 mg/20,000 mL or 1 mg/20 mL

1:50,000 dilution = 1 g/50,000 mL = 1000 mg/50,000 mL or 1 mg/50 mL

1:100,000 dilution = 1 g/100,000 mL = 1000 mg/100,000 mL or 1 mg/100 mL

1:200,000 dilution = 1 g/200,000 mL = 1000 mg/200,000 mL or 1 mg/200 mL

Maximum recommended dose calculation for the vasoconstrictor is not weight dependent; it is dependent on healthy patients versus patients with significant cardiovascular disease or patients needing treatment modifications.

This small variance will not alter the calculation formula. Therefore 1.8 mL will be used in all dosing formulas even for cartridges labeled as containing 1.7 mL. Some regional local anesthesia board examinations are currently requiring the candidate to calculate drug doses based on 1.7 mL rather than the recommended 1.8 mL, although others are using 1.8 mL. A special appendix has been included at the end of this chapter to assist licensure candidates who will be taking board examinations requiring the calculation based on 1.7 mL. As a student dental hygienist, it is important to thoroughly review the candidate's guide before taking any written or clinical examination. The candidate's guide will

TABLE 8.2 Summary of Steps for Calculating Maximum Recommended Dose of Local Anesthetic Agents in Milligrams, Number of Cartridges, and Milliliters

Step 1	Obtain necessary patient information.
Step 2	***Determine the Number of Milligrams in One Cartridge of Anesthetic*** Take the percentage of the drug and multiply by 10. Take the answer and multiply by 1.8 = **milligrams of anesthetic per cartridge.** (See Table 8.3.)
Step 3	***Calculate Patient's MRD of Anesthetic in Milligrams*** Convert pounds to kilograms if using this unit of measurement: lb ÷ 2.2 = kg. Multiply pounds by mg/lb or kilograms by mg/kg (memorize Table 8.1). This number may be different for each anesthetic and provides **the MRD in milligrams** for the patient, based on his or her weight.
Step 4	***Convert Maximum Recommended Dose of Anesthetic to Cartridges*** Divide the MRD (step 3) by the number of mg of the selected anesthetic per cartridge (step 2) = **maximum number of cartridges.**
Step 5	***Convert Maximum Cartridges of Anesthetic to Milliliters*** Multiply maximum number of cartridges (step 4) by 1.8 (mL in one cartridge) = **maximum number of milliliters.** (This unit of measurement is not always needed.)

MRD, Maximum recommended dose.

provide you with the information you need to successfully pass the examination. If you are unsure which guidelines an examination will be testing you on, contact the examination agency for clarification (Box 8.3 and Appendix 8.3).

All anesthetics are labeled with a percentage concentration. A 100% local anesthetic solution contains 1 g (1000 mg) of anesthetic per milliliter of solution, a 10% local anesthetic solution contains 0.1 g (100 mg) of anesthetic per milliliter of solution, and a 1% local anesthetic solution contains 0.01 g (10 mg) of local anesthetic per milliliter of solution. You can therefore calculate the number of milligrams of local anesthetic drug per milliliter of solution by multiplying the percent concentration of local anesthetic drug by 10 mg. A 2% lidocaine solution contains 2 × 10 mg/mL = 20 mg/mL of lidocaine and a 3% mepivacaine solution contains 3 × 10 mg/mL = 30 mg/mL of mepivacaine. Because there is 1.8 mL of solution in one cartridge, the dental hygienist should multiply the number of milligrams in 1 mL of solution by 1.8 to determine the number of milligrams of the selected anesthetic in one cartridge.

2% lidocaine: 2 × 10 mg/mL = 20 mg/mL × **1.8 mL per cartridge** = 36 mg (in one cartridge of a 2% solution)

Table 8.3 lists the local anesthetic concentrations in percentage of solution, milligrams per milliliter, and total number of milligrams per cartridge.

Step 3: Calculate Patient's Maximum Recommended Dose of Anesthetic in Milligrams

The patient's MRD is the dose in milligrams that can be delivered to a patient in one appointment. For most dental hygiene procedures requiring anesthesia, this dose will most likely never be reached. The dosage calculation for the MRD is based on the patient's weight and can be calculated based on maximum milligrams per pound (mg/lb) or maximum milligrams per kilogram (mg/kg) (see Table 8.1). To calculate the number of milligrams the patient can receive of the chosen anesthetic, multiply the patient's weight (lb or kg) by the MRD (mg/lb or mg/kg) listed in Table 8.1 (see Box 8.4 for dosage calculation example). The absolute MRD is the absolute maximum dose that any patient can receive per appointment, regardless of his or her weight. For example, a 200-lb patient can receive only 500 mg of 2% lidocaine even though the calculated number based on the patient's weight is higher. (Table 8.1 lists MRDs for each local anesthetic drug.)

BOX 8.3 Volume of Local Anesthetic per Cartridge

Most standard local anesthetic cartridges distributed in North America are designed to contain 1.8 mL of solution, and drug calculations are based upon this amount. Some manufacturers market their anesthetics as 1.7 mL of solution. This variation is in compliance with the U.S. Food and Drug Administration (FDA) regulations stating that manufacturers must label their anesthetics with a guaranteed amount of solution, even if this amount is lower than the actual amount in the cartridge. Although the standard local anesthetic cartridge can contain 1.8 mL of solution, the average dental cartridge in the United States contains 1.76 mL of solution. The reason for this discrepancy is that local anesthetic solutions are filled by a machine on a conveyor belt, causing slight solution variations of +/− 0.1. Therefore some manufacturers will guarantee and label their anesthetics with a *minimum* of 1.7 mL of solution. This will not alter the calculation formula of an anesthetic labeled as 1.7 mL and will provide a margin of safety if 1.8 mL of solution is actually in the cartridge. All drug calculations in this chapter and throughout the text will be based upon 1.8 mL of solution in one cartridge of anesthetic.

Although 1.8 mL is the recommended unit for the drug calculation, some regional local anesthesia board examinations are currently requiring candidates to calculate drug doses based upon the labeled amount of solution: 1.7 mL depending on the manufacturer. Licensure candidates must be prepared to alter the calculation formulas with the specified amount of solution identified on the examination. Therefore a special appendix has been included with this chapter that will provide calculation information and dosage tables to assist dental hygiene local anesthesia licensure candidates who will be taking examinations that require dosage calculations based on 1.7 mL of solution in one cartridge. Licensure candidates should thoroughly read the examination candidate's guide to determine the expected dose requirements for that particular examination (see Appendix 8.3).

TABLE 8.3 Calculation of Milligrams per Cartridge for Varying Local Anesthetic Concentrations

Local Anesthetic Concentration (%)	Number of mg/mL	Multiply by Milliliters in One Cartridge of Anesthetic (mg/mL x 1.8)	Number of mg/Cartridge
2%	20	1.8	36
3%	30	1.8	54
4%	40	1.8	72
0.5%	5	1.8	9

Step 4: Convert Maximum Recommended Dose of Anesthetic to Cartridges

Because local anesthetic agents are administered in single-use cartridges, the dental hygienist must convert the MRD in milligrams

BOX 8.4 Dosage Calculation of Maximum Recommended Dose for Lidocaine 2% for a 120-Pound Patient

Maximum recommended dose (MRD) can be calculated based on mg/lb or mg/kg as listed in Table 8.1.

To calculate milligrams of drug per unit of body weight, *milligrams per pound (mg/lb)*

120 lb × **3.2 (mg/lb)** = 384 mg (MRD)

To calculate milligrams of drug per unit of body weight, *milligrams per kilogram (mg/kg)*

To convert pounds to kilograms, divide the pounds by 2.2.

120 ÷ **2.2** = 54.5 kg × **7 (mg/kg)** = 381.5 mg (MRD)

BOX 8.5 Dosage Calculation of Maximum Number of Cartridges for 2% Lidocaine for a 120-Pound Patient

2% = 36 mg/cartridge (see Table 8.3 and Box 8.2)

Maximum recommended dose (MRD) = 381.5 mg (see Box 8.4)

Divide MRD (381.5 mg) by the number of mg per cartridge of lidocaine (36 mg):

381.5 mg ÷ **36 mg** = 10.5 cartridges

BOX 8.6 Dosage Calculation of Maximum Number of Milliliters for 2% Lidocaine for a 120-Pound Patient

Calculating this dose is not always needed.

2% = 36 mg/cartridge (see Table 8.3 and Box 8.2)

Maximum recommended dose (MRD) = 381.5 mg (see Box 8.4)

Maximum cartridges = 10.5 cartridges (see Box 8.5)

Multiply number of cartridges (10.5) by 1.8 mL of solution in one cartridge:

10.5 × **1.8 mL** = 18.9 mL

(described in step 3) to the maximum number of cartridges to make this clinically practical. This is accomplished by dividing the MRD in milligrams (step 3) by the number of milligrams per cartridge of anesthetic (step 2, see Box 8.5 for dosage calculation example).

Step 5: Convert Maximum Cartridges of Anesthetic to Milliliters

In one cartridge of solution there is 1.8 mL. To convert the maximum number of cartridges to maximum number of milliliters, multiply the number of cartridges by 1.8 (see Box 8.6 for dosage calculation example).

To convert milliliters to cartridges divide the milliliters by 1.8. This step is useful when calculating milligrams administered when less than an entire cartridge was administered (discussed next).

CALCULATING MILLIGRAMS OF ANESTHETIC ADMINISTERED

To calculate the milligrams of anesthetic administered, multiply the number of cartridges administered by the number of milligrams of anesthetic in each cartridge. If the dental hygienist administered two cartridges of a 3% drug (mepivacaine):

2 (cartridges 3% mepivacaine) × **54 mg/cartridge** (see Table 8.3) = 108 mg of 3% mepivacaine administered

Then, the number of milligrams administered is the measurement that should be used for chart documentation. Therefore the dental hygienist should document that the patient received 108 mg of 3% mepivacaine.

Calculating Milligrams of Anesthetic Administered of Less Than an Entire Cartridge

If the dental hygienist administered less than an entire cartridge, the dental hygienist should determine how much of the cartridge was administered in mL, then convert mL to cartridges and multiply the number of cartridges administered by the number of milligrams of anesthetic in each cartridge. Helpful tips include the following:

- Some manufacturers place volume indicators on the anesthetic cartridges, allowing the clinician to deposit precise volumes of anesthetic or to determine precisely how much anesthetic was delivered (Fig. 8.1).
- If the cartridge does not have a volume indicator label, the clinician can determine the local anesthetic volume administered by the width of the rubber stopper. Each rubber stopper width deposits approximately 0.2 mL of solution from a 1.8-mL cartridge (Fig. 8.2).
- If the dental hygienist deposited two cartridges and three stopper widths of the third cartridge of 3% mepivacaine, the calculation of administered drug would be as follows (see Table 8.4 for summary of steps):

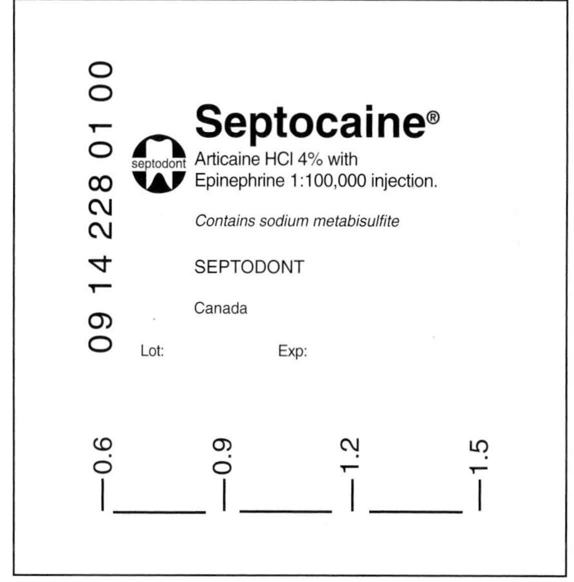

Fig. 8.1 Volume indicator label. (Courtesy Septodont, New Castle, DE.)

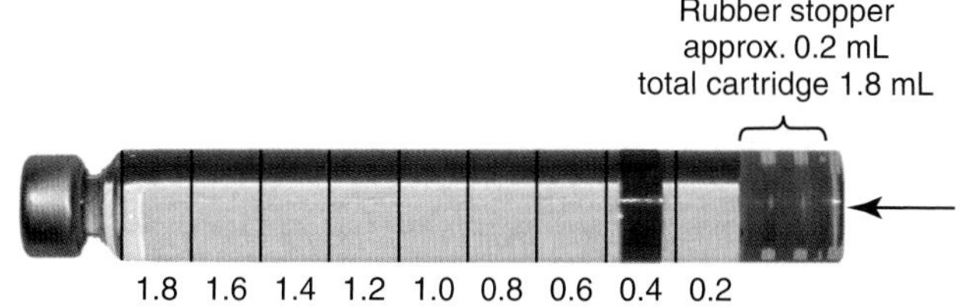

Fig. 8.2 Volume of anesthetic deposited by the width of the rubber stopper.

TABLE 8.4 Calculating Milligrams of Local Anesthetic Administered of Less Than an Entire Cartridge

Step 1	***Determine How Many Milliliters of the Cartridge was Administered.*** Number of stopper widths administered x 0.2 mL
Step 2	***Add the Number of Milliliters of Full Cartridge(s) Administered (if applicable) to the Number of Milliliters Calculated Above in Step 1.*** Number of cartridges x 1.8 = mL + number of mL calculated from step 1 = total number of mL administered (If only a partial amount of one cartridge was administered, then this step is not necessary)
Step 3	***Convert Milliliters Administered to Cartridges.*** Total number of milliliters administered in step 2 ÷ 1.8 = total cartridges administered
Step 4	***Convert Cartridges to Milligrams.*** Total cartridges administered x mg of selected anesthetic or vasoconstrictor in one cartridge = milligrams administered (see Tables 8.2 and 8.3).

Step 1: Determine how many milliliters of the third cartridge was administered:

$$3 \text{ stoppers widths} \times \mathbf{0.2\ mL} = 0.6 \text{ mL of the third cartridge was administered of } 3\% \text{ mepivacaine}$$

Step 2: Add the number of milliliters of full cartridge(s) administered to the number of milliliters calculated in step 1. If only a partial amount of one cartridge was administered, then this step is not necessary:

$$\begin{aligned} &1.8 \text{ mL (in one cartridge)} \\ &\times 2 \text{ (cartridges administered)} \\ &= 3.6 \text{ mL} + \mathbf{0.6\ mL} \text{ (of third cartridge)} \\ &= 4.2 \text{ mL administered} \end{aligned}$$

Step 3: Convert milliliters administered to cartridges:

$$4.2 \text{ mL} \div \mathbf{1.8} = 2.33 \text{ cartridges administered of } 3\% \text{ mepivacaine}$$

Step 4: Convert cartridges to milligrams:

$$2.33 \text{ cartridges} \times \mathbf{54\ mg} = 125.8 \text{ mg administered of } 3\% \text{ mepivacaine}$$

CALCULATING ADDITIONAL DOSES OF THE SAME DRUG

If the patient weighs 120 lb, and the dental hygienist will be administering 3% mepivacaine, the patient's MRD is 360 mg.

$$120 \times \mathbf{3.0\ mg/lb} = 360 \text{ mg MRD}$$
or
$$120 \div 2.2 = 54.5 \text{ kg} \times \mathbf{6.6\ mg/kg} = 360 \text{ mg MRD}$$

As discussed earlier, if the dental hygienist administered two cartridges of 3% mepivacaine, the patient received 108 mg of the MRD of 360 mg. To determine how many more milligrams of drug (mepivacaine) this patient can receive, subtract the MRD (360 mg) by the dose administered (108 mg).

$$360 \text{ mg} - 108 \text{ mg} = 252 \text{ mg}$$

The patient can receive 252 mg more of 3% mepivacaine.

To determine how many more cartridges this patient can receive, divide 252 mg by 54 mg (3% mepivacaine in one cartridge):

$$252 \text{ mg} \div \mathbf{54\ mg/cartridge} = 4.6 \text{ cartridges}$$

The patient can receive 4.6 additional cartridges of 3% mepivacaine.

CALCULATING ADDITIONAL DOSES OF DIFFERENT LOCAL ANESTHETIC DRUGS

In some instances, the dental hygienist may need to administer a different anesthetic drug to a patient after a drug has already been administered. Although this is uncommon, the situation may arise, and the dental hygienist must know how to calculate the amount of the new drug he or she can safely administer. There is no guaranteed formula to calculate this number.[2] However, a commonly used method to ensure that the total dose of the two drugs does not exceed the MRD of the most toxic drug is as follows: The lower of the two individual MRDs should be used to calculate the amount of the second drug.[2] The following steps describe this method for a 130-lb healthy patient using 2% lidocaine as drug number one (two cartridges already administered) and switching to 4% prilocaine as drug number two, as an example (see Table 8.5 for summary of steps):

Step 1: Determine a second anesthetic drug that the patient may safely receive. Consider the patient's medical history to ensure that the patient does not have any contraindications to the new drug (for this example, prilocaine is drug number two).

Step 2: Determine how much anesthetic of drug number one (2% lidocaine) has been administered. In this example, two cartridges of 2% lidocaine were administered.

$$\begin{aligned} 2\% \text{ solution} &= 20 \text{ mg/mL} \times \mathbf{1.8\ mL\ per\ cartridge} \\ &= 36 \text{ mg in one cartridge of } 2\% \text{ lidocaine} \end{aligned}$$

$$\begin{aligned} &2 \text{ cartridges already administered:} \\ &2 \times \mathbf{36\ mg/cartridge} \\ &= 72 \text{ mg of } 2\% \text{ lidocaine was administered} \end{aligned}$$

TABLE 8.5 Summary of Steps to Calculating Additional Doses of Different Local Anesthetic Drugs

Step 1	Review patient's medical history to determine appropriateness of new drug (drug number two).
Step 2	Calculate how many milligrams of drug number one have been administered (number of mg in one cartridge [Table 8.3] × number of cartridges administered).
Step 3	Calculate MRD of drug number two. Compare with MRD of drug number one (already determined) and use the lower of the two MRDs for the calculation in step 4.
Step 4	Subtract the lower of the two MRDs (step 3) by the total number of milligrams of drug number one already administered (step 2). This gives you the new MRD of drug number two.
Step 5	Calculate how many milligrams are in one cartridge of drug number two (Table 8.3). Divide the new MRD (step 4) by the number of milligrams in one cartridge of drug number two to determine how many cartridges of drug number two can be safely administered.

MRD, Maximum recommended dose.

Step 3: Calculate the MRD of drug number two (4% prilocaine) and use the lower of the two MRDs as the new MRD. The MRD for lidocaine (413 mg for the 130-lb patient) should have already been determined. This example will be using maximum mg/kg to determine MRD.

130 lb ÷ 2.2 = 59 kg × **8.0 mg/kg (for prilocaine)**
= 472 mg MRD

130 lb ÷ 2.2 = 59 kg × **7.0 mg/kg (for lidocaine)**
= 413 mg MRD

Lidocaine is the lower of the two MRDs and will be used for the remainder of the calculation.

Step 4: Subtract the MRD (413 mg, step 3) by the number of milligrams already administered (step 2):

413 mg − 72 mg = **341 mg** of prilocaine may be administered

Step 5: To make this clinically practical, the number of cartridges of prilocaine that can be administered should be calculated. Therefore divide the new MRD (341 mg) by the number of milligrams in one cartridge of 4% prilocaine:

4% solution = 40 mg/mL × **1.8 mL per cartridge**
= 72 mg in one cartridge of prilocaine

341 mg ÷ **72 mg** = 4.7 cartridges of 4% prilocaine may be administered

Although it is usually uncommon to switch anesthetic drugs during treatment, the following are a few examples of when a different drug may be required:

- A cardiac patient may be receiving treatment with 2% lidocaine 1:100,000 epinephrine using the cardiac dose described in Chapter 7 for epinephrine. More anesthetic is needed for treatment, but the MRD for epinephrine for this medically compromised patient (0.04 mg) has been exceeded. The dental hygienist may safely switch to a local anesthetic drug without a vasoconstrictor (such as 3% mepivacaine or 4% prilocaine).
- The dental hygienist administers a local anesthetic drug but has no more on hand for another dose. The dental hygienist should select a different anesthetic to complete treatment.
- Inadequate anesthesia caused by a "bad batch" of anesthetic. This is highly unlikely to occur. Inadequate anesthesia is usually the result of improper technique, anatomic variations, or a too low volume of administered anesthetic. The dental hygienist should attempt to readminister the anesthetic, adjusting his or her technique using troubleshooting procedures described in Chapters 12 and 13.

MAXIMUM RECOMMENDED DOSE OF ANESTHETIC FOR MEDICALLY COMPROMISED PATIENTS AND ELDERLY PATIENTS

MRDs of the local anesthetic agent should be decreased for patients with medically compromised situations (see Chapter 7) and elderly patients.

Certain medical conditions described in Chapter 7 may significantly increase the half-life of the administered drug, causing an increase in blood plasma levels of the drug, thus increasing the risk of an overdose. Moreover, older patients' organ functions may be reduced, decreasing the effectiveness of the organs to biotransform the administered anesthetic, also increasing the risk of overdose. There is no guaranteed formula to calculate this number. Therefore the lowest effective dose should be administered, significantly lowering the MRD based on body weight. The dental hygienist should review the dental hygiene care plan, taking into consideration the necessity of lowering the patient's MRD.[2]

The care plan should minimize the extent of treatment completed in one appointment. For example, an appointment for NSPT for two quadrants that could normally be completed in one appointment could be completed in two shorter appointments rather than one longer appointment. This would decrease the amount of local anesthetic needed per appointment, providing safer treatment to the medically compromised or elderly patient.

MAXIMUM RECOMMENDED DOSE OF ANESTHETIC FOR PEDIATRIC PATIENTS

Considerable attention must be given to local anesthetic drug administration to children. Toxic effects may be caused by the administration of large volumes of the drug. Overdose reactions are a particular risk in treating children. Local anesthetic systemic toxicity (LAST) is dose-related and occurs more frequently in small children than adults.[3,4] LAST has a greater tendency to occur in pediatric patients due to important physiologic differences between children and adults (see Chapter 14). To prevent the overestimation of body weight in a child, a standard scale should be used to provide the clinician with accurate body weight. In addition, LAST occurs more frequently when the patient is administered concomitant central nervous system depressants, such as opioid/sedative medications.[2-4] The practice of multiple-quadrant dentistry and the concomitant use of sedatives in children increase their risk of LAST. Adhering to MRDs for children and only anesthetizing the quadrants currently being treated will decrease the possibility of LAST.[4] It is suggested that the dose of a local anesthetic be adjusted downward when the child is sedated with opioids.[5] Moreover, when considering MRDs for children, consider that children's organ function may be immature. This decreases the effectiveness of the organs to biotransform the administered anesthetic, increasing the risk of overdose. In addition, calculating the child's MRD based on his or her weight may indicate that an overweight child could receive 500 mg (approximately a 156-lb child) of lidocaine. This amount of anesthetic may not be biotransformed effectively due to immature organs. Therefore the lowest effective dose should be administered in this situation, significantly lowering the MRD based on body weight.

Local anesthetic selection is equally important when treating children. Studies have shown that using a local anesthetic with a vasoconstrictor will decrease the possibility of LAST and will provide equal anesthetic soft tissue duration as a plain anesthetic such as 3% mepivacaine (see Chapter 14).[3,6–8]

The need for local anesthesia to be administered by the dental hygienist to a pediatric patient is rare because these patients typically do not require NSPT. However, in some instances, the dentist performing restorative work on children may ask the dental hygienist to administer the local anesthetic. Moreover, if a pediatric patient has back-to-back appointments, first with the dental hygienist and second with the dentist for restorative work, it may be more time efficient for the dental hygienist to administer the local anesthesia for the restorative work before moving the patient into the dentist's chair. The dental hygienist should review the care plan, taking into consideration the necessity of lowering the child's MRD.[3] The care plan should minimize the extent of treatment completed in one appointment.

TABLE 8.6 American Academy of Pediatric Dentistry Maximum Recommended Doses of Local Anesthetic Agent per Appointment for Healthy Patients

Anesthetic	mg/lb	mg/kg	Maximum Milligrams per Appointment
Lidocaine	2.0	4.4	300 mg
Mepivacaine	2.0	4.4	300 mg
Prilocaine	2.7	6.0	400 mg
Articaine	3.2	7.0	500 mg
Bupivacaine	0.6	1.3	90 mg

MRDs, Maximum recommended doses.
American Academy of Pediatric Dentistry adopted MRD values (2009). These values are current as of 2020.

Calculating Pediatric Doses

The calculation of drug dosages for children follows the same principles as adult dosages as previously described. However, as of 2020, the American Academy of Pediatric Dentistry (AAPD) recommends lower MRDs compared with the FDA-approved MRDs. The dose calculation is the same, but lower values for mg/lb or mg/kg are used (see Table 8.6 for AAPD MRDs). In addition to the calculation method already described in this chapter, another approach can be used to calculate pediatric doses for patients with lean body mass and normal body development.

The maximum dose may be determined by the application of one of the standard formulas termed *Clark's rule.*[3,6] Clark's rule determines the dose suitable for a child based on the typical adult weight of 150 lb (or 70 kg). The procedure is to take the child's weight in pounds and divide it by 150 lb, then multiply the fractional result by the AAPD dose (Table 8.6) to find the equivalent child's dosage. See Table 8.7 for a calculation example of determining the MRD using Clark's rule.[3,6] Determining the MRD based on the standard tables and using Clark's rule will not apply to children who are obese. It has been suggested that in situations with children who are obese, an ideal body weight (IBW) index should be used in the Clark's rule calculation rather than actual body weight.[8,9] IBW tables can be easily found online as a reference.

VASOCONSTRICTOR DOSES

When administering local anesthetics with vasoconstrictors, the local anesthetic solution will have two potentially limiting drugs: (1) the dose of local anesthetic drug and (2) the dose of the accompanying vasoconstrictor. Either of these agents may be the limiting drug in determining the maximum dose of any particular local anesthetic depending on the patient's medical status (see Box 8.1).

When calculating vasoconstrictor doses, the dental hygienist must have an understanding of the following:

- Dilution ratios or percentages
- Standard cartridge volume (1.8 mL of solution in one cartridge)
- MRDs for epinephrine and levonordefrin
- Health status of the patient

Local anesthetics are expressed as percentages and vasoconstrictors are expressed as dilution ratios. For example, 2% lidocaine with 1:100,000 epinephrine means that the concentration of lidocaine in the cartridge is 2% and the dilution of epinephrine is 1 gram (g) in 100,000 mL of solution. These two different drugs are in no way related and each must be considered independently.

Vasoconstrictor Dilutions

Vasoconstrictor dilutions are always expressed as a ratio. It is necessary to be able to convert this ratio to the number of milligrams of vasoconstrictor per milliliter of solution because the maximum doses are expressed in milligram amounts. For example, the maximum dose of epinephrine for a healthy adult is 0.2 mg (discussed next). It is necessary to understand that 1:1000 means that there is 1 g (1000 mg) of vasoconstrictor in 1000 mL of solution or 1 mg of vasoconstrictor in 1 mL of solution. A 1:10,000 solution contains 1 mg vasoconstrictor in 10 mL of solution or 0.1 mg of vasoconstrictor in 1 mL of solution, and a 1:100,000 solution contains 0.01 mg of vasoconstrictor in 1 mL of solution (Table 8.8).

Maximum Recommended Dose for Vasoconstrictor Drugs

The maximum doses for vasoconstrictor drugs are based on recommendations from the 1954 Special Committee of the New York Heart Association, and afterward the American Heart Association recommended the restriction of epinephrine in patients with ischemic heart

TABLE 8.7 Dosage Calculation of Maximum Recommended Dose Using Clark's Rule for Lidocaine 2% for a 50-Pound Child

The dose of local anesthetic should be reduced by the ratio of the child's weight to an adult weight of 150 lb. The following example will illustrate this calculation:

Step 1	Divide the child's weight by 150 (for this example we will be using 50 lb as the child's weight).	50 ÷ 150 = 0.33
Step 2	Multiply the MRD from Table 8.6 (American Academy of Pediatric Dentistry dosage recommendations) by the answer in step 1. For this example, 2% lidocaine will be the drug of choice.	300 mg x **0.33** = 100 mg (MRD for 50-lb child)
Step 3	Calculate the number of cartridges by dividing the number of milligrams in one cartridge of the selected anesthetic by the MRD from step 2.	100 ÷ **36** = 2.7 cartridges of 2% Lidocaine

MRD, Maximum recommended dose.

TABLE 8.8 Volume of Vasoconstrictor Drug

Concentration 1 g/mL of Solution (Dilution)	Milligrams per Milliliter	Multiply by mL in One Cartridge of Anesthetic (mg/mL x 1.8)	Number of Milligrams per Cartridge
1:20,000	0.05	1.8	0.09
1:50,000	0.02	1.8	0.036
1:100,000	0.01	1.8	0.018
1:200,000	0.005	1.8	0.009

TABLE 8.9 Maximum Recommended Doses of Vasoconstrictors

Concentration (Dilution)	Maximum Recommended Dose per Appointment: Healthy Patient	Number of Cartridges: Healthy Patient (ASA I)	Maximum Recommended Dose per Appointment: Patient With Cardiovascular Disease (ASA III or IV) or Patients Needing Treatment Modifications	Number of Cartridges: Patient With Cardiovascular Disease or Patients Needing Treatment Modifications
1:50,000 Epinephrine	0.2 mg	5.5	0.04 mg	1.1
1:100,000 Epinephrine	0.2 mg	11.1	0.04 mg	2.2
1:200,000 Epinephrine	0.2 mg	22.2	0.04 mg	4.4
1:20,000 Levonordefrin	1.0 mg	11.1	0.2 mg	2.2

disease.[2,10] Maximum doses of vasoconstrictors are calculated based on the recommended dose for a "healthy" individual and a "compromised" individual and are not dependent on the patient's weight as determined in the calculation of MRDs for the local anesthetic drug. For healthy individuals, the MRD for epinephrine is 0.2 mg per appointment and 1.0 mg per appointment for levonordefrin. When limits of vasoconstrictors are needed for patients with significant cardiovascular disease, this is referred to as the cardiac dose. The cardiac dose for epinephrine is 0.04 mg per appointment and 0.2 mg per appointment for levonordefrin. (See Table 8.9 for the MRDs of vasoconstrictors and Chapter 7 for information on "healthy" vs "compromised" conditions affecting the selection and dosage of local anesthetics and vasoconstrictors, as well as dosage modifications due to epinephrine drug–drug interactions.)

Calculating Vasoconstrictor Drug Doses

Several easy steps to follow in calculating drug doses for vasoconstrictors are described in the following sections (Box 8.7 and Table 8.10).

Step 1: Obtain Necessary Patient Information

The dental hygienist must first obtain the necessary patient information before beginning the drug calculation. The selection of the drug to be administered will be determined by the treatment to be rendered and the patient's medical history (see Chapter 7). From the patient's medical history, the dental hygienist determines whether the patient requires the cardiac dose of vasoconstrictor or the dose for a healthy patient. Once this is determined, the dental hygienist can calculate the safe dose of the selected vasoconstrictor.

BOX 8.7 Dosing Facts for Vasoconstrictors

1 cartridge = 1.8 mL of solution

Some cartridges are marketed as a minimum of 1.7 mL of solution. In these cases, 1.8 mL will be used in all formulas.

1 cc = 1 mL

1.8 cc = 1.8 mL

1 g = 1000 mg

Maximum recommended dose (MRD) calculation for the vasoconstrictor is not weight dependent.

Maximum dose of epinephrine for a healthy patient = 0.2 mg

Maximum dose of epinephrine for a patient with significant cardiovascular disease = 0.04 mg (cardiac dose)

Maximum dose of levonordefrin for a healthy patient = 1.0 mg

Maximum dose of levonordefrin for a patient with significant cardiovascular disease = 0.2 mg (cardiac dose)

TABLE 8.10 Summary of Steps for Calculating Maximum Recommended Dose for Vasoconstrictors in Milligrams, Number of Cartridges, and Milliliters

Step 1	Obtain necessary patient information utilizing the patient's medical history form.
Step 2	Calculate the milligrams (mg) of vasoconstrictor in one cartridge of the anesthetic (see Table 8.8).
Step 3	Obtain the MRD, healthy vs cardiac dose (Table 8.9).
Step 4	Convert the MRD to cartridges. Divide the MRD (step 3) by the number of mg per cartridge (step 2) = maximum number of cartridges.
Step 5	Convert maximum cartridges to milliliters. Multiply maximum number of cartridges (step 4) by 1.8 (mL per cartridge) = maximum number of mL. This step is not always needed, but is useful when calculating milligrams administered when less than an entire cartridge was administered (see Table 8.4).

MRD, Maximum recommended dose.

Step 2: Calculate Milligrams of Vasoconstrictor in One Cartridge of Anesthetic

Using a 1:100,000 epinephrine dilution as an example, this ratio contains 1 g, or 1000 mg, of vasoconstrictor diluted in 100,000 mL of solution. The ratio must be converted to the amount of vasoconstrictor per milliliter of solution because the maximum doses are expressed in milligram amounts. Because there is 1.8 mL of solution in one cartridge, this number must be multiplied by 1.8 to calculate the number of milligrams in one cartridge. In this example there is 0.018 mg of vasoconstrictor drug per cartridge (see Table 8.8). Calculation and unit conversions for each of the vasoconstrictor dilutions used in dentistry are listed in Table 8.11.

Step 3: Obtain Maximum Recommended Dose of Vasoconstrictor

Because the dose calculation for vasoconstrictors is not dependent on the patient's weight, there is no need to calculate the MRD as shown earlier in step 3 of the anesthetic drug calculation. There are only two MRDs for vasoconstrictors: (1) ***healthy patient:*** MRD 0.2 mg for epinephrine and 1.0 mg for levonordefrin, per appointment and (2) ***compromised patient:*** individuals with significant cardiovascular disease or other compromised health conditions that effect the use of vasoconstrictors, as well as dosage modifications due to epinephrine drug–drug interactions—MRD 0.04 mg for epinephrine and 0.2 mg for levonordefrin, per appointment (see Table 8.9 for maximum doses

TABLE 8.11 Calculation and Unit Conversions of Vasoconstrictor Dilutions

Ratio	Unit Conversion to mg/mL	Milligrams per Cartridge
1:20,000	$\frac{1000\,mg}{20{,}000\,mL} = \frac{1\,mg}{20\,mL} = \frac{1/20\,mg}{20/20\,mL} = \frac{0.05\,mg}{1\,mL}$ of solution	0.05 mg/mL × 1.8 mL = 0.09 mg
1:50,000	$\frac{1000\,mg}{50{,}000\,mL} = \frac{1\,mg}{50\,mL} = \frac{1/50\,mg}{50/50\,mL} = \frac{0.02\,mg}{1\,mL}$ of solution	0.02 mg/mL × 1.8 mL = 0.036 mg
1:100,000	$\frac{1000\,mg}{100{,}000\,mL} = \frac{1\,mg}{100\,mL} = \frac{1/100\,mg}{100/100\,mL} = \frac{0.01\,mg}{1\,mL}$ of solution	0.01 mg/mL × 1.8 mL = 0.018 mg
1:200,000	$\frac{1000\,mg}{200{,}000\,mL} = \frac{1\,mg}{200\,mL} = \frac{1/200\,mg}{200/200\,mL} = \frac{0.005\,mg}{1\,mL}$ of solution	0.005 mg/mL × 1.8 mL = 0.009 mg

1 gram = 1000 mg

of vasoconstrictors, and see Chapter 7 for detailed explanations of vasoconstrictor precautions).

Step 4: Convert Maximum Recommended Dose of Vasoconstrictor to Cartridges

Because local anesthetic solutions with vasoconstrictors are administered in single-use cartridges, the dental hygienist must convert the MRD in milligrams (described in step 3) to the maximum number of cartridges to make this application clinically practical. This is accomplished by dividing the MRD in milligrams (step 3) by the number of milligrams of vasoconstrictor per cartridge of anesthetic (step 2).

For a healthy patient receiving 1:100,000 epinephrine:
0.2 mg (**MRD**) ÷ 0.018 mg/cartridge = 11.1 cartridges

For patients with significant cardiovascular disease receiving 1:100,000 epinephrine:
0.04 mg (**MRD**) ÷ 0.018 mg/cartridge = 2.2 cartridges

Table 8.12 lists dosage calculations of each vasoconstrictor dilution. Because these calculations are not dependent on the patient's weight, these numbers should be memorized for the healthy and cardiac doses.

Step 5: Convert Maximum Cartridges of Vasoconstrictor to Milliliters

In one cartridge of solution, there is 1.8 mL. To convert the maximum number of cartridges to milliliters, multiply the number of cartridges by 1.8 (example 1:100,000 epinephrine healthy patient: 11.1 cartridges maximum × 1.8 mL = 19.98 mL maximum).

TABLE 8.12 Conversion of Maximum Recommended Doses of Vasoconstrictors to Maximum Number of Cartridges

Conversion of MRD (Healthy Patient = 0.2 mg) of Epinephrine to Maximum Number of Cartridges

Concentration (Dilution)	mg/Cartridge	Conversion to Maximum Number of Cartridges MRD ÷ mg per Cartridge
1:50,000	0.036	0.2 mg ÷ 0.036 mg = 5.5 cartridges
1:100,000	0.018	0.2 mg ÷ 0.018 mg = 11.1 cartridges
1:200,000	0.009	0.2 mg ÷ 0.009 mg = 22.2 cartridges

Conversion of MRD (Cardiac Dose = 0.04 mg) of Epinephrine to Maximum Number of Cartridges

Concentration (Dilution)	mg/Cartridge	Conversion to Maximum Number of Cartridges MRD ÷ mg per Cartridge
1:50,000	0.036	0.04 mg ÷ 0.036 mg = 1.1 cartridges
1:100,000	0.018	0.04 mg ÷ 0.018 mg = 2.2 cartridges
1:200,000	0.009	0.04 mg ÷ 0.009 mg = 4.4 cartridges

Conversion of MRD (Healthy Patient = 1.0 mg) of Levonordefrin to Maximum Number of Cartridges

Concentration (Dilution)	mg/Cartridge	Conversion to Maximum Number of Cartridges MRD ÷ mg per Cartridge
1:20,000	0.09	1.0 mg ÷ 0.09 mg = 11.1 cartridges

Conversion of MRD (Compromised Patient = 0.2 mg) of Levonordefrin to Maximum Number of Cartridges

Concentration (Dilution)	mg/Cartridge	Conversion to Maximum Number of Cartridges MRD ÷ mg per Cartridge
1:20,000	0.09	0.2 mg ÷ 0.09 mg = 2.2 cartridges

MRD, Maximum recommended dose.

CALCULATING MILLIGRAMS OF VASOCONSTRICTOR ADMINISTERED

Calculating the milligrams of vasoconstrictor administered uses the same principles as for calculating the milligrams administered for the anesthetic. Multiply the number of cartridges administered by the number of milligrams of vasoconstrictor in each cartridge (see Table 8.8). If the dental hygienist administered two cartridges of 2% lidocaine 1:100,000, then:

2 (cartridges) × **36 mg/cartridge**
= 72 mg of lidocaine administered

2 (cartridges) × **0.018 mg/cartridge**
= 0.036 mg of epinephrine administered

If the dental hygienist administered less than an entire cartridge, the dental hygienist should determine how much of the cartridge was administered in milliliters, then convert milliliters to cartridges and multiply the number of cartridges administered by the number of milligrams of anesthetic in each cartridge (see previous section Calculating Milligrams of Anesthetic Administered of Less Than an Entire Cartridge and Table 8.5).

Calculating Additional Doses of the Same Vasoconstrictor

If the patient's MRD of epinephrine is 0.2 mg and the dental hygienist administered two cartridges of 2% lidocaine 1:100,000 epinephrine, then the patient received 0.036 mg of the MRD of 0.2 mg. To determine how many more milligrams of drug this patient can receive, subtract the MRD by the total dose delivered:

0.2 mg − **0.036 mg** = 0.164 mg

The patient can receive 0.164 mg more of epinephrine 1:100,000.

To determine how many more cartridges this patient can receive, divide the remaining amount of epinephrine the patient can receive (0.164 mg) by the number of milligrams of vasoconstrictor in one cartridge (0.018 mg):

0.164 mg ÷ **0.018 mg** = 9.1 cartridges

The patient can receive 9.1 additional cartridges of 1:100,000 epinephrine.

DETERMINING THE LIMITING DRUG

As previously discussed, when a local anesthetic agent and a vasoconstrictor are combined in an anesthetic cartridge, the dental hygienist must determine which of the two drugs is the limiting drug. The limiting drug will be the drug that limits the amount of agent that can be safely administered based on the patient's medical status. For example, the absolute MRD of 2% lidocaine 1:100,000 epinephrine for a healthy patient is 500 mg or 13.8 cartridges of lidocaine and 0.2 mg or 11.1 cartridges of epinephrine. Because 11.1 cartridges of vasoconstrictor is the lower number, in this example the vasoconstrictor is the limiting drug. For a patient with significant cardiovascular disease, the MRD for epinephrine is 0.04 mg or 2.2 cartridges and for lidocaine is 500 mg or 13.8 cartridges. Because 2.2 cartridges is the lower number, in this example the vasoconstrictor is also the limiting drug.

DENTAL HYGIENE CONSIDERATIONS

- The maximum recommended dose (MRD) of an anesthetic containing a vasoconstrictor is dependent on which of the two drugs reaches its MRD first.
- The limiting drug is the drug that limits the total amount of volume delivered.
- The dental hygienist must obtain necessary medical history information before determining the MRD.
- The MRD for epinephrine for a healthy patient is 0.2 mg per appointment and 0.04 mg per appointment for patients with significant cardiovascular disease or dosage modifications due to epinephrine systemic disease and drug–drug interactions.
- The MRD for levonordefrin for a healthy patient is 1.0 mg per appointment and 0.2 mg per appointment for patients with significant cardiovascular disease or dosage modifications due to levonordefrin systemic disease and drug–drug interactions.
- When calculating the maximum number of cartridges for levonordefrin for a healthy or compromised patient, the calculation result will always be identical to the epinephrine 1:100,000 dilution for a healthy or compromised patient.
- The MRD of local anesthetic drugs should be decreased for patients with medically compromised health and older adults. There is no guaranteed formula; therefore the minimal effective dose should be administered.
- The MRD of local anesthetic drugs should be decreased for obese children, and considerable attention must be given to drug administration to all children.
- Clark's rule is a standard formula that may be used when calculating the MRD in children with lean or normal body weight.
- The use of ideal body weight (IBW) index is recommended when calculating the MRD for obese children.
- The calculation of the MRD for the local anesthetic is based on the patient's weight and is calculated based on mg/kg or mg/lb.
- The calculation of the MRD for vasoconstrictor is not weight dependent. It is a given value of 0.2 mg for "healthy patient" and 0.04 mg for "significant cardiovascular disease" for epinephrine, or 1.0 mg for "healthy patient" and 0.2 mg for "significant cardiovascular disease" for levonordefrin.
- Local anesthetic drugs are expressed in percentages, and vasoconstrictor drugs are expressed in ratios.

CASE STUDY 8.1 The Dentist Asks the Dental Hygienist to Switch Anesthetics

A patient is in your office for restorative work. The dentist you work for cannot achieve numbness in the patient because he says the anesthetic is "bad." He asks the dental hygienist for assistance. He administered two cartridges of 4% prilocaine 1:200,000 and tells you to switch to 2% lidocaine 1:100,000. The patient's blood pressure is 128/90 mm Hg and her weight is 140 lb. She had a history of hepatitis B 10 years ago.

Critical Thinking Questions

- What medical history issues should be considered for lidocaine?
- How many more milligrams and cartridges of lidocaine can be safely administered to this patient?
- Should the dental hygienist switch the anesthetic? Why or why not?

CHAPTER REVIEW QUESTIONS

1. What is the cardiac dose of epinephrine?
   A. 0.02 mg
   B. 0.04 mg
   C. 0.2 mg
   D. 0.4 mg
   E. 2 mg
2. A 2% local anesthetic solution means all of the following EXCEPT one. Which one is the EXCEPTION?
   A. 2 g per 100 mL
   B. 2000 mg per 100 mL
   C. 20 mg per 1 mL
   D. 2000 mg per 10 mL
3. The dental hygienist administered 2.3 cartridges of 3% mepivacaine. How many cc's were administered?
   A. 3.24 cc
   B. 4.80 cc
   C. 4.14 cc
   D. 3.98 cc
4. What is the MRD dose of 4% prilocaine for a 130-lb patient?
   A. 355 mg
   B. 370 mg
   C. 381 mg
   D. 472 mg
5. The dental hygienist administers 4 stopper widths of 2% lidocaine 1:100,000; how many milligrams was administered?
   A. 10 mg
   B. 16 mg
   C. 20 mg
   D. 25 mg
6. How many cartridges of 4% prilocaine can a healthy 150-lb patient receive?
   A. 6.8
   B. 7.5
   C. 8.0
   D. 8.3

To answer questions 7 to 13, use the following information. A 140-lb healthy patient received 2.5 cartridges of 2% lidocaine 1:100,000 epinephrine. The dental hygienist reaches for another cartridge and realizes there is no more 2% lidocaine. The dental hygienist decides to switch to 3% mepivacaine.

7. What is the maximum recommended dose for lidocaine?
   A. 420 mg
   B. 445 mg
   C. 485 mg
   D. 500 mg
8. How many milligrams of lidocaine did the dental hygienist administer?
   A. 80 mg
   B. 90 mg
   C. 75 mg
   D. 85 mg
9. What is the maximum recommended dose for mepivacaine?
   A. 400 mg
   B. 450 mg
   C. 490 mg
   D. 500 mg
10. How many more milligrams of 3% mepivacaine can be administered to this patient?
    A. 310 mg more
    B. 330 mg more
    C. 420 mg more
    D. 450 mg more
11. How many more cartridges of 3% mepivacaine can be administered to this patient?
    A. 5.7
    B. 6.8
    C. 7.3
    D. 8.0
12. How many more milliliters of 3% mepivacaine can be administered?
    A. 10.2 mL
    B. 11 mL
    C. 11.5 mL
    D. 12 mL
13. Since 2.5 cartridges of 2% lidocaine 1:100,000 was administered, how many milligrams of epinephrine was administered to this patient?
    A. 0.045 mg
    B. 0.099 mg
    C. 0.068 mg
    D. 0.088 mg
14. What is the cardiac dose for levonordefrin?
    A. 0.2 mg
    B. 0.04 mg
    C. 0.02 mg
    D. 1.0 mg
15. How many milligrams are in one cartridge of 4% articaine?
    A. 72 mg
    B. 68 mg
    C. 54 mg
    D. 9 mg
16. What is the absolute maximum dose of bupivacaine?
    A. 80 mg
    B. 70 mg
    C. 100 mg
    D. 90 mg
17. How many cartridges of 2% mepivacaine with levonordefrin can a 130-lb patient with significant cardiovascular disease receive?
    A. 2.2
    B. 1.1
    C. 4.4
    D. 5.9
18. The dental hygienist administered four cartridges of mepivacaine 2% 1:20,000 levonordefrin to a 170-lb patient. How many more cartridges of 2% mepivacaine can the dental hygienist administer to complete the treatment?
    A. 4.8 more
    B. 5.5 more
    C. 6.0 more
    D. 7.1 more

19. What is the absolute number of milligrams of epinephrine 1:200,000 a patient with significant cardiovascular disease can receive?
A. 0.072 mg
B. 0.029 mg
C. 0.039 mg
D. 0.049 mg

20. What is the maximum recommended dose for 0.5% bupivacaine for a 102-lb patient?
A. 70 mg
B. 60 mg
C. 80 mg
D. 90 mg

REFERENCES

1. American Dental Association. *ADA/PDR guide to dental therapeutics.* ed 5. Montvale: Thompson PDR; 2009.
2. Malamed SF. *Handbook of local anesthesia.* ed 7. St Louis: Elsevier; 2020.
3. Saraghi M, Moore PA, Hersh EV. Local anesthetic calculations: avoiding trouble with pediatric patients. *Gen Dent.* 2015;63(1):48–52.
4. Tarsitano JJ. Children, drugs and local anesthesia. *J Am Dent Assoc.* 1965;70(5):1153–1158.
5. Moore PA. Adverse drug reactions in dental practice: interactions associated with local anesthetics, sedatives, and anxiolytics. *J Am Dent Assoc.* 1999;130(4):541–544.
6. Moore PA, Hersh EV. Local anesthesia: pharmacology and toxicity. *Dent Clin North Am.* 2010;54(4):587–599.
7. Goebel WM, Allen G, Randall F. The effect of commercial vasoconstrictor preparations on the circulating venous serum level of mepivacaine and lidocaine. *J Oral Med.* 1980;35(4):91–96.
8. Bouillon T, Shafer SL. Does size matter? *Anesthesiology.* 1998;89:557–560.
9. Leykin Y, Pellis T, Lucca M, Lomangino G, Marzano B, Gullo A. The pharmacodynamic effects of rocuronium when dosed according to real body weight or ideal body weight in morbidly obese patients. *Anesth Analg.* 2004;99:1056–1089.
10. Special Committee of the New York Heart Association. Use of epinephrine with procaine in dental procedures. *J Am Dent Assoc.* 1955;50:108.

APPENDIX 8.1: Summary of Local Anesthetic Agents and Vasoconstrictors

Anesthetic	Concentration of Anesthetic Agent (Expressed in Percentage)	Amount of Anesthetic Agent per Cartridge	Maximum Dose of Anesthetic Agent (mg/lb)	Maximum Dose of Anesthetic Agent (mg/kg)	Maximum Recommended Dose (MRD) Anesthetic per Appointment	Number of Cartridges Needed to Reach MRD of Anesthetic	Vasoconstrictor Formulations (Expressed in Ratios)	Number of Cartridges Needed to Reach MRD of Vasoconstrictor for Healthy Adult	Number of Cartridges Needed to Reach MRD of Vasoconstrictor for Patients with Ischemic Heart Disease (ASA III or IV) or Patients Needing Treatment Modifications
Lidocaine (Xylocaine, Lignospan, Octocaine)	2%	36 mg	3.2	7.0	500 mg	13.8	1:50,000 epinephrine	5.5	1.1
						13.8	1:100,000 epinephrine	11.1	2.2
Mepivacaine (Carbocaine, Polocaine Arestocaine, Isocaine, Scandonest)	2%	36 mg	3.0	6.6	400 mg	11.1	1:20,000 Levonordefrin or Neo-Cobefrin	11.1	2.2
Mepivacaine (Carbocaine, Polocaine, Arestocaine, Isocaine, Scandonest)	3%	54 mg	3.0	6.6	400 mg	7.4	Plain	No vasoconstrictor	No vasoconstrictor
Prilocaine (Citanest, Citanest Forte)	4%	72 mg	3.6	8.0	600 mg	8.3	Plain	No vasoconstrictor	No Vasoconstrictor
						8.3	1:200,000 (Citanest Forte)	22.2	4.4
Articaine (Septocaine, Zorcaine, Articadent)	4%	72 mg	3.2	7.0	None listed**	**	1:100,000 epinephrine	11.1	2.2
						**	1:200,000 epinephrine	22.2	4.4
Bupivacaine (Marcaine, Vivacaine)	0.5%	9 mg	0.9*	2.0*	90 mg	10	1:200,000 epinephrine	22.2	4.4

*Canadian recommendations; no US recommendations available.
**No U.S. Food and Drug Administration (FDA) maximum recommended dose listed.

APPENDIX 8.2: COMPARISON OF PREVIOUS AND CURRENT MAXIMUM RECOMMENDED DOSES OF ANESTHETIC DRUGS PER APPOINTMENT FOR HEALTHY PATIENTS

Previous (Conservative) Recommendations				Current FDA* Approved Recommendations			
Anesthetic	**mg/lb**	**mg/kg**	**Maximum mg per Appointment**	**Anesthetic**	**mg/lb**	**mg/kg**	**Maximum mg per Appointment**
Lidocaine	2.0	4.4	300 mg	Lidocaine	3.2	7.0	500 mg
Mepivacaine	2.0	4.4	300 mg	Mepivacaine	3.0	6.6	400 mg
Prilocaine	2.7	6.0	400 mg	Prilocaine	3.6	8.0	600 mg
Articaine	3.2	7.0	500 mg	Articaine	3.2	7.0	None listed
Bupivacaine	0.6	1.3	90 mg	Bupivacaine	0.9**	2.0**	90 mg

Maximum recommended dose (MRD) listed for the local anesthetic drug is determined for anesthetic drug only, not the vasoconstrictor; dosages must be reduced for children, the elderly, and medically compromised patients.
*U.S. Food and Drug Administration
**Canadian recommendations; no US recommendations available.

APPENDIX 8.3: DOSING INFORMATION FOR REGIONAL LOCAL ANESTHESIA BOARD EXAMINATIONS REQUIRING CALCULATIONS BASED ON 1.7 mL OF SOLUTION

Local anesthesia dosage calculations should be based on 1.8 mL of solution (see Box 8.4). Although not recommended by this author, some regional local anesthesia board examinations are currently requiring candidates to calculate drug doses based on the labeled amount of solution: 1.7 mL depending on the manufacturer. Licensure candidates taking these dental hygiene local anesthesia board examinations must be prepared to alter the calculation formulas with the specified amount of solution identified on the examination. Drug dosing information for regional local anesthesia board examinations requiring calculations based on 1.7 mL of solution are provided in this appendix. Appendix Table 8.1 provides step-by-step drug calculation information, and Appendix Table 8.2 provides a drug calculation example.

Board examination testing requirements are reviewed annually by examination committees, and changes are made annually for local anesthetic board examinations. The companion Evolve website will provide updated information in the *content update section* and the *board examinations section* of the website. Licensure candidates should review the website periodically for new updates.

As described in the chapter content for local anesthetic agents that contain a vasoconstrictor, an additional calculation to determine the maximum number of cartridges based on the vasoconstrictor needs to be determined. When administering local anesthetics with vasoconstrictors, the local anesthetics will have two potentially limiting drugs: (1) the dose of local anesthetic agent and (2) the dose of the accompanying vasoconstrictor. Either of these agents may be the limiting drug in determining the maximum dose of any particular local anesthetic depending on the patient's medical status. Appendix Table 8.4 provides the volume of vasoconstrictor drug in each concentration based on 1.7 mL of solution. Appendix Table 8.5 provides recommended doses of vasoconstrictors for healthy and cardiovascularly involved patients and maximum number of cartridges for each based on 1.7 mL of solution.

APPENDIX TABLE 8.1 Steps for Calculating Maximum Recommended Dose of Local Anesthetic Agents in Milligrams, Number of Cartridges, and Milliliters Based on 1.7 mL of Solution

Step 1	Determine the number of milligrams in one cartridge of solution Take the percentage of solution and multiply by 10 Take the answer and multiply by 1.7 = mg per cartridge (See also Appendix Table 8.3)
Step 2	Convert pounds to kilograms if using this unit of measurement lb ÷ 2.2 = kg Multiply pounds by mg/lb or kilograms by mg/kg (memorize Table 8.1). This number may be different for each anesthetic and gives the MRD in milligrams
Step 3	Divide the MRD (step 2) by the number of mg per cartridge (step 1) = maximum number of cartridges
Step 4	Multiply maximum number of cartridges (step 3) by 1.7 (mL in one cartridge) = maximum number of milliliters

MRD, Maximum recommended dose.

APPENDIX TABLE 8.2 Example Dosing Calculation of MRD in Milligrams, Number of Cartridges, and Milliliters Based on 1.7 mL of Solution for Lidocaine 2% for a 120-Pound Patient

Step 1	Determine the number of milligrams in one cartridge of solution	2% solution = 2 × 10 = 20 mg/mL × **1.7** = 34 mg in one cartridge (see Appendix Table 8.3)
Step 2	Calculate the MRD MRD can be calculated based on mg/lb or mg/kg as listed in Table 8.1	
	To calculate milligrams of drug per unit of body weight, *milligrams per pound (mg/lb), then multiply the patient's weight in kg by the mg/kg of the selected drug*	120 lb × **3.2 (mg/lb)** = 384 mg (MRD)
	To calculate milligrams of drug per unit of body weight, *milligrams per kilogram (mg/kg), then multiply the patient's weight in kg by the mg/kg of the selected drug*	First, convert pounds to kilograms by dividing the pounds by 2.2. 120 ÷ 2.2 = 54.5 kg × **7 (mg/kg)** = 381.5 mg (MRD)
Step 3	Determine the maximum number of cartridges Divide MRD (384 mg) by number of milligrams per cartridge (34 mg)	384 mg ÷ **34 mg** = 11.2 cartridges
Step 4	(Optional) Determine the maximum number of milliliters Multiply number of cartridges (11.2) by number of milliliters in one cartridge (1.7)	11.2 × **1.7 mL** = 19.07 mL

MRD, Maximum recommended dose.

APPENDIX TABLE 8.3 Calculation of Milligrams per Cartridge for Varying Local Anesthetic Concentrations Based on 1.7 mL of Solution

Local Anesthetic Concentration (%)	Number of mg/mL	Multiply by mg in One Cartridge of Anesthetic	Number of mg/Cartridge
2%	20	1.7	34
3%	30	1.7	51
4%	40	1.7	68
0.5%	5	1.7	8.5

APPENDIX TABLE 8.4 Volume of Vasoconstrictor Drug

Concentration of 1 g/mL of Solution	Milligrams per Milliliter	Milligrams per Cartridge mg/mL × 1.7
1:20,000	0.05	0.085
1:50,000	0.02	0.034
1:100,000	0.01	0.017
1:200,000	0.005	0.008

APPENDIX TABLE 8.5 Maximum Recommended Doses of Vasoconstrictors Based on 1.7 mL of Solution

Concentration (Dilution)	Maximum Recommended Dose (MRD) per Appointment: Healthy Patient	Number of Cartridges: Healthy Patient (ASA I)	Maximum Recommended Dose (MRD) per Appointment: Patient With Cardiovascular Disease (ASA III or IV) or Patients Needing Treatment Modifications	Number of Cartridges: Patient With Cardiovascular Disease or Patients Needing Treatment Modifications
1:50,000 Epinephrine	0.2 mg	5.8	0.04 mg	1.2
1:100,000 Epinephrine	0.2 mg	11.7	0.04 mg	2.3
1:200,000 Epinephrine	0.2 mg	25	0.04 mg	5
1:20,000 Levonordefrin	1.0 mg	11.7	0.2 mg	2.3

PART 4

Pain Control Techniques

CHAPTER 9 Armamentarium/Armamentarium Preparation, 131

CHAPTER 10 Anatomic Considerations for Local Anesthesia Administration, 184

CHAPTER 11 Basic Injection Techniques, 209

APPENDIX 11.1 Sharps Management: Centers for Disease Control and Prevention Guidelines for Infection Control in the Dental Health Care Setting, 229

APPENDIX 11.2 Safe and Unsafe Needle Recapping Techniques, 230

CHAPTER 12 Maxillary Anesthesia, 233

APPENDIX 12.1 Summary of Maxillary Injections, 277

CHAPTER 13 Mandibular Anesthesia, 280

APPENDIX 13.1 Summary of Mandibular Injections, 321

SPECIAL APPENDIX Summary of Maxillary and Mandibular Injection Techniques With Distribution of Anesthesia, 325

CHAPTER 14 Local Anesthesia for the Child and Adolescent, 326

CHAPTER 15 Nitrous Oxide/Oxygen Administration, 335

9

Armamentarium/Armamentarium Preparation

Demetra Daskalos Logothetis, RDH, MS

LEARNING OBJECTIVES

1. Name and discuss the three main components to the armamentarium of anesthetic equipment and supplies.
2. Discuss the criteria for acceptance of local anesthetic syringes.
3. Name and discuss the components of the anesthetic syringe.
4. List and describe the seven types of syringes used in anesthetic procedures and the advantages and disadvantages of each.
5. Discuss routine maintenance of reusable syringes.
6. Name and discuss the components of the needle, as well as recognize manufacturer color codes for needle gauge.
7. Discuss proper care and handling of needles to minimize the risk of cross contamination.
8. Discuss problems relative to the needle, which may occur during anesthetic procedures.
9. Discuss the benefits and use of training needles.
10. Name and discuss the components of an anesthetic cartridge, as well as recognize the American Dental Association standard color codes for anesthetic cartridges.
11. Discuss the proper care and handling of the cartridge.
12. Discuss the problems that can be associated with local anesthetic cartridges.
13. List and describe necessary supplemental equipment.
14. List and describe the steps necessary to assemble, as well as disassemble, the breech-loading aspirating syringe.
15. List and describe the steps necessary to assemble, as well as disassemble, the safety syringe.
16. List and describe the steps necessary to assemble and disassemble the Wand STA Computer-Controlled Local Anesthetic Delivery System.
17. Describe how to buffer local anesthetics using the Onset buffering system.

INTRODUCTION

The administration of safe and effective local anesthesia depends on the anesthetic delivery devices. There are three main components to the armamentarium of anesthetic equipment and supplies: the aspirating syringe, the disposable hypodermic needle, and the single-dose anesthetic cartridge. When handled correctly, this equipment will ensure that the dental hygienist can precisely administer the local anesthetic agent to the patient without risk of intravascular injection and cross contamination. In addition to the syringe, needle, and cartridge, supplemental equipment includes topical antiseptic, topical anesthetic, applicator sticks, gauze, hemostat or cotton pliers, and needle capping aids, all of which are also important to the effective delivery of local anesthetic agents (Fig. 9.1).

SYRINGES

The first intraoral local anesthetic syringe was introduced by Cook Laboratories in 1921, and considerable improvements have been made since then, with the most important improvement being the addition of the aspirating harpoon. The harpoon allows the anesthetic syringe to engage the silicone rubber stopper of the anesthetic cartridge. This addition introduced the important concept of aspirating before injecting local anesthetic agents to assess whether the location of the needle tip is within a blood vessel. Intravascular injections rapidly produce high blood levels of drugs, potentially resulting in an anesthetic overdose, but can be prevented by performing an aspiration test. Aspiration tests are accomplished by pulling back on the thumb ring of the syringe to create negative pressure within the cartridge. This action determines whether the needle tip rests within a blood vessel, as observed by the absence or entry of blood into the cartridge.[1,2]

Certain criteria have been developed by the Council on Dental Material and Devices of the American Dental Association for the acceptance of local anesthetic syringes that include the following:[3,4]

- Syringes must be durable and able to withstand repeated sterilization without damage. (If the unit is disposable, it should be packaged in a sterile container.)
- Syringes should be capable of accepting a wide variety of cartridges and needles of different manufacturers and permit repeated use.
- Syringes should be inexpensive, self-contained, lightweight, and simple to use with one hand.
- Syringes should provide for effective aspiration and be constructed so that blood may be easily observed in the cartridge.

Components of the Anesthetic Syringe

Needle Adaptor

The needle adaptor (Fig. 9.2A) is located at the top of the syringe and is attached to the barrel of the syringe. The threaded tip allows the attachment of the needle to the barrel of the syringe. The needle is attached by passing it through the needle adaptor to the barrel and properly screwing it to the adaptor. The needle then penetrates the diaphragm at the top of the local anesthetic cartridge. Care should be taken when removing the needle from the needle adaptor. The needle adaptor can be easily unscrewed when the needle is removed and can be inadvertently disposed of with the contaminated needle into the sharps container (Fig. 9.3).

Syringe Barrel

The breech-loading syringe barrel (Fig. 9.2B) allows the glass anesthetic cartridge to be inserted into the syringe through the side of the barrel. The barrel has a "large window" and a "small window" on

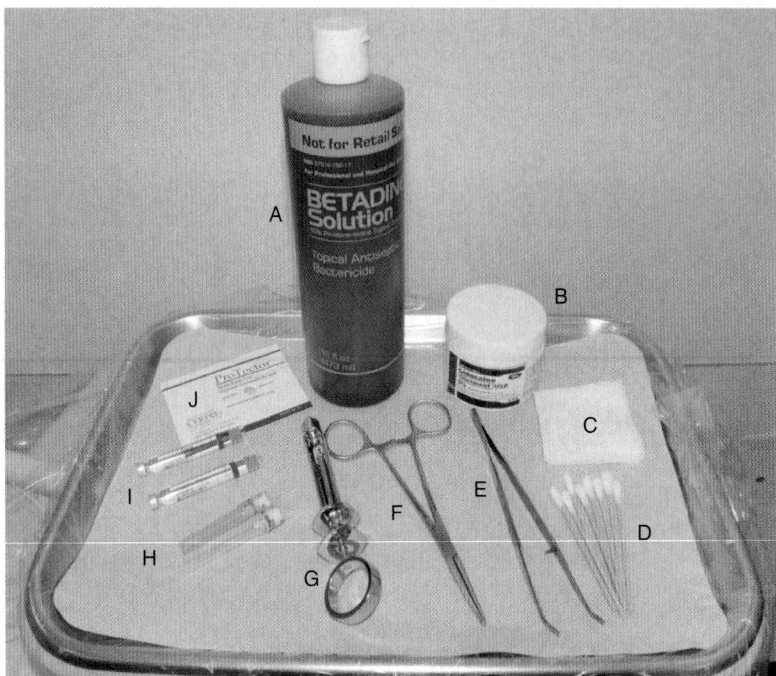

Fig. 9.1 Local anesthetic armamentarium. (A) Betadine antiseptic. (B) Topical anesthetic. (C) Gauze. (D) Cotton-tipped applicators. (E) Cotton pliers. (F) Hemostat. (G) Aspirating syringe. (H) Long and short needles. (I) Anesthetic cartridges. (J) Needle sheath prop.

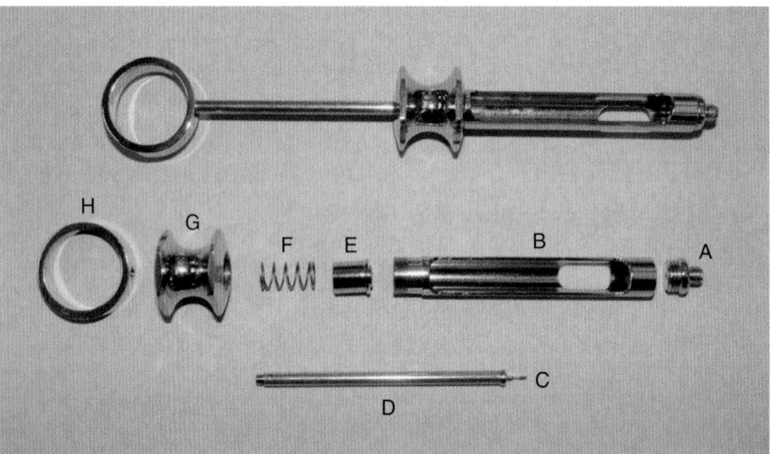

Fig. 9.2 Components of a standard local anesthetic syringe. (A) Needle adaptor. (B) Syringe barrel. (C) Harpoon. (D) Piston. (E) Guide gearing. (F) Spring. (G) Finger grip. (H) Thumb ring.

opposite sides (Fig. 9.4). The large window provides adequate room for breech-loading cartridges to be inserted into the syringe and provides the clinician with direct vision of the cartridge during anesthetic administration. This is an important feature because any positive aspiration that occurs during the injection can be seen. The large window should always be in view of the clinician during administration of local anesthetics (see Chapter 11).

Piston and Harpoon

The piston (Fig. 9.2D) passes through the finger grip and attaches to the thumb ring of the syringe. The spring (Fig. 9.2F) allows the piston to be pulled back during the insertion of the cartridge and during aspiration tests. The harpoon (Fig. 9.2C) of the aspirating syringe is a sharp tip attached to the internal end of the piston. Advancing the piston allows the clinician to embed the harpoon into the silicone rubber stopper at the bottom of the cartridge. The advantage and purpose of the harpoon is to provide negative pressure inside the anesthetic cartridge when the thumb ring is pulled back, causing the rubber stopper to retract and produce an aspiration test. If the tip of the needle is within a blood vessel, blood will enter the cartridge, signaling a positive aspiration to the clinician. (See Chapter 11.)

Finger Grip

The finger grip (Fig. 9.2G) attaches to the barrel of the syringe and allows the piston to pass through and attach to the thumb ring. Clinicians hold the syringe using the finger grip with the index and middle fingers, providing the clinician stability and control of the syringe. There are two basic types of finger grips: winged and wingless;

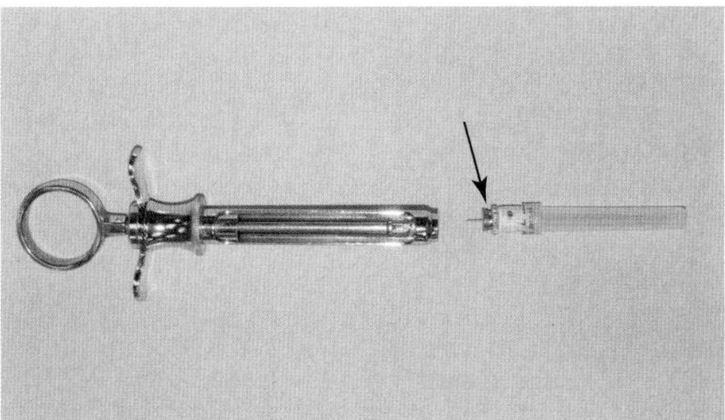

Fig. 9.3 Needle adaptor can be inadvertently disposed of in sharps container.

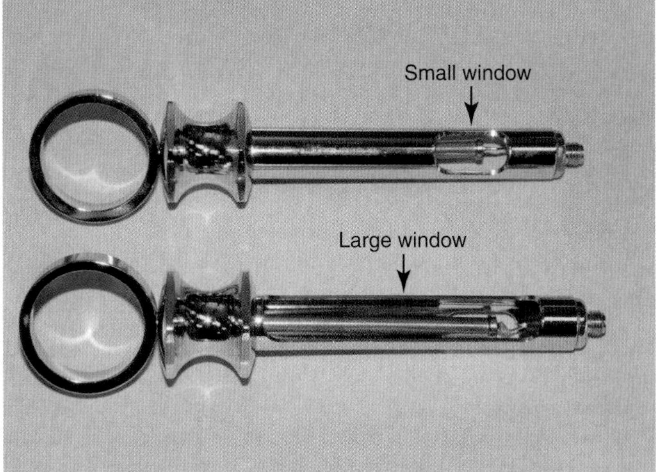

Fig. 9.4 Small and large windows of the anesthetic syringe. The large window should be facing up toward the clinician during the administration of the local anesthetic.

these may be silicone-coated to aid in establishing a firm grip (Fig. 9.5 and Fig. 9.6).

Thumb Ring

The purpose of the thumb ring (Fig. 9.2H) is to add control over the syringe and to advance or retract the piston. The thumb ring is attached to the external end of the piston. Applying pressure to the thumb ring advances the piston to embed the harpoon into the silicone rubber stopper and pushes the anesthetic agent out of the cartridge through the needle. Pulling back on the thumb ring provides negative pressure by retracting the silicone rubber stopper and producing an aspiration. Syringes are available with different sizes of thumb rings to accommodate varying hand sizes (Fig. 9.7). The dental hygienist must be able to stretch his or her fingers to effectively pull back on the thumb ring and should select an appropriate syringe to fit his or her hand size. In addition, some manufacturers are providing thumb ring designs with a textured silicone coating to enhance the clinician's grip and to prevent slipping (Fig. 9.6).

TYPES OF LOCAL ANESTHETIC SYRINGES

There are several styles of syringes manufactured to be used for local anesthetic administration (Fig. 9.8) with different sizes of thumb rings to accommodate various hand sizes, and personal preference dictates the size and type of thumb ring to use (see Fig. 9.7). They are as follows:[2]

- Reusable breech-loading metallic cartridge-type aspirating syringe
- Reusable breech-loading metallic cartridge-type self-aspirating syringe
- Reusable breech-loading plastic cartridge-type aspirating syringe

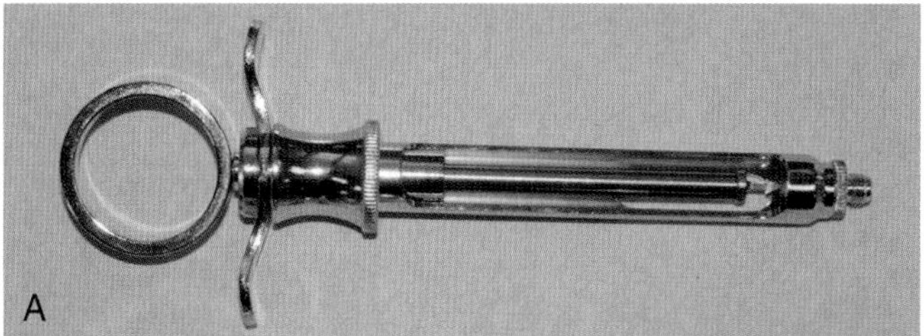

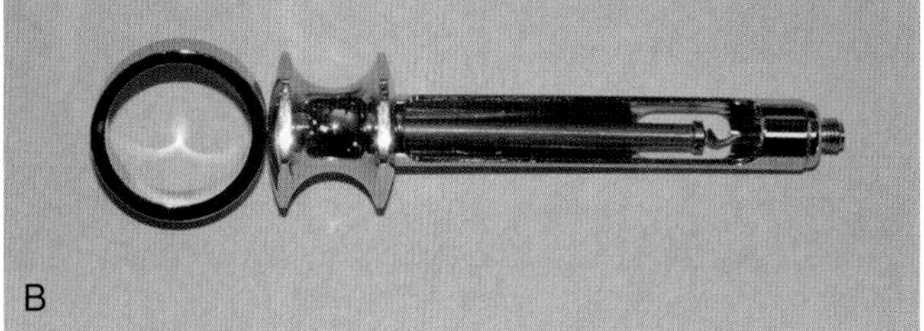

Fig. 9.5 Finger grips. (A) Winged. (B) Wingless.

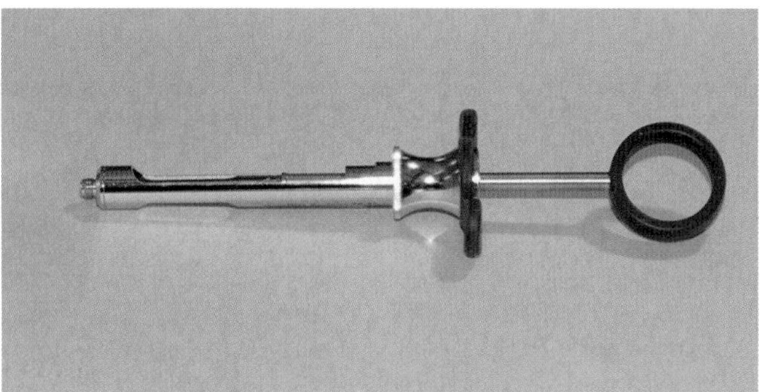

Fig. 9.6 Silicone coated finger grips and thumb ring aid in providing the clinician with a firm grip and reduce "slipping" during aspiration tests. They are available on standard or petite syringes.

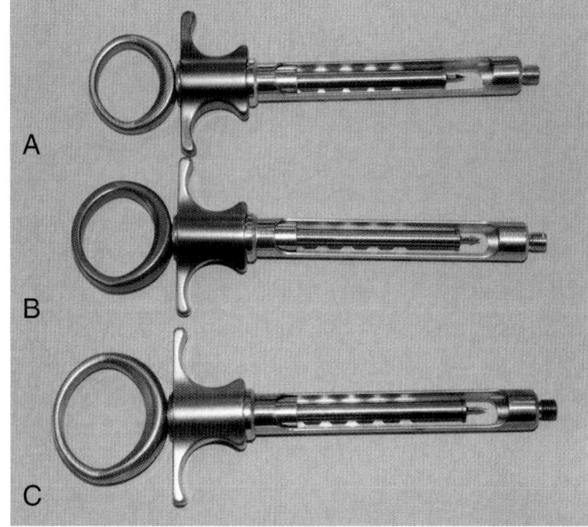

Fig. 9.7 Thumb ring sizes. (A) Small (petite). (B) Medium. (C) Large. The contoured thumb rings maximize control during aspiration.

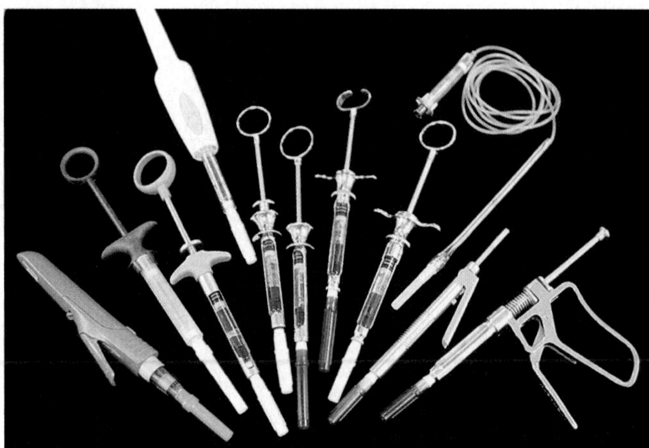

Fig. 9.8 Variations of local anesthetic delivery syringes. Styles are numerous: metal, plastic, computerized, pressurized, and topical anesthetic delivery. (From Daniel S, Harfst S, Wilder R, et al: *Dental hygiene concepts, cases and competencies,* ed 2, St Louis, 2008, Mosby.)

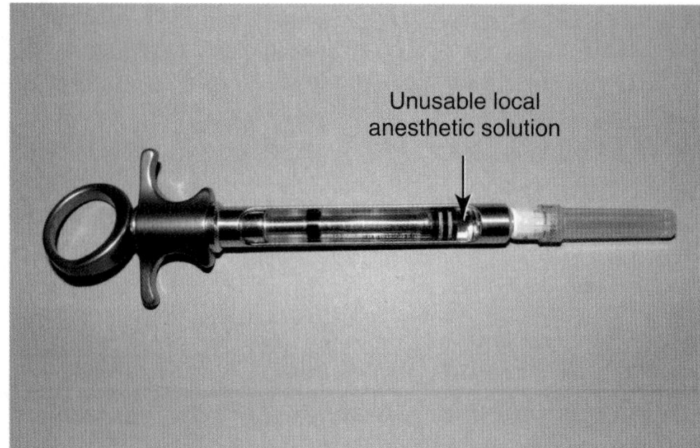

Fig. 9.9 Petite syringe is manufactured with a shorter piston that does not allow complete removal of anesthetic agent from the cartridge compared with the standard syringe. Unusable remaining anesthetic is enough to administer buccal block to achieve complete anesthesia of a quadrant after the inferior alveolar block.

TABLE 9.1 Advantages and Disadvantages of Metallic, Breech-Loading, Aspirating Syringe

Advantages	Disadvantages
Readily visible cartridge through large window to detect positive aspirations and to observe the rate of anesthetic deposition	Heavy weight of the syringe (for standard size)
	Size may be too large for smaller hands (for standard size)
Ease of aspiration with one hand	Harpoon disengagement may occur during aspiration, necessitating the clinician to remove the syringe, reengage the harpoon, and repeat the procedure
Autoclavable	
Rust resistant	
Long-lasting	

- Pressure syringe for periodontal ligament injection
- Jet injector
- Computer-controlled local anesthetic delivery devices
- Disposable safety syringes

Reusable Breech-Loading Metallic Cartridge-Type Aspirating Syringe

The most commonly used syringe for the administration of intraoral local anesthetics is the reusable breech-loading metallic cartridge-type aspirating syringe (see Fig. 9.2). Single-use cartridges of anesthetic are inserted into the syringe through the large window. The harpoon is embedded in the silicone rubber stopper, and the needle is affixed to the needle adaptor. The device is then ready to be used.

The advantages and disadvantages of using the metallic breech-loading aspirating syringe are listed in Table 9.1. To help accommodate the differences in hand sizes, newer syringes have been manufactured to include choices of smaller syringes with smaller contoured thumb rings to facilitate the smaller-handed clinician in performing sufficient aspiration techniques (Fig. 9.7). The advantages of these syringes are that they are lightweight and made of surgical grade aluminum and stainless steel, which reduces weight and hand stress, providing better ergonomic control during injection without compromising durability. The contoured thumb rings maximize control during aspiration. In addition, they contain no removable parts, so the needle adaptor cannot be loosened or removed. The disadvantage of the smaller syringe is that the entire cartridge of anesthetic cannot be deposited because of the shorter length of the piston. A small portion of the anesthetic remains in the cartridge and is unusable (Fig. 9.9).

Disengagement of the harpoon during injection can occur when the clinician retracts the thumb ring to achieve an aspiration. This can be caused by a dull harpoon, excessive pull on the thumb ring, or improper engagement of the harpoon during syringe setup. This frequently produces a "popping" noise, alerting the clinician to the disengagement. However, the dental hygienist should ensure that the harpoon is fully engaged during aspiration to make certain that the proper technique has been accomplished. If the harpoon becomes disengaged during the aspiration, the negative aspiration cannot be guaranteed and the dental hygienist must remove the syringe from the patient's mouth, remove the needle, and reengage the harpoon into the silicone rubber stopper. The needle must be placed back on the syringe, and the injection repeated.

Reusable Breech-Loading Metallic Cartridge-Type Self-Aspirating Syringe

The importance of aspirating before anesthetic deposition and the potential hazards associated with intravascular injections are widely known and accepted. The breech-loading metallic cartridge-type self-aspirating syringe aids the clinician in performing this procedure without difficulty (Fig. 9.10).

The self-aspirating syringe achieves the negative pressure necessary for an aspiration without a harpoon (Fig. 9.11A). Instead, the negative pressure is achieved by a metallic sleeve at the base of the syringe that surrounds the needle-penetrating end and rests on the rubber diaphragm in the cartridge (Fig. 9.11B). There are two types of thumb rings available: one with a half-moon and one with a thumb ring (see Fig. 9.12A). When the dental hygienist exerts pressure on the thumb ring, the entire cartridge moves forward, causing the elasticity of the rubber diaphragm to come in contact with the metallic sleeve and stretch the diaphragm. When the thumb ring is released, the cartridge springs back slightly, producing negative pressure within the cartridge to achieve an aspiration (Fig. 9.12B). An alternative method, using a self-aspirating syringe, uses a thumb disk that, when pressed and released, produces the negative pressure in a similar fashion as the thumb ring (Fig. 9.12C). Table 9.2 lists the advantages and disadvantages of a self-aspirating syringe.

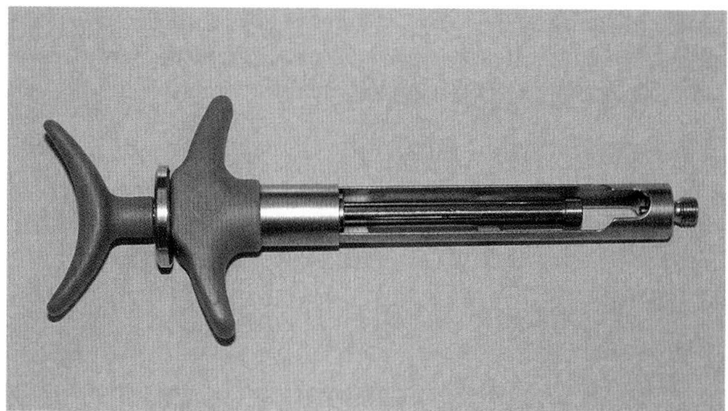

Fig. 9.10 Self-aspirating syringe.

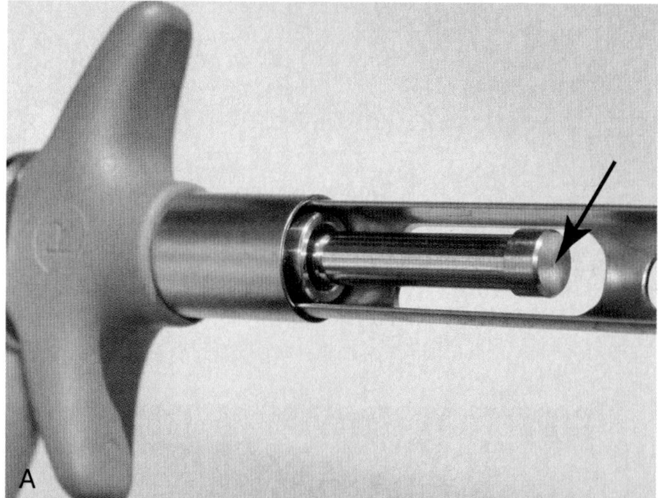

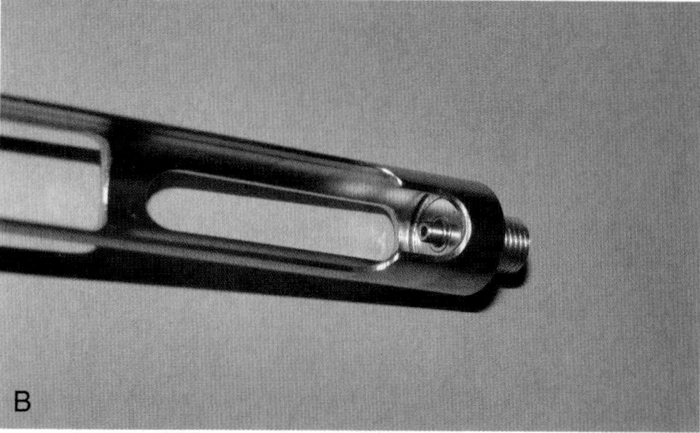

Fig. 9.11 (A) Self-aspirating syringe does not have a harpoon attached to the piston. (B) Metallic sleeve of self-aspirating syringe is located at the base of the syringe and comes in contact with the diaphragm of the cartridge, stretching it to produce the necessary negative pressure within the cartridge to produce an aspiration test.

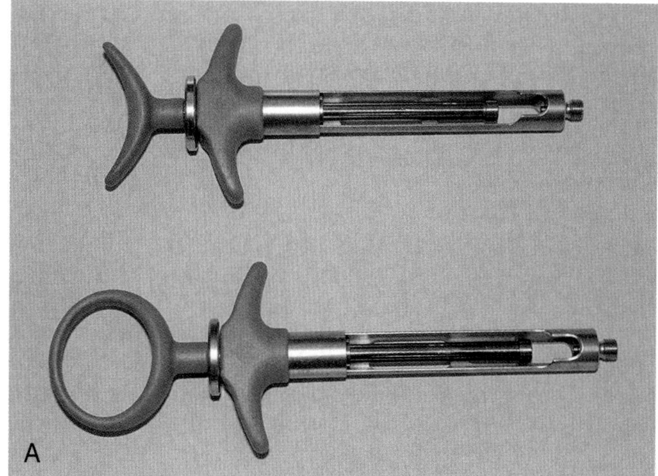

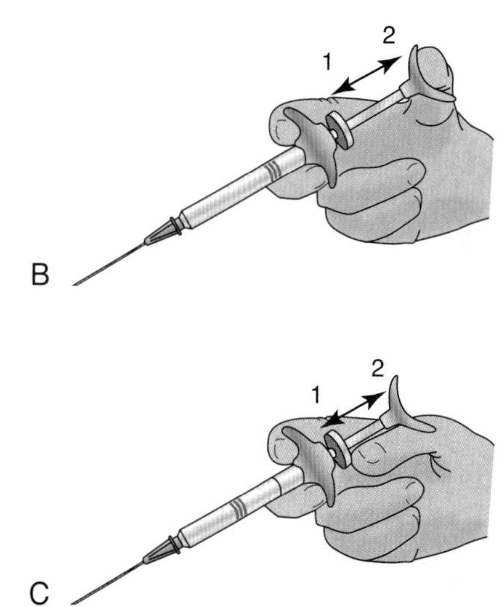

Fig. 9.12 (A) Self-aspirating syringe with half-moon and thumb ring. (B) Aspiration using thumb ring. (1, Apply pressure on thumb ring. 2, Release thumb ring.) (C) Aspiration using thumb disk. (1, Apply pressure on the thumb disk. 2, Release the thumb disk.)

TABLE 9.2 Advantages and Disadvantages of Metallic, Self-Aspirating Syringe

Advantages	Disadvantages
Readily visible cartridge through large window to detect positive aspirations and to observe the rate of anesthetic deposition	Heavy weight of the syringe
Ease of aspiration with small hands	Size may be too large for smaller hands
No disengagement of harpoon from rubber stopper can occur	Thumb must be moved from thumb ring to thumb disk
Autoclavable	Insecurity of clinician accustomed to harpoon-type syringe
Rust resistant	
Long-lasting	

Reusable Breech-Loading Plastic Cartridge-Type Aspirating Syringe

A plastic version of the cartridge-type aspirating syringe is available for intraoral administration of local anesthetics. The syringe is autoclavable and chemically sterilizable. The same concepts apply as for the metallic version. Advantages and disadvantages are listed in Table 9.3.

Pressure-Type Syringes

The pressure-type syringe is used for periodontal ligament (PDL) or intraligamentary injections, and it provides reliable anesthesia for one tooth in the mandible (Fig. 9.13). This allows the clinician to achieve anesthesia of a single tooth in the mandible where supraperiosteal injections are unsuccessful because of bone density, and an inferior alveolar (IA) block, or Gow-Gates mandibular block, anesthetizes more teeth than needed for the procedure (see Chapter 13). Standard syringes can be used for this injection, but the tissue resistance necessitates more muscle strength to administer. Pressure syringes can also be used for intraseptal injections (see Chapter 12). The advantage of a pressure syringe is that it administers a measured dose of 0.2 mL of anesthetic, making it easier to express the solution against the tissue resistance. The disadvantage is the higher cost, and it may cause trauma to surrounding tissues when anesthetic is delivered under pressure.

Jet Injector Syringe

The dental hygienist may encounter the jet injector syringe (Fig. 9.14), which is used primarily for topical anesthesia of soft tissues before needle insertion or mucosal anesthesia of the palate. The jet injection technology is based on the principle of using a mechanical energy source to create a release of pressure sufficient to push a liquid medication through very small orifices called *jets,* creating enough force (2000 psi) that it can penetrate into the subcutaneous tissue without a needle. The jet injector syringe delivers the anesthesia in measured doses of 0.05 to 0.2 mL to the mucous membranes. Because of the high pressure associated with the anesthetic administration, the patient may be startled by the force by which the anesthetic is delivered. The jet injector is not intended to replace the needle and syringe. For complete pulpal anesthesia, nerve blocks or supraperiosteal injections must be administered after the jet injector is used. Topical anesthetics can accomplish the same result as the jet injector at a fraction of the cost.[2]

TABLE 9.3 Advantages and Disadvantages of Plastic, Breech-Loading, Aspirating Syringe

Advantages	Disadvantages
Readily visible cartridge through large window to detect positive aspirations and to observe the rate of anesthetic deposition	Size may be too large for smaller hands
Lighter weight	Harpoon disengagement may occur during aspiration, necessitating the clinician to remove the syringe, reengage the harpoon, and repeat the procedure
The look may be less threatening to the patient than the metallic version	
Ease of aspiration with one hand	Discoloration of plastic from autoclave
Autoclavable	
Rust resistant	
Long-lasting with proper maintenance	
Lower cost	

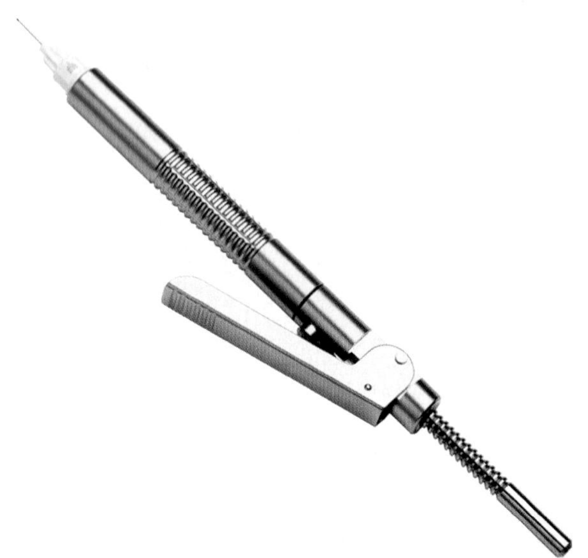

Fig. 9.13 Pressure-type syringe. (Courtesy Septodont, New Castle, DE.)

Computer-Controlled Local Anesthetic Delivery Devices

In 1997, Milestone Scientific Inc. introduced the first computer-controlled local anesthetic delivery (C-CLAD) system as the CompuDent Wand System (Fig. 9.15). This model is no longer marketed by Milestone Scientific. The device was designed to replace the standard

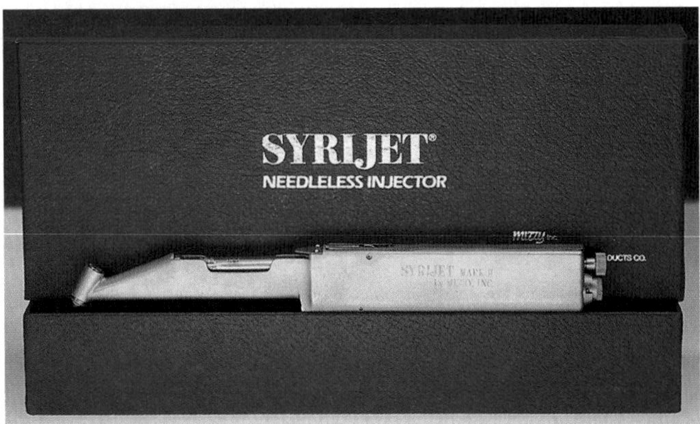

Fig. 9.14 Jet injector. (From Malamed S: *Handbook of local anesthesia,* ed 6, St Louis, 2013, Mosby.)

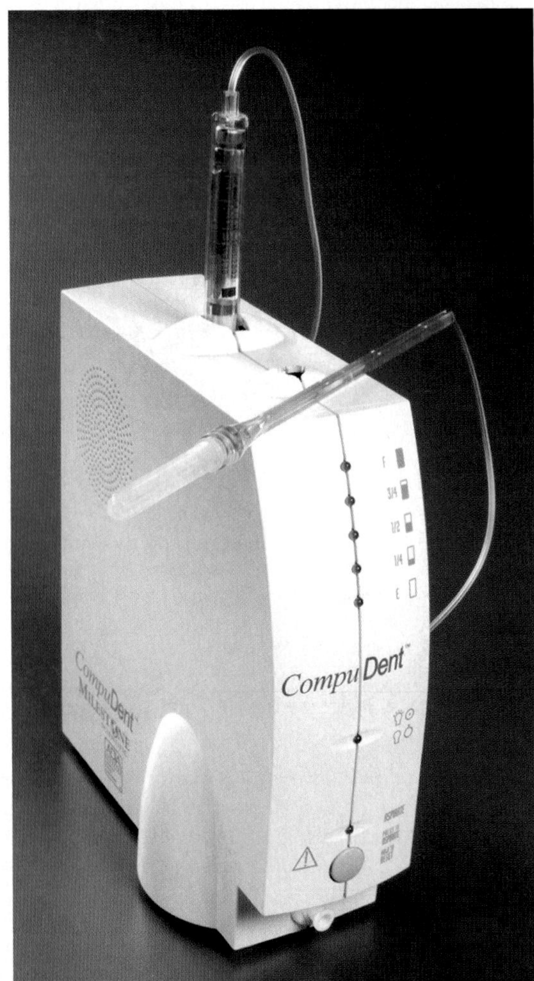

Fig. 9.15 Wand CompuDent. (Courtesy Milestone Scientific.)

breech-loading aspirating syringe that requires the clinician to attempt to control the variables of drug infusion and needle movement in soft tissue. The difficulty in controlling these variables utilizing the standard syringe can compromise the injection technique and patient comfort. Moreover, the standard syringe is held with a palm up grasp that is not designed for needle control during tissue penetration and proper ergonomics. The large syringe can also be difficult for clinicians with small hands. The C-CLAD was designed to improve ergonomics and precision of local anesthetic delivery. The drug is administered at a preprogrammed flow rate, allowing the clinician to focus on the needle positioning and insertion while providing the injection of local anesthetic.[5,6]

Currently, there are several C-CLAD systems available in North America, including the Wand STA, Calaject, EZ-Flow, Dentapen, and Anaeject.

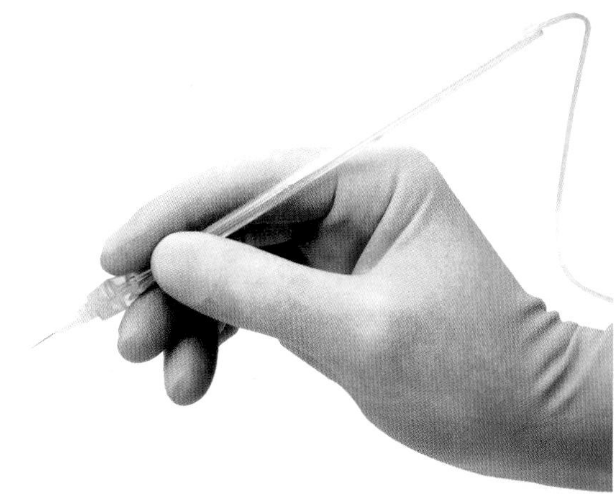

Fig. 9.17 Feather-light handpiece provides ergonomic control.

The Wand STA System

Milestone Scientific Inc. introduced the next generation to C-CLAD systems as the Wand STA (Fig. 9.16). The clinician holds a featherlight "Wand" handpiece as if holding a pen (Fig. 9.17), which gives superior ergonomic control. Clinicians with small hands may find the Wand headpiece easier to use because of the design and ultralightweight features. A pen-like grasp allows clinicians to rotate the handpiece back and forth, using a birotational insertion technique that eliminates needle deflection during needle penetration into tissue, resulting in accurate needle placement[5,6] (Fig. 9.18). Because of the "slim line" design of the handpiece, dental hygienists find it easy to grasp and handle during the injection. In addition, the handpiece can be modified to any preferable length by snapping off portions of the plastic handpiece at any of the preformed indentations (see Procedure Box 9.1). This modification is particularly useful for clinicians with small hands and when administering palatal injections. Moreover, the handpiece can be less intimidating for the patient and can help alleviate the patient's fear associated with the standard large metal syringe.

The Wand STA system incorporates dynamic pressure-sensing (DPS) technology to provide real-time continuous pressure feedback during the injection. Fluid pressure at the tip of the needle is used to identify location or specific tissue type. The Wand STA system guides the clinician by the fluid exit pressure with spoken and/or audible sounds and visual feedback[2] (Fig. 9.19), enabling him or her to identify accurate needle placement in the PDL space for intraligamentary injections. The Wand STA system can be used to perform all the standard dental injections for all routine dental treatments, including nonsurgical periodontal therapy and newer-described injections such as the anterior middle superior alveolar (AMSA), palatal approach anterior superior alveolar (P-ASA), and STA-intraligamentary (see Chapters 12 and 13). For added patient comfort, Milestone Scientific has developed a three-stage technique: prepuncture, penetration, and delivery (see Chapter 11 for technique steps). The unit accommodates any local anesthetic cartridge, a single patient–use disposable handpiece, and a variety of needle sizes and gauges (Fig. 9.20).

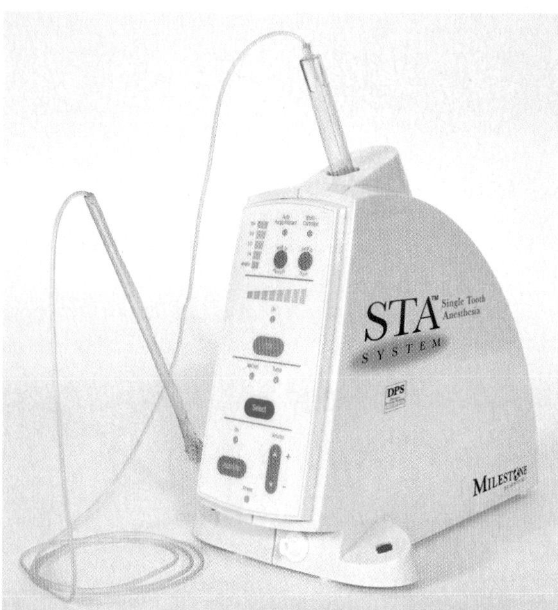

Fig. 9.16 Computer-controlled local anesthetic delivery device. *Wand STA,* Wand single tooth anesthesia (STA) system. (Courtesy Milestone Scientific.)

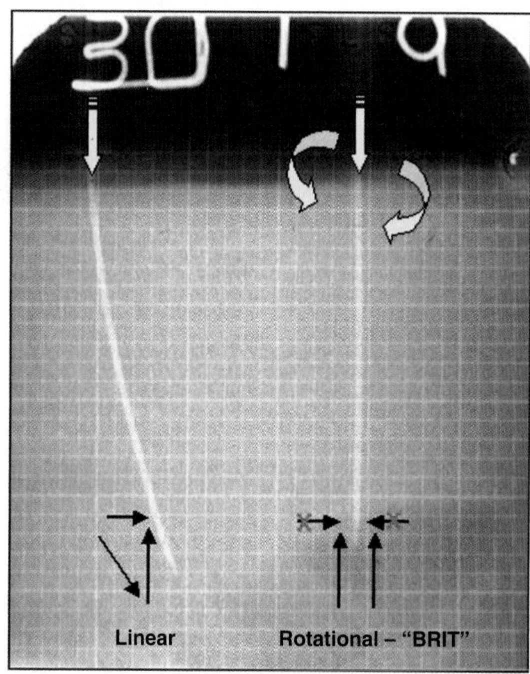

Fig. 9.18 Birotational insertion technique (BRIT) eliminates needle deflection during needle penetration of tissue to accurately reach the target. (From Malamed S: *Handbook of local anesthesia,* ed 6, St Louis, 2013, Mosby.)

The Wand STA and Wand CompuDent systems precisely regulate the flow rate of the local anesthetic agent administered via a computer-controlled module. In addition, the DPS technology regulates and monitors the pressure of the anesthetic agent. These systems are activated by foot control (Fig. 9.21), allowing the clinician to delicately hold the Wand handpiece (see Fig. 9.17). The rate of flow can be set as precisely as one drop every other second (slow rate), or the clinician can use the foot pedal to set the control rate at various settings, including "cruise control." Patients typically experience painless injections. Although there is still a minimal sensation of the needle insertion, the actual anesthetic administration is precisely controlled and painless. The advantages and disadvantages of this system are listed in Table 9.4.

Dentapen

The Dentapen (Fig. 9.22) is a battery operated, handheld C-CLAD device for the routine administration of local anesthesia. The device allows the clinician the option of two different handles to be used

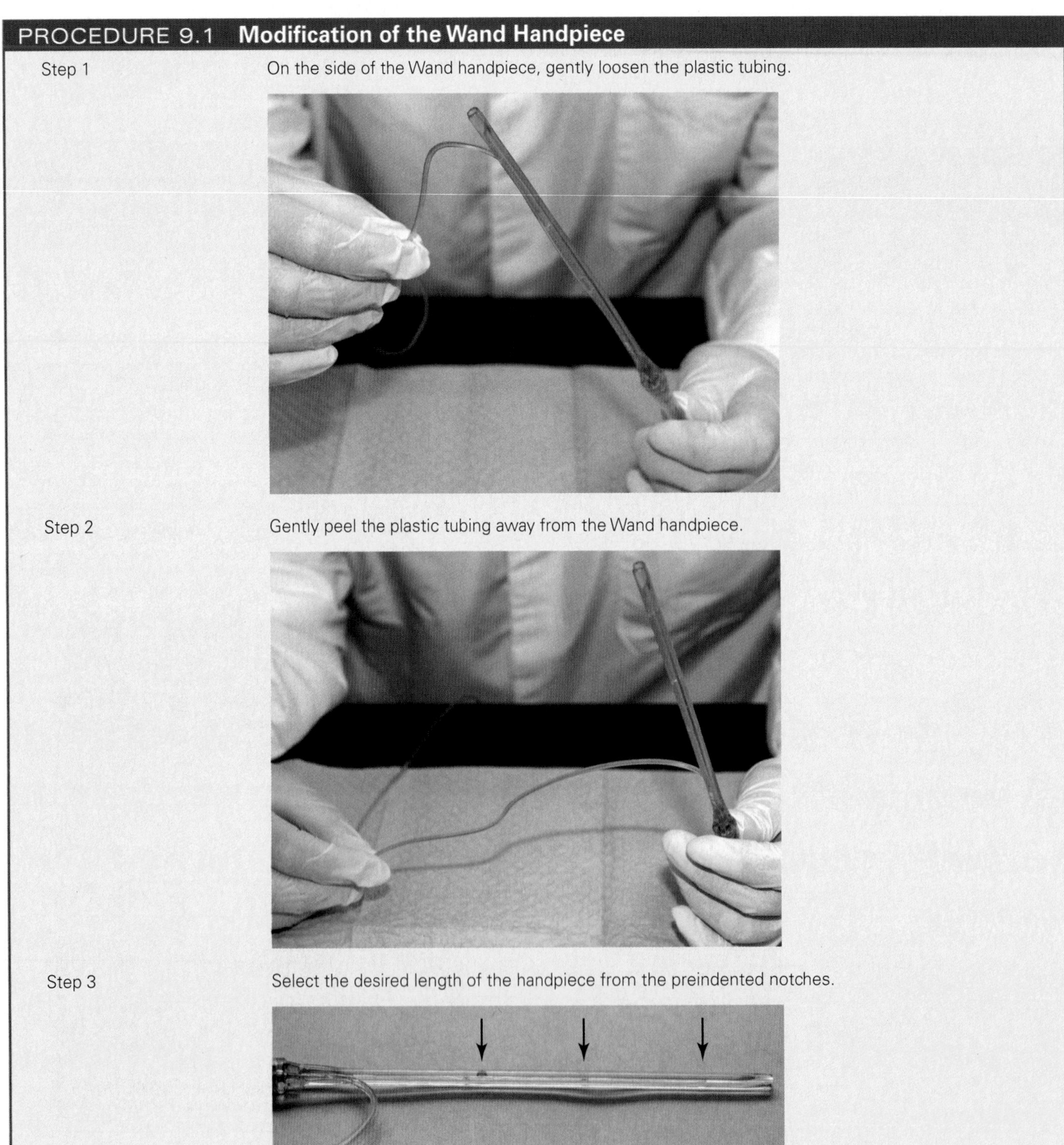

PROCEDURE 9.1 Modification of the Wand Handpiece

Step 1 — On the side of the Wand handpiece, gently loosen the plastic tubing.

Step 2 — Gently peel the plastic tubing away from the Wand handpiece.

Step 3 — Select the desired length of the handpiece from the preindented notches.

(Continued)

PROCEDURE 9.1 Modification of the Wand Handpiece (*Cont.*)

Step 4

Gently rock the handpiece back and forth at the indentation.

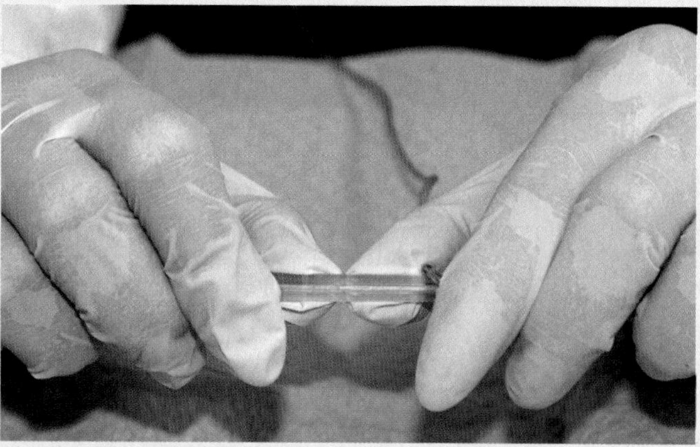

Step 5

The slim handle will snap off at the desired length.

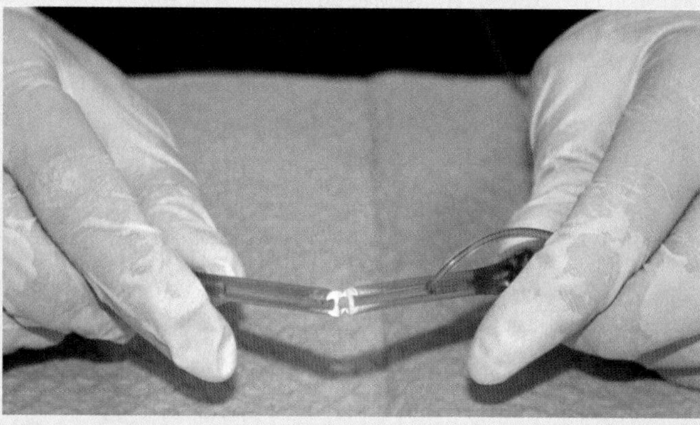

Step 6

The modified handpiece is ready for use.

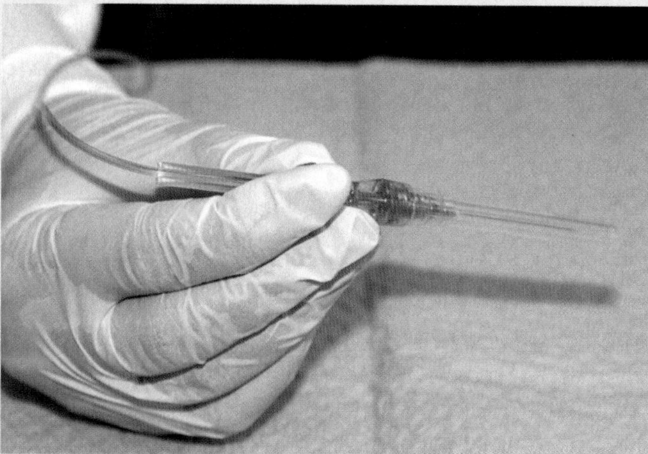

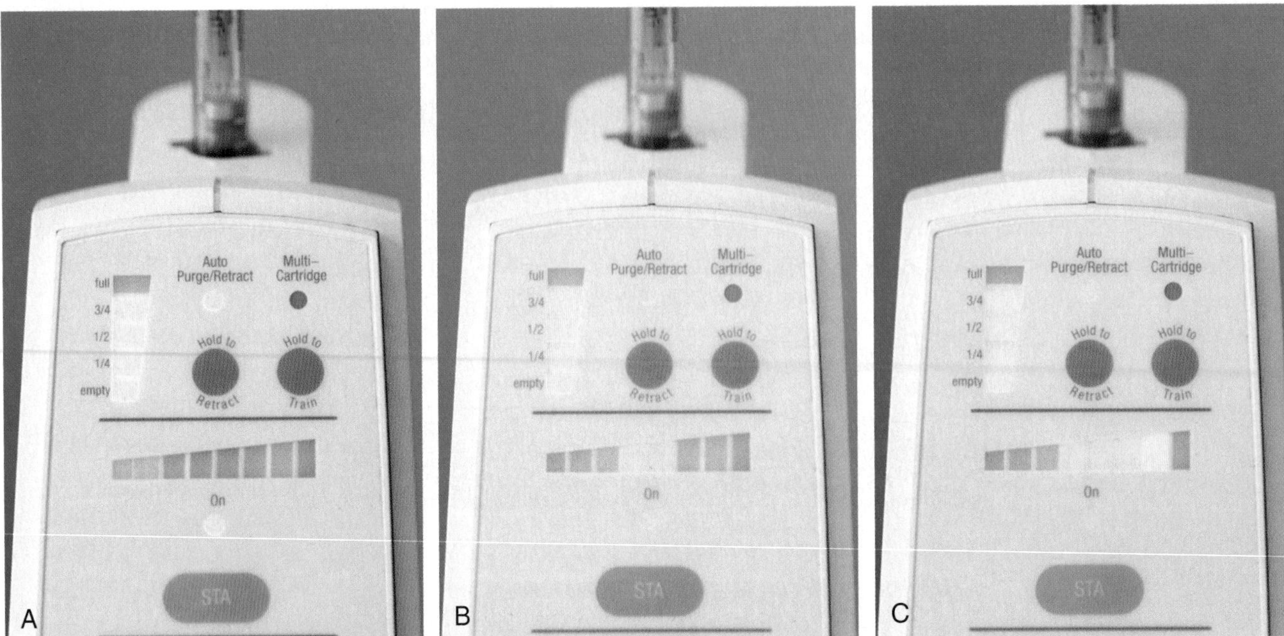

Fig. 9.19 Dynamic pressure sensing (DPS) on the Wand STA computer-controlled local anesthetic delivery (C-CLAD) device provides both visual and audible feedback regarding placement of the needle tip during the periodontal ligament (PDL) injection. Horizontal color bars indicate pressure at the tip of the needle. (A) Red; pressure is too low. (B) Orange and dark yellow; increasing pressure but not yet adequate. (C) Light yellow; correct pressure for PDL injection. At this point the Wand STA unit will also provide an audible clue "PDL, PDL, PDL" that the needle tip is properly situated. (From Malamed S: *Handbook of local anesthesia,* ed 6, St Louis, 2013, Mosby.)

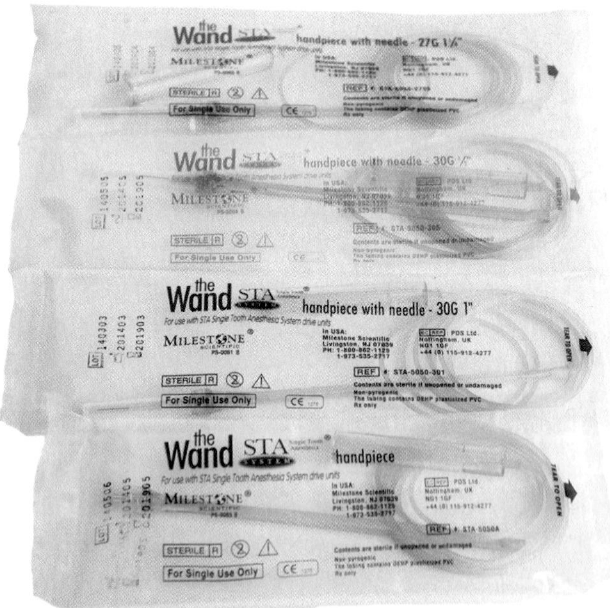

Fig. 9.20 Wand STA handpieces are presterilized, single use, and are available in a variety of lengths and gauges.

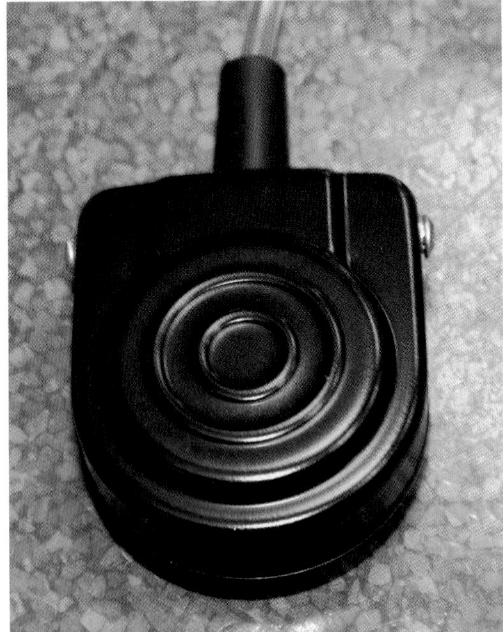

Fig. 9.21 Wand STA foot control.

either as a traditional syringe or as a pen-style grasp. It permits three injection speeds: fast (30 seconds/mL), medium (50 seconds/mL), and slow (90 seconds/mL). It offers two modes of flow: continuous flow or gradual increase. The gradual increase flow is excellent for PDL injections where the anesthetic flow will gradually increase to provide a more painless PDL injection.[7]

DISPOSABLE SAFETY SYRINGES

Because of concerns regarding the risk of accidental exposure to the clinician from contaminated needles after the administration of local anesthetics, the safety syringe was developed as an alternative to the standard breech-loading aspirating syringe. Examples include the

TABLE 9.4 Advantages and Disadvantages of Computer-Controlled Local Anesthetic Delivery System

Advantages	Disadvantages
Precise control of anesthetic flow and pressure	Cost
Provides setting for slow (1 drop every other second) flow rate to create a numbing pathway for the needle	
Automatic aspiration	
Lightweight handpiece requires activation of fine muscles of the hand rather than larger muscles, resulting in less hand fatigue	
Birotational needle insertion minimizes needle deflection for more accurate deposition at target site	

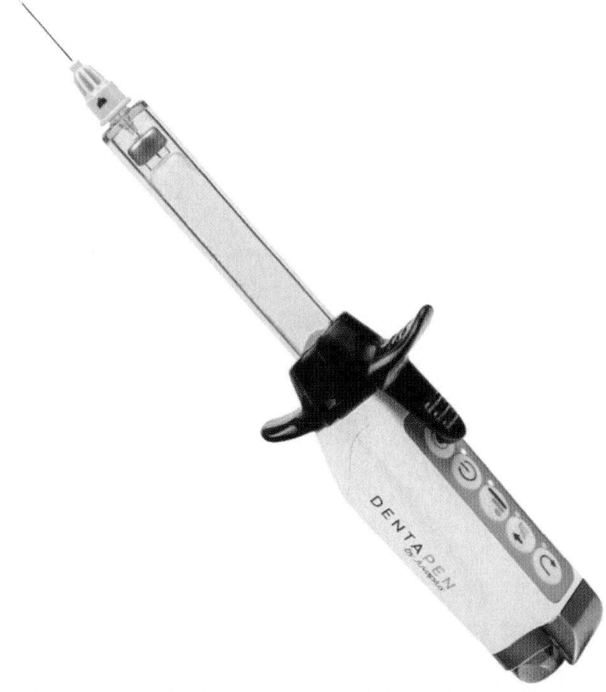

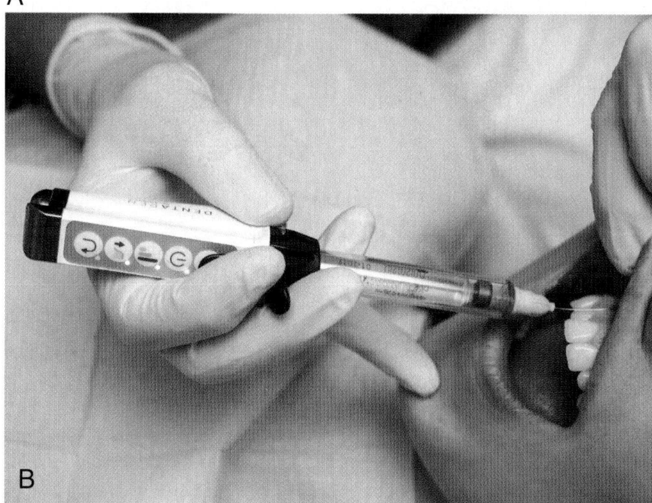

Fig. 9.22 (A) Computer-controlled local anesthetic delivery (C-CLAD) device, Dentapen. (B) Dentapen uses a palm-thumb grasp to hold and operate. (Images courtesy Dentapen.)

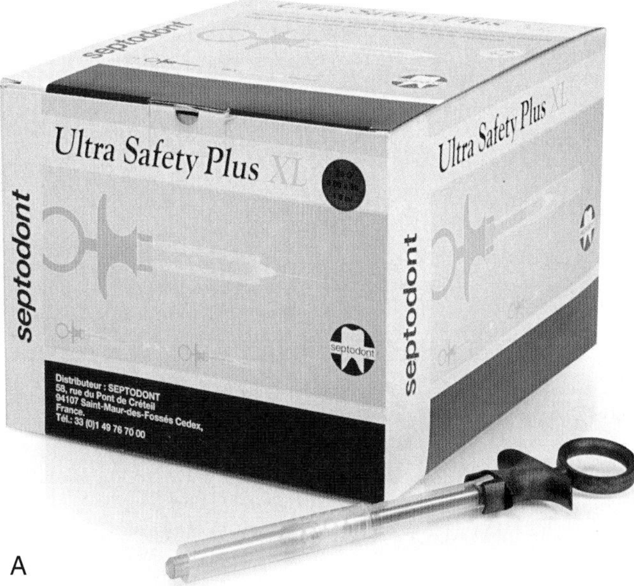

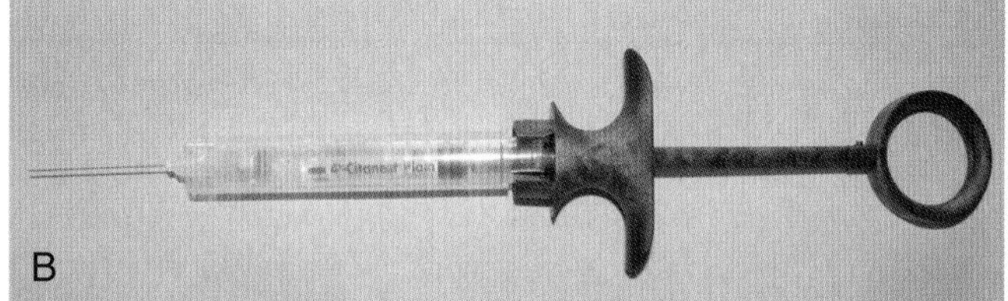

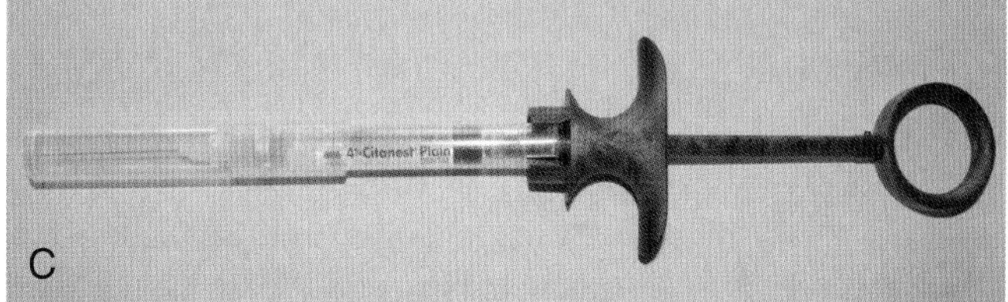

Fig. 9.23 (A) Ultra Safety Plus XL, aspirating syringe. (Ultra Safety Plus System Courtesy Septodont, New Castle, DE.) (B) Ultra Safety Plus XL, aspirating syringe ready for injection. (C) Ultra Safety Plus XL, aspirating syringe sheathed to prevent needlestick injury.

Ultra Safety Plus XL (Fig. 9.23A). The safety syringe is a plastic, single-use, or partially disposable syringe with short and long needle lengths. A plastic sheath on the syringe is retracted when the clinician is ready to administer an injection (Fig. 9.23B), and the sheath locks over the needle upon removal from the tissue; the mechanism is easily activated by the clinician with one hand (Fig. 9.23C). The safety syringe is designed as a single-use item that allows for reinjection using the same cartridge and reloading the syringe for additional anesthetic cartridges if needed. This provides an added advantage over standard syringes by decreasing the risk of accidental exposure. See Procedure Box 9.4 for syringe assembly and Procedure Box 9.5 for syringe disassembly.

ROUTINE MAINTENANCE OF REUSABLE SYRINGES

Routine maintenance of reusable syringes is required to ensure the long-term efficiency of the device. Manufacturer recommendations include:

- Reusable syringes should be thoroughly cleaned and sterilized using appropriate infection control guidelines after each patient.
- After repeated autoclaving, the dental hygienist should dismantle and lubricate all the threaded joints with a light oil.

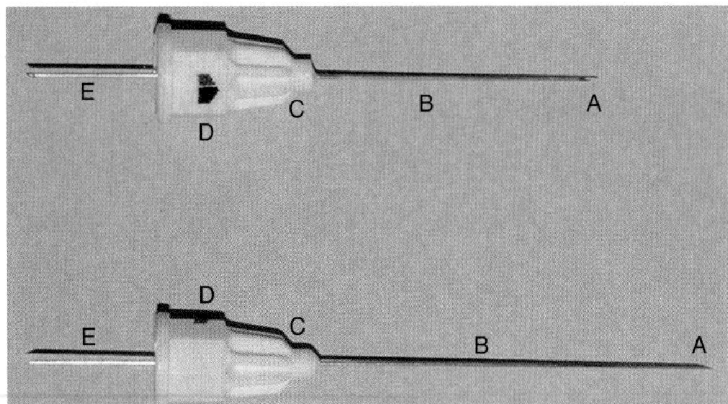

Fig. 9.24 Components of the needle. (A) Bevel. (B) Needle shaft. (C) Hub. (D) Syringe adaptor. (E) Cartridge-penetrating end.

- To ensure reliable aspiration, the piston and harpoon should be replaced if the harpoon loses its sharpness and readily disengages from the rubber stopper of the cartridge or if the harpoon is bent.

NEEDLE

The needle delivers the anesthetic agent from the cartridge to the surrounding tissue through its lumen. The type of injection, how much tissue needs to be penetrated, and individual preference will determine whether an extra-short, short, or long needle should be used and which gauge is appropriate. All needles manufactured for dentistry are stainless steel, presterilized, and disposable.

Needle Components

Bevel

The bevel of the needle (Fig. 9.24A) is the angled surface of the needle tip that is directed into the tissue to provide a cutting surface that offers little resistance to mucosa as the needle penetrates and withdraws from the tissue. The sharper the bevel, the less tissue resistance to the needle, and patient discomfort can be minimized. The bevels may be configured by manufacturers as short, medium, long, multi, and scalpel (Fig. 9.25). Although several bevel configurations are available for use in dentistry, the multibeveled point is considered to produce the most effective puncture while eliciting the least amount of tissue trauma.[1] The newer scalpel design can only be used for maxillary and PDL injections and is not recommended for any injection procedures in which a nerve may be directly contacted. The scalpel design, similar to a surgical scalpel-like point (see Fig. 9.25), has been reported to allow for needle insertion with less tissue displacement, thus requiring less force to penetrate the mucosa.[8] The angle of the bevel in relation to the long axis of the needle may have an effect on the amount of needle deflection when significant tissue is penetrated, such as with the IA block. The greater the angle of the bevel, the greater the degree of needle deflection[2] (Fig. 9.26). To increase patient comfort during injections that are administered in close proximity to the periosteum, the bevel of the needle should be turned toward the bone (Fig. 9.27). To assist the clinician in determining the location of the bevel, several manufacturers are placing indicators of the bevel location on the hub of the needle (Fig. 9.28).

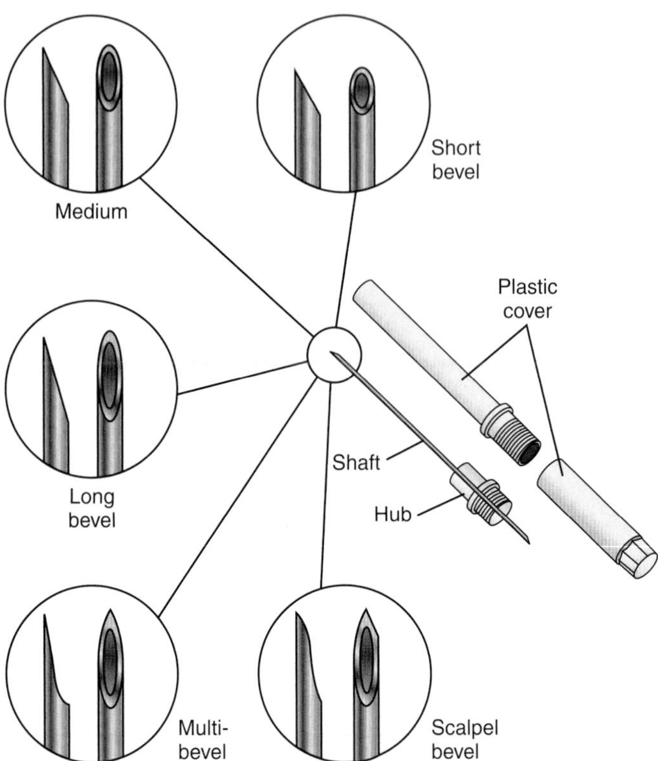

Fig. 9.25 Types of bevels on disposable needles.

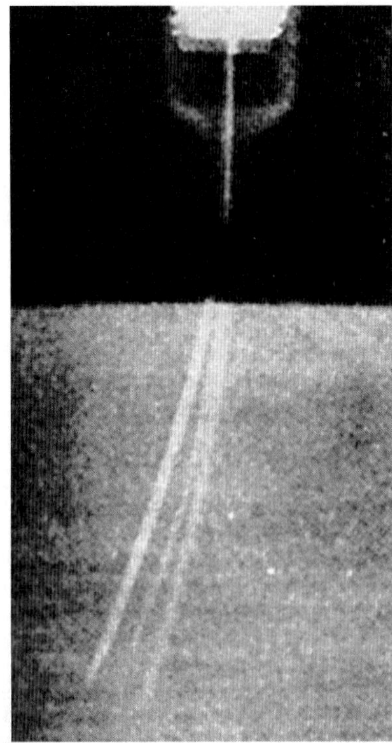
Fig. 9.26 Deflection of needle. (From Robison SE, et al: Comparative study of deflection characteristics and fragility of 25-, 27-, and 30-gauge short dental needles, *J Am Dent Assoc* 109:920–924, 1984.)

Shaft

The shaft of the needle (see Fig. 9.24B) is the length of the needle that consists of long tubular metal extending from the tip of the needle through the hub (discussed next) to the piece (cartridge-penetrating end) that penetrates the diaphragm of the cartridge. Needle breakage is rare; however, needle breakage usually occurs when the entire shaft of the needle is inserted up to the hub. This primarily occurs from exerted lateral pressure against the shank or sudden movement of the syringe or patient.

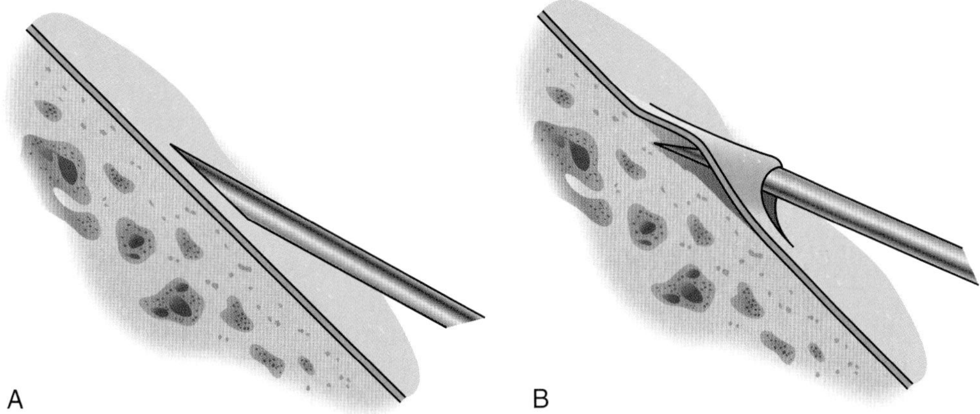

Fig. 9.27 (A) Correct bevel placement against bone. (B) Incorrect placement of bevel, causing the tip to scrape the bone.

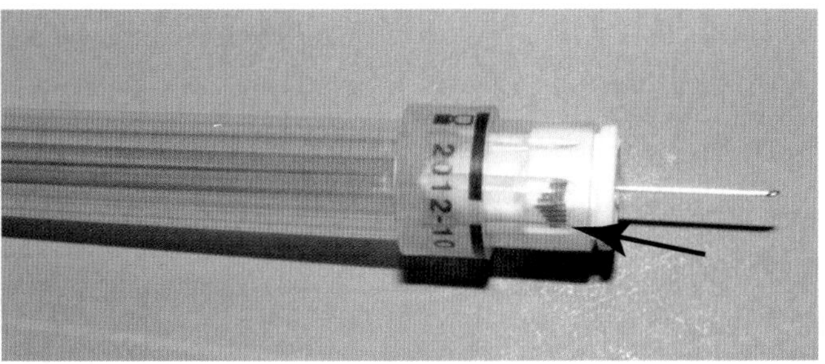

Fig. 9.28 Manufacturer placed arrow indicating location of bevel.

The significant components of the shaft are the length and the gauge. The gauge is the diameter of the needle, and the size tubular lumen (channel) of the needle is related to the gauge (discussed later).

Hub

The hub and syringe adaptor (see Fig. 9.24C–D) are made of plastic or metal and provide a means to attach the needle to the syringe (Fig. 9.29). The syringe adaptor and hub are frequently referred to as *the hub.* The metal syringe adaptor has a prethreaded interior that allows for easy attachment to the syringe. A disadvantage to the metal syringe adaptor is that it can easily be unscrewed and when fully screwed is seated in one position, securing the bevel of the needle in one direction and making it difficult to properly align the bevel toward the bone. The plastic syringe adaptor is not prethreaded, and the dental hygienist must simultaneously push and screw the needle onto the syringe. The advantages of the plastic syringe adaptor include easy adaptation and bevel alignment with most syringes. The hub of the needle is the point where the shaft of the needle joins and secures the needle to the syringe adaptor. The needle shank should never be inserted into tissue up to the hub of the needle.

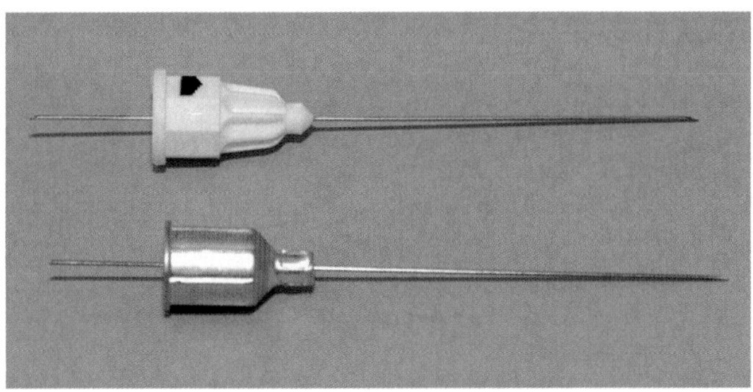

Fig. 9.29 Needle hub variations.

Cartridge-Penetrating End

The cartridge-penetrating end (see Fig. 9.24E) is the part of the shaft that passes through the hub and penetrates the rubber diaphragm of the cartridge, lying within the anesthetic agent of the cartridge.

Needle Shields

Needle shields protect the needle that is inserted in the tissue, as well as the cartridge-penetrating end of the needle. Various colors are used by manufacturers to determine the designated length and gauge of the needle that is inserted in the tissue. The shield that covers the cartridge-penetrating end is clear. There are no uniform guidelines for the color of needle shields. However, manufacturers are consistent with their own color-coding system (Fig. 9.30). Needle shields have an important role in protecting the clinician from needlestick injuries.

Gauge

Needles used for intraoral injection are available in gauge sizes of 25, 27, and 30. The gauge is the diameter of the needle, and the lumen is the hollow portion of the needle. The smaller the gauge number, the larger the diameter of the needle and the lumen. Therefore the 25-gauge needle has the largest needle and lumen diameter, followed by the 27-gauge, and so on. The needle with the smallest diameter and lumen is the 30-gauge (Fig. 9.31 and Table 9.5). Some manufacturers color code the needle hubs to easily identify the gauge of the needle (Fig. 9.32). The gauge selection is determined by the depth of tissue penetration and the risk of intravascular injection. The 25-gauge needle is the recommended needle for areas of high risk for positive aspiration, such as the IA block and posterior superior alveolar block. A common belief among practitioners is that the 30-gauge needle causes less needle insertion discomfort to the patient than the 25-gauge needle. However, numerous comparisons over the years have demonstrated that patients cannot discern the difference between a 25-gauge needle and a 30-gauge needle.[9-11] However, the correlation between the lumen size and patient comfort is related to the amount of pressure needed to inject the anesthetic agent into the tissue. Injection pressure is created when the rubber stopper in the cartridge is depressed, creating a flow of anesthetic agent into the tissue. Injection pressure has been found to directly influence the patient's perceived pain and anxiety level.[12] The lumen of a 30-gauge needle is smaller than a lumen of

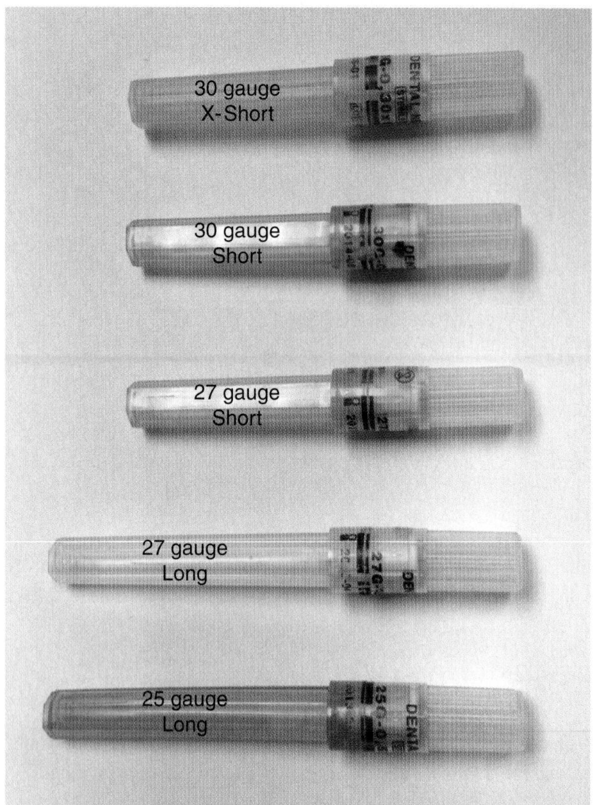

Fig. 9.30 Color coding by needle length and gauge. (Courtesy Septodont, New Castle, DE.)

a 25-gauge needle and therefore requires more pressure to be placed on the rubber stopper to inject the anesthetic agent into the tissue, causing tissue injury and pain.[13] In contrast, it has been demonstrated that a needle with a larger lumen, such as with a 25-gauge needle, will reduce pain and tissue injury during anesthetic administration due to decreased pressure necessary to depress the rubber stopper.[13] In addition, the 25-gauge needle is safer for the patient because the lumen is larger, providing easier access for blood to enter the cartridge during the aspiration procedure.

Larger gauge needles (25-gauge) have several significant advantages over smaller gauge needles (30-gauge). Because of the rigidity of the larger gauge needles, less deflection occurs during significant tissue penetration (Fig. 9.26). This provides greater accuracy to the target location and increases the likelihood of success of the injection. This is of particular importance for the IA block. Moreover, because the shaft of the 25-gauge needle is significantly stronger than its thinner counterparts, needle breakage is considerably minimized. An injection technique to help reduce needle deflection is called birotational insertion technique (BRIT). This technique, which is similar to acupuncture, uses a back-and-forth rotational movement of the handpiece or needle to advance the needle into the tissue. This technique can completely eliminate needle deflection regardless of needle length or gauge[2] (Fig. 9.18). Because conventional dental syringes must be held with a palm-thumb grasp (Fig. 9.33A–B), a linear insertion technique is necessary and is not permitted for this type of technique. However, the C-CLAD system, as discussed previously, works ideally for the BRIT as the handpiece is lightweight and held with a pen-like grasp that can be easily rotated (Fig. 9.33C–D).

Although it is possible to aspirate with smaller gauge needles (30-gauge), the smaller lumen does significantly impede blood flow into the cartridge. It also requires more pressure by the clinician to adequately

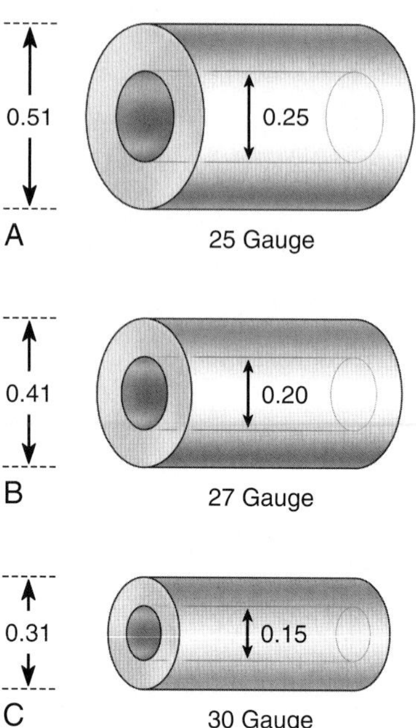

Fig. 9.31 Magnified view of the different needle gauges illustrates the difference in the measurements of the outer diameter and lumen (hollow area) in millimeters between 25-gauge, 27-gauge, and 30-gauge needles. (A) 25-Gauge needles have a thicker wall and the largest lumen compared with the other needle gauges used in dentistry, allowing for less needle deflection during insertion, increased reliability during aspiration tests, and decreased pressure needed to administer the anesthetic agent. (B) 27-Gauge needles have a slightly thinner wall and a smaller lumen than 25-gauge needles, and (C) 30-gauge needles have the thinnest wall and the smallest lumen compared with 25- and 27-gauge needles, causing more needle deflection during insertion, decreased reliability during aspiration tests, and increased pressure needed to administer the anesthetic agent.

TABLE 9.5 Common Needle Gauges Used for Intraoral Injections

Gauge	Outside Diameter (mm)	Lumen Diameter (mm)
25	0.51	0.25
27	0.41	0.20
30	0.31	0.15

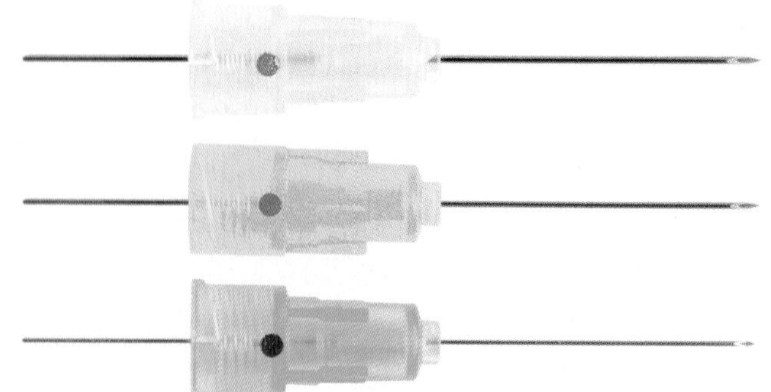

Fig. 9.32 Gauge indicators are placed by the manufacturer to easily identify the gauge of the needle. Clear hubs = 25-gauge needles, yellow hubs = 27-gauge needles, and blue hubs = 30-gauge needles. (Courtesy Dentsply Pharmaceutical, York, PA.)

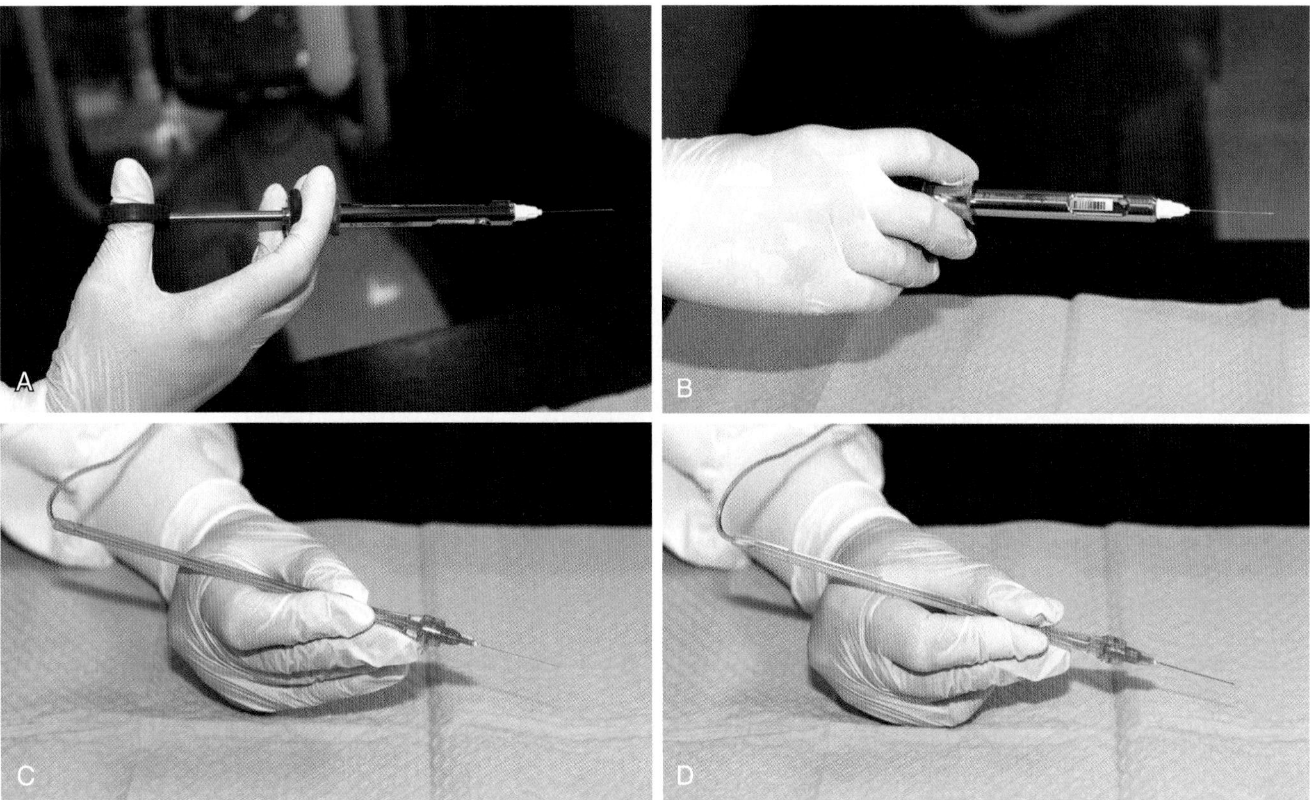

Fig. 9.33 (A) Holding a standard syringe. (B) Demonstrating the difficulty of birotational needle insertion; the entire hand must rotate back and forth. (C) Holding a Wand handpiece. (D) Demonstrating the ease of birotational needle insertion with the Wand handpiece by using the fingers to roll the handpiece back and forth.

BOX 9.1 Advantages of Larger-Gauge Needles Over Smaller-Gauge Needles

- Less deflection from intended path as needle penetrates significant tissue
- Greater accuracy in achieving target location
- Increased success of the injection
- Less chance of needle breakage
- Aspiration is easier to achieve and more reliable
- No difference in patient comfort as needle penetrates the tissue
- Less pressure needed to administer the anesthetic agent, resulting in decreased pain and tissue injury

aspirate through the narrow lumen of smaller gauge needles. This makes it difficult to achieve a reliable aspiration, increases the possibility of needle movement away from the target location, and increases the likelihood that the harpoon will disengage from the rubber stopper during aspiration. Therefore it is recommended that the dental hygienist use a 25-gauge needle for injections that pose an increased risk for positive aspirations such as the IA, posterior superior alveolar, and mental and incisive blocks. However, the 27-gauge needle may be more readily available and is also acceptable. The 30-gauge needle is not recommended. See Box 9.1 for the advantages of larger gauge needles.

Length

There are three commonly used needle lengths for intraoral injection: long, short, and extra-short. Despite manufacturer claims that there is uniformity of needle lengths, differences may be found. The following are approximate needle lengths: the extra-short needle is 12 mm, the short needle is 20 mm, and the long needle is 32 mm, as measured from the hub to the tip of the needle (Fig. 9.34).[2,14] Extra-short needles are available only in a 30-gauge. The needle length selection is based on the gauge needed and the amount of tissue that needs to be penetrated to reach the target location and to deposit the anesthetic successfully. Long needles are required for injections that require significant needle penetration of thick tissue to reach the nerve, such as the IA block, Gow-Gates mandibular block, Vazirani-Akinosi block, and infraorbital block (see Chapters 12 and 13). Short needles are preferred for injections that require less soft tissue penetration to reach the target location, such as supraperiosteal injections. Needles used with the Wand handpiece are also available in the standard lengths: 30-gauge ½-inch, 30-gauge 1-inch, and 27-gauge 1¼-inch lengths (Fig. 9.35). Needles are prebonded onto the handpiece for single use (per patient visit). In addition to the prebonded Wand handpieces, Milestone Scientific also offers Wand handpieces without preattached needles. This handpiece requires Luer-Lok needles to be attached to the handpiece. All standard needle lengths and gauges are available as Luer-Lok (Fig. 9.36). When performing STA PDL injections, preattached needles are recommended because of the pressure involved in these injections.

For safety reasons, the needle should never be inserted to the hub. Although needle breakage is rare, a sufficient length of the shaft for any length must be visible in the oral cavity during insertion to permit retrieval of the needle fragment in case of breakage. Long needles are required for the IA block, the Gow-Gates mandibular block, and the Vazirani-Akinosi block, and they are preferred for the infraorbital block. This allows for adequate tissue penetration to reach the target and for sufficient length of the shaft to be visible.

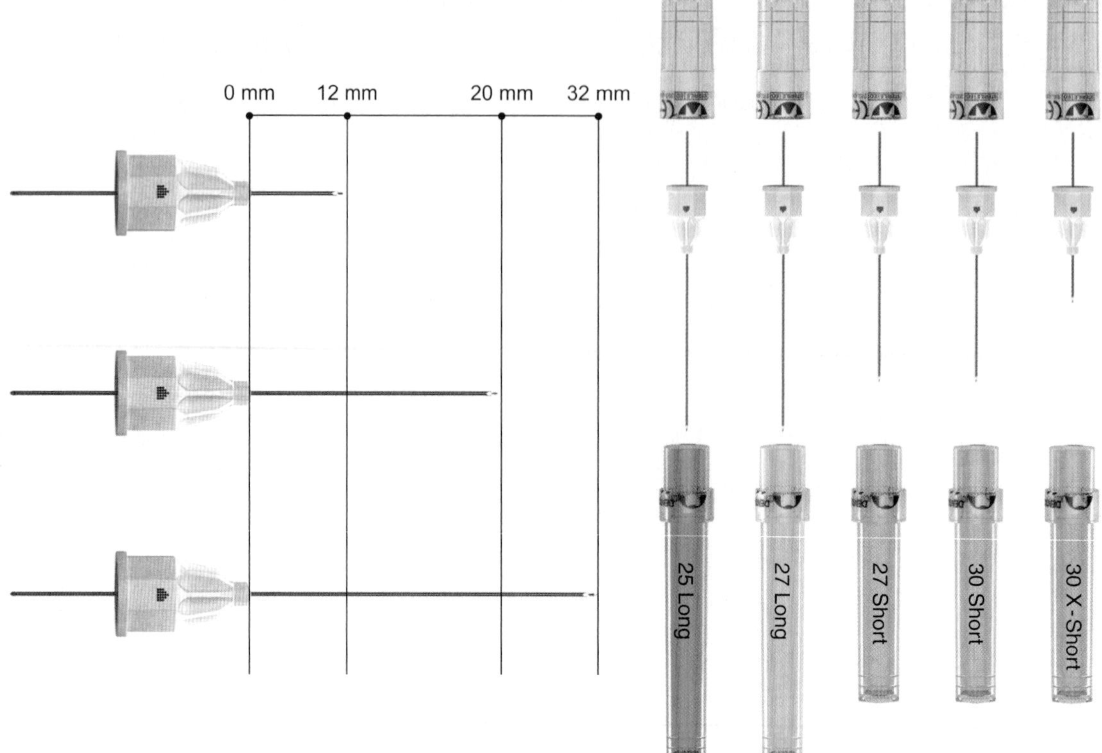

Fig. 9.34 (A) Approximate length of dental needles: extra-short, short, and long. (B) Various needle lengths according to gauge. (Courtesy Septodont, New Castle, DE.)

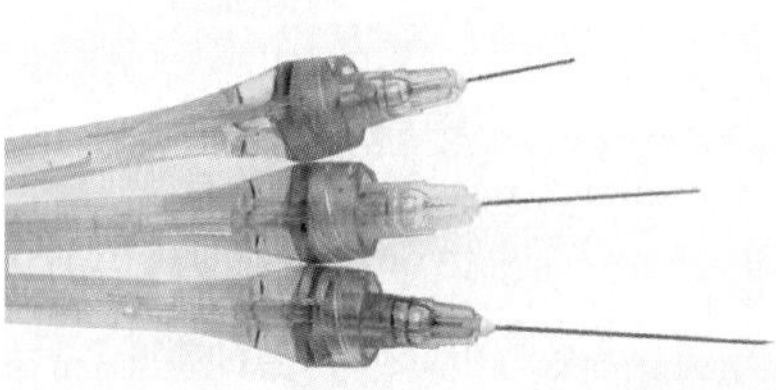

Fig. 9.35 Wand STA handpiece needle lengths. 30-Gauge ½-inch, 30-gauge 1-inch, and 27-gauge 1¼-inch lengths.

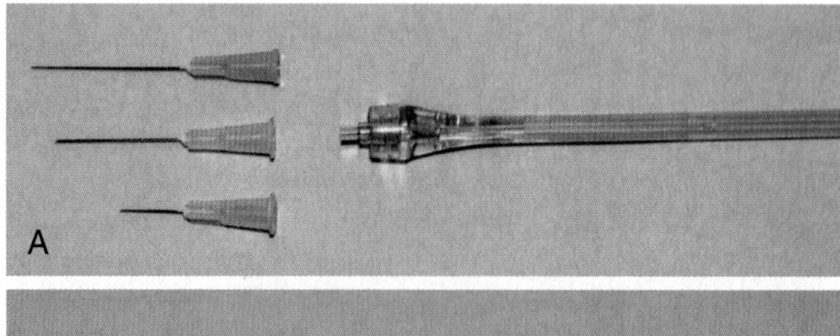

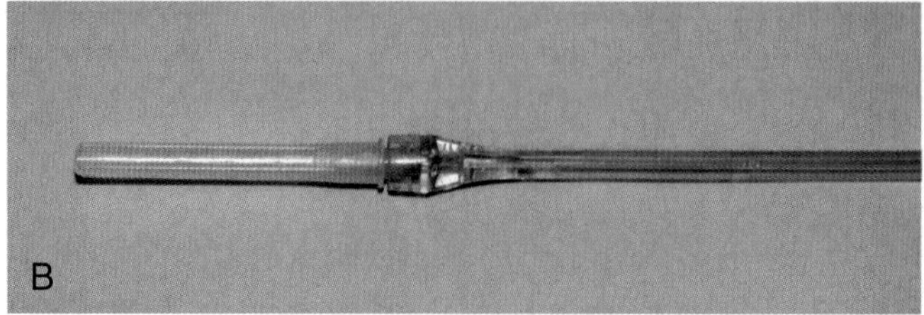

Fig. 9.36 (A) Luer-Lok needles for Wand STA handpiece in extra-short, short, and long lengths. (B) Luer-Lok long needle attached to the Wand handpiece.

Care and Handling of Needles

Proper care and handling of contaminated needles will reduce the risk of needle exposure to the patient and clinician. The following recommendations should be followed by the dental hygienist to minimize the risk of cross contamination:

- Needles are presterilized by the manufacturer and are disposable. They should never be used on more than one patient.
- For patient comfort, the needle should be changed after approximately three to four injections in the same patient. The stainless steel of the needle becomes dull after three to four needle penetrations, causing tissue trauma and pain on insertion with each subsequent injection. The patient may also experience soreness when sensation returns.
- Needles should be immediately covered by the protective shield, using the one-handed scoop method with a needle sheath prop or other recapping aids after the administration of the injection to prevent accidental needlestick with the contaminated needle.
- Several recapping devices are available to assist the dental hygienist in recapping the contaminated needle (Fig. 9.37).
- The dental hygienist should scoop the contaminated needle into the shield using one hand, as demonstrated in Fig. 9.38.
- The dental hygienist should know the location of the uncovered needle tip at all times, whether inside or outside of the patient's mouth. This will prevent needle injury to both the patient and clinician. It will also prevent accidental needle contamination by the clinician in case the needle tip touches any nonsterile extraoral surface. If needle contamination occurs, the dental hygienist should recap the needle using the method described above and discard it in the appropriate sharps container. A new sterilized needle should be placed to complete the injection.

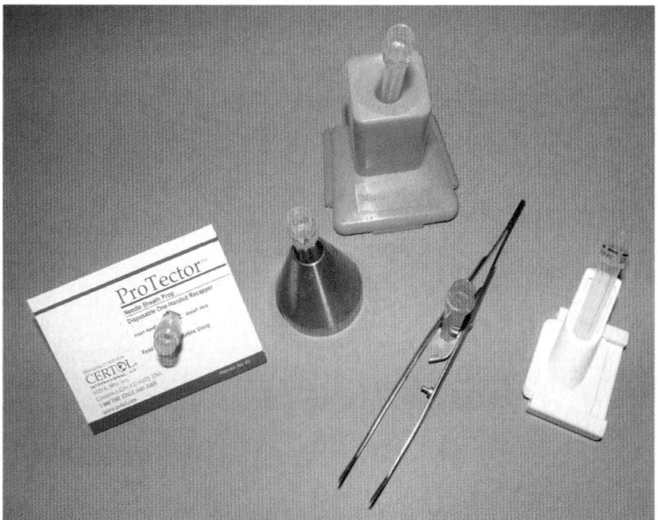

Fig. 9.37 Recapping devices. Needle capping devices are available in many forms to assist the dental hygienist to safely cap the contaminated needle using a one-handed technique.

- Contaminated needles should be properly disposed of after use in an approved sharps container (Fig. 9.39). The sharps container should be properly disposed of according to federal, state, and local regulations.

Needle Problems

The dental hygienist should be aware that several needle problems can occur during or after the injection.

Pain on Insertion

Patients may complain of pain during needle insertion. This is usually caused by dull needles after repeated needle penetrations. To prevent this problem, the dental hygienist should change the needle after three to four needle penetrations.

Pain on Withdrawal

The patient may complain of pain when the needle is withdrawn from the tissue. This is usually caused by barbs on the needle tip. Barbs can occur during manufacturing but are most likely to occur if the needle contacts bone forcefully during the injection. To prevent this, the needle should never be forced against any hard surface during the injection.

Needlestick Exposure to the Clinician

To prevent accidental needlestick exposure to the clinician, the one-handed scoop method with needle sheath prop should be used immediately after the injection to cap the needle in the protective shield. Needlestick injuries typically occur from inattention by the clinician or unexpected patient movement (see Chapter 18 for needlestick protocol).

Needle Breakage

Although needle breakage is rare when needles are properly used, the incidence of needle breakage is increased in the following situations:

- *Bending the needle before the injection.* If the injection is administered properly, there is no need to bend the needle to reach the target location. Bending the needle compromises the integrity of the needle and increases the risk of breakage. Therefore the needle

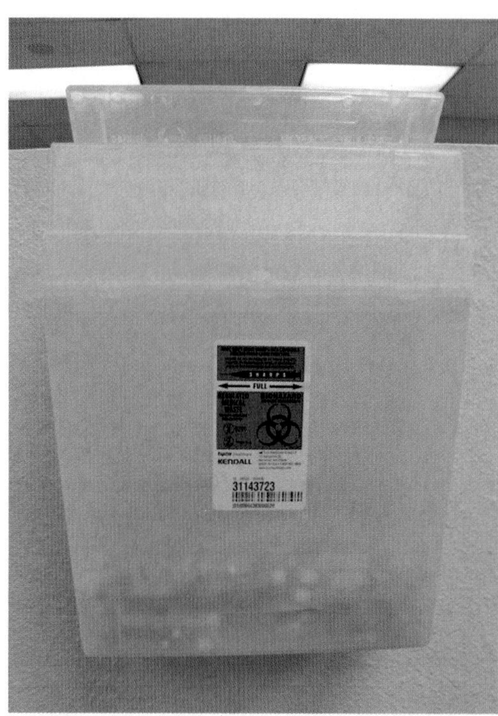

Fig. 9.39 Needle disposal in approved sharps containers.

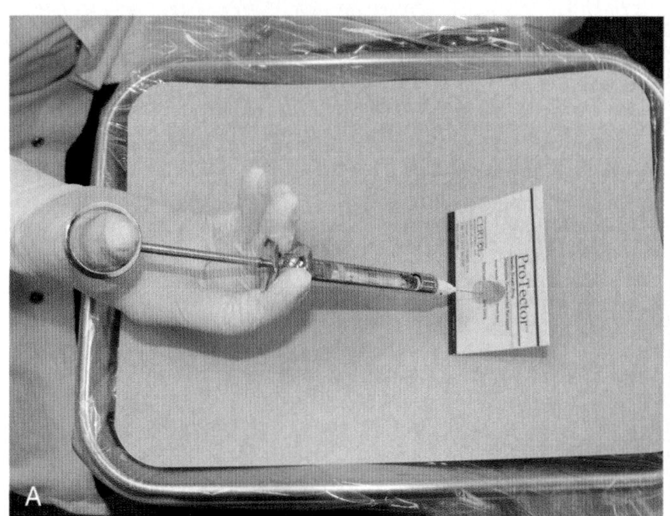

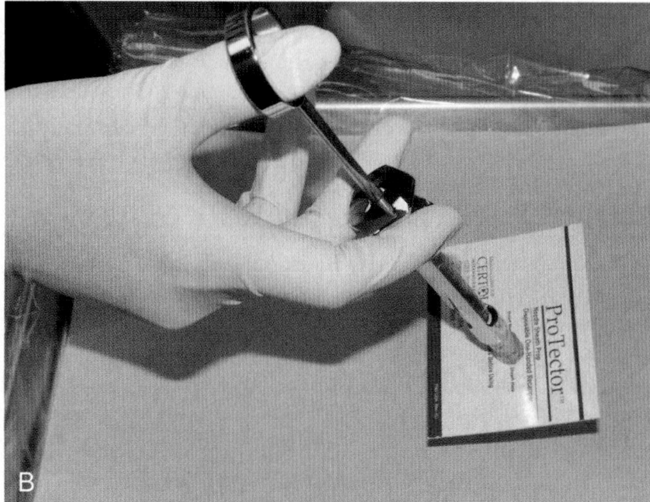

Fig. 9.38 Scoop method with a needle sheath prop to safely cap contaminated needle. (A) One-handed scoop technique. (B) Secure the needle using one hand.

should never be bent by the dental hygienist. The only exception is for intraligamentary injection techniques because the needle will not be in deep tissue.

- *Sudden direction changes.* Needle breakage can occur if sudden direction changes are made during the administration of the anesthetic, especially when the needle is deeply embedded in tissue. If the needle must be redirected during the injection (e.g., troubleshooting the IA block; see Chapter 13), the needle should be withdrawn almost completely from the tissue and the change in direction can be safely made. The needle can then be readvanced to the target location.
- *Forcing the needle against resistance.* Needles are not designed to penetrate bone and should never be forced against resistance.
- *Inserting the needle to the hub.* Breakage of the needle is more likely to occur at the hub (the weakest portion of the needle) if sudden movement of the syringe or patient occurs. The likelihood of needle breakage increases when the needle is inserted into tissue all the way to the hub. Moreover, if the needle breaks at the hub during the injection, the needle fragment will be embedded in tissue and impossible to retrieve.
- *Using 30-gauge needles.* The majority of needle breakage incidences have occurred with 30-gauge short or ultrashort needles.[2] It is recommended that the dental hygienist use 25-gauge needles for all injections that penetrate significant soft tissue (see Chapters 12 and 13).

Local Anesthetic Training Needles

Learning to administer local anesthesia can be challenging and frightening. Research[15] has shown that the novice clinician experiences significant anxiety during local anesthesia training. The local anesthetic training needle known as the *Safe-D-Needle* was developed as a simple, safe, effective teaching aid for clinical instruction of local anesthesia. It is available in short and long needle lengths and resembles a standard dental local anesthetic needle with a safety ball tip that can be set up on a standard syringe (Fig. 9.40A–B). This needle offers students the real-life experience of holding and manipulating a set-up syringe while practicing on real patients. While duplicating the touch and feel of the actual syringe and the standard dental anesthetic needle, the smooth round-ball modification of the tip of the needle allows for unlimited noninvasive practice on patients for the student to gain confidence prior to proceeding to the actual administration of local anesthesia. The clinician is able to practice hand positioning on the syringe, safe entry and exit of the oral cavity, effective positioning of the syringe and syringe stabilization, effective retraction, determination of the insertion point and correct needle angulation, and simulated rotation and aspiration techniques (Fig. 9.41). Additionally, an instructor can make adjustments to the hand and arm of the clinician during practice without concern over a possible needle-inflicted trauma. The needles are for single use and should be discarded in the sharps container utilizing usual protocol (see Chapter 11).

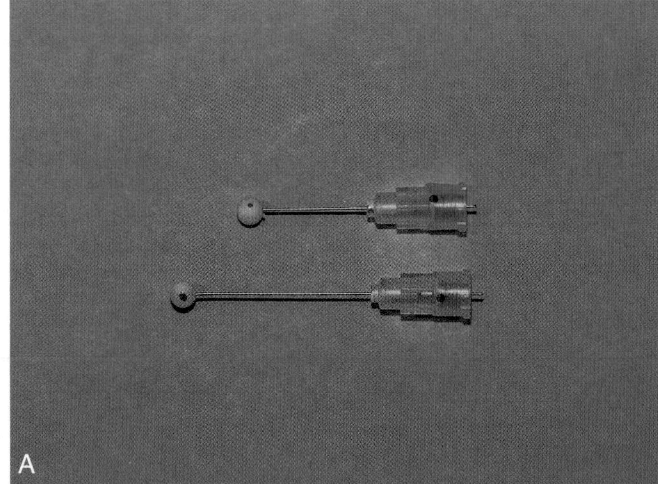

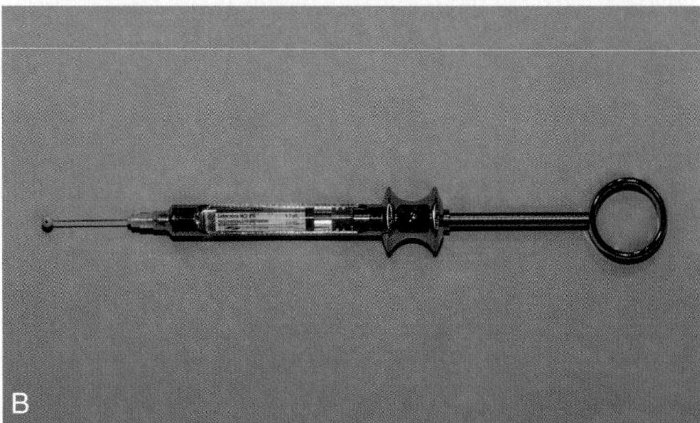

Fig. 9.40 (A) Safe-D-Needles are available in short and long needle lengths and designed with a safety ball tip. The red dot on the ball tip is an indicator of where the bevel of the needle would be to allow the student to practice setting up the needle properly on the syringe. (B) The Safe-D-Needle can be set up on a standard dental syringe.

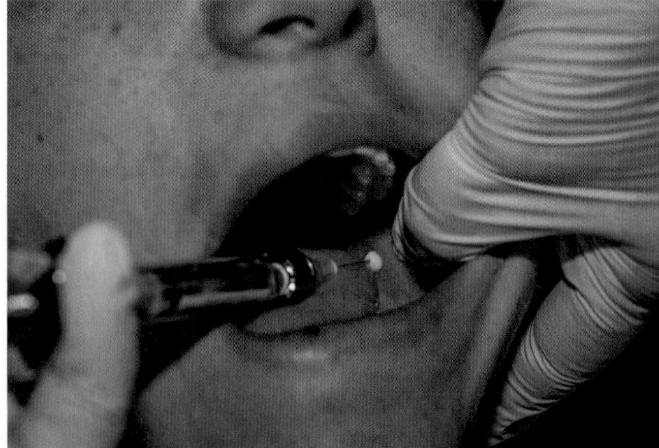

Fig. 9.41 Intraoral image of the Safe-D-Needle in use to aid in noninvasive clinical instruction and practice prior to proceeding to the actual administration of local anesthesia.

ANESTHETIC CARTRIDGES

The glass local anesthetic cartridge contains the sterile local anesthetic drug and other contents in a convenient single-use dose. Each cartridge consists of a glass cylinder with a rubber diaphragm enclosed in a metal cap at the top of the cartridge (Fig. 9.42B) and a silicone rubber stopper at the bottom of the cartridge (Fig. 9.42D). The glass tube allows the dental hygienist adequate visibility of delivered doses and aspiration tests.

Cartridge Components

The standard local anesthetic cartridge is prefilled with up to 1.8 mL of sterile anesthetic agent and consists of several components.

The Glass Cylinder

The glass cylinder (Fig. 9.42A) is the body of the cartridge and contains the anesthetic agent (see Chapter 5 for the composition of the local anesthetic agents). The glass cylinder is capable of containing 2.0 mL of agent. However, once the rubber stopper is added, the net

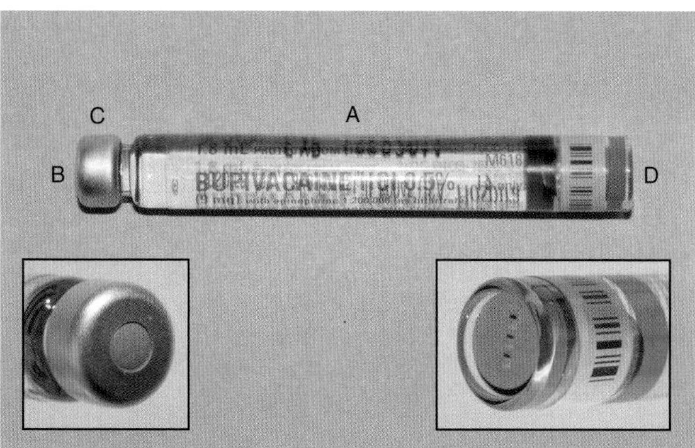

Fig. 9.42 Components of local anesthetic cartridge. (A) Glass cylinder containing anesthetic agent. (B) Diaphragm. (C) Aluminum cap. (D) Silicone rubber stopper slightly indented from glass rim.

volume of anesthetic is reduced to a maximum 1.8 mL for all local anesthetic agents.

Cartridge Labeling

On the body of the glass cylinder, a Mylar plastic label is applied by the manufacturer that lists the contents of the cartridge, trade and generic drug names, drug concentrations, vasoconstrictor dilutions, expiration date, and manufacturer's name (Fig. 9.43A). Some manufacturers may include volume indicators on the label to assist in determining the amount of agent deposited (Fig. 9.44). A color-coded band on the Mylar plastic label on the glass cylinder also identifies the anesthetic drug contained in the cartridge. The standardized color-coded bands are required by the American Dental Association (ADA) for all local anesthetic cartridges to receive the ADA Seal of Approval (Table 9.6 and Fig. 9.43B). The Mylar plastic label also serves as protection to the patient and administrator in the event of glass breakage during the administration of anesthetic.

Silicone Rubber Stopper

The silicone rubber stopper (or plunger) is located at the bottom of the anesthetic cartridge and is slightly indented from the rim of the glass barrel (see Fig. 9.42D). This is an important feature for the dental hygienist to observe when examining the cartridges before syringe setup. Cartridges that have rubber stoppers that are not indented slightly should be discarded because sterility of the anesthetic agent cannot be guaranteed. The harpoon of the aspirating syringe is embedded into the rubber stopper, providing the clinician a means to aspirate. Recently many manufacturers have been using nonlatex materials for the rubber stoppers and rubber diaphragms (discussed next) because latex allergies are becoming more common. The local anesthetic agent is administered by pressure on the thumb ring, creating a forward movement of the rubber stopper into the glass cylinder. The width of each rubber stopper expels approximately 0.2 mL of solution, providing a means to determine the amount of anesthetic deposited when an entire cartridge is not administered (Fig. 9.45).

Diaphragm

The rubber diaphragm is made of semipermeable material and is located at the top of the cartridge where the needle is inserted into the center of the rubber (Fig. 9.42B). Because the rubber is semipermeable, if the cartridge is improperly stored (e.g., in disinfecting solution), the anesthetic agent can be contaminated by diffusion of the disinfecting solution into the cartridge.

Aluminum Cap

The silver-colored aluminum cap fits securely around the rubber diaphragm, keeping it in place (Fig. 9.42C).

Care and Handling of the Cartridge

Local anesthetic cartridges are packaged in boxes containing *blister packs* of 5 or 10 units of 10 sealed cartridges (Fig. 9.46). Local anesthetic cartridges should be stored in their original container at room temperature in a dark place. This keeps the cartridges clean and uncontaminated and prevents premature deterioration of the solution, particularly the oxidation of the vasoconstrictor drug caused by prolonged exposure to heat or direct sunlight.

Commercially available cartridge warmers keep the local anesthetic agent at body temperature. It has been assumed by many dental professionals that this promotes patient comfort during the administration of the anesthetic agent. These warmers are not necessary or recommended. Overheating of the cartridge can cause a burning sensation during injection of the anesthetic agent and destroy the heat-sensitive vasoconstrictor drug and decrease the duration of action.[2,13]

The local anesthetic cartridge does not need to be prepared before use if stored properly. The anesthetic agent is presterilized during manufacturing, and bacterial cultures taken from the exterior cartridge immediately after opening the container have not demonstrated any

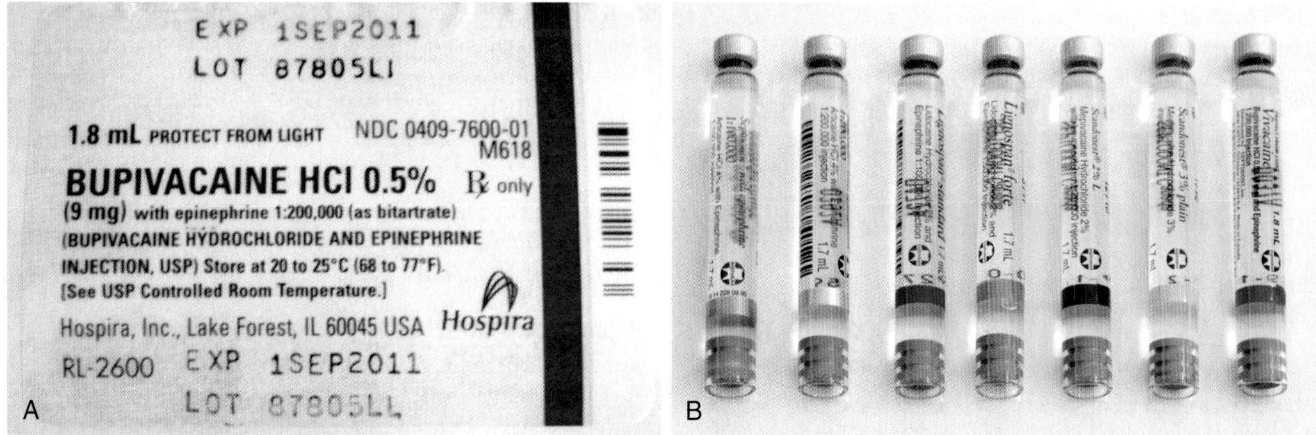

Fig. 9.43 (A) American Dental Association (ADA) Mylar label standard. (B) ADA color coated bands on anesthetic cartridge identify the drug.

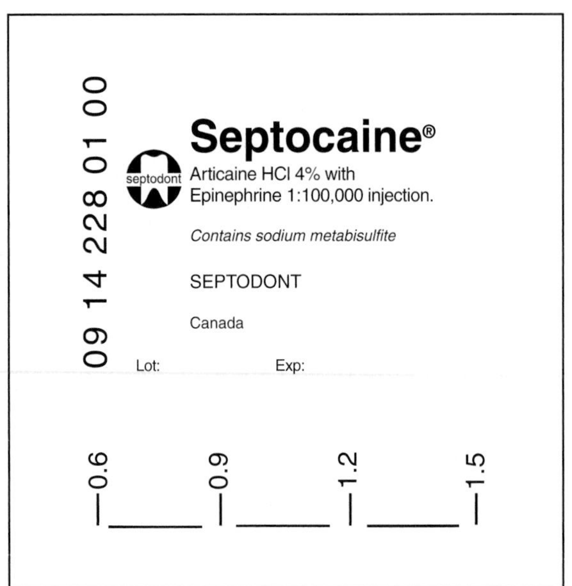

Fig. 9.44 Volume indication label. (From Malamed S: *Handbook of local anesthesia,* St Louis, 2004, Mosby. Courtesy Septodont, New Castle, DE.)

TABLE 9.6 American Dental Association Color Coding of Local Anesthetic Cartridges

Local Anesthetic Drug	ADA Color-Coded Band
Lidocaine 2% 1:50,000 epinephrine	Green
Lidocaine 2% 1:100,000 epinephrine	Red
Mepivacaine 3%	Tan
Mepivacaine 2% 1:20,000 levonordefrin	Brown
Prilocaine 4%	Black
Prilocaine 4% 1:200,000 epinephrine	Yellow
Articaine 4% 1:100,000 epinephrine	Gold
Articaine 4% 1:200,000 epinephrine	Silver
Bupivacaine 0.5% 1:200,000 epinephrine	Blue

ADA, American Dental Association.
Modified from American Dental Association June 2003 color coding of local anesthetic cartridges.

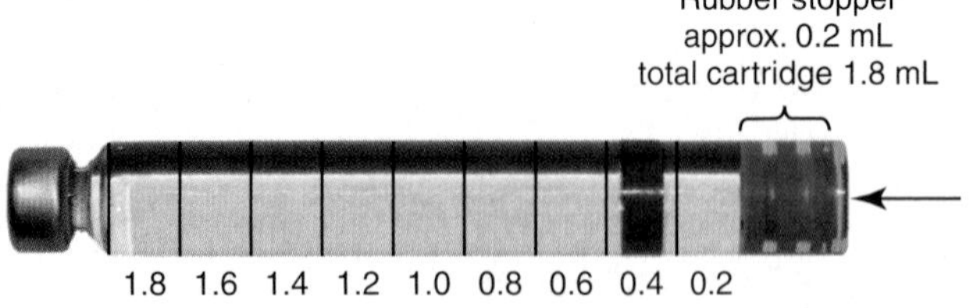

Fig. 9.45 Volume of anesthetic deposited by the width of the rubber stopper.

bacterial growth.[2] If the dental hygienist is concerned about the exterior surfaces of the cartridge, he or she can wipe all the surfaces with an approved ADA disinfectant. The local anesthetic cartridge should never be placed in alcohol or sterilizing solutions because the rubber diaphragm is permeable. This can cause contamination of the local anesthetic agent and corrode the aluminum cap.

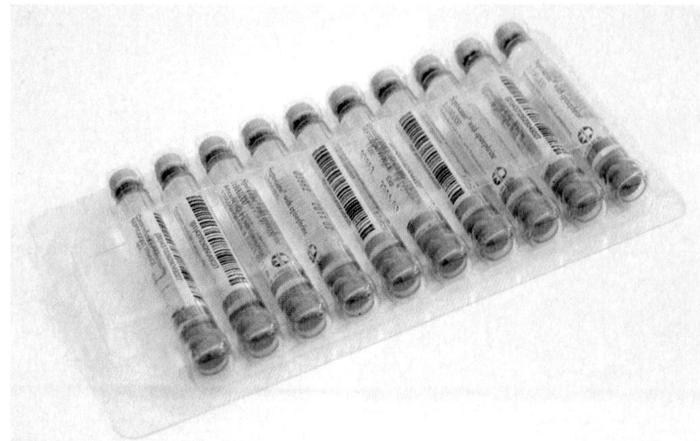

Fig. 9.46 Blister pack of cartridges. (Courtesy Septodont, New Castle, DE.)

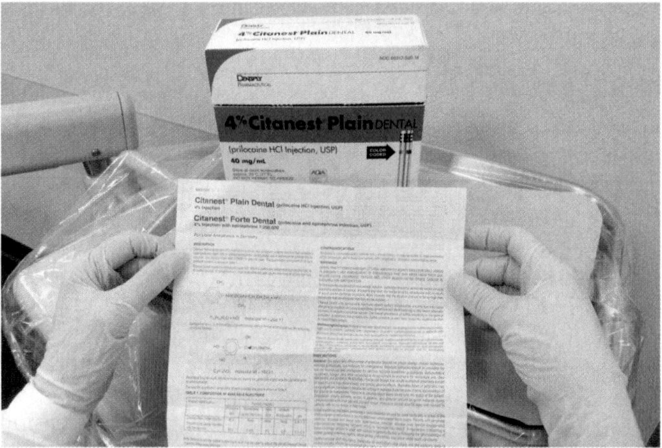

Fig. 9.47 Product insert; the dental hygienist should review for drug information.

The expiration date of the anesthetic is located on the box or canister and is also located on each individual cartridge. Local anesthetic cartridges should be discarded and not used past the expiration date. The reliability of the anesthetic agent cannot be guaranteed, and the administration of an expired anesthetic agent may result in patient discomfort.

The manufacturer inserts product identification information in every local anesthetic container. This provides the clinician with important information concerning the anesthetic agent, including dosages, warnings, precautions, care and handling, and more. Practitioners should review the product inserts periodically as this information can change (Fig. 9.47).

Cartridge Problems

Problems with the cartridge are rarely observed; however, the dental hygienist may encounter the following.

Bubble in the Cartridge

During manufacturing, bubbles can be trapped in the cartridge and are either small or large.

- *Small bubble.* Nitrogen gas is used during manufacturing of the anesthetic agent to prevent oxygen from being trapped in the cartridge, potentially destroying the vasoconstrictor. Small bubbles

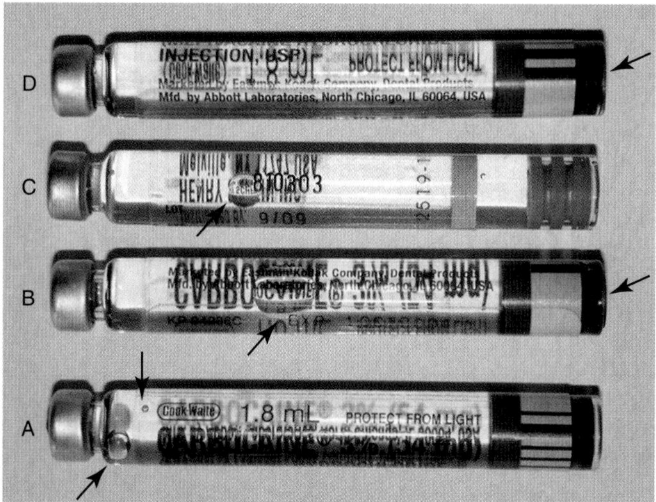

Fig. 9.48 (A) Insignificant small nitrogen bubbles. (B) Large bubble with extruding stopper indicating the cartridge has been frozen and should be discarded. (C) Large bubble without extruded stopper indicating the cartridge has been frozen and should be discarded. (D) Extruded stopper without a bubble indicates the cartridge has been placed in disinfecting solution and should be discarded.

(1–2 mm in diameter) are harmless and produced by nitrogen gas bubbled into the solution during this process (Fig. 9.48A).

- *Large bubble.* Bubbles in the cartridge that are larger than 2 mm are a warning that the anesthetic cartridge has been frozen. They can be present in the cartridge with or without the rubber stopper extended beyond the glass rim. These cartridges should not be used and should be discarded because the sterility of the anesthetic agent cannot be guaranteed (Fig. 9.48B–C).

Extruded Stopper

If the rubber stopper is extruded beyond the glass rim and accompanied with a large bubble, it is an indication the cartridge has been frozen and should not be used (see Fig. 9.48B). An extruded stopper without a large bubble is an indication that the cartridge has been placed in disinfecting solution (see Fig. 9.48D). The disinfecting solution can be diffused through the diaphragm into the anesthetic agent, causing the stopper to extrude past the glass rim. The sterility of the anesthetic agent cannot be guaranteed. These cartridges should not be used and should be discarded.

Sticky Stopper

A sticky stopper is caused by paraffin being employed during manufacturing. This has become less of a problem because most manufacturers are currently treating the rubber stopper with silicone. Storing cartridges at room temperature can minimize this problem.

Burning on Injection

Burning sensations can be experienced by the patient for the following reasons:

- *pH of the drug.* This is a normal reaction to the anesthetic agent having a lower pH (5–6) than the tissues (7.4) in which it is administered. The sensation only lasts a couple of seconds until the anesthetic takes effect and is noted primarily on sensitive patients and when the anesthetic is deposited on anterior teeth.
- *Cartridge contains a vasoconstrictor drug.* The use of a vasoconstrictor and the sodium bisulfite preservative lowers the pH of the anesthetic even further than the anesthetic without a vasoconstrictor to between 3.0 and 5.5, which causes a burning sensation.
- *Overheated cartridges.* Overheating of cartridges causes burning sensations upon administration. Warmers are not recommended, and local anesthetic agent should be kept at room temperature.
- *Expired agents.* The burning sensation from local anesthetic agents, especially those that contain a vasoconstrictor, is enhanced when an expired agent is used. This can be avoided by carefully checking the expiration date before use.
- *Cartridge containing disinfecting solution.* Cartridges contaminated with disinfecting solution and subsequently injected into the mucous membranes can produce an intense burning sensation. This can also cause other problems such as paresthesia and tissue edema (see Chapter 16). Cartridges should never be placed in disinfecting solution.

Corroded Cap

The dental hygienist may observe a corroded aluminum cap (white debris) if it has been immersed in quaternary compounds such as benzalkonium chloride used for "cold sterilization." Disinfection of the cartridge can be accomplished by using an approved ADA disinfectant lightly applied to a gauze square. Never immerse the cartridge into disinfecting solutions.

Rust on Cap

Red rust on the cartridge is an indication that a cartridge contained in the metal container has broken, depositing the anesthetic agent on the other cartridges within the container. This cartridge should not be used and should be discarded, and all other cartridges within the same container should be evaluated for rust.

Leakage During Injection

This is caused by a bent needle or the off-center perforation of the needle-penetrating end into the rubber diaphragm of the anesthetic cartridge, producing an oval puncture. When the anesthetic agent is administered, leakage through the diaphragm may occur. The dental hygienist should carefully examine the needle before syringe setup and insert the needle straight into the diaphragm to avoid this problem.

Broken Cartridge

A broken cartridge can be a result of the following situations:

- *Breakage during shipping and handling.* Cartridges arriving in damaged containers should be examined carefully for possible fractures or chips in the cartridges. Hairline fractures may not be easily identified. However, the Mylar plastic label also serves as a protective shield by reinforcing the glass in case the cartridge fractures during administration.
- *Excessive force during harpoon engagement.* The harpoon should be gently engaged into the rubber stopper during syringe setup. Exerting excessive force may fracture the cartridge.

OTHER ANESTHETIC DEVICES

Onset Mixing Pen

As discussed in Chapter 3, all local anesthetic solutions are acidic prior to injection, causing a slower than desired onset of pulpal anesthesia, stinging or burning sensation on injection, postinjection tissue injury, and poor reliability of local anesthetic action in the presence of infection and inflammation. Anesthetic buffering provides a way to neutralize the anesthetic immediately before the injection to bring the pH of the anesthetic toward physiologic values to improve patient comfort by eliminating the sting, reduce tissue injury and anesthetic latency, and provide more effective anesthesia in the area of infection.[16-19] The buffering process uses a sodium bicarbonate solution that is mixed via

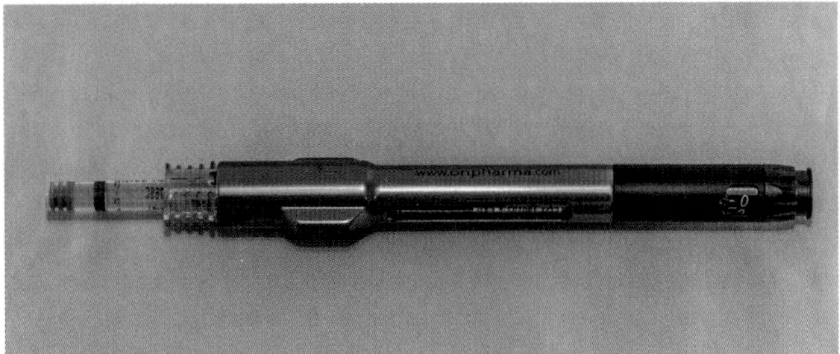

Fig. 9.49 Assembled Onset Mixing Pen.

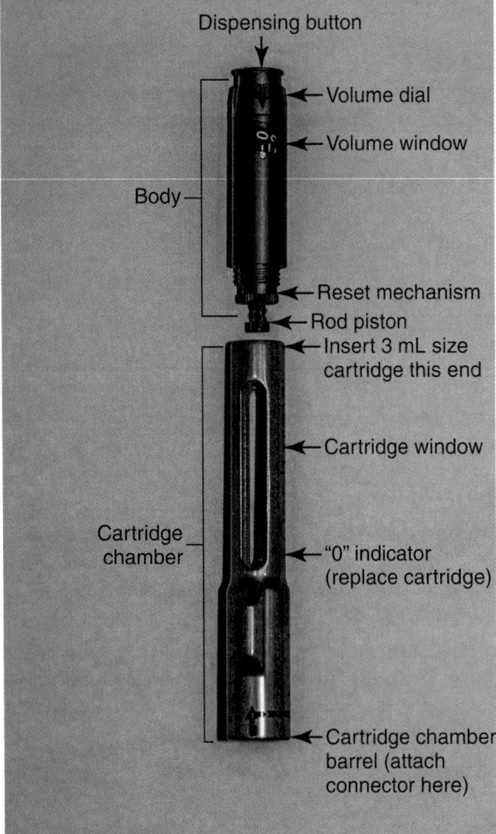

Fig. 9.50 Onset Mixing Pen parts.

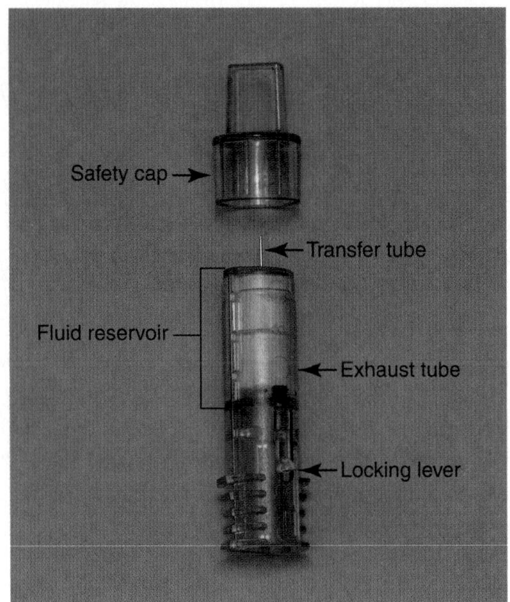

Fig. 9.51 Onset Cartridge Connector parts. The cartridge connector transfers sterile fluids from one sealed container into a second sealed container.

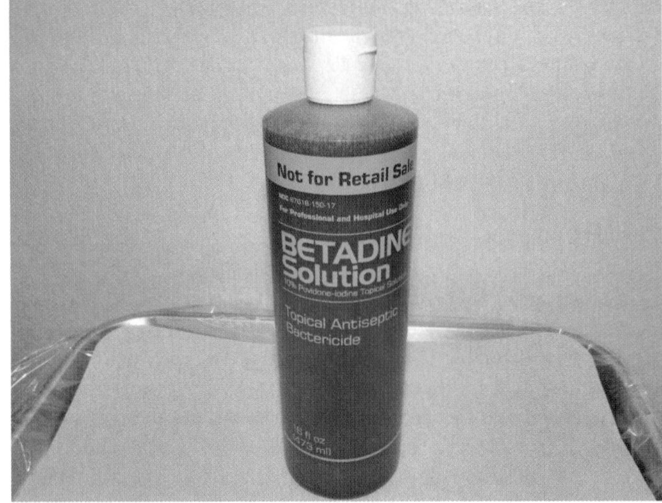

Fig. 9.52 Topical antiseptic.

the Onset Mixing Pen device with the cartridge of local anesthetic. The Onset Mixing Pen (Fig. 9.49) is a dispensing device used for mixing two solutions together during the buffering process. It dispenses a standard 3 mL cartridge of sodium bicarbonate 8.4% USP buffer solution to a standard 1.8 mL cartridge of anesthetic with vasoconstrictor to mix the solutions (Fig. 9.50). The Mixing Pen is designed to be used with an Onset Cartridge Connector (Fig. 9.51) for the transfer of sterile fluids from one sealed container into a second sealed container. The connector provides a reservoir for collecting waste fluid displaced from the second container during the transfer process. For information on how to buffer local anesthetics using the Onset Mixing Pen, see Procedure Box 9.8.

SUPPLEMENTARY ARMAMENTARIUM

In addition to the syringe, needle, and cartridge, supplemental equipment includes topical antiseptic, topical anesthetic, applicator sticks, gauze, and hemostat or cotton pliers, and needle capping aids.

TOPICAL ANTISEPTIC

A topical antiseptic (Betadine or Merthiolate) may be applied to the tissue to reduce the possibility of surface microorganisms from entering the soft tissue, which could result in a postinjection infection[2] (Fig. 9.52). This step is optional, and before application the patient must be first screened for a possible allergy to iodine. However, the use of topical antiseptic before the administration should be considered for patients who are immunosuppressed.[2] Other methods to reduce surface bacteria before the injection include wiping the surface with gauze or having the patient preprocedural rinse with 0.2% chlorhexidine.

Topical Anesthetic

Topical anesthetic agents are applied to the mucous membranes before needle insertion to provide soft tissue anesthesia of the terminal nerve endings for patient comfort. They are most effective if applied to the

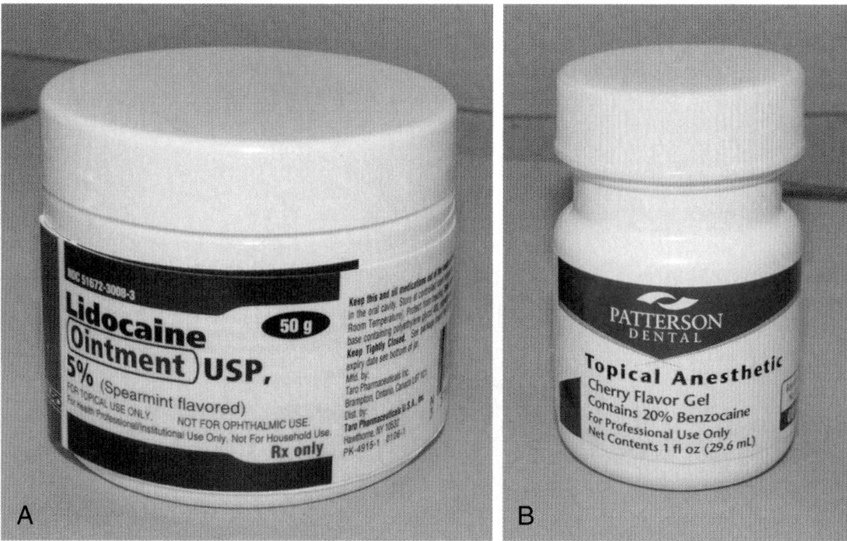

Fig. 9.53 Topical anesthetic. (A) Lidocaine (amide). (B) Benzocaine (ester).

dry mucous membrane for 1 to 2 minutes. Topical anesthetics do not contain vasoconstrictors and are absorbed rapidly when applied to the mucous membrane. The concentration of topical anesthetics is high compared with injectable anesthetics to facilitate diffusion through the mucous membranes (approximately 2–3 mm).[9] Because of the rapid absorption and higher concentrations, only small amounts should be used and caution should be taken to avoid toxic reactions from surface applications (Fig. 9.53 and see Chapter 6).

Applicator Sticks

Cotton-tipped applicator sticks are used in the application of topical antiseptics and anesthetics. They are also recommended to provide pressure anesthesia during palatal injections (Fig. 9.54).

Gauze

Gauze 2 × 2 squares are used to dry the mucous membranes before the application of topical antiseptic and anesthetic. They are also used to dry the tissue before needle insertion, and although not as effective, can serve as an alternative to the application of topical antiseptic. The gauze squares can assist in retraction, visibility, and stabilization.

Hemostat or Cotton Pliers

Hemostat or cotton pliers should be a part of the local anesthetic armamentarium in the rare incidence of a needle breakage. The hemostat, or cotton pliers, can aid in the retrieval of the needle fragment (Fig. 9.55).

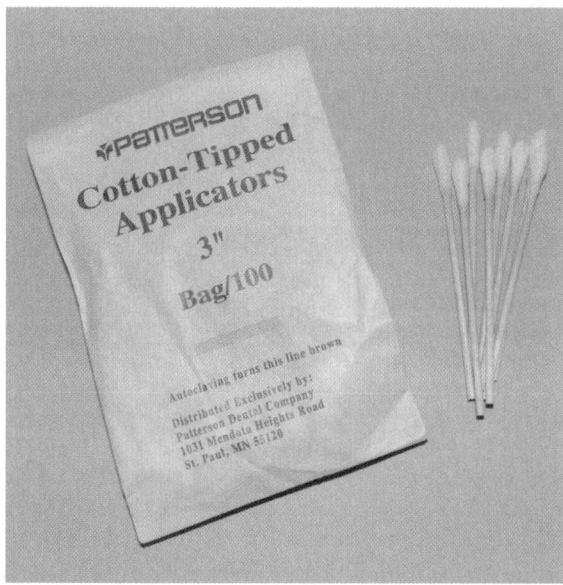

Fig. 9.54 Cotton-tipped applicator sticks.

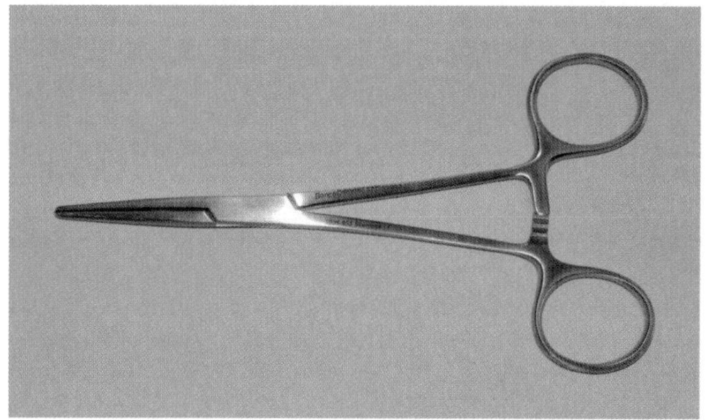
Fig. 9.55 Hemostat.

PROCEDURE 9.2 Preparation of the Breech-Loading Aspirating Syringe

Step 1

Based on the treatment to be performed and the patient's medical history, the appropriate local and topical anesthetics should be selected, and the appropriate equipment should be assembled.

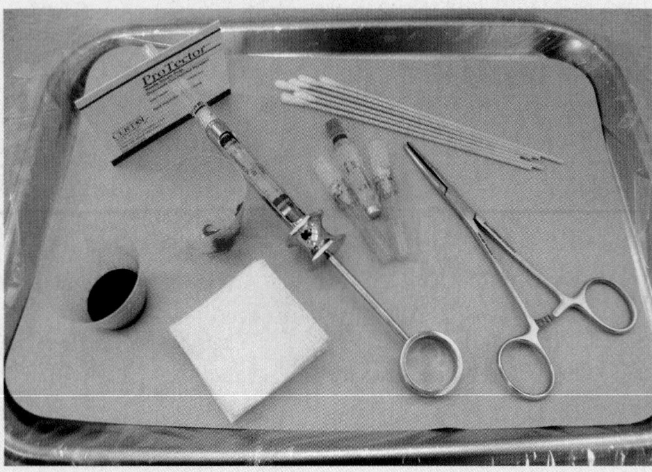

The equipment should include:

- Personal protective equipment
- Anesthetic syringe
- Anesthetic cartridge
- Needle (length and gauge selected according to injection to be administered)
- Topical antiseptic (optional)
- Topical anesthetic
- Gauze
- Cotton-tipped applicators
- Hemostat or cotton pliers

Step 2

The dental hygienist should carefully evaluate the local anesthetic cartridge:

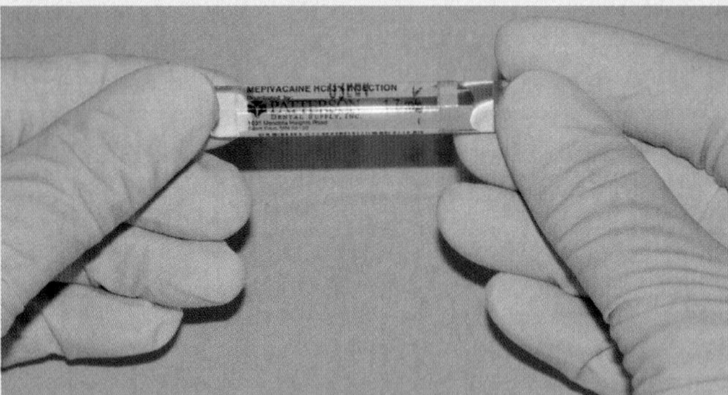

Check the selected anesthetic to ensure that the proper drug has been selected.
Check that anesthetic drug is not outdated.
Check for large bubbles that might be present in the cartridge.
Check for an extruded stopper that extends beyond the glass rim.
Check for any corrosion or rust on the cartridge.
Check the cartridge for any hairline fractures or chipped glass.

(Continued)

PROCEDURE 9.2 Preparation of the Breech-Loading Aspirating Syringe (*Cont.*)

Step 3 (Optional)

If the dental hygienist feels it is necessary, he or she can wipe the rubber diaphragm with a disinfectant applied to a gauze square.

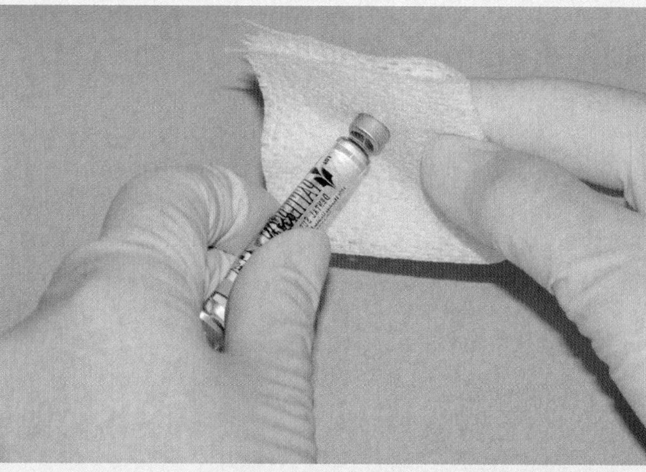

Step 4

Retract the piston of the syringe by pulling back on the thumb ring.

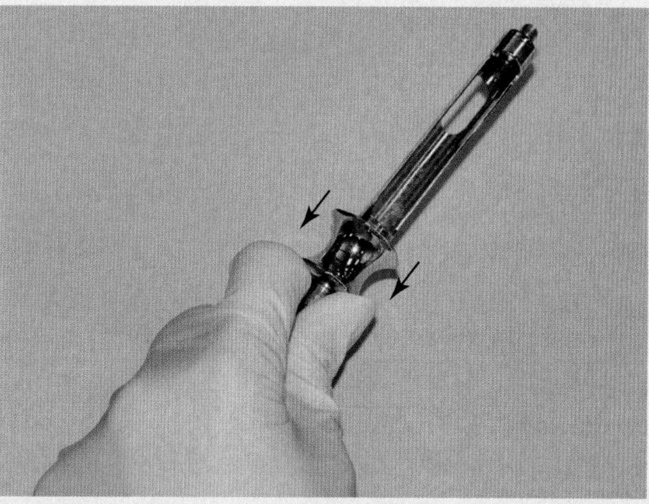

Step 5

Insert the cartridge with the rubber stopper going into the syringe first, toward the piston.

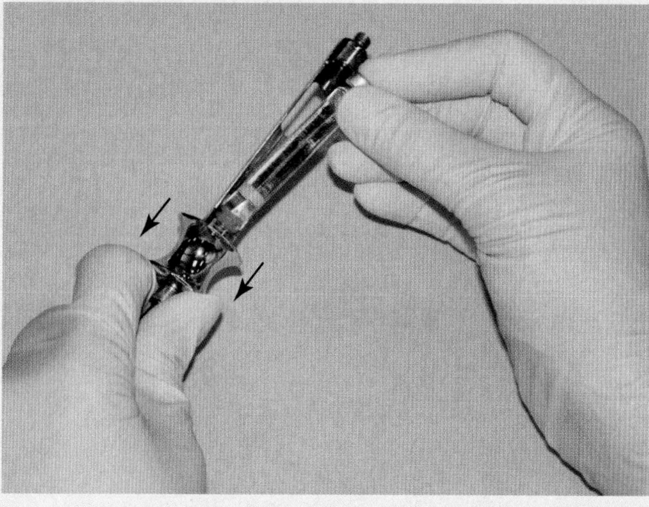

PROCEDURE 9.2 Preparation of the Breech-Loading Aspirating Syringe (*Cont.*)

Step 6

Engage the harpoon into the plunger with gentle finger pressure exerted on the thumb ring.

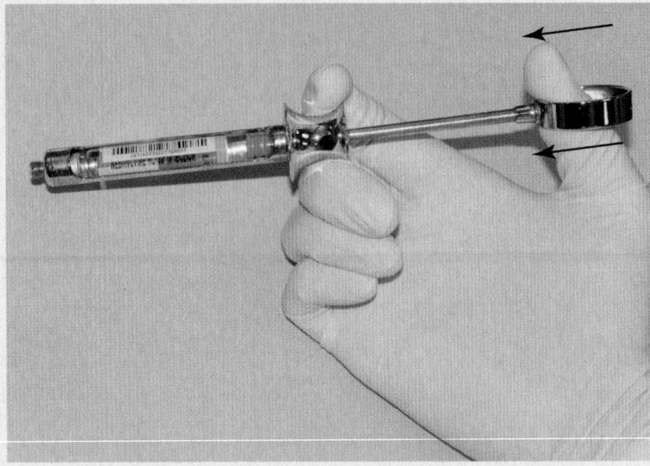

Do NOT exert extreme force on the rubber stopper; the glass cartridge may break.

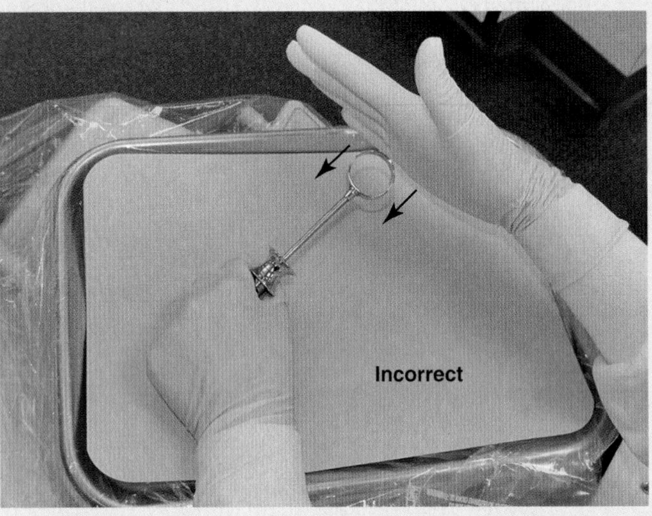

(*Continued*)

PROCEDURE 9.2 Preparation of the Breech-Loading Aspirating Syringe (*Cont.*)

Step 7

Attach the needle. Remove the shield from the needle penetrating end. If the seal is intact, it should require snapping the seal as the shield is twisted. Seals that are not intact should be discarded.

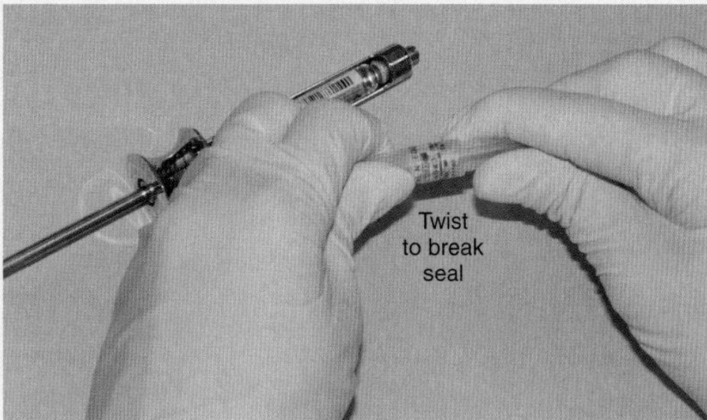

Attach the needle to the metal needle adaptor of the syringe. If a plastic hub is being used, the dental hygienist must simultaneously push and screw the needle into position. The needle should always be attached to the syringe after the cartridge has been inserted. It is too difficult to engage the harpoon into the rubber stopper when the needle is already in place, causing excessive force to be applied to the thumb ring to engage the harpoon.

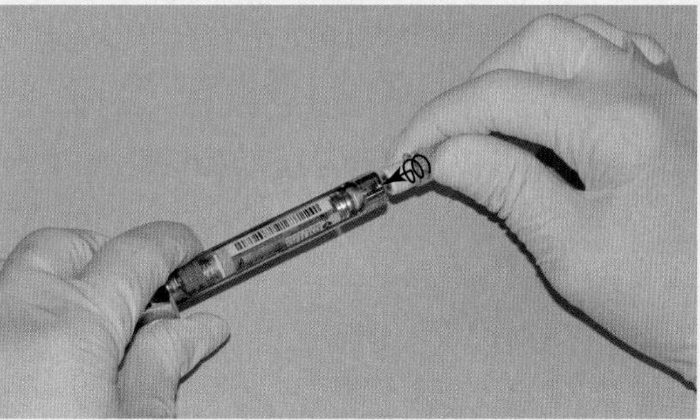

Step 8

Carefully uncap the colored plastic shield on the needle and expel a few drops of anesthetic to ensure the proper flow of the agent.

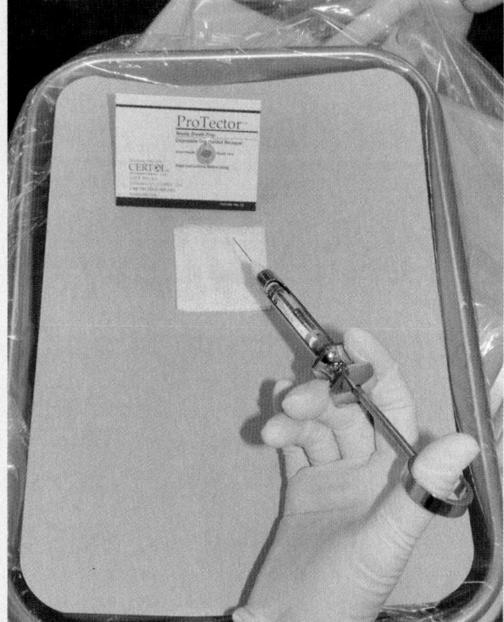

PROCEDURE 9.2 Preparation of the Breech-Loading Aspirating Syringe (*Cont.*)

Step 9	Scoop the protective shield back onto the needle using the one-handed scoop technique with a needle sheath prop to protect the needle until it is ready for use. The one-handed scoop technique should be used whether or not the needle is contaminated. Needle capping devices are available in many forms (see Fig. 9.37). Individual preference will determine the aid that is appropriate. 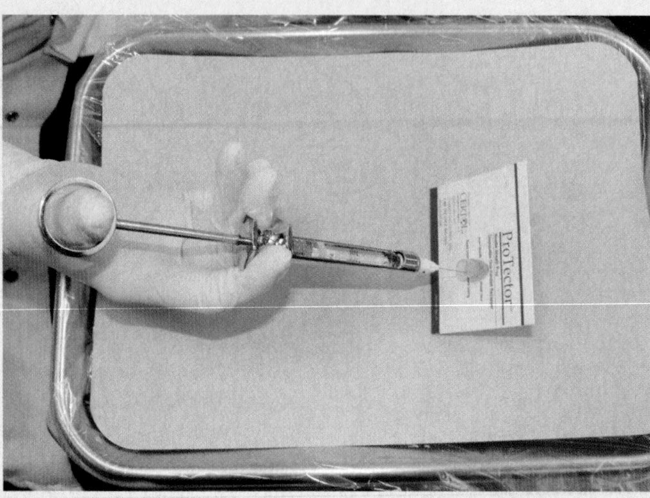
Step 10	The protective shield should remain on the needle at all times when the syringe is not in use. 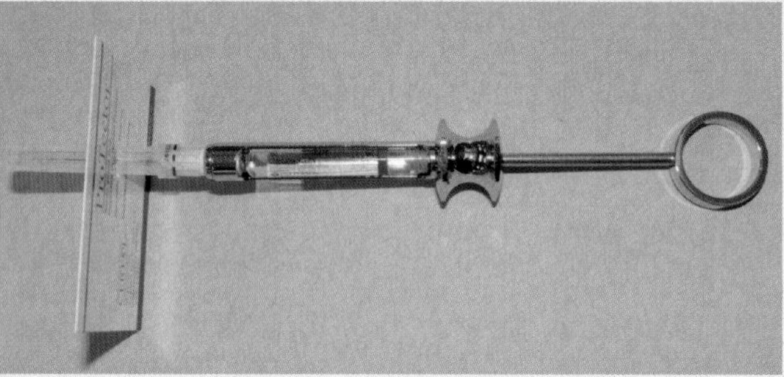

PROCEDURE 9.3 Unloading the Breech-Loading Aspirating Syringe

Step 1

Take the syringe to the appropriate sharps container. Carefully remove the needle.

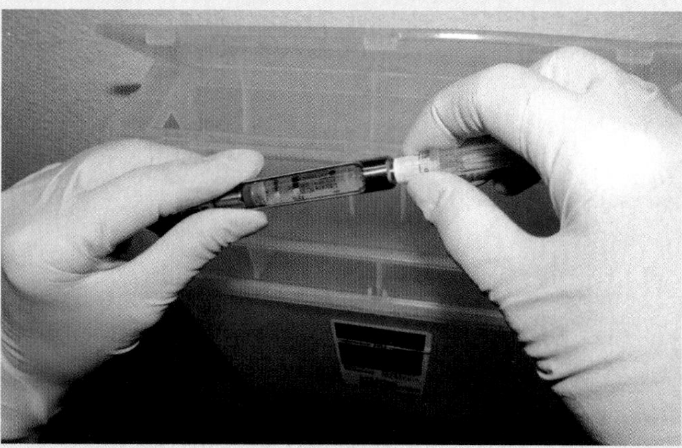

Immediately discard in the approved sharps container.

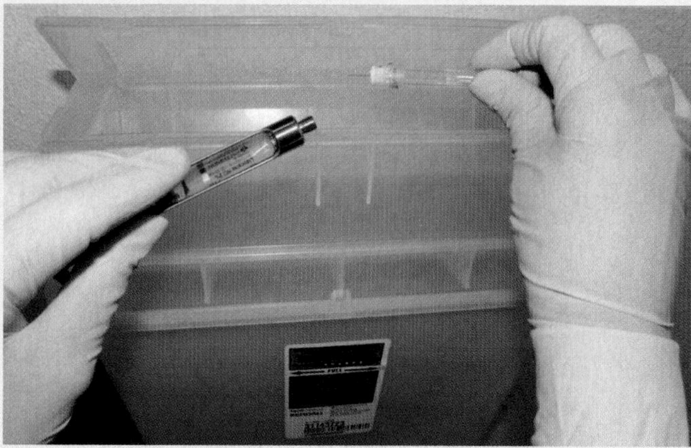

If using a cardboard needle sheath prop, hold the needle from the back of the sheath and gently push the needle through the sheath until it drops into the sharps container.

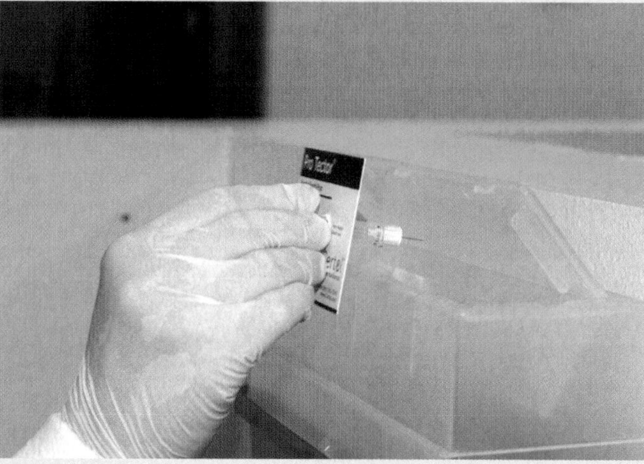

PROCEDURE 9.3 Unloading the Breech-Loading Aspirating Syringe (*Cont.*)

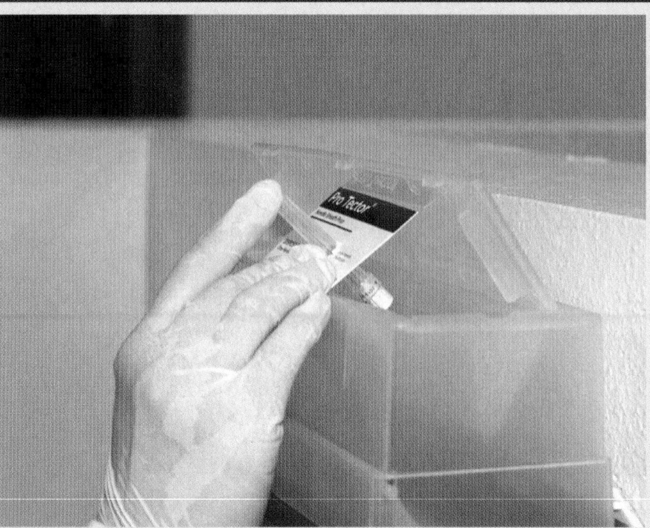

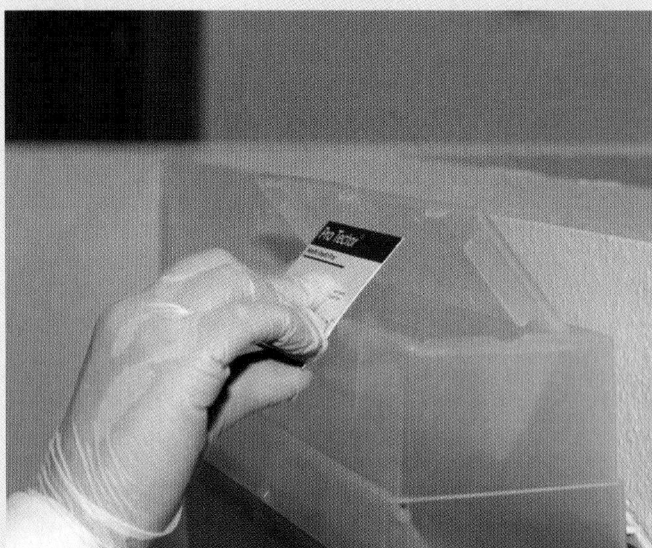

It is recommended that the cartridge-penetrating end of the needle not be recapped and left on the anesthetic tray before discarding because there is the possibility that the used needle could be mistaken for an unused needle and be reused on another patient. This technique ensures that the needle cannot accidentally be used on another patient and protects the clinician from needlestick exposure from the needle-penetrating end.

When discarding the needle, care should be taken to avoid inadvertently discarding the needle adaptor.

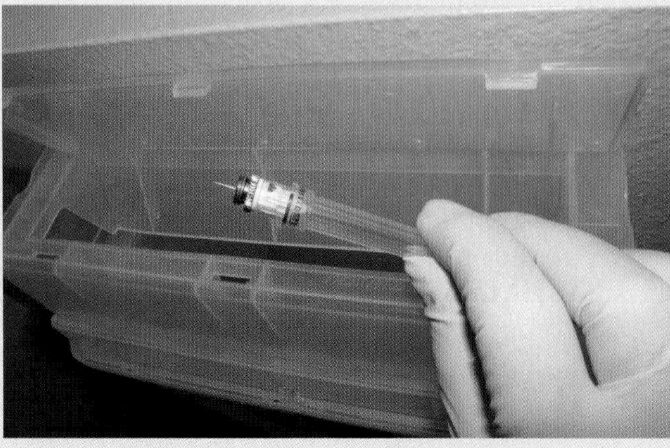

(*Continued*)

PROCEDURE 9.3 Unloading the Breech-Loading Aspirating Syringe (*Cont.*)

If the needle adaptor remains on the needle, it can be safely removed with cotton pliers.

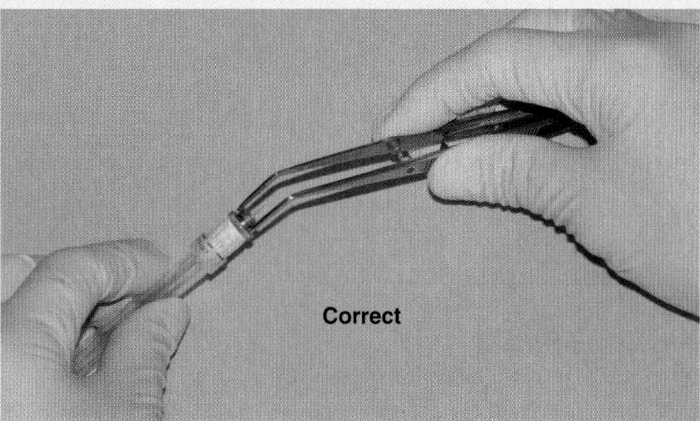

Never attempt to remove the needle adaptor with unprotected hands.

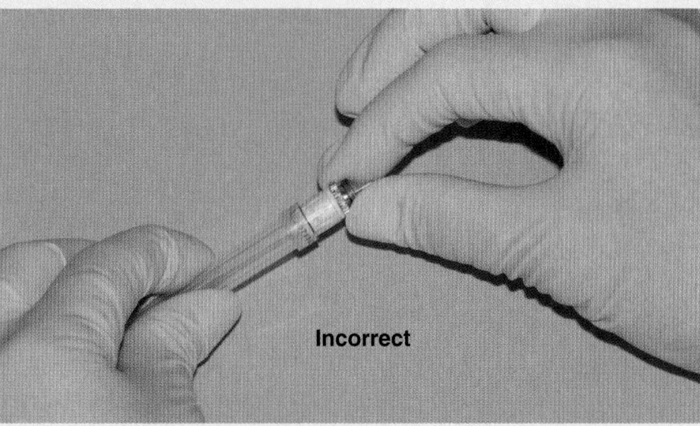

Step 2 Retract the piston by pulling back on the thumb ring.

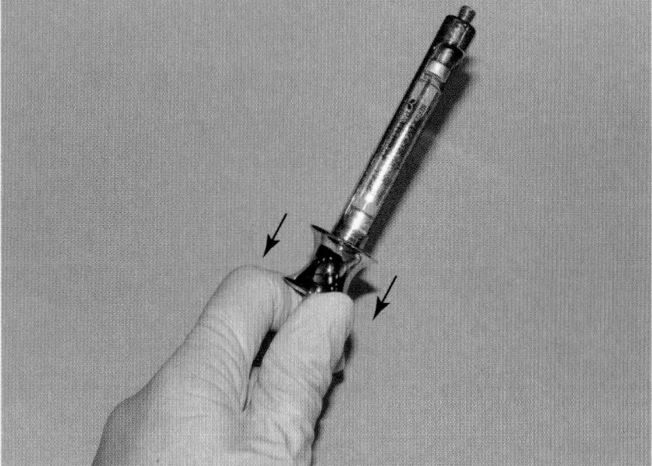

PROCEDURE 9.3 Unloading the Breech-Loading Aspirating Syringe (*Cont.*)

Step 3

Remove the cartridge.

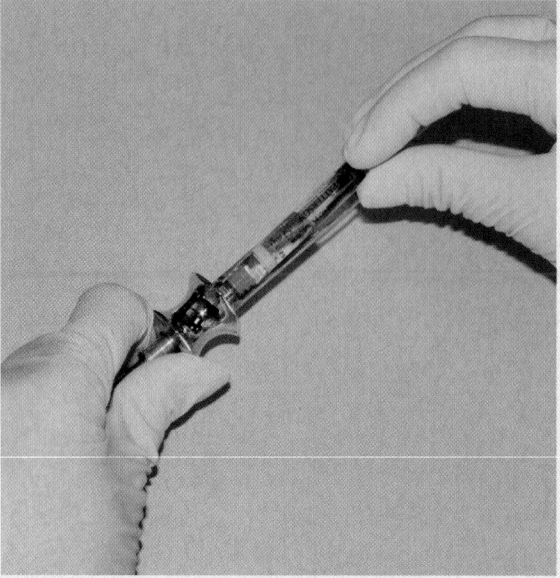

Dispose of in separate sealed container or in approved sharps container.

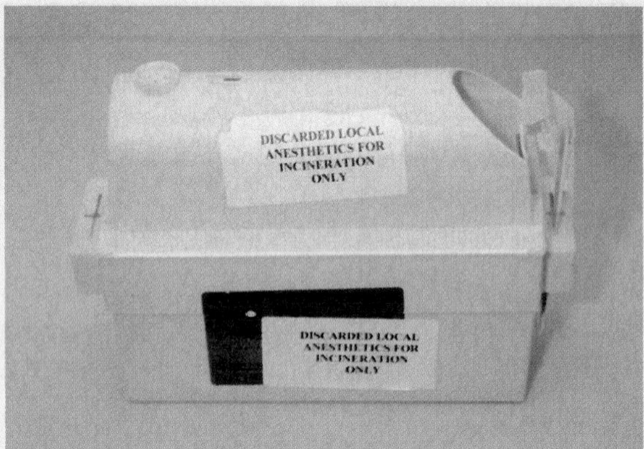

Occasionally the rubber stopper may be lodged on the harpoon. It can be safely removed with cotton pliers.

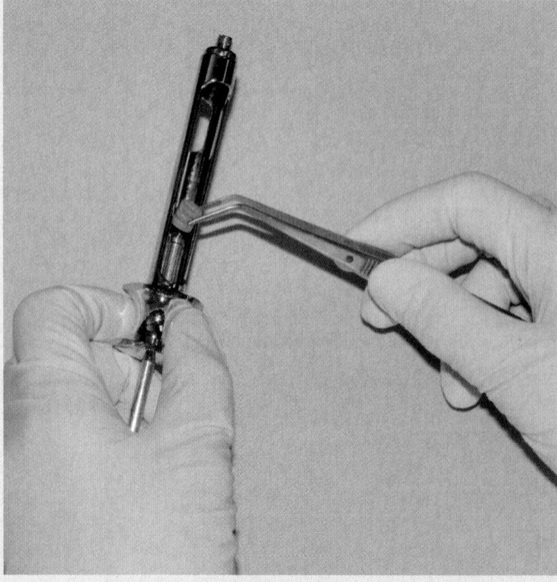

PROCEDURE 9.4 Preparation and Use of the Ultra Safety Plus XL Aspirating Syringe

Step 1

Review Procedure 9.2 steps 1-3.
Remove the syringe by tearing open the sterile package.

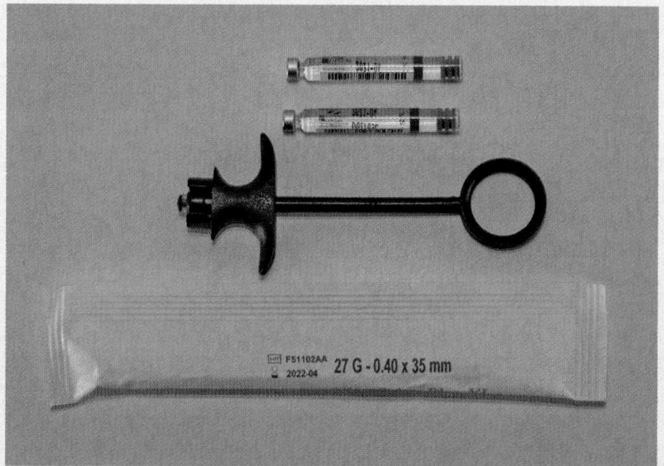

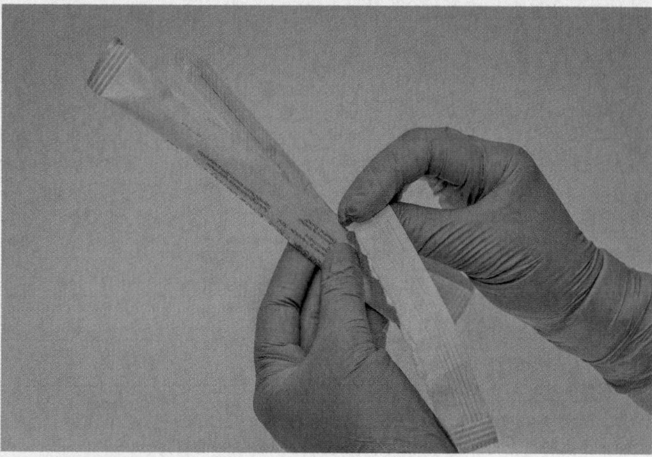

Step 2

Insert the cartridge into the barrel of the safety syringe.

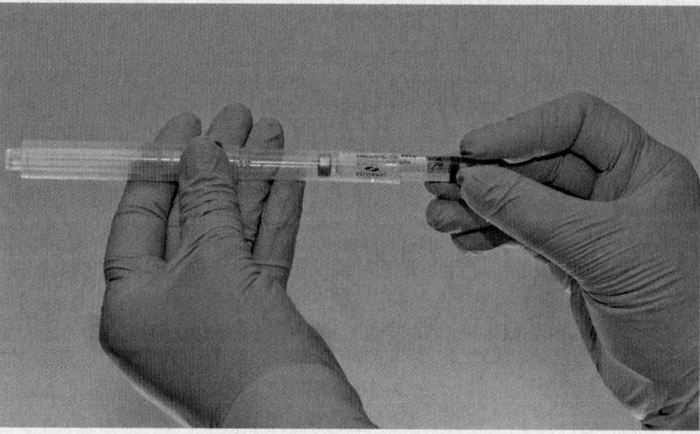

PROCEDURE 9.4 Preparation and Use of the Ultra Safety Plus XL Aspirating Syringe (*Cont.*)

Step 3

Retract the thumb ring of the handle backward so the piston is fully retracted, and introduce the handle tip into the barrel of the injectable system behind the cartridge. Push forward to lock the handle in place.

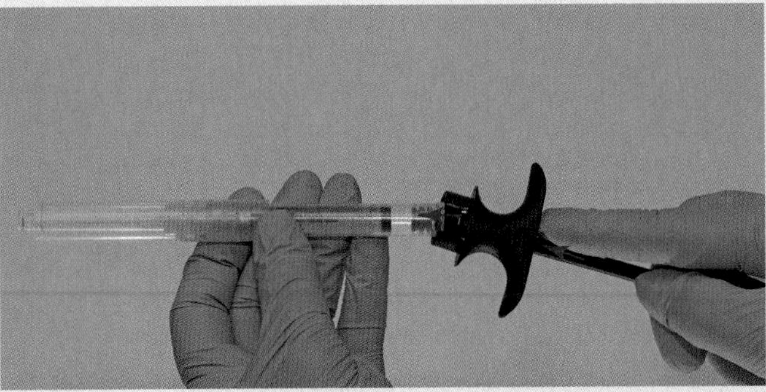

Step 4

With your thumb and forefinger on the finger grips, pull down the protective sheath until it clicks and locks on the handle.

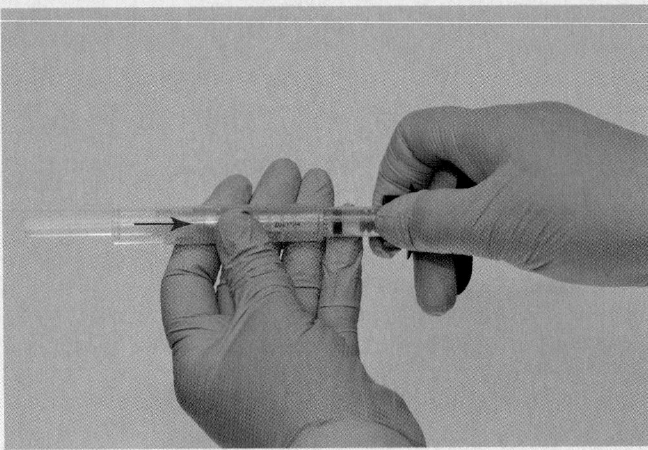

Step 5

Remove the needle cap and discard it. The Ultra Safety Plus has a bevel indicator, and the bevel should be positioned to be facing the bone during the injection.

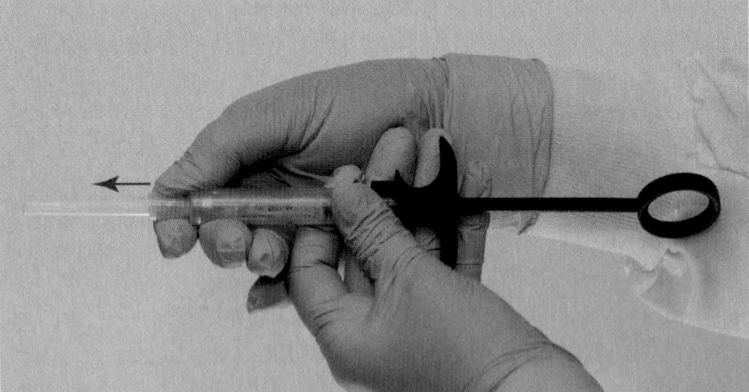

The syringe is now ready for use.

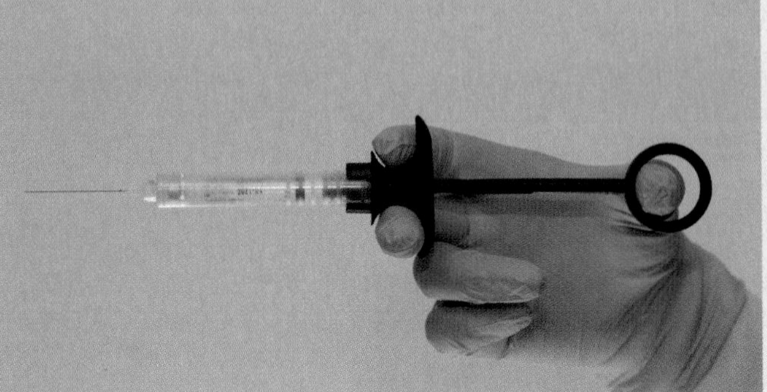

(*Continued*)

PROCEDURE 9.4 Preparation and Use of the Ultra Safety Plus XL Aspirating Syringe (*Cont.*)

Step 6

Aspiration

Passive aspiration (self-aspiration):

The small protuberance at the base of the cartridge barrel penetrates the diaphragm of the cartridge when inserted. At the start of the injection when the dental hygienist exerts pressure on the thumb ring, the diaphragm is pressed and stretched against the protuberance. When the thumb ring is released, the diaphragm moves back away from the protuberance and aspiration occurs.

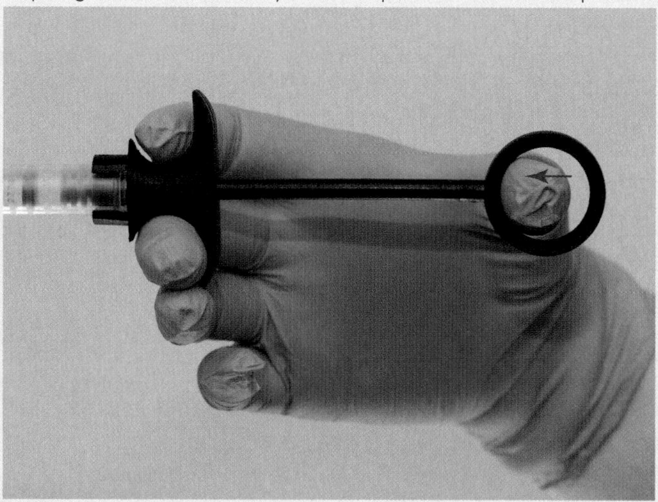

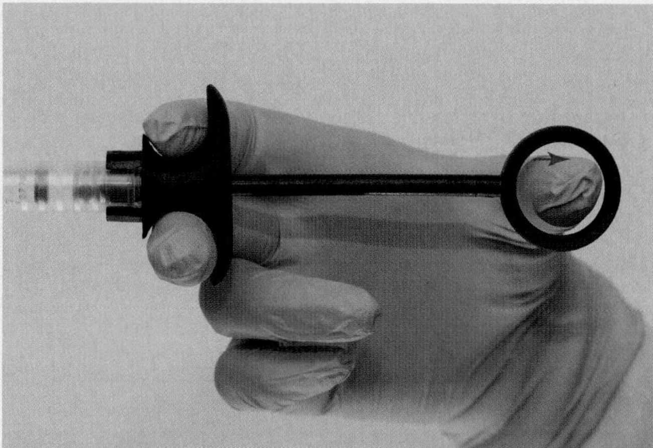

Active aspiration:

The clinician pulls back on the thumb ring, pulling the rubber stopper in the cartridge backward, creating negative pressure in the cartridge and causing an active aspiration.

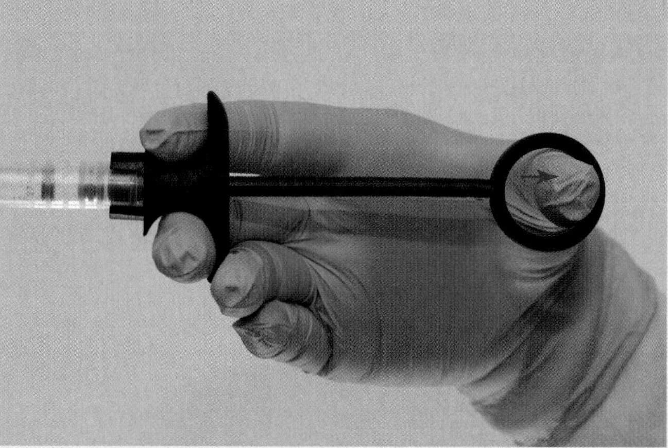

After a negative aspiration, the clinician can inject the solution.

PROCEDURE 9.4 Preparation and Use of the Ultra Safety Plus XL Aspirating Syringe (*Cont.*)

Step 7

When the determined amount of anesthetic has been deposited, carefully withdrawal the needle from the patient's mouth. Release your hand from the handle and place your thumb and forefinger on the finger grips. With your other hand, carefully move the sheath toward the needle until it reaches the holding position so that the needle can be used again. At this point, the Ultra Safety syringe can be placed on the instrument tray in case a second injection needs to be performed using the same cartridge.

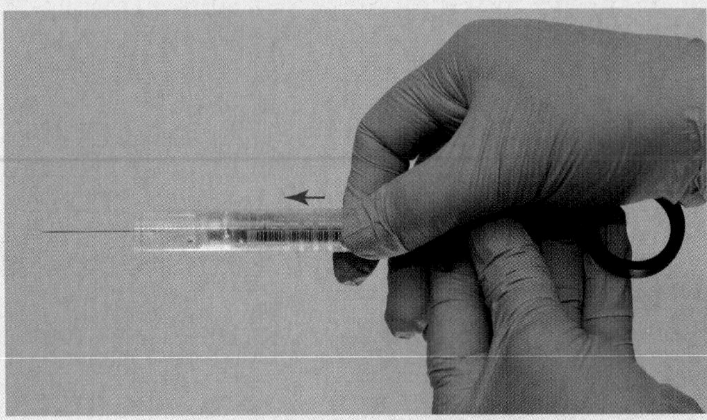

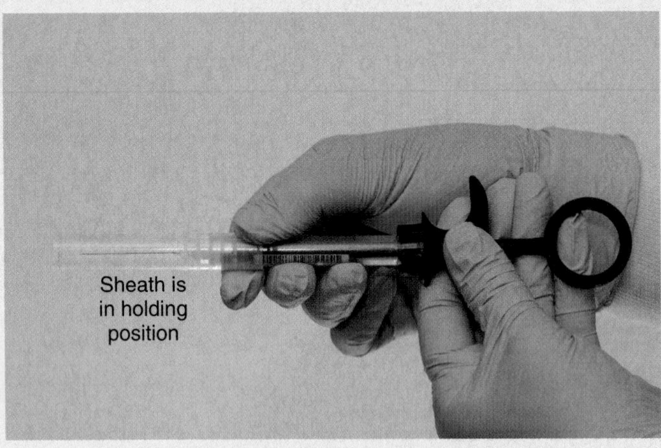

(*Continued*)

PROCEDURE 9.4 Preparation and Use of the Ultra Safety Plus XL Aspirating Syringe (*Cont.*)

Step 8

Use of a second cartridge

Should you need to insert a second cartridge, lock the injectable system as demonstrated in Step 7 into the holding position. To remove the handle, hold the syringe of the injectable system with one hand, and while using the other hand on the ring of the handle, pull the plunger backward until it is fully retracted.

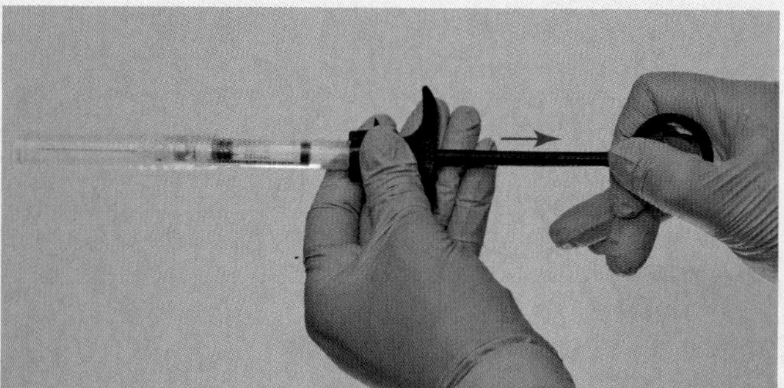

After you have fully retracted the plunger, peel off the handle in one movement.

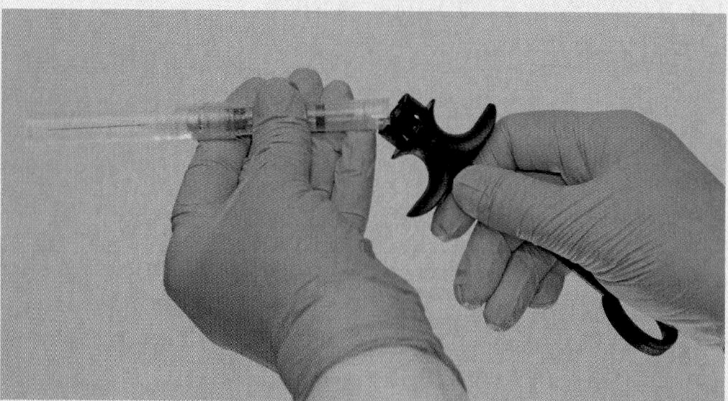

Use the silicone ring on the piston of the handle and insert into the anesthetic cartridge, pulling the used anesthetic cartridge out.

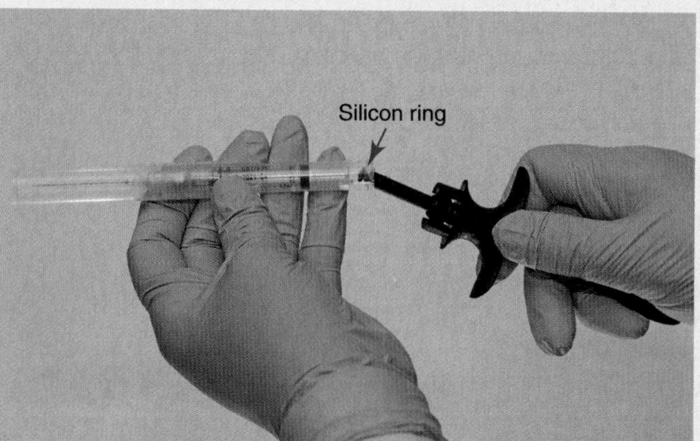

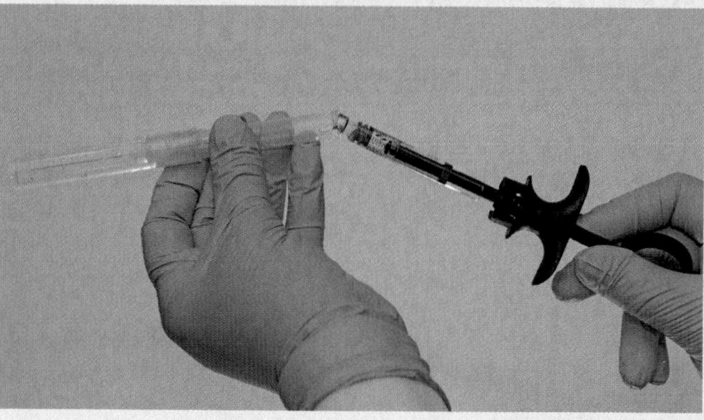

Replace with a new cartridge following steps 2–7, and complete the administration of local anesthetic.

PROCEDURE 9.5 Unloading the Ultra Safety Plus XL Aspirating Syringe

Step 1 When the clinician has finished administering local anesthesia, slide the protective sheath into the holding position and then push one more time until a loud "click" is heard.

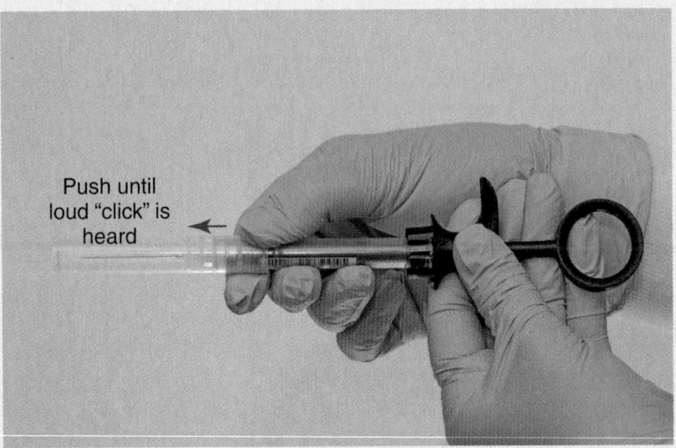

Step 2 To remove the plunger handle, hold the syringe of the injectable system with one hand while using the other hand to pull the plunger backward until it is fully retracted.

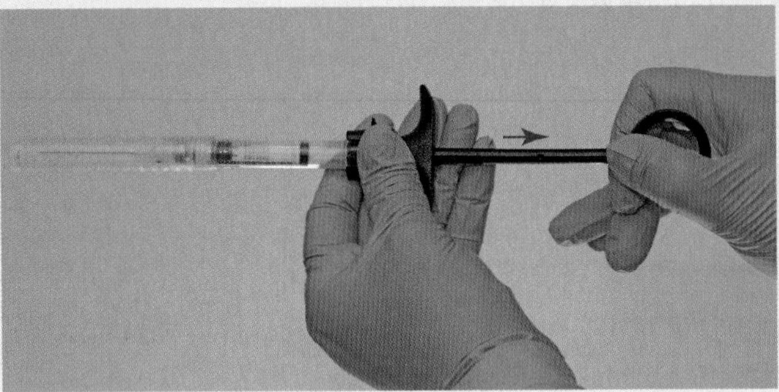

Step 3 After you have fully retracted the plunger, peel off the handle in one movement.

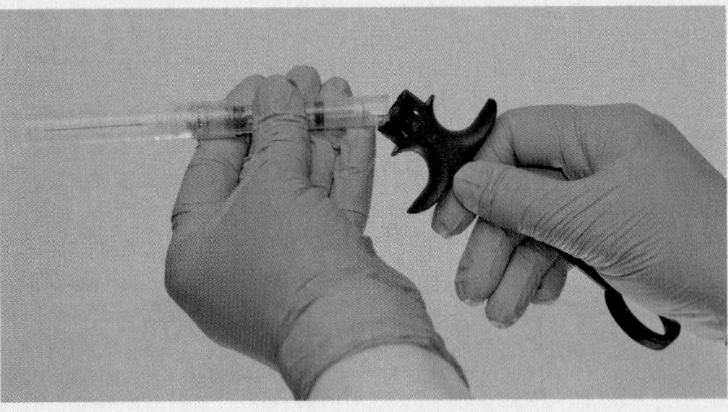

(*Continued*)

PROCEDURE 9.5 Unloading the Ultra Safety Plus XL Aspirating Syringe (*Cont.*)

Step 4 Safely dispose of the barrel and used cartridge into an approved sharps container. The handle should be bagged and autoclaved for future use.

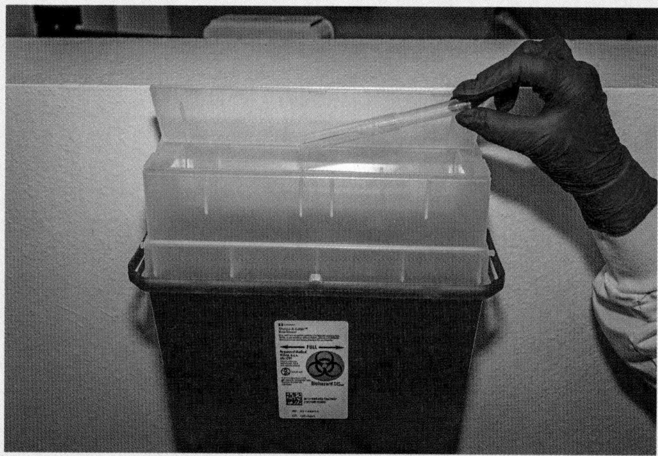

PROCEDURE 9.6 Assembly of the Wand STA Computer-Controlled Local Anesthetic Delivery System

Step 1 Connect the foot pedal to the front of the unit.

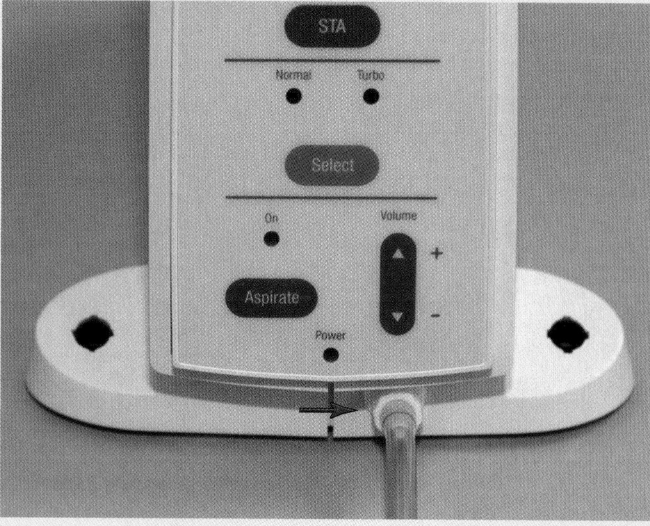

PROCEDURE 9.6 Assembly of the Wand STA Computer-Controlled Local Anesthetic Delivery System (*Cont.*)

Step 2

Connect the power cord to the back of the unit.

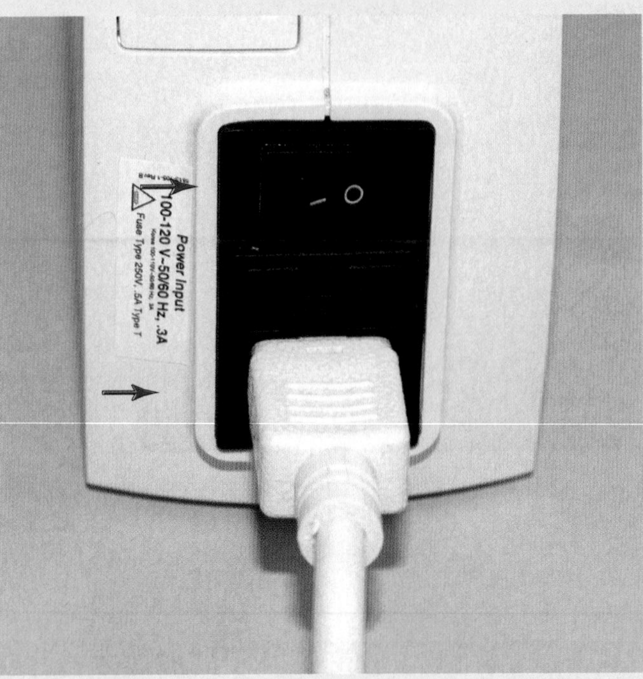

Turn the unit on using the on/off switch on the back of the unit and wait 5 seconds to allow the unit to go through warm up and calibration.

Step 3

Activate the training mode feature by holding the "Hold to Train" button for 4 seconds; this activates the spoken voice prompts that are available throughout the injection. This will assist the new user. You can deactivate the training mode at any time by again pressing the button for 4 seconds.

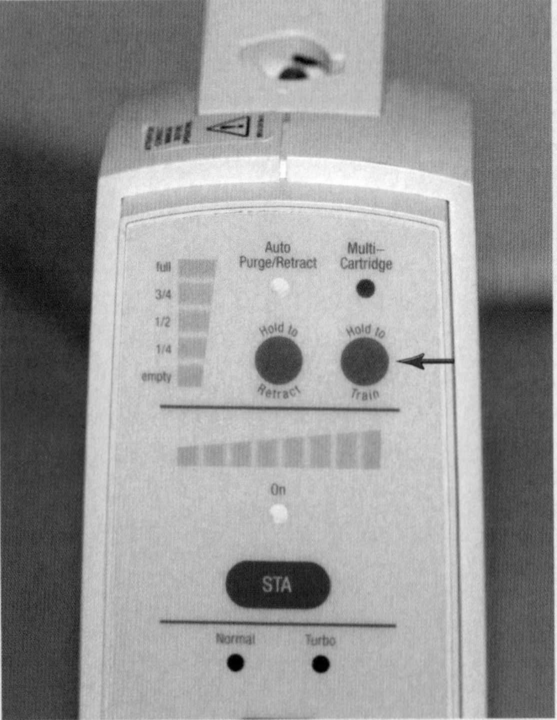

(*Continued*)

PROCEDURE 9.6 Assembly of the Wand STA Computer-Controlled Local Anesthetic Delivery System (*Cont.*)

Step 4

Open the sterile handpiece package.

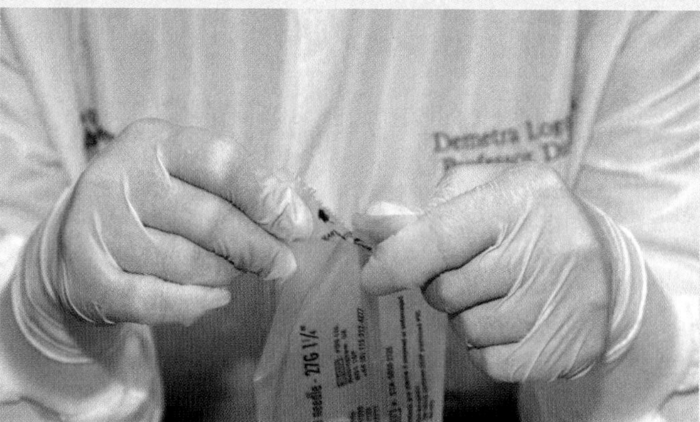

Step 5 (Optional)

If preferred, break off the handpiece at any of the preformed indentations to your desired length (see Procedure 9.1).

Step 6

Attach the Wand handpiece to the Wand STA system by inserting an anesthetic cartridge into the cartridge holder by pushing and rotating the cartridge. This will ensure that the spike within the cartridge holder will thoroughly penetrate the diaphragm of the cartridge. The spike should completely enter the cartridge.

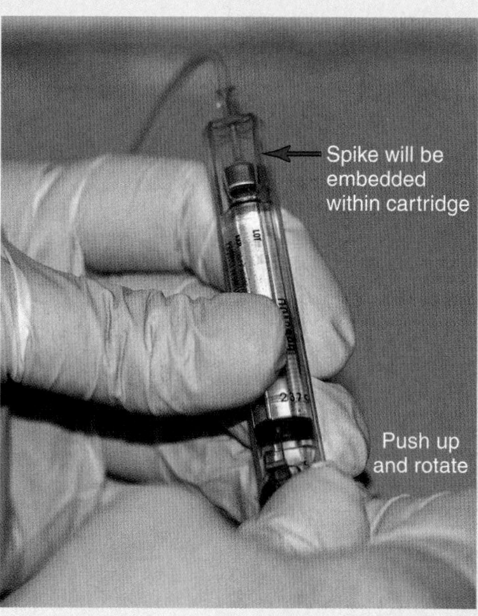

PROCEDURE 9.6 Assembly of the Wand STA Computer-Controlled Local Anesthetic Delivery System (*Cont.*)

Step 7

Connect the cartridge holder to the top of the Wand STA system. Insert the cartridge into the slot at the top of the Wand STA drive unit with a counterclockwise one-quarter turn until it locks into place. This will signal the Wand STA to automatically purge air and a slight amount of anesthetic from the needle tip of the handpiece.

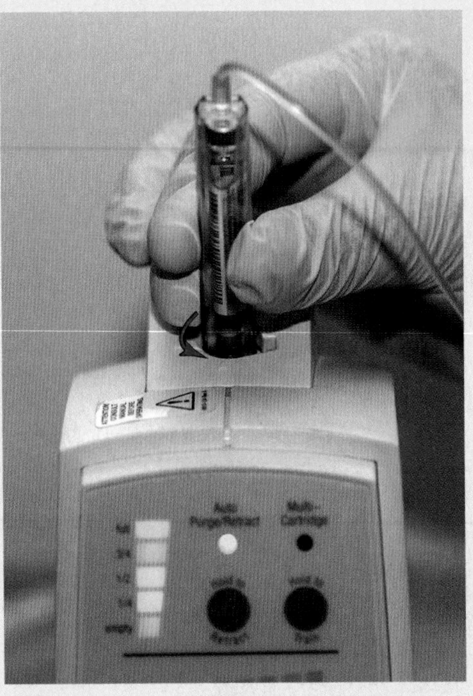

Step 8

Rest the handpiece in the holder. The unit is now ready for use.

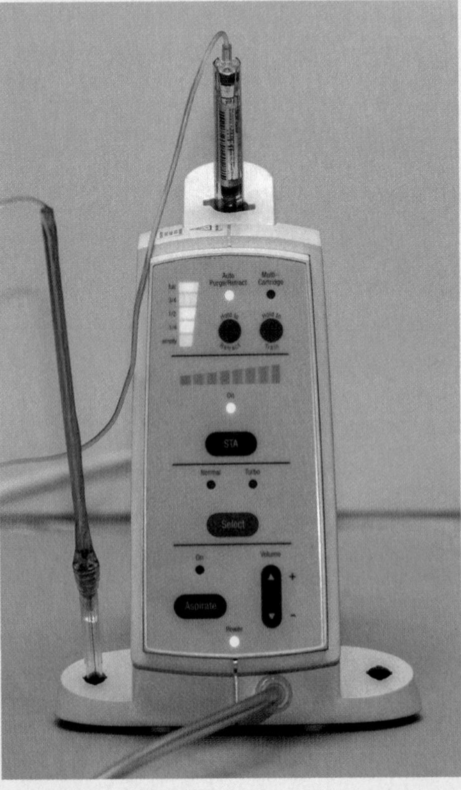

(*Continued*)

PROCEDURE 9.7 Disassembly of the Wand STA Computer-Controlled Local Anesthetic Delivery System

Step 1

Remove the used cartridge from the top of the Wand STA unit by rotating the cartridge holder clockwise by one-quarter turn. The auto purge/retract light will appear, and the plunger will automatically retract. Wait until the plunger completely retracts back into the unit before removing the cartridge holder from the top of the unit.

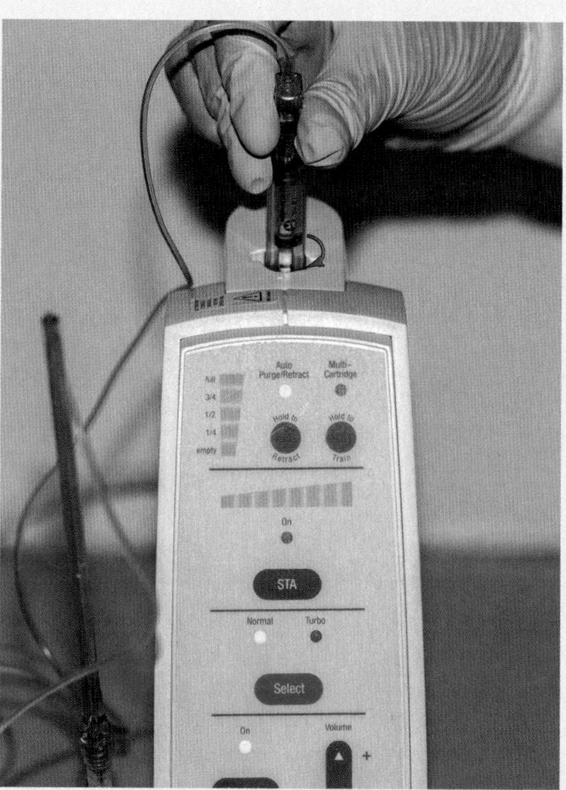

Step 2

Remove the cartridge holder from the top of the Wand STA unit.

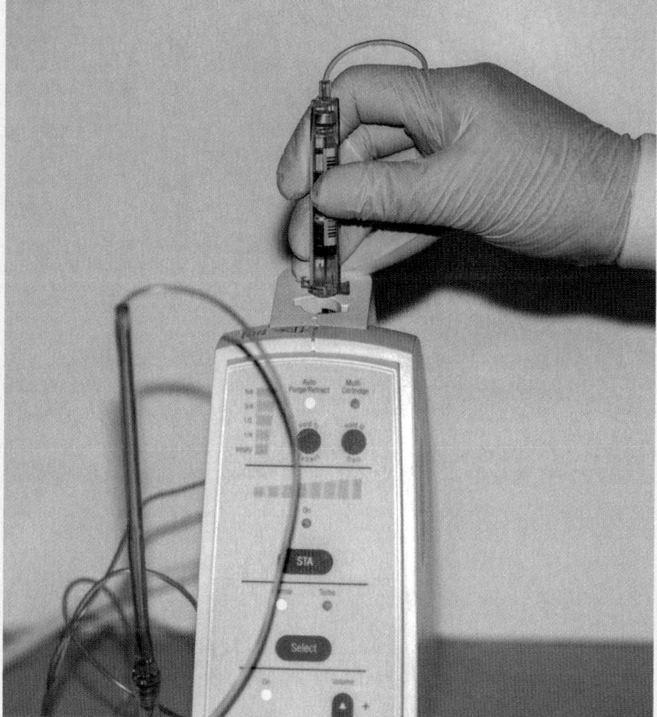

PROCEDURE 9.7 Disassembly of the Wand STA Computer-Controlled Local Anesthetic Delivery System (*Cont.*)

Step 3

To remove the cartridge from the cartridge holder, use the two small access windows at the top of the holder.

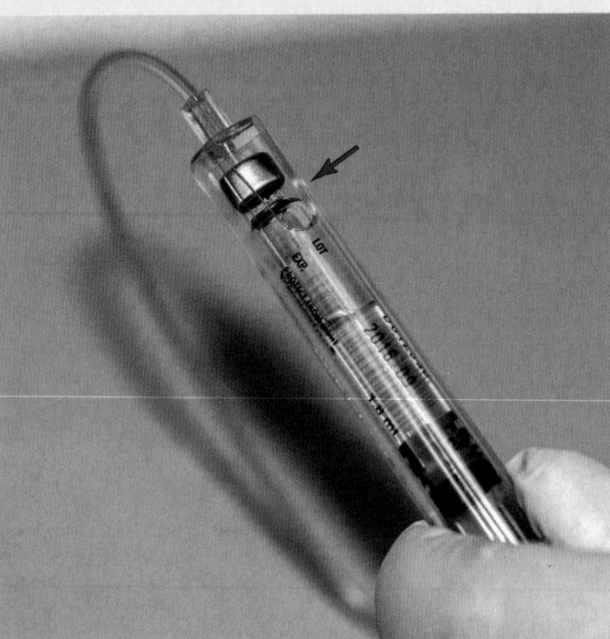

Using your fingertip, push the cartridge out of the cartridge holder.

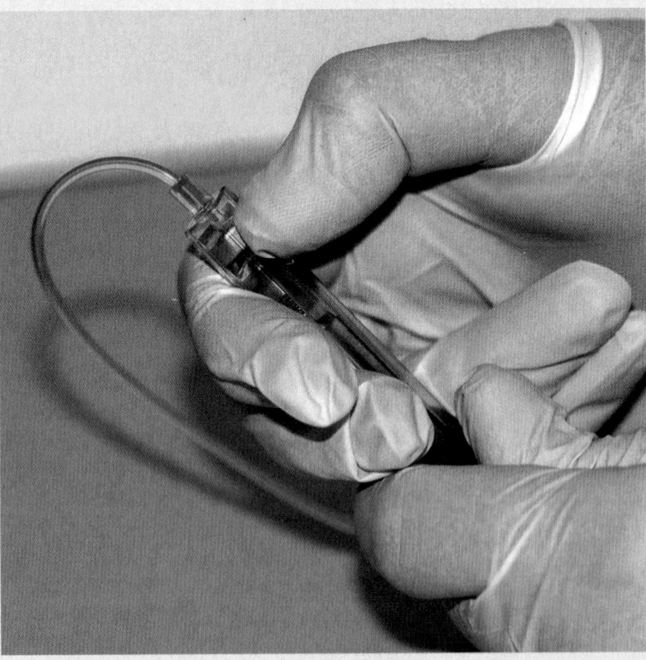

(*Continued*)

PROCEDURE 9.7 Disassembly of the Wand STA Computer-Controlled Local Anesthetic Delivery System (*Cont.*)

Step 3

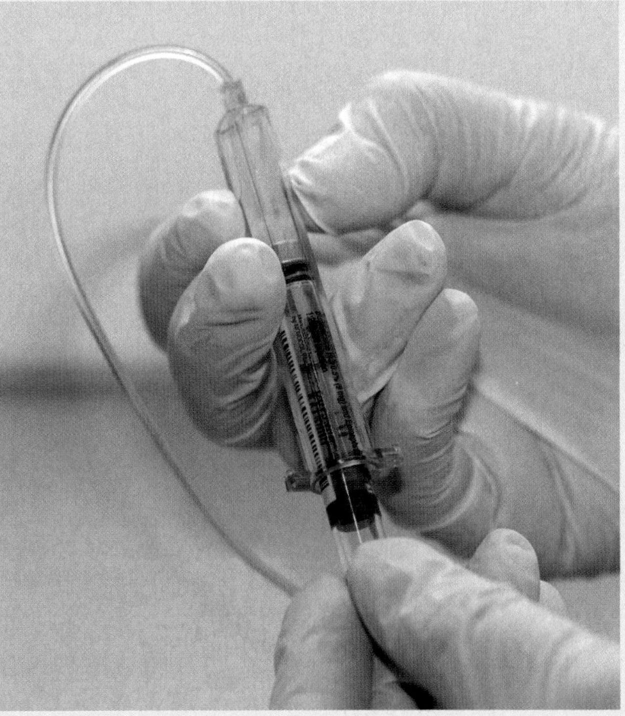

Dispose of the needle and cartridge in an approved sharps container.

Warning — Do not turn the unit on or off when a cartridge is installed at the top of the unit, as this will damage the system.

PROCEDURE 9.8 How to Buffer Local Anesthetics Using the Onset Buffering System

Step 1: Reset the piston rod — Unscrew the dosing mechanism (body) from the cartridge chamber and check to make sure the piston rod is fully retracted.

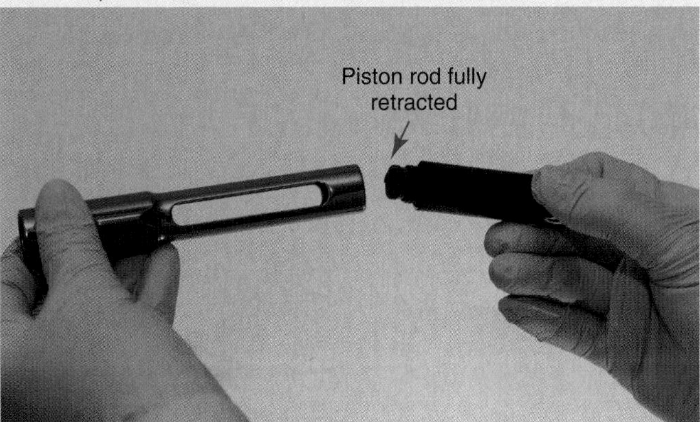

If the piston rod is not fully retracted, grip the red reset mechanism with your thumb and forefinger and turn the dosing mechanism counterclockwise until the piston rod is fully retracted.

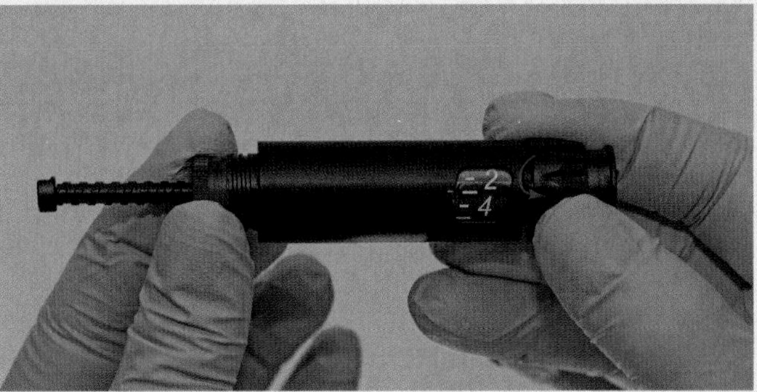

PROCEDURE 9.8	How to Buffer Local Anesthetics Using the Onset Buffering System (*Cont.*)
Step 2: Insert a 3 mL cartridge	Insert a 3 mL cartridge (such as sodium bicarbonate 8.4% pH buffer solution) into the small end of the pen's cartridge chamber with the septum entering first, then screw the pen back together. 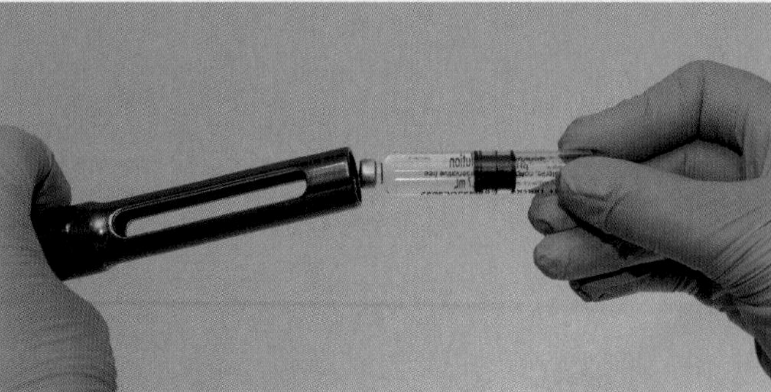
Step 3: Prime the Onset Mixing Pen	After loading a new 3 mL cartridge, you must first prime the pen to ensure the piston rod makes contact with the 3 mL cartridge of sodium bicarbonate. Dial the pen to any number. 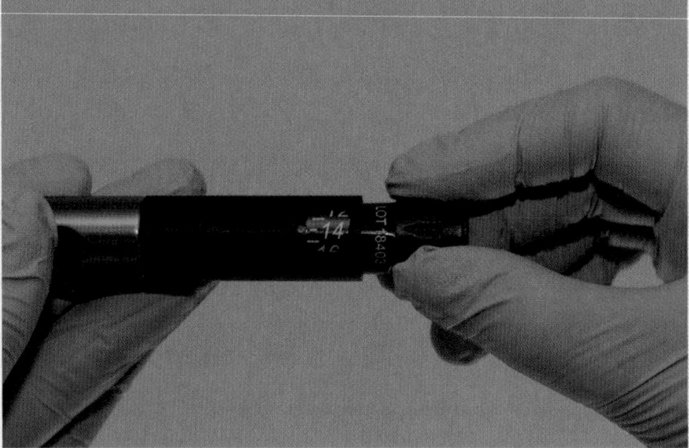 Then gently push the center of the dispensing button straight down. You many need to repeat this step a few times until the piston rod makes contact with the 3 mL cartridge. 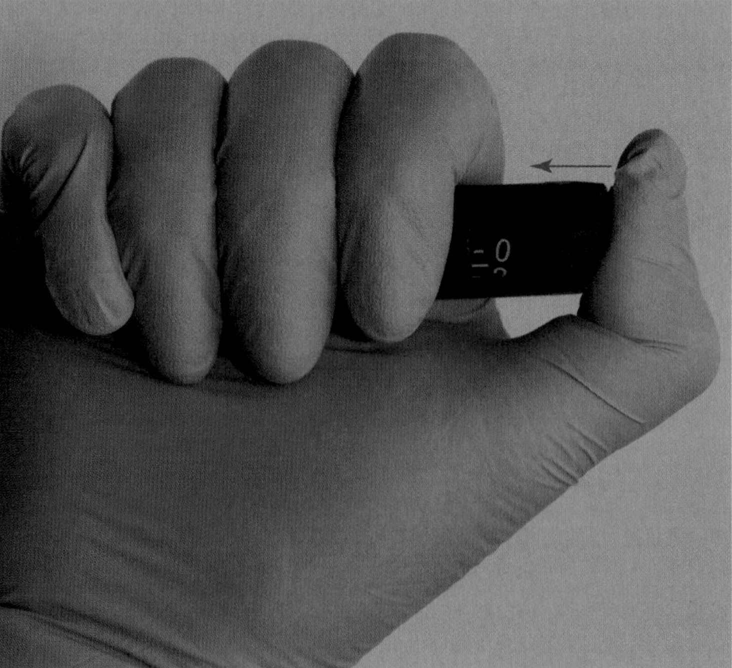 When the piston rod is in the proper position after priming successfully, the dial will not go all the way to the 0 setting. Turn the volume dial back to 0 before mixing your first cartridge.

(*Continued*)

PROCEDURE 9.8 How to Buffer Local Anesthetics Using the Onset Buffering System (*Cont.*)

Step 4: Attach an Onset Cartridge Connector

Remove the Onset Cartridge Connector from its sterile pouch and, using aseptic technique, carefully remove the safety cap. Align the arrow on the cartridge connector with the #1 position on the pen's chamber.

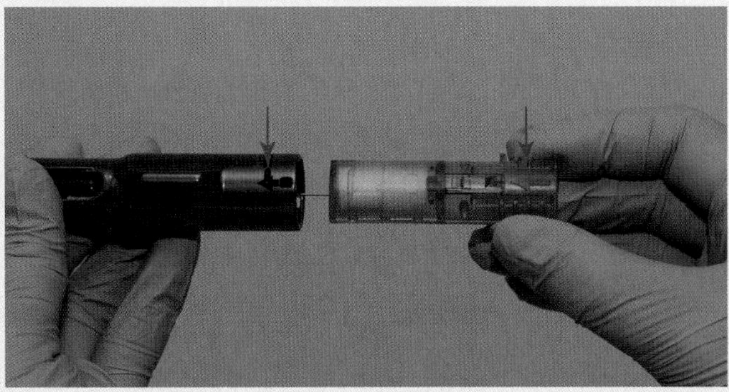

Push the cartridge connector in approximately one-quarter inch until you hear a "click."

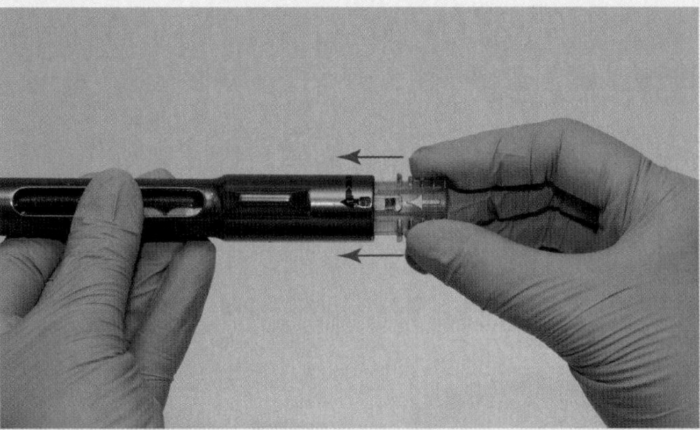

Step 5: Dial volume to be dispensed

Dial the desired volume of solution to be mixed. For example, you may dial the pen to "9" (0.09 mL) to mix sodium bicarbonate 8.4% pH buffer solution with a standard cartridge of lidocaine with epinephrine. This represents a 19:1 ratio of lidocaine with epinephrine to sodium bicarbonate.

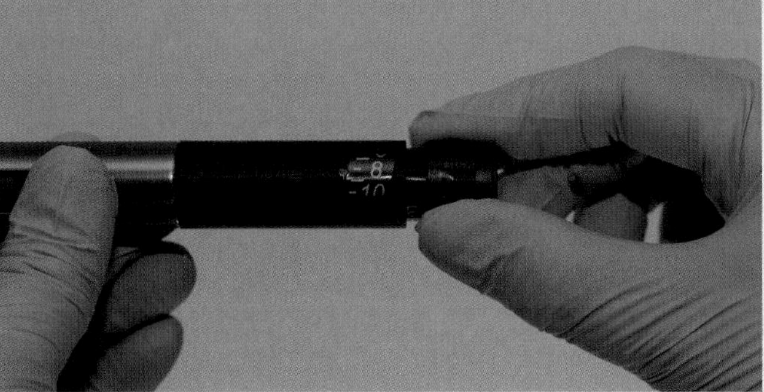

PROCEDURE 9.8 How to Buffer Local Anesthetics Using the Onset Buffering System (*Cont.*)

Step 6: Load 1.8 mL cartridge	Before loading the 1.8 mL cartridge of anesthetic into the cartridge connector, check to make sure the arrow on the cartridge connector is aligned with the #1 position on the pen. Load a 1.8 mL cartridge into the Onset Cartridge Connector with the septum entering first, pushing straight and firmly into place. Check that the 1.8 mL cartridge is fully seated by making sure the metal cap is hidden from view in the pen. You will feel a slight resistance. 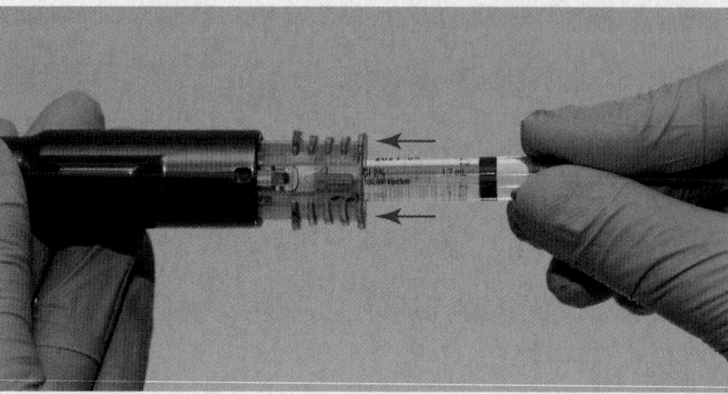
Step 7: Lock the cartridge in place	Lock the 1.8 mL cartridge in place by gripping the cartridge connector with your thumb and forefinger and rotating it clockwise to position #2, approximately one-quarter turn. 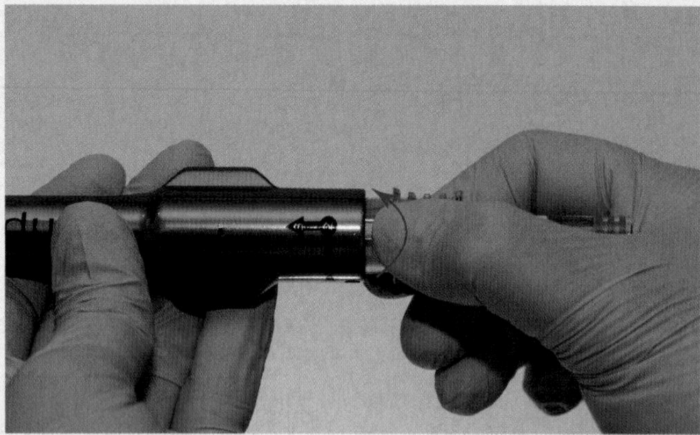 Push the cartridge connector straightforward into position #3. The anesthetic cartridge is now locked in place. This establishes a sterile fluid path between the 1.8 mL anesthetic cartridge and the 3 mL sodium bicarbonate cartridge. 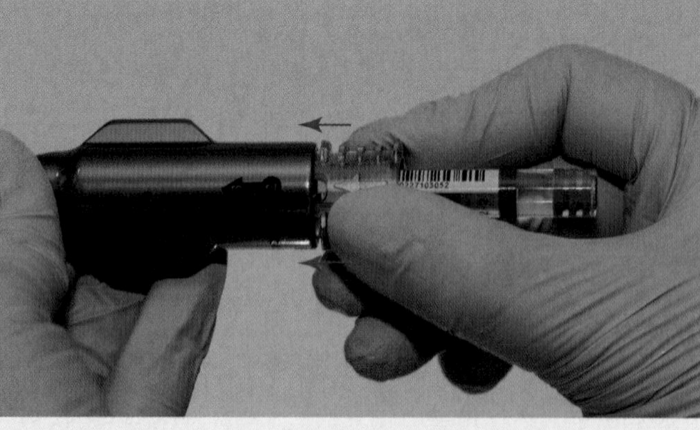

(*Continued*)

PROCEDURE 9.8 How to Buffer Local Anesthetics Using the Onset Buffering System (*Cont.*)

Step 8: Dispense solution to mix

The amount of sodium bicarbonate to be mixed was dialed in Step 5.
Depress the center of the dispensing button all the way down to dispense the sodium bicarbonate into the anesthetic cartridge. Do not force the button. Press gently along the pen axis until the volume window returns to 0.

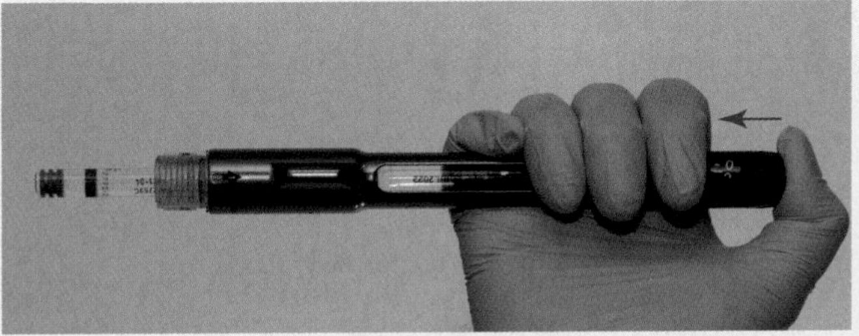

Once the solutions are mixed, start your injection within 1 minute for best results.

Step 9: Unlock the 1.8 mL cartridge

To unlock the mixed 1.8 mL anesthetic cartridge, pull the Onset Cartridge Connector straight out, approximately one-quarter inch to position #2.

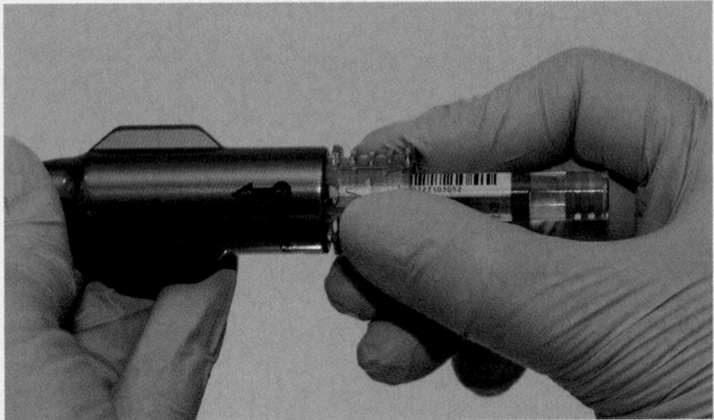

Turn the connector counterclockwise back to position #1, about a one-quarter turn.

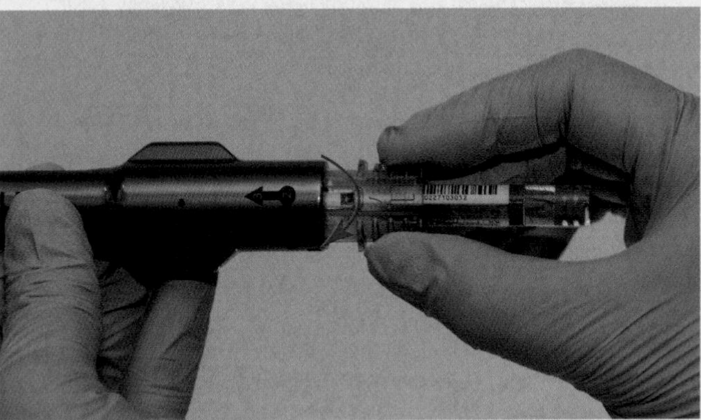

Step 10: Remove mixed cartridge

Remove the mixed 1.8 mL anesthetic cartridge by pulling it straight out. Use the cartridge immediately.
Note: Always inspect any solution prior to use. Do not use if solution is cloudy. Use combined solutions immediately. **Do not store.**

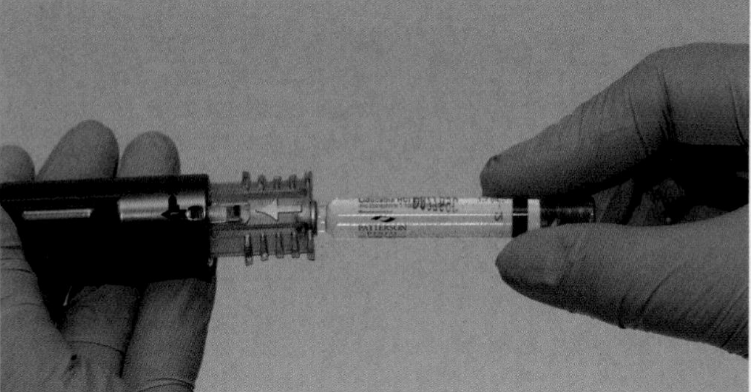

Should another cartridge need to be buffered repeat steps 5–10.

PROCEDURE 9.8 How to Buffer Local Anesthetics Using the Onset Buffering System (*Cont.*)

Step 11: Replacing or removing the 3 mL cartridge	To determine when to replace the 3 mL cartridge, check the pen's chamber window. When the plunger of the 3 mL cartridge reaches the bottom of the cartridge chamber, the 3 mL cartridge is empty and needs to be replaced. Another indication the 3 mL cartridge needs to be replaced is if the volume dial on the pen will not dial to the desired amount of solution to be mixed. The cartridge connector should always be replaced at the same time as the 3 mL cartridge. 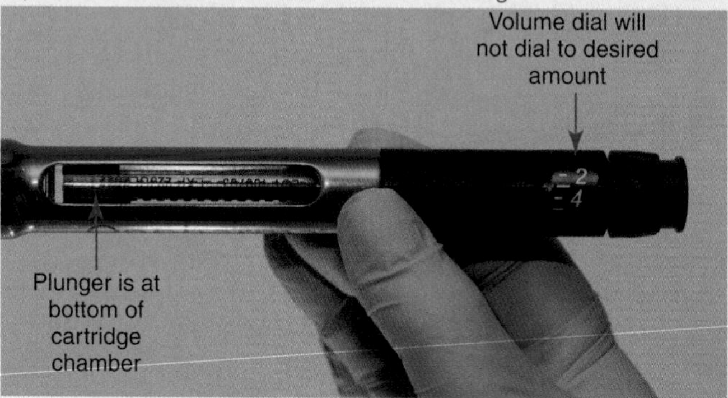
Step 12: Remove the Onset Cartridge Connector	Check to make sure the Onset Cartridge Connector arrow is in position #1, then push in the two locking levers with your thumb and forefinger and carefully pull the cartridge connector out. Dispose of in a sharps container. 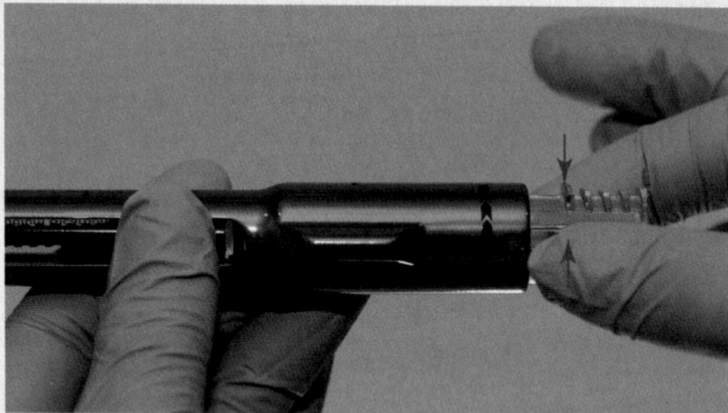
Step 13: Remove the 3 mL cartridge	Unscrew the dosing mechanism from the cartridge chamber and remove the empty 3 mL cartridge. If the sodium bicarbonate cartridge is not completely used at the end of a 5-day period, it should be removed and disposed of. To ensure best results, a new sodium bicarbonate cartridge must be used after the 5-day period. 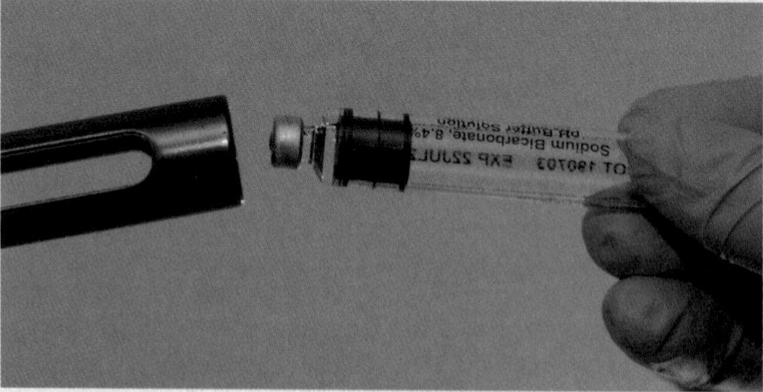
Step 14: Cleaning the Onset Mixing Pen	The mixing pen should not be sterilized in the autoclave. Clean the inside of the cartridge chamber with warm water and soap using the cleansing brush included with the pen. Use a disinfectant wipe to clean the dosing mechanism.

https://onpharma.com/pages/training.

DENTAL HYGIENE CONSIDERATIONS

- It is critical for the dental hygienist to administer local anesthetics with an aspirating syringe. If the tip of the needle is within a blood vessel, blood will enter the cartridge through the lumen of the needle after a successful aspiration, informing the dental hygienist of a positive aspiration.
- The dental hygienist should select a syringe that accommodates his or her hand size for ease of aspiration and stability of the syringe.
- Disengagement of the harpoon during aspiration frequently produces a "popping" noise. Should this occur, the dental hygienist must remove the needle from the tissue, reengage the harpoon, and redo the procedure.
- The bevel of the needle should be toward the bone when administering injections in close proximity to the periosteum.
- The smaller the gauge number, the larger the diameter of the lumen.
- A 30-gauge needle has the smallest lumen diameter, causing more needle deflection during insertion, decreased reliability during aspiration tests, and increased pressure needed to administer the anesthetic agent. It may cause increased pain and tissue trauma.
- A 25-gauge needle is recommended for areas of high risk for positive aspiration (inferior alveolar block, posterior superior alveolar block, mental and incisive blocks) as it provides the most reliable results from an aspiration test, less needle deflection during insertion, and less pressure needed to administer the anesthetic agent. It will also decease pain and tissue trauma.
- Long needles should be used when penetrating significant thick tissue (inferior alveolar, Gow-Gates mandibular block, Vazirani-Akinosi mandibular block, and infraorbital blocks).
- The dental hygienist should know the location of an uncovered needle at all times, whether the needle is inside or outside the mouth. If needle contamination occurs, recap the needle and discard it in the appropriate sharps container.
- Using the one-handed scoop method with a needle sheath prop, the dental hygienist should immediately cap the needle after the injection.
- The dental hygienist should never bend the needle before use except for intraligamentary injections.
- The dental hygienist should never insert the needle to the hub and should not make any sudden direction changes while the needle is embedded in tissue.
- The dental hygienist should not use cartridges that contain large bubbles, extruded stoppers, corroded caps, rust on the cap, or expired agents.
- The dental hygienist should discard contaminated needles in an approved sharps container.

CASE STUDY 9.1 The Patient Experiences Burning During the Injection

A patient is in the office today for nonsurgical periodontal therapy. The dental hygienist is assembling the equipment when she drops the anesthetic cartridges on the floor. Concerned that she has contaminated the cartridges, she drops them into the disinfecting solution to clean them before she loads a cartridge in the syringe. Approximately 30 minutes later, the dental hygienist removes the cartridges from the disinfecting solution and loads the syringe without inspecting the cartridge. She administers an anterior superior alveolar (ASA) block to the patient, who immediately demonstrates signs of extreme discomfort. The dental hygienist removes and safely caps the needle and questions the patient regarding the discomfort. The patient expresses that she has never experienced such an intense burning sensation before when she received a local anesthetic. A few minutes later, the dental hygienist notices some swelling in the area of the injection.

Critical Thinking Questions

- Why was the patient experiencing burning during the injection?
- How could the dental hygienist have avoided this response?
- Why did the swelling occur?

CHAPTER REVIEW QUESTIONS

1. What is the most important improvement that has been made to the local anesthetic syringe?
   A. Recapping devices to prevent needlesticks
   B. The addition of the aspirating harpoon
   C. Adding weight for better grasp
   D. Various thumb ring sizes
2. Which of the following are important criteria for an acceptable local anesthetic syringe?
   A. Inexpensive, self-contained, and able to withstand repeated sterilization without damage
   B. Able to withstand repeated sterilization, lightweight, and expensive
   C. Not self-contained, inexpensive, and able to withstand repeated sterilization without damage
   D. Not self-contained, heavy in weight, and able to withstand repeated sterilization without damage
3. What is the purpose of applying negative pressure to the harpoon?
   A. To ensure the rubber stopper does not move
   B. To advance the piston
   C. To evaluate whether the needle is within a blood vessel
   D. To evaluate whether the needle is within a nerve
4. Computer-controlled local anesthetic devices are beneficial because they deliver exact amounts of local anesthetic at a controlled rate. They are less ergonomic for the clinician.
   A. Both statements are correct.
   B. Both statements are NOT correct.
   C. The first statement is correct; the second statement is NOT correct.
   D. The first statement is NOT correct; the second statement is correct.
5. What is the definition of the needle bevel?
   A. The diameter of the needle lumen
   B. The lumen of the needle
   C. The angled point or tip of the needle
   D. The plastic or prethreaded metal adaptor
6. Which of the following intraoral needle gauges used in dentistry are listed from smallest to largest?
   A. 16, 20, 30
   B. 25, 27, 30
   C. 30, 27, 16
   D. 30, 27, 25

7. It is safe to insert the needle to the hub. The hub of the needle is the strongest part of the needle.
   A. Both statements are correct.
   B. Both statements are NOT correct.
   C. The first statement is correct; the second statement is NOT correct.
   D. The first statement is NOT correct; the second statement is correct.
8. Larger gauge needles have what advantages over smaller gauge needles?
   A. More deflection
   B. Greater accuracy
   C. Increased injection success
   D. B and C
9. The bevel of the needle should:
   A. Never touch the bone
   B. Be turned away from the bone
   C. Be turned toward the bone
   D. Does not matter where the bevel is
10. What are the two COMMONLY used needle lengths for intraoral injections?
    A. 16 mm, 24 mm
    B. 20 mm, 30 mm
    C. 30 mm, 32 mm
    D. 20 mm, 32 mm
11. All are acceptable ways to recap a needle EXCEPT one. Which one is the EXCEPTION?
    A. The use of recapping devices
    B. Single-handed scoop method
    C. Using cotton pliers to recap the needle
    D. Using fingers to recap the needle when the needle has not entered the patient's mouth
12. All are ways that increase the risk of needle breakage EXCEPT one. Which one is the EXCEPTION?
    A. Using a 25-gauge needle
    B. Inserting into the hub
    C. Bending the needle
    D. Sudden directional changes
13. The color-coded band on the anesthetic cartridges identifies what?
    A. Anesthetic drug inside the cartridge
    B. Amount of anesthetic agent
    C. Expiration date
    D. Location of the bevel
14. Warming the anesthetic agent is recommended for patient comfort because it can activate the vasoconstrictor. This can cause an increase in the duration of action.
    A. Both statements are correct.
    B. Both statements are NOT correct.
    C. The first statement is correct; the second statement is NOT correct.
    D. The first statement is NOT correct; the second statement is correct.
15. Which of the following indicates that the cartridge should be used?
    A. Small bubbles less than 2 mm
    B. Large bubbles more than 2 mm
    C. Extruded stopper
    D. Extruded stopper with a large bubble
16. All of the following cause a burning sensation when the anesthetic is injected into the tissue EXCEPT one. Which one is the EXCEPTION?
    A. The anesthetic is more acidic than the tissue
    B. The low pH
    C. Vasoconstrictors
    D. Buffered anesthetic
17. What are characteristics of topical anesthetics?
    A. Provide soft tissue anesthesia
    B. Diffuse 5 mm into the mucous membrane
    C. Less concentrated than injectable anesthetic solutions
    D. A and B
18. What is optional when preparing to give an intraoral injection?
    A. Personal protective equipment
    B. Anesthetic syringe, cartridge, and needle
    C. Topical antiseptic
    D. Hemostat
19. How should a clinician properly dispose of anesthetic needles?
    A. Recapping using the one-handed scoop method and placing in the garbage
    B. Bending the needle, recapping, and disposing of in an approved sharps container
    C. Recapping using the one-handed scoop method and disposing of in an approved sharps container
    D. Bending the needle, recapping, and disposing of in a biohazard container
20. Which of the following is a way to decrease pain during injections?
    A. Change needle after three to four tissue penetrations
    B. Withdraw the needle quickly
    C. Use a vasoconstrictor
    D. Advance the needle quickly

REFERENCES

1. Jastak T, Yagiela J, Donaldson D. *Local anesthesia of the oral cavity.* St Louis: Saunders; 1995.
2. Malamed S. *Handbook of local anesthesia.* ed 7. St Louis: Elsevier; 2020.
3. Council on Dental Materials and Devices. New American National Standard Institute/American Dental Association specification No. 34 for dental aspirating syringes. *J Am Dent Assoc.* 1978;97:236–238.
4. Council on Dental Materials. Instruments, and Equipment. Addendum to American National Standard Institute/American Dental Association Specification No. 34 for Dental Aspirating Syringes. *J Am Dent Assoc.* 1982;104:69–70.
5. Friedman MJ, Hochman MN. 21st century computerized injection for local pain control. *Compend Contin Educ Dent.* 1997;18:995–1003.
6. Hochman MN, Chiarello D, Hochman CB, et al. Computerized local anesthesia delivery vs. traditional syringe technique. *NYS Dent J.* 1997;63(24):29.
7. Kwak EJ, Pang NS, Cho JH, Jung BY, Kim KD, Park W. Computer-controlled local anesthetic delivery for painless anesthesia. *J Dent Anesth Pain Med.* 2016;16(2):81–88.
8. Steele AC, German MJ, Haas J, et al. An in vitro investigation of the effect of bevel design on the penetration and withdrawal forces of dental needles. *J Dent.* 2013;41(2):164–169.
9. Fuller NP, Menke RA, Meyers WJ. Perception of pain to three different intraoral penetrations of needles. *J Am Dent Assoc.* 1979;99:822–824.
10. Brownbill JW, Walker PO, Bourcy BD, Keenan KM. Comparison of inferior dental nerve block injections in child patients using 30 gauge and 25 gauge short needles. *Anesth Prog.* 1987;34:215–219.

11. Flanagan T, Wahl MJ, Schmitz MM, Wahl JA. Size doesn't matter: needle gauge and injection pain. *Gen Dent.* 2007;55(3):216–217.
12. Pashley EL, Nelson R, Pashley DH. Pressures created by dental injections. *J Dent Res.* 1981;60(10):1742–1748.
13. Diggle L, Deeks JJ, Pollard AJ. Effects of needle size on immunogenicity and reactogenicity of vaccines in infants: a randomized controlled trial. *BMJ.* 2006;333(7568):571.
14. Delgado-Molina E, Tamarit-Borrás M, Berini-Aytés L, Gay-Escoda C. Evaluation and comparison of 2 needle models in terms of blood aspiration during truncal block of the inferior alveolar nerve. *J Oral Maxillofac Surg.* 2003;61:1011–1015.
15. Aboytes D, Calleros C. Effects of a training needle on dental hygiene student anxiety. *JDH.* 2018;92(2):57–61.
16. Malamed S. Buffering local anesthetics in dentistry. *The Pulse.* 2011;44(1):7–9.
17. Bowles WH, Frysh H, Emmons R. Clinical evaluation of buffered local anesthetic. *Gen Dent.* 1995;43(2):182.
18. Stewart JH, Cole GW, Klein JA. Neutralized lidocaine with epinephrine for local anesthesia. *J Dermatol Surg Oncol.* 1989;15(10):1081.
19. Catchlove RFH. The influence of CO_2 and pH on local anesthetic action. *J Pharmacol Exp Ther.* 1972;181(2):208.

10

Anatomic Considerations for Local Anesthesia Administration

Margaret Fehrenbach, RDH, MS

LEARNING OBJECTIVES

1. Locate and identify the skull bones that are relevant to the administration of local anesthesia.
2. Indicate and describe in detail the various landmarks of the maxillae, palatine bones, and mandible that are relevant to the administration of local anesthesia on a diagram, skull, peer, and patient.
3. Discuss the importance of the trigeminal nerve in relation to administration of local anesthesia and name the three divisions of the sensory root.
4. Identify and trace the branches of the trigeminal nerve that are relevant to the administration of local anesthesia on a diagram, skull, peer, or patient.
5. Discuss the importance of the facial nerve and the surrounding parotid salivary gland when administering local anesthetics.
6. Identify and trace the routes of the blood vessels of the head and neck that are relevant to the administration of local anesthesia on a diagram, skull, peer, and patient.

INTRODUCTION TO ANATOMIC CONSIDERATIONS

The management of pain with hemostatic control through local anesthesia during dental hygiene care requires a thorough understanding by the dental hygienist of the anatomy of the relevant regions of the skull and the trigeminal and facial nerves as well as adjacent structures. This chapter discusses the anatomic considerations for the administration of local anesthesia within the oral cavity.

OROFACIAL SKULL BONES

The skull bones involved in local anesthetic administration are the maxillae, palatine bones, and mandible. Soft tissue of the face and oral cavity may serve the dental hygienist as initial landmarks to visualize and then palpate before local anesthesia administration as discussed further in Chapters 12 and 13. However, there are many variations in soft tissue surface anatomy among patients. Thus to increase the reliability of the local anesthesia, the dental hygienist must learn to rely mainly on the visualization and palpation of the bony as well as dental landmarks while injecting patients.

The prominences and depressions on the bony surface of the skull are landmarks for the attachments of associated muscles, tendons, and ligaments as well as for the administration of local anesthesia. A general term for any prominence on a bony surface is a **process**. One specific type of prominence located on the bony surface is a **condyle**, which is usually involved in joints. Another large, often rough prominence is a **tuberosity**. A **line** is a small straight ridge.

One type of depression on the bony surface is a **notch**, an indentation at the edge of the bone. Another depression on a bony surface is a **sulcus**, which is a shallow depression or groove that usually marks the course of blood vessels or nerves. A generally deeper depression on a bony surface is a **fossa** (plural, **fossae**).

The openings in the bone are also landmarks where various nerves and blood vessels enter or exit, which is important when administering local anesthesia. A **foramen** (plural, **foramina**) is a short windowlike opening in the bone. A **canal** is a longer narrow tubelike opening in the bone. Another opening in a bone is a **fissure**, which is a narrow cleftlike opening.

Maxillae

The upper jaw or maxillae consists of two maxilla (or maxillary bones), which are fused together at the intermaxillary suture (Fig. 10.1). Each maxilla includes a body and four processes: the frontal, zygomatic, palatine, and alveolar processes. The body of the maxilla has orbital, nasal, infratemporal, and facial surfaces. The bodies contain air-filled spaces or paranasal sinuses, the maxillary sinuses.

From an anterior view, each frontal process of the maxilla articulates with the frontal bone. The zygomatic process of the maxilla forms the medial part of the infraorbital (IO) rim, with the maxillary process of the zygomatic bone providing the lateral part on its anterior surface; both processes also form the zygomatic arch (Figs. 10.2 and 10.3). Clinicians can palpate a "notch" or more correctly described as a depression in the midpoint of the IO rim created by the more vertical zygomaticomaxillary suture located between the maxilla and the zygomatic bone. Each maxilla's orbital surface is separated from the sphenoid bone by the inferior orbital fissure (Table 10.1; Fig. 10.1). The inferior orbital fissure carries the IO nerve, zygomatic nerve, IO artery, and inferior ophthalmic vein (see later discussion). The groove in the floor of the orbital surface is the IO sulcus.

The IO sulcus becomes the IO canal and then terminates on the facial surface of each maxilla as the IO foramen (see Figs. 10.3 and 10.19 and Table 10.1). The IO foramen is located approximately 10 mm inferior to the midpoint of the IO rim and is in a linear relationship on the ipsilateral (or same) side of the face with the more superior supraorbital notch of supraorbital rim as well as the pupil of the eye and corner of the mouth (or labial commissure) (see Fig. 12.9 in Chapter 12).

The IO foramen transmits the IO nerve and blood vessels (discussed later). Palpation of the IO foramen will cause transient soreness

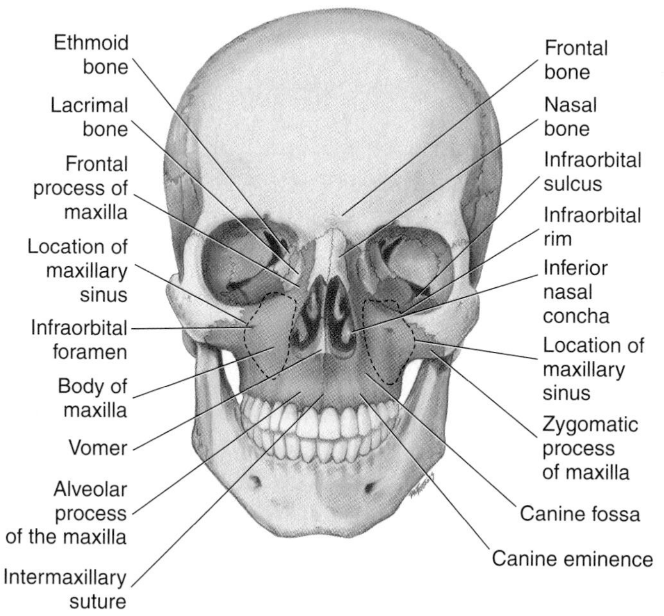

Fig. 10.1 Anterior view of the skull with the maxillae highlighted and its bony articulations and features noted such as the location of the maxillary sinuses *(dashed lines).* (From Fehrenbach MJ, Herring SW: *Illustrated anatomy of the head and neck,* ed 6, St Louis, 2021, Saunders/Elsevier.)

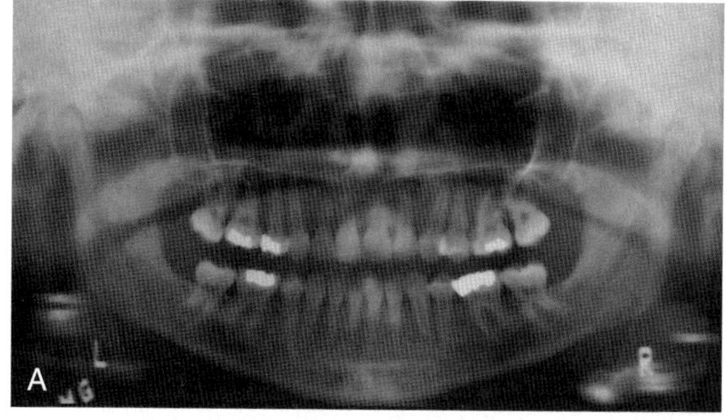

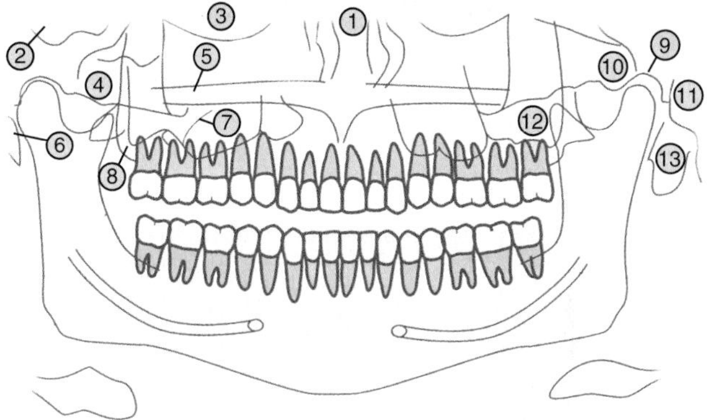

Fig. 10.2 Panoramic radiograph (A) and associated anatomy of the midface (B). (A, Fehrenbach MJ, Popowics T: *Illustrated dental embryology, histology, and anatomy,* ed 5, St Louis, 2020, Saunders/Elsevier; B, from Fehrenbach MJ, Herring SW: *Illustrated anatomy of the head and neck,* ed 6, St Louis, 2021, Saunders/Elsevier.)

to the area in a patient due to the presence of the nerve (see Fig. 12.8 in Chapter 12). The opening of the IO foramen is a landmark for the administration of the IO block (see Chapter 12). Inferior to the IO foramen on each maxilla is an elongated depression, the canine fossa. The canine fossa is just posterosuperior to each of the roots of the maxillary canines.

Also present is a facial and palatal cortical plate as part of the alveolar process of the maxilla. The root of each tooth of the maxillary arch is covered by a prominent facial ridge of bone, another part of the alveolar process of the maxilla (Table 10.2; Figs. 10.3 and 10.19). The facial ridge over each of the roots of the maxillary canines, the canine eminence, is especially prominent, which is a landmark for the administration of the anterior superior alveolar (ASA) block (see Chapter 12).

The alveolar process of the maxilla usually contains the roots of the maxillary teeth within the tooth sockets (or alveoli) (see Figs. 10.2 and 10.4 and Table 10.2). The apices of these roots between both the facial and palatal cortical plates of the alveolar process of the maxilla are landmarks for the administration for the majority of the maxillary injections (see Chapter 12). The alveolar process of the maxilla can become resorbed in a patient who is completely edentulous in the maxillary arch; resorption occurs to a lesser extent in partially edentulous cases. However, the more superiorly located body of the maxilla is not resorbed with tooth loss, but its walls may become thinner in this case.

In general, the alveolar process of the maxillary teeth is less dense and more porous than the alveolar process of similar mandibular teeth as demonstrated on a panoramic radiograph (see Fig. 10.2). These differences in bone density allow a greater incidence of clinically effective local anesthesia for the maxillary arch when the local anesthetic agent is administered as a supraperiosteal injection or local infiltration than would occur with similar teeth on the mandibular arch (see Chapters 12 and 13).

From the lateral view, each zygomatic process of the maxilla articulates with the zygomatic bone and its maxillary process laterally, completing the medial part of the IO rim and helping also form the zygomatic arch as was discussed earlier (Figs. 10.2 and 10.3 and Table 10.2). On the posterior part of the body of the maxilla is a rounded rough elevation, the maxillary tuberosity, just posterior to the most distal maxillary molar (Figs. 10.2–10.4).

Posterosuperior on the maxillary tuberosity are the posterior superior alveolar (PSA) foramina that perforate the infratemporal surface of the maxilla multiple times. These foramina are where the PSA nerve branches and blood vessel branches enter the bone from the posterior and then open up onto the infratemporal surface of the maxilla. Both the maxillary tuberosity and the openings of the PSA foramina are landmarks for the administration of the PSA block (see Chapter 12). The maxillary tuberosity also serves as a landmark for the administration of the Vazirani-Akinosi (V-A) mandibular block (see Chapter 13).

From an inferior view, each palatine process of the maxilla articulates with the other to form the anterior hard palate (see Figs. 10.2 and 10.4 and Table 10.2). The anterior part of the median palatine suture is noted between these two palatine processes of the maxilla (Table 10.3). In the patient, this suture is covered by the median palatine raphe, a midline tendinous band of tissue that serves as a landmark for the administration for both the greater palatine (GP) block and anterior middle superior alveolar (AMSA) block (see Chapter 12).

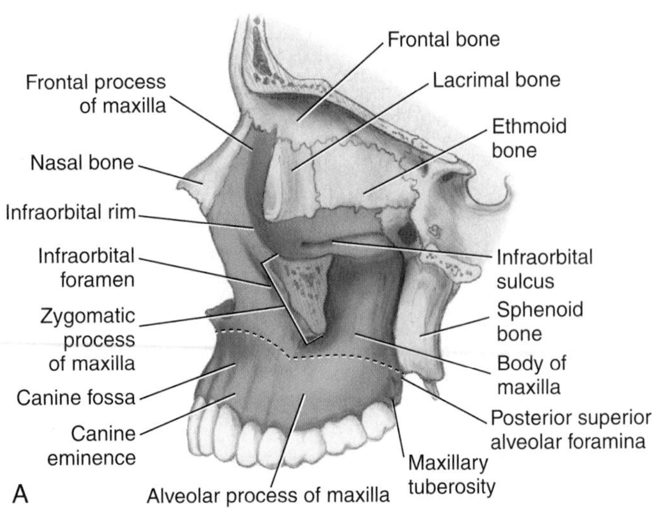

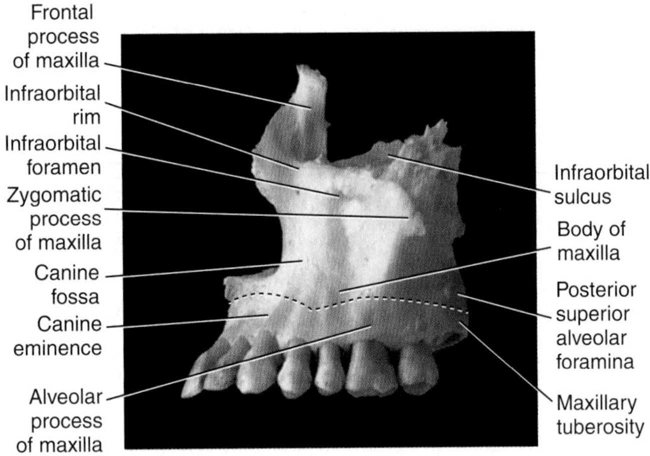

Fig. 10.3 Lateral cutaway view of the skull with the maxilla highlighted and the bony articulations and features noted such as the approximate junction between the alveolar process and the body of the maxilla *(dashed lines)* (A) and the disarticulated bone (B). (From Fehrenbach MJ, Herring SW: *Illustrated anatomy of the head and neck,* ed 6, St Louis, 2021, Saunders/Elsevier.)

In addition, on the inferior surface there are a number of small pores in each maxilla of the anterior hard palate that will allow for some diffusion of local anesthetic agent during the administration of the AMSA block.

In the anterior midline between the two articulating palatine processes of the maxillae, just palatal to the maxillary central incisors, is the incisive foramen (see Table 10.1 and Fig. 10.20). This foramen carries branches of both the right and left nasopalatine nerves as well as branches of the sphenopalatine artery from the nasal cavity to the anterior hard palate (see later discussion). The incisive papilla is the small soft tissue bulge over the opening of the incisive foramen. Both the incisive foramen and its incisive papilla are landmarks for the administration of the nasopalatine (NP) block (see Chapter 12).

Palatine Bones

The palatine bones are paired bones, each consisting of two plates: the horizontal and vertical plates. Both the horizontal and vertical plates can be seen from a posterior view of the palatine bone (Fig. 10.5). The horizontal plates of the palatine bones form the posterior hard palate.

TABLE 10.1 Bony Openings in the Skull Related to the Trigeminal Nerve and With Contents

Bony Opening	Location	Contents
Foramen ovale	Sphenoid bone	Mandibular nerve of the fifth cranial or trigeminal nerve and blood vessels
Foramen rotundum	Sphenoid bone	Maxillary nerve of the fifth cranial or trigeminal nerve and blood vessels
Greater palatine foramen	Palatine bone	Greater palatine nerve and blood vessels
Incisive foramen	Maxillae	Right and left nasopalatine nerves and branches of the sphenopalatine artery
Inferior orbital fissure	Between sphenoid bone and maxilla	Infraorbital and zygomatic nerves, infraorbital artery, and inferior ophthalmic vein
Infraorbital foramen and canal	Maxilla	Infraorbital nerve and blood vessels
Lesser palatine foramen	Palatine bone	Lesser palatine nerve and blood vessels
Mandibular foramen	Mandible	Inferior alveolar nerve and blood vessels
Mental foramen	Mandible	Mental nerve and blood vessels
Superior orbital fissure	Sphenoid bone	Ophthalmic nerve of the fifth cranial or trigeminal nerve and blood vessels

TABLE 10.2 Processes of Maxillae and Mandible With Associated Structures

Processes of Skull	Skull Bones	Associated Structures
Alveolar process	Mandible	Contains roots of mandibular teeth within alveoli
Alveolar process	Maxillae	Contains roots of maxillary teeth within alveoli
Coronoid process	Mandible	Part of mandibular ramus
Frontal process	Maxilla	Articulates with frontal bone
Palatine processes	Maxillae	Form anterior hard palate
Zygomatic process	Maxilla	Form medial part of infraorbital rim (lateral part is from maxillary process of zygomatic bone)

The vertical plates of the palatine bones form a part of the lateral walls of the nasal cavity, and each plate contributes a small part of bone to the orbital apex.

The palatine bones serve as a link between the maxillae and the sphenoid bone with which they articulate, in addition to articulating with each other. The two horizontal plates articulate with each other at the posterior part of the median palatine suture underlying the median palatine raphe (as discussed earlier) and more anteriorly with the palatine processes of the maxillae at the transverse palatine suture (see Fig. 10.4 and Table 10.3).

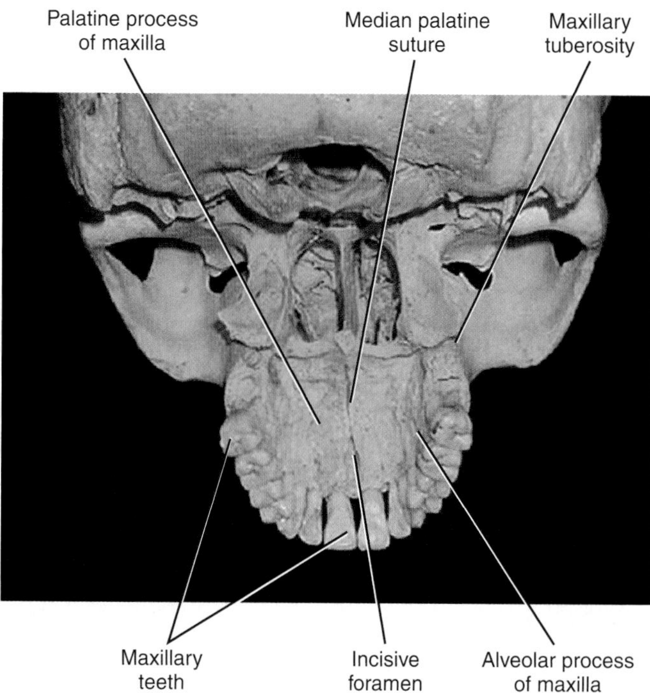

Fig. 10.4 Posteroinferior view of the skull with the maxillae and hard palate features noted. (From Fehrenbach MJ, Herring SW: *Illustrated anatomy of the head and neck,* ed 6, St Louis, 2021, Saunders/Elsevier.)

TABLE 10.3 Sutures of Maxillae and Palatine Bones

Suture	Bony Articulations
Intermaxillary suture	Maxillae
Median palatine suture	Anterior part: Maxillae Posterior part: Palatine bones
Transverse palatine suture	Maxillae and palatine bones
Zygomaticomaxillary suture	Maxilla and zygomatic bone

There are two main foramina in each of the palatine bones: the GP and lesser palatine (LP) foramina (discussed later) (Fig. 10.6; see Fig. 10.20 and Table 10.1). The larger GP foramen is located in the posterolateral region of each horizontal plate of the palatine bones, usually superior to the apices of the maxillary second (in children) or third molars (in adults). The GP foramen is approximately 10 mm medial and directly superior to the palatal gingival margin. The GP foramen is also midway between the median palatine raphe overlying the median palatine suture and the palatal gingival margin of the maxillary molar. The GP foramen transmits the GP nerve and blood vessels, and its opening is a landmark for the administration of the GP block (see Chapter 12).

The smaller opening nearby, the LP foramen, transmits the LP nerve and blood vessels to the soft palate and tonsils. Both foramina are openings of the pterygopalatine canal that carries the descending palatine nerves and blood vessels from the pterygopalatine fossa to the palate.

The pterygopalatine fossa is a cone-shaped paired depression posterior to the maxilla on each side of the skull. This smaller skull fossa is located between the sphenoid bone and the maxillary tuberosity as well as being close to the apex of the orbit. The pterygopalatine fossa communicates via fissures and foramina within its walls with the cranial cavity, orbit, nasal cavity, and oral cavity.

Mandible

The lower jaw or mandible is the only freely movable bone of the skull (Figs. 10.7 and 10.8). The mandible has its movable articulation with the temporal bones at each temporomandibular joint (TMJ). The single mandible also occludes with the maxillae by way of their contained respective mandibular and maxillary dental arches.

From an anterior view of the mandible, there are prominent landmarks to note (Figs. 10.9 and 10.11). The mental protuberance, the bony prominence of the chin, is located inferior to the roots of the mandibular incisors. In the midline on the anterior surface of the mandible is a faint ridge, an indication of the mandibular symphysis, where the mandibular bone was formed by the fusion of right and left processes.

Farther posteriorly on the lateral surface of the mandible is the opening of the mental foramen, which is usually inferior to the apices of the mandibular premolars as recently noted dental cone-beam computed tomography (CBCT) studies (see Figs. 10.2, 10.9, 10.10,

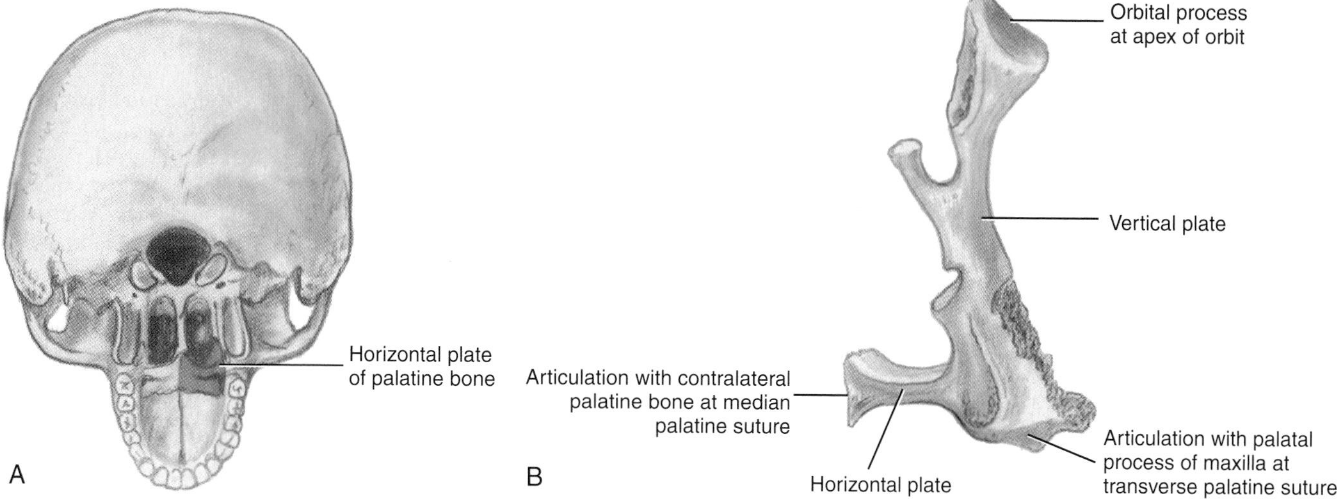

Fig. 10.5 Posteroinferior view of the skull with the right palatine bone highlighted as it articulates with the left palatine bone (A) and the posterolateral view of the disarticulated right palatine bone with its features noted (B). (From Fehrenbach MJ, Herring SW: *Illustrated anatomy of the head and neck,* ed 6, St Louis, 2021, Saunders/Elsevier.)

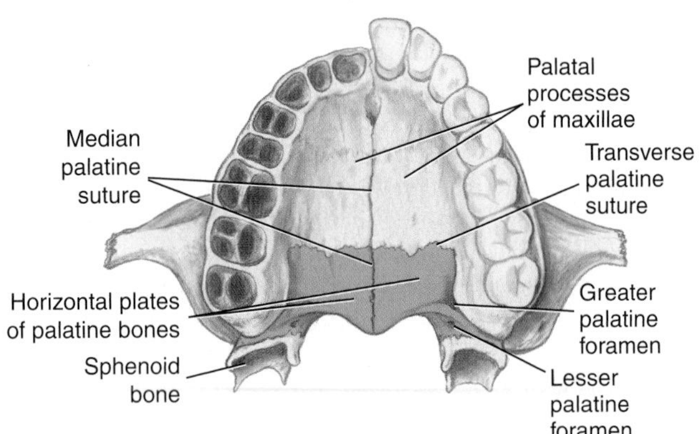

Fig. 10.6 Inferior view of the hard palate with the horizontal plates of the palatine bones highlighted and features noted. (From Fehrenbach MJ, Herring SW: *Illustrated anatomy of the head and neck,* ed 6, St Louis, 2021, Saunders/Elsevier.)

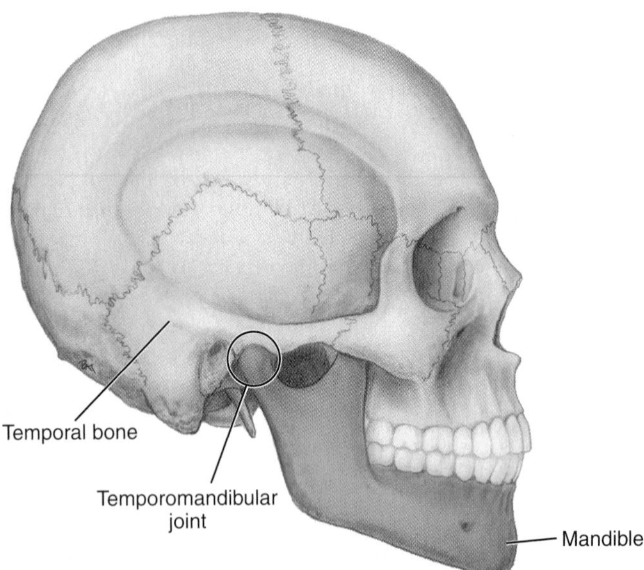

Fig. 10.7 Lateral view of the skull showing the mandible highlighted and the temporomandibular joint *(circle)* and its articulating bones noted. (From Fehrenbach MJ, Herring SW: *Illustrated anatomy of the head and neck,* ed 6, St Louis, 2021, Saunders/Elsevier.)

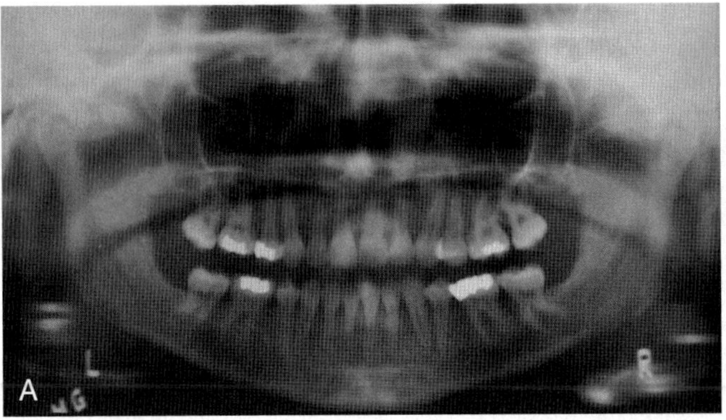

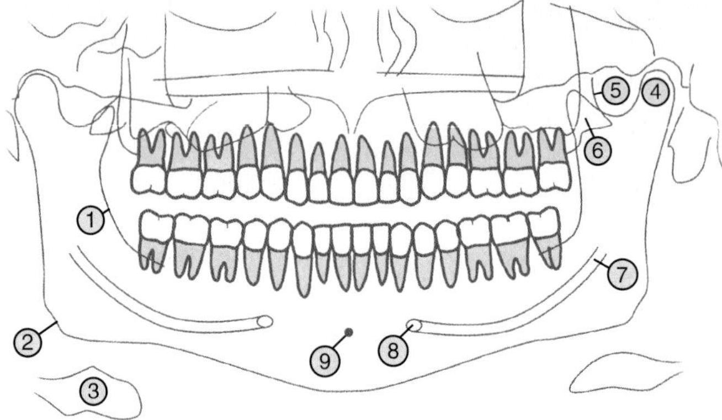

Fig. 10.8 Panoramic radiograph (A) and associated anatomy of the lower face (B). (A from Fehrenbach MJ, Popowics T: *Illustrated dental embryology, histology, and anatomy,* ed 5, St Louis, 2020, Saunders/Elsevier; B from Fehrenbach MJ, Herring SW: *Illustrated anatomy of the head and neck,* ed 6, St Louis, 2021, Saunders/Elsevier.)

and 10.25 and Table 10.1). As mandibular growth proceeds in children, the mental foramen alters in direction from anterior to posterosuperior. The mental foramen allows the entry of the mental nerve and blood vessels into the mandibular canal to merge with the incisive nerve and blood vessels (discussed later).

The mental foramen's posterosuperior opening in adults signifies the changed direction of the emerging mental nerve. This opening of the mental foramen onto the bony lateral surface of the mandible is an important landmark to note intraorally and on a radiograph before administration of both the mental and incisive blocks (see Chapter 13, Table 13.6, Figure L). Studies show that the mental foramen can be as far posterior as the apex of the mandibular first molar or as far anterior as the apex of the mandibular canine. Palpation of the mental foramen before an administration of a local anesthetic agent will cause transient soreness to the area in a patient due to the presence of the nerve.

The heavy horizontal part of the lower jaw inferior to the mental foramen is the body of the mandible (see Figs. 10.9 and 10.10). Superior to this, the part of the lower jaw that usually contains the roots of the mandibular teeth within the tooth sockets (or alveoli) is the alveolar process of the mandible (see Table 10.2). Also present is a facial and lingual cortical plate, which is also part of the alveolar process of the mandible.

The alveolar process of the mandible can become resorbed if a patient becomes completely edentulous in the mandibular arch; resorption occurs to a lesser extent in partially edentulous cases. This resorption can occur to such an extent that the mental foramen is virtually on the superior border of the mandible instead of opening on the lateral surface, changing its relative position. However, the more inferiorly located body of the mandible is not affected and remains thick and rounded. This resorption can possibly alter the landmarks when administering both the mental or incisive blocks as well as the inferior alveolar (IA) block (see Chapter 13).

In general, the alveolar process of the mandibular anterior teeth is also less dense and more porous than the alveolar process of the mandibular posterior teeth as demonstrated with a panoramic radiograph (see Fig. 10.8). These differences in bone density allow a supraperiosteal injection or local infiltration of the mandibular anterior teeth by a local anesthetic agent to have greater incidence of clinically effective local anesthesia than the mandibular posterior teeth but always with less clinically effective overall anesthesia of the mandibular teeth than the maxillary teeth (see Chapters 12 and 13).

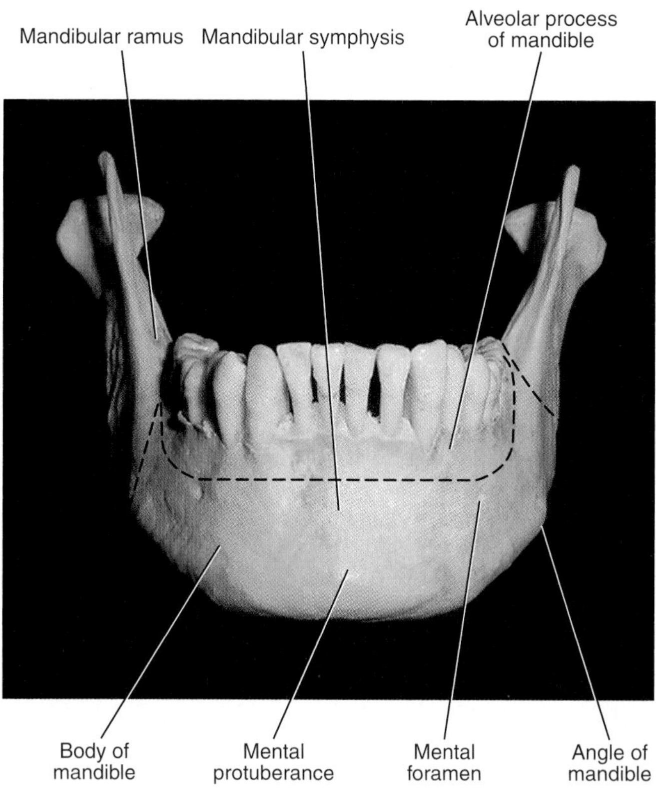

Fig. 10.9 Anterior view of the disarticulated mandible and its associated features such as the approximate junction between the alveolar process and the body of the mandible *(dashed lines)*. (From Fehrenbach MJ, Herring SW: *Illustrated anatomy of the head and neck,* ed 6, St Louis, 2021, Saunders/Elsevier.)

The sharp bent of the lower jaw inferior to the ear's lobule is the angle of the mandible. On the lateral surface (or outer surface) of the mandible, the stout flat plate of the mandibular ramus rises up from the angle and extends superiorly and posteriorly from the body of the mandible on each side (see Fig. 10.10). Each mandibular ramus serves as the primary area for the attachment of the muscles of mastication.

At the anterior border of the mandibular ramus is a thin sharp margin that terminates in the coronoid process (see Figs. 10.11 and 10.12 and Table 10.2). The main part of the anterior border of the mandibular ramus forms a concave anterior curve, the coronoid notch. This notch is the greatest depression on the anterior border of the mandibular ramus. The anterior border of the mandibular ramus is a landmark for the administration of the buccal block and the coronoid notch is a landmark for the administration of the IA block (see Chapter 13).

Inferior to the coronoid notch, the anterior border of the mandibular ramus becomes the external oblique ridge. The external oblique ridge is where the mandibular ramus joins the body of the mandible on its lateral surface. The external oblique ridge is noted as a radiopaque line on a radiograph superior to the mylohyoid line or internal oblique ridge (discussed next); clinicians may also palpate this line extraorally to help locate the coronoid notch as well as the posterior border of the mandibular ramus (see Fig. 10.8).

The posterior border of the mandibular ramus is thickened and extends from the angle of the mandible to the projection of the mandibular condyle with its neck (see Figs. 10.7–10.12). The anteromedial border of the neck of the mandibular condylar is a landmark for the administration of the Gow-Gates (G-G) mandibular block (see Chapter 13). The articulating surface of the condyle is an oval head

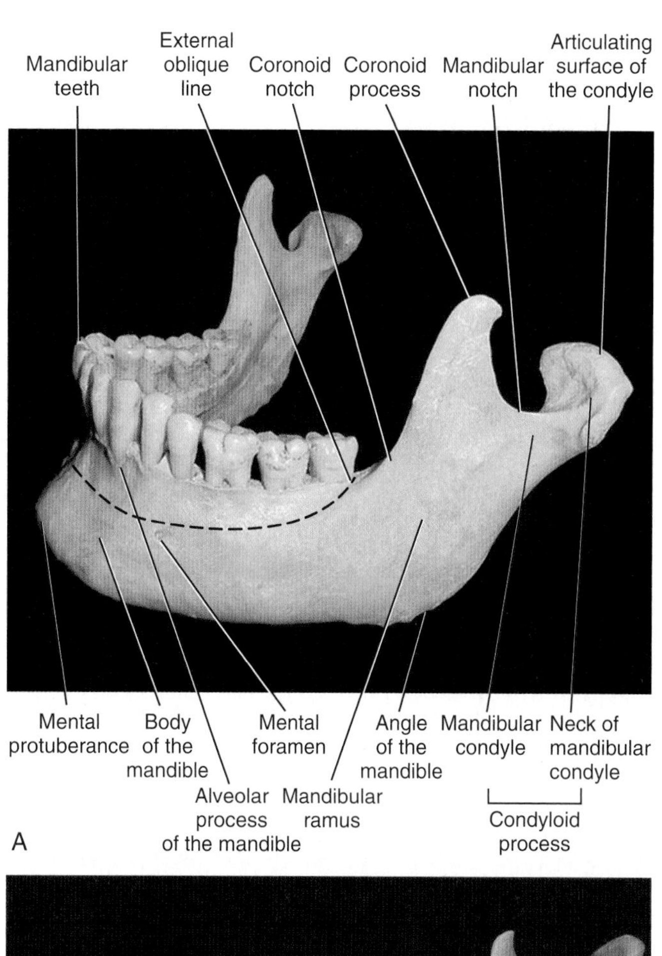

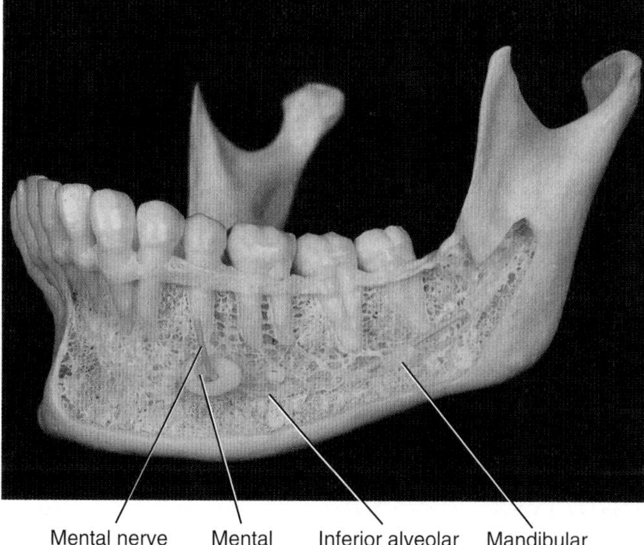

Fig. 10.10 Slight anterolateral view of the disarticulated mandible and its associated features. Note the approximate junction between the alveolar process and the body of the mandible *(dashed lines)* (A) with a slight anterolateral cutaway view demonstrating the pathway of the inferior alveolar nerve *(yellow marker)* as it forms from a merger of the mental and incisive nerves (not shown here) and travels within the mandibular canal and then exits by way of the mandibular foramen (B). (A from Fehrenbach MJ, Herring SW: *Illustrated anatomy of the head and neck,* ed 6, St Louis, 2021, Saunders/Elsevier; B from Logan BM, Reynold PA, Hutching RT: *McMinn's color atlas of head and neck anatomy,* ed 4, London, 2010, Mosby Ltd. In: Fehrenbach MJ, Herring SW: *Illustrated anatomy of the head and neck,* ed 6, St Louis, 2021, Saunders/Elsevier.)

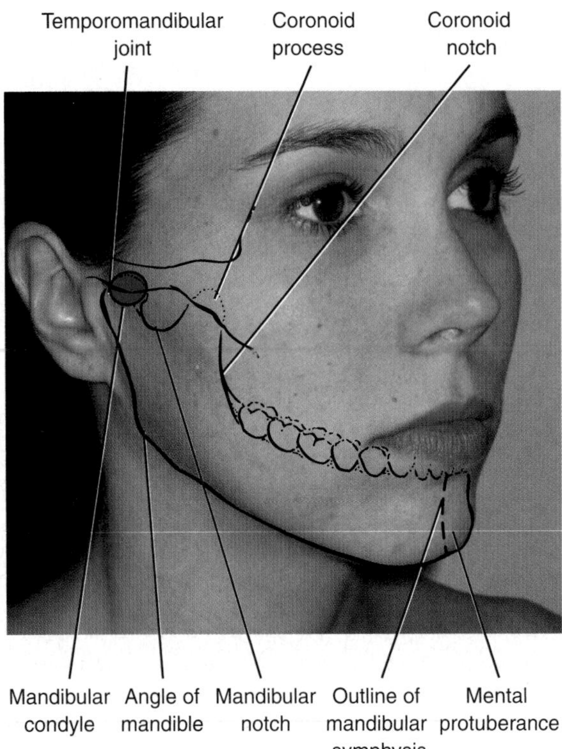

Fig. 10.11 Anterolateral view of the face with a superimposition of the bony landmarks of mandible noted such as the temporomandibular joint *(colored in circle)* and the mandibular symphysis *(dashed lines)*. (From Fehrenbach MJ, Herring SW: *Illustrated anatomy of the head and neck*, ed 6, St Louis, 2021, Saunders/Elsevier.)

involved in the TMJ. Between the coronoid process and the condyle is a deep concavity, the mandibular notch.

Visible on the medial surface (or inner surface) of the mandible are the body of the mandible, alveolar process of the mandible, and the mandibular ramus on each side (see Table 10.2 and Fig. 10.12). The medial surface of the mandibular ramus is a landmark for the administration of the IA block and the V-A block (see Chapter 13).

At the posterior edge of each alveolar process of the mandible is a rounded roughened area, the retromolar triangle, just posterior to the most distal mandibular molar. When covered with soft tissue, the retromolar triangle is seen in the oral cavity as the retromolar pad and is a bony landmark for the administration of the buccal block (see Chapter 13).

The pterygomandibular space associated with the mandible is a small cleft containing mostly loose connective tissue and is bordered by the medial surface of the mandibular ramus laterally and by the medial pterygoid muscle medially (see Chapter 13). Posteriorly, the parotid salivary gland curves medially around the posterior border of the mandibular ramus, while anteriorly the buccinator and superior constrictor muscles come together to form the medially located pterygomandibular raphe (discussed next).

The pterygomandibular raphe associated with the pterygomandibular space is seen in the oral cavity as the pterygomandibular fold, which is a tendinous band located posterior to the most distal mandibular molar as it spans the area between the mandible. This raphe is located at the point at which the hard and soft palates meet to designate the posterior border of the mandibular ramus. The pterygomandibular fold becomes accentuated as the mouth is opened and is another landmark for administration of the IA block (see Chapter 13).

The pterygotemporal depression associated with the pterygomandibular space is the hollow between the medial pterygoid muscle and the laterally located temporalis muscle tendon (hence the name). Thus this depression exists between the pterygomandibular raphe and the coronoid notch. The pterygotemporal depression serves as a visible landmark for needle entry into the depth of the pterygomandibular space for both the IA block and the V-A block. The temporalis muscle attaches onto the coronoid process and it is important to avoid this sensitive structure when inserting the needle.

Along each medial surface of the body of the mandible is the mylohyoid line or *internal oblique ridge* that extends posteriorly and superiorly, becoming more prominent as it moves superiorly on the body of the mandible. The mylohyoid line is the point of attachment of the mylohyoid muscle that forms the floor of the mouth. The posterior border of the mylohyoid line also provides for attachment of the pterygomandibular raphe. The roots of the mandibular posterior teeth often extend internally inferior to the mylohyoid line. The mylohyoid line can be noted on a radiograph as the radiopaque line inferior to the external oblique ridge (see Fig. 10.8).

On the medial surface of the ramus is also the opening of the mandibular canal, the mandibular foramen (see Fig. 10.12 and Table 10.1). Most skulls show the mandibular foramen position as approximately two-thirds to three-fourths the distance from the coronoid notch to the posterior border of the mandibular ramus; this variance can be noted in reference textbooks depending on their currency. The opening of the mandibular foramen is a landmark for the administration of the IA block as well as the V-A block (see Chapter 13).

The IA nerve and blood vessels exit the mandible through the mandibular foramen after traveling in the mandibular canal and after the merging of the mental and incisive nerves and blood vessels (see later discussion). The incisive nerve was initially located within the mandibular incisive canal, which is an anterior continuation of the mandibular canal bilaterally between the two mental foramina.

With age and tooth loss, the alveolar process of the mandible is resorbed (as discussed earlier) so that the mandibular canal is nearer the superior border. Sometimes with excessive alveolar process resorption, the mandibular canal disappears entirely and leaves the IA nerve without its bony protection, although it is still covered by soft tissue. The height of the mandibular foramen can also seem to be more superior without the presence of teeth in the mandibular posterior sextant.

Rarely there may be present a bifid IA nerve, in which case a second mandibular foramen more inferiorly located exists and can be detected by noting a doubled mandibular canal upon radiographic assessment such as with CBCT. Keeping this anatomic variant of the mandibular foramen in mind is important when administering an IA block along with any changes resulting from bony resorption (see Chapter 13).

Overhanging the mandibular foramen on each side is a bony spine, the lingula, which serves as an attachment for the sphenomandibular ligament associated with the TMJ. The lingula is also a landmark for the IA block. A small groove, the mylohyoid groove, passes anteriorly and inferiorly from the mandibular foramen. The mylohyoid nerve and blood vessels travel in the mylohyoid groove (discussed later), which in some cases can have an unusual pathway that may cause difficulty with the clinical effectiveness of an IA block (see Chapter 13).

TRIGEMINAL NERVE

The fifth cranial (V) or trigeminal nerve provides sensory information for the teeth and associated tissue as well as most of the skin of the face and head (Table 10.4; see Chapter 2). It is the orofacial divisions of the trigeminal nerve that are anesthetized before most possibly painful

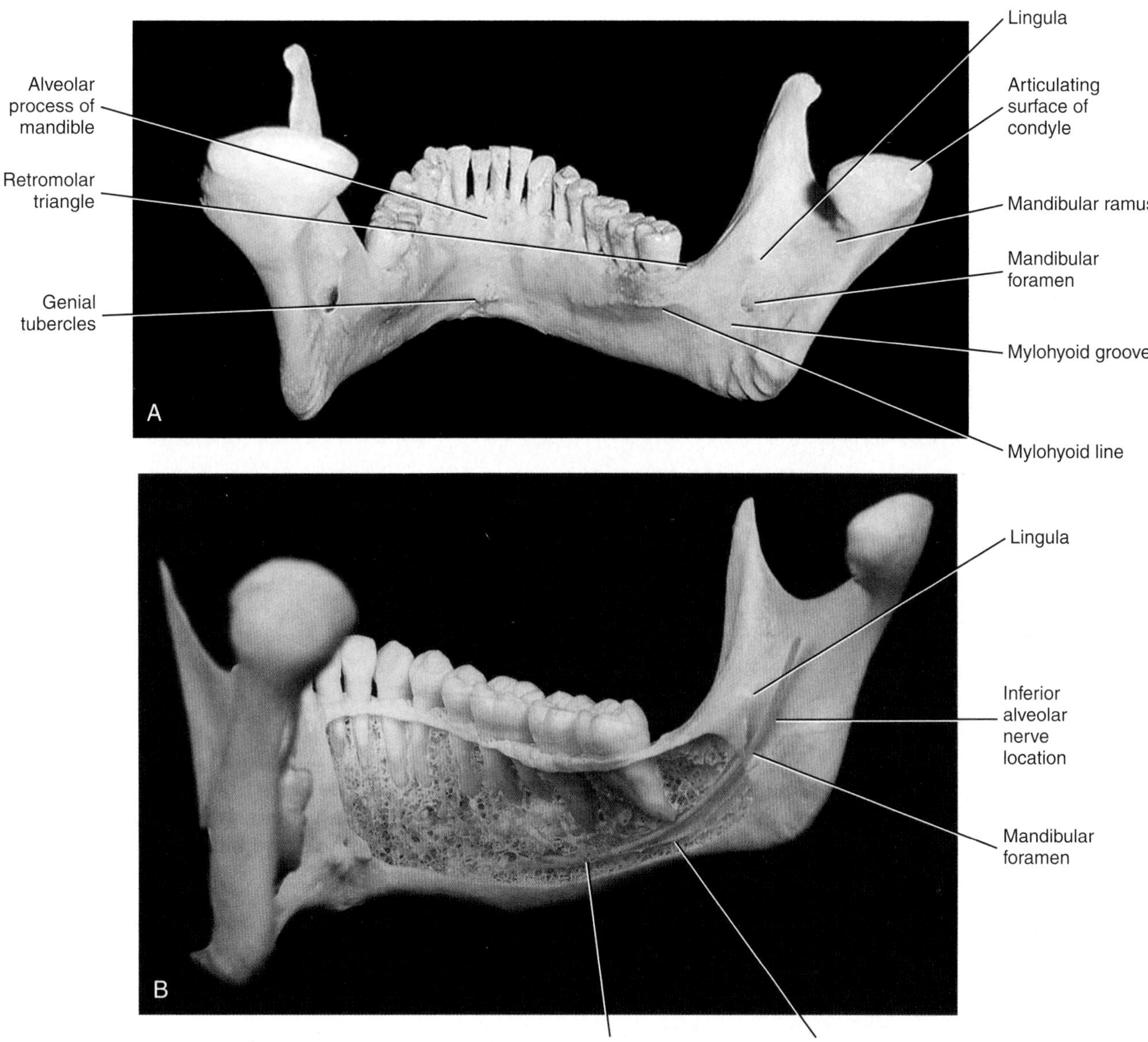

Fig. 10.12 Medial view of the disarticulated mandible and its associated features (A) and a medial cutaway view demonstrating the pathway of the inferior alveolar nerve *(yellow marker)* within the mandibular canal as it forms from a merger of the mental and incisive nerves (not shown here) and exits by way of the mandibular foramen (B). (A from Fehrenbach MJ, Herring SW: *Illustrated anatomy of the head and neck,* ed 6, St Louis, 2021, Saunders/Elsevier; B from Logan BM, Reynold PA, Hutching RT: *McMinn's color atlas of head and neck anatomy,* ed 4, London, 2010, Mosby Ltd. In: Fehrenbach MJ, Herring SW: *Illustrated anatomy of the head and neck,* ed 6, St Louis, 2021, Saunders/Elsevier.)

dental procedures (see Chapters 12 and 13). Thus the dental hygienist must have a thorough understanding of these divisions of the trigeminal nerve to effectively and safely administer local anesthetics to patients.

Each trigeminal nerve is a short nerve trunk composed of two closely adapted roots (Figs. 10.13 and 10.14). These roots of the nerve consist of a thicker sensory root and thinner motor root.

Within the skull, a bulge can be noted in the sensory root of the trigeminal nerve. This bulge is the trigeminal ganglion, which is located on the anterior surface of the temporal bone. Anterior to the trigeminal ganglion, the sensory root begins from three divisions that pass into the skull by way of three different openings in the sphenoid bone.

These divisions of the sensory root are the ophthalmic, maxillary, and mandibular nerves. The ophthalmic and maxillary nerves of the sensory root carry only afferent nerves (see Chapter 2). In contrast, the mandibular nerve off the sensory root runs together with the motor root and thus carries both afferent and efferent nerves. Important to note is that the commonly used terms V_1, V_2, and V_3 (pronounced "vee one," "vee two," and "vee three") are simply shorthand notation for these nerves or divisions of the fifth cranial (or trigeminal nerve) since it uses the notation "V," which means five (see Fig. 10.14). This chapter will discuss mainly the orofacial divisions of the trigeminal nerve, which are the maxillary and mandibular nerves as well as their branches.

Ophthalmic Nerve

The first nerve division or V_1 of the sensory root of the trigeminal nerve is the ophthalmic nerve (Figs. 10.15 and 10.16). This smallest

TABLE 10.4 Orofacial Structures and Trigeminal Nerve Innervation

Orofacial Structures	Nerves and Fiber Type
Maxillary anterior teeth and associated labial periodontium and gingiva	Anterior superior alveolar of V_2: afferent
Maxillary posterior teeth and associated buccal periodontium and gingiva as well as maxillary sinus	Middle superior alveolar and posterior superior alveolar of V_2: afferent
Anterior hard palate and associated palatal periodontium and gingiva of the maxillary anterior teeth as well as nasal septum	Nasopalatine of V_2: afferent
Posterior hard palate and associated palatal periodontium and gingiva of maxillary posterior teeth	Greater palatine of V_2: afferent
Mandibular teeth and associated facial periodontium and gingiva of mandibular anterior teeth and premolars as well as labial mucosa	Inferior alveolar and its incisive and mental branches of V_3: afferent
Associated buccal periodontium and gingiva of mandibular molars as well as buccal mucosa	Buccal of V_3: afferent
Associated lingual periodontium and gingiva of mandibular teeth as well as floor of mouth	Lingual of V_3: afferent
Muscles of mastication	Muscle branches of V_3: medial pterygoid, deep temporal, masseteric, and lateral pterygoid: efferent

V2, Maxillary nerve; *V3,* mandibular nerve.

division serves as an afferent nerve for the conjunctiva, cornea, eyeball, orbit, forehead, ethmoidal, and frontal sinuses plus a part of the dura mater and parts of the nasal cavity and nose. The nerve carries this sensory information toward the brain by way of the superior orbital fissure of the sphenoid bone. The ophthalmic nerve begins from three major nerves: the frontal, lacrimal, and nasociliary nerves.

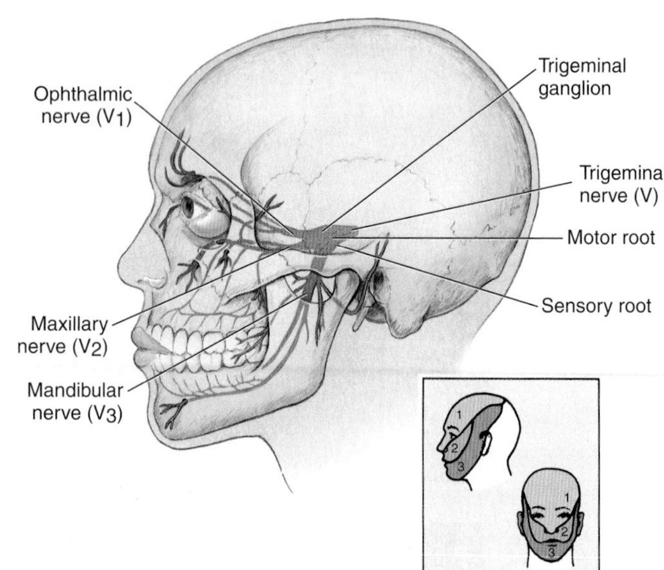

Fig. 10.14 General pathway of the trigeminal or fifth cranial nerve and its motor and sensory roots and three divisions or nerves; note the innervation coverage for each nerve division *(see inset).* (From Fehrenbach MJ, Herring SW: *Illustrated anatomy of the head and neck,* ed 6, St Louis, 2021, Saunders/Elsevier.)

Maxillary Nerve

The second nerve division or V_2 from the sensory root of the trigeminal nerve is the maxillary nerve, which is set between the other two divisions both in size and location (Figs. 10.17 and 10.18). The afferent nerve branches of the maxillary nerve carry sensory information by afferent nerve fibers for the maxillae and its overlying tissue and skin, maxillary sinuses, nasal cavity, palate, nasopharynx, and a part of the dura mater (see Table 10.4 and Chapter 2).

The maxillary nerve is a nerve trunk formed within the pterygopalatine fossa by the convergence of many nerves; the largest contributor is the IO nerve. Tributaries of the IO nerve or maxillary nerve trunk include the zygomatic, anterior, middle and PSA, GP and LP, and NP nerves.

After all these branches come together within the pterygopalatine fossa to form the maxillary nerve, the nerve enters the skull through

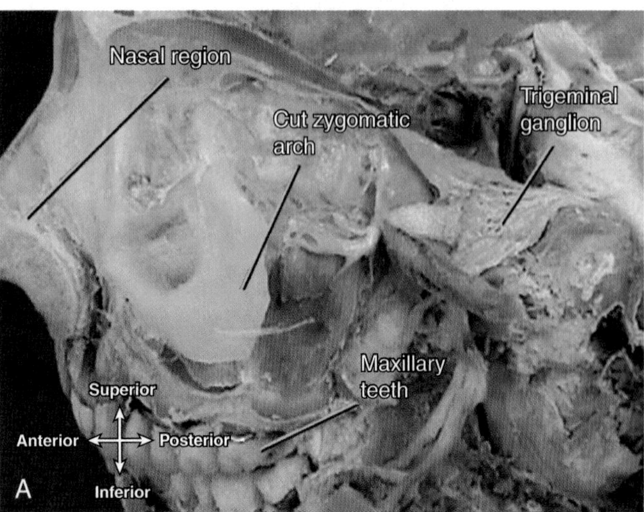

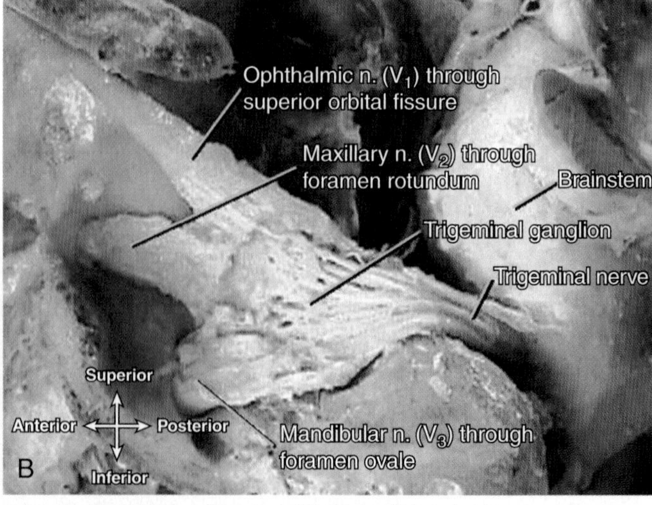

Fig. 10.13 Dissection of the trigeminal ganglion (A) and the three divisions or nerves (B). (From Fehrenbach MJ, Herring SW: *Illustrated anatomy of the head and neck,* ed 6, St Louis, 2021, Saunders/Elsevier.)

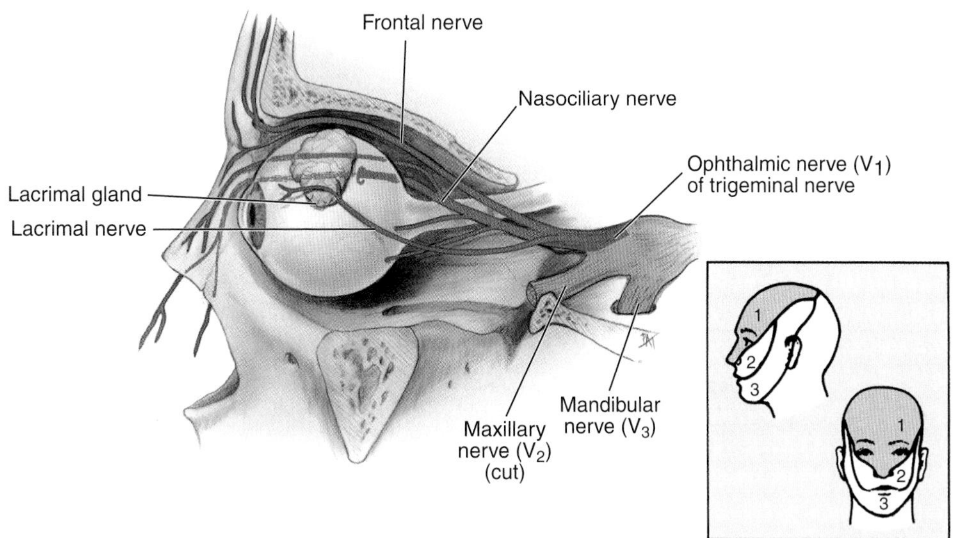

Fig. 10.15 Lateral cutaway view of the orbit with the pathway of the ophthalmic nerve (V_1) of the trigeminal nerve highlighted with only its major branches noted; note also the innervation coverage for the ophthalmic nerve *(see inset)*. (From Fehrenbach MJ, Herring SW: *Illustrated anatomy of the head and neck,* ed 6, St Louis, 2021, Saunders/Elsevier.)

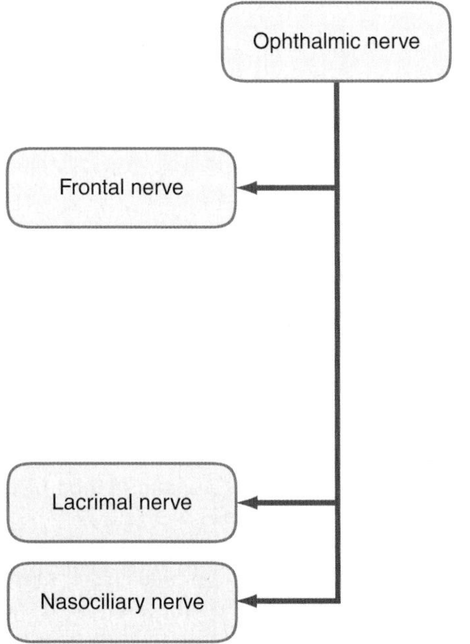

Fig. 10.16 Ophthalmic nerve (V_1) and its major branches to the facial region. (From Fehrenbach MJ, Herring SW: *Illustrated anatomy of the head and neck,* ed 6, St Louis, 2021, Saunders/Elsevier.)

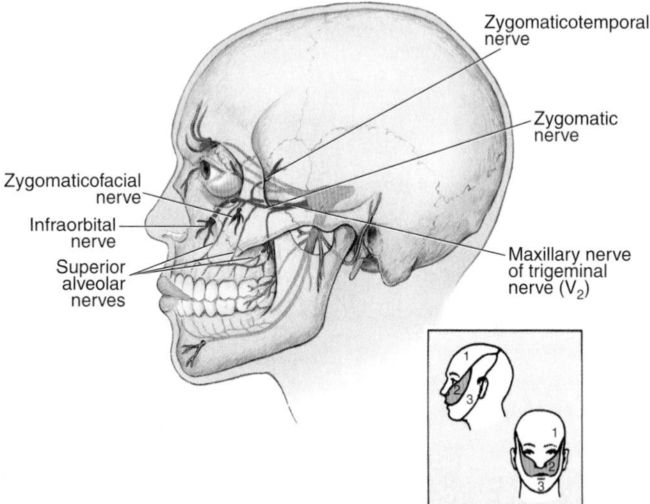

Fig. 10.17 Pathway of the maxillary nerve (V_2) of the trigeminal nerve is highlighted; note the innervation coverage for the maxillary nerve *(see inset)*. (From Fehrenbach MJ, Herring SW: *Illustrated anatomy of the head and neck,* ed 6, St Louis, 2021, Saunders/Elsevier.)

the foramen rotundum of the sphenoid bone. Small afferent meningeal branches from parts of the dura mater join the maxillary nerve as it enters the trigeminal ganglion.

Zygomatic Nerve

The zygomatic nerve is an afferent nerve composed of the merger of the zygomaticofacial nerve and the zygomaticotemporal nerve in the orbit. This nerve also conveys the postganglionic parasympathetic fibers for the lacrimal gland to the lacrimal nerve. The zygomatic nerve courses posteriorly along the lateral orbit floor and enters the pterygopalatine fossa through the inferior orbital fissure, which is located between the sphenoid bone and maxilla, to finally join the maxillary nerve or V_2.

The rather small zygomaticofacial nerve serves as an afferent nerve for the skin of the cheek. This nerve pierces the frontal process of the zygomatic bone and enters the orbit through its lateral wall. The zygomaticofacial nerve then turns posteriorly to join with the zygomaticotemporal nerve (Figs. 10.17 and 10.18).

The other nerve, the zygomaticotemporal nerve, serving as an afferent nerve for the skin of the temporal region, pierces the temporal surface of the zygomatic bone and traverses the lateral wall of the orbit to join the zygomaticofacial nerve to go on to form the zygomatic nerve.

Infraorbital Nerve

The IO nerve is an afferent nerve formed from the merger of cutaneous branches from the upper lip, medial part of the cheek, side of nose, and lower eyelid (Fig. 10.19; see Figs. 10.1 and 10.3). The IO nerve then

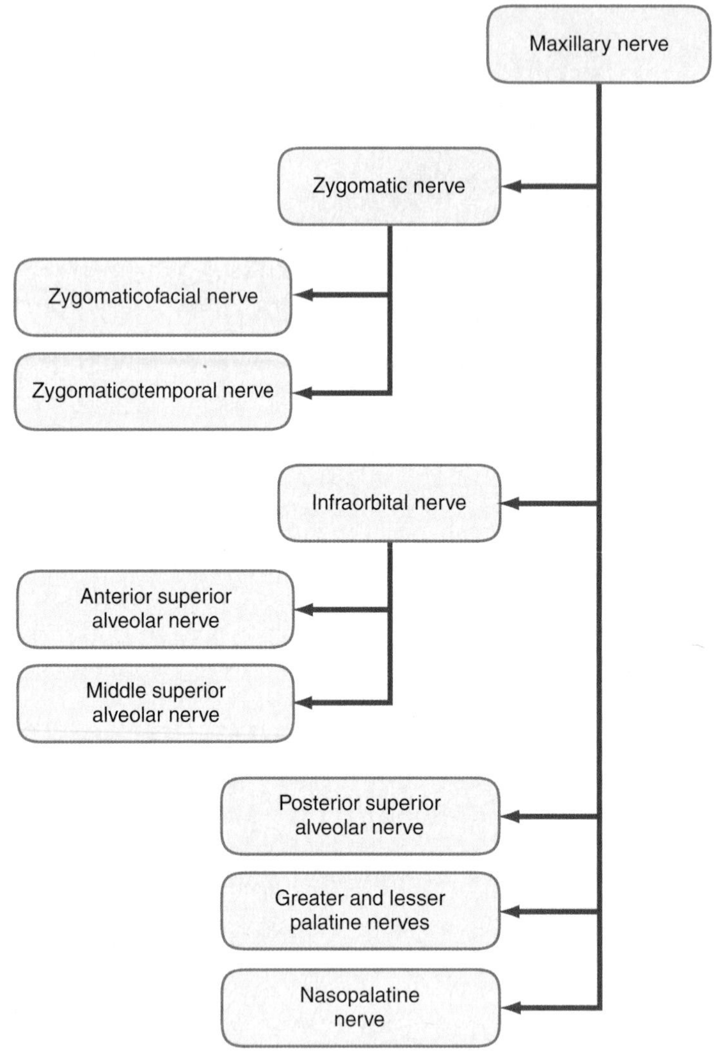

Fig. 10.18 Maxillary nerve (V_2) and its branches to the oral cavity. (From Fehrenbach MJ, Herring SW: *Illustrated anatomy of the head and neck,* ed 6, St Louis, 2021, Saunders/Elsevier.)

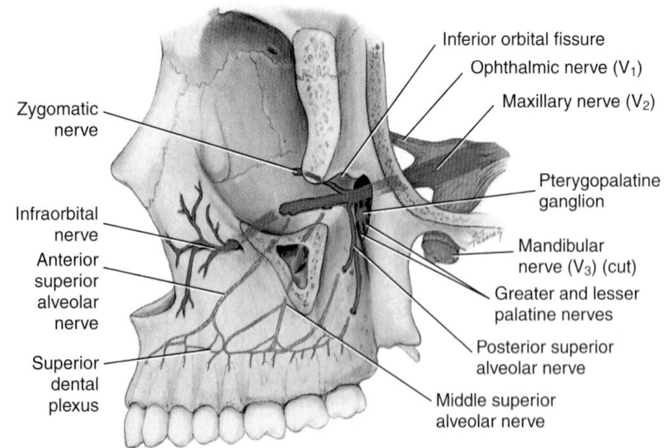

Fig. 10.19 Lateral cutaway view of the skull with part of lateral wall of the orbit removed; the branches of the maxillary nerve are highlighted. (From Fehrenbach MJ, Herring SW: *Illustrated anatomy of the head and neck,* ed 6, St Louis, 2021, Saunders/Elsevier.)

passes into the IO foramen of each maxilla and travels posteriorly through the IO canal along with the IO blood vessels where it is joined by the ASA nerve. The IO nerve is anesthetized by the IO block as well as both the ASA nerve and middle superior alveolar (MSA) nerve at the site of the IO foramen with the administration of the IO block (discussed next) (see also Chapter 12).

From the IO canal and groove, the IO nerve passes into the pterygopalatine fossa through the inferior orbital fissure. After it leaves the IO groove and within the pterygopalatine fossa, the IO nerve receives the PSA nerve and joins with it or directly with the maxillary nerve or V_2.

Anterior Superior Alveolar Nerve

The ASA nerve serves as an afferent nerve for the maxillary anterior teeth and associated labial periodontium and gingiva to the midline in one maxillary quadrant (see Table 10.4).

The ASA nerve originates from dental branches in the pulp of these teeth that exit through the apical foramina (see Figs. 10.3 and 10.19). The ASA nerve also receives interdental branches from the surrounding periodontium, which together become part of the superior dental plexus within the maxillary arch. A **dental plexus** is a network of nerves within both the maxillary and mandibular dental arches (see later discussion on the inferior dental plexus within the mandibular arch). The superior dental plexus within the maxillary arch also receives interdental branches from other branches of the maxillary nerve or V_2, including both the MSA and PSA nerves (discussed later). The apex of the maxillary canine and canine eminence are both landmarks for the ASA block that anesthetizes the ASA nerve (see Chapter 12).

The ASA nerve then moves superiorly along the anterior wall of the maxillary sinus to join the IO nerve in the IO canal. Thus the ASA nerve can be anesthetized by either the ASA block at the site or along with the MSA nerve by the IO block (discussed earlier). The ASA nerve can also be anesthetized with the AMSA block along with other maxillary nerve branches using a palatal technique.

The ASA nerve can also involve crossover-innervation to the contralateral (or opposite) side in a patient. Crossover-innervation is the overlap of terminal nerve fibers from the contralateral side of the dental arch. Crossover-innervation is important to consider when administering local anesthesia for the maxillary anterior teeth and associated tissue with the ASA nerve as well as for the mandibular anterior teeth with the incisive nerve (mandibular association discussed later) (see also Chapters 12 and 13).

Middle Superior Alveolar Nerve

The MSA nerve serves as an afferent nerve for the maxillary premolars and the mesiobuccal root of the maxillary first molar and associated buccal periodontium and gingiva in one maxillary quadrant if the nerve is present (see Table 10.4).

The MSA nerve if present originates from dental branches in the pulp that exit the teeth through the apical foramina as well as interdental and interradicular branches from the surrounding periodontium (see Figs. 10.2, 10.3, and 10.19). The MSA nerve, like the ASA and PSA nerves, is part of the superior dental plexus within the maxillary arch. The MSA nerve then moves superiorly to join the IO nerve by running in the lateral wall of the maxillary sinus. The apex of the maxillary second premolar is the landmark for the administration of the MSA block that anesthetizes the MSA nerve (see Chapter 12).

Thus the MSA nerve if present can be anesthetized by either the MSA block (as discussed) or by the IO block along with the ASA nerve (see Chapter 12). The MSA nerve can also be anesthetized with the AMSA block along with other maxillary nerve branches using a palatal technique.

However, the MSA nerve is not always present in all patients; it is present only in approximately 28% of the population. If the MSA nerve is not present, the area is innervated by both the ASA and PSA nerves but mainly by the ASA nerve. If the MSA nerve is present, there is communication between the MSA nerve and both the ASA and PSA nerves. These considerations are important when administering local anesthesia for the maxillary posterior teeth and associated tissue; however, the administration of both the PSA block as well as the MSA block will provide complete coverage to the maxillary posterior teeth (see Chapter 12).

Posterior Superior Alveolar Nerve

The PSA nerve joins the IO nerve (or the maxillary nerve directly in some cases) within the pterygopalatine fossa (see Figs. 10.2, 10.5, and 10.19). The PSA nerve serves as an afferent nerve for the maxillary molars and associated buccal periodontium and gingiva as well as the maxillary sinus in one maxillary quadrant in most cases unless the MSA nerve is present (see Table 10.4).

Thus some branches of the PSA nerve remain external to the posterior surface of the maxilla. These are the external branches that provide afferent innervation for the maxillary molars. Other afferent nerve branches of the PSA nerve originate from dental branches in the pulp of each of the maxillary molars that exit the teeth by way of the apical foramina as well as the interdental branches and interradicular branches from the surrounding periodontium. The PSA nerve, like the ASA and MSA nerves, is part of the superior dental plexus within the maxillary arch.

All these internal branches of the PSA nerve enter from the multiple PSA foramina on the infratemporal surface of the maxilla. The PSA foramina are posterosuperior on the maxillary tuberosity (as discussed earlier) as well as posterosuperior to the apex of the maxillary second molar. The PSA blood vessels from the maxillary artery also travel through these same foramina. The openings of the PSA foramina as well as the maxillary tuberosity are landmarks for the administration of the PSA block (see Chapter 12).

Both these external and internal branches of the PSA nerve then move superiorly together along the maxillary tuberosity, which forms the posterolateral wall of the maxillary sinus to join either the IO nerve or maxillary nerve.

Greater and Lesser Palatine Nerves

Both palatine nerves join with the maxillary nerve from the palate (Fig. 10.20; see Fig. 10.6). The GP nerve is located in the deepest part of the interface between the mucoperiosteum and bone of the posterior hard palate. The GP nerve serves as an afferent nerve for the posterior hard palate and associated palatal periodontium and gingiva of the maxillary posterior teeth in the maxillary posterior sextant (see Table 10.4). Communication also occurs with the NP nerve terminal fibers in the associated palatal periodontium and gingiva of the maxillary first premolar, which may complicate the use of local anesthesia in the region (see Chapter 12).

Posteriorly, the GP nerve enters the GP foramen in the palatine bone superior to the apices of the maxillary second or third molar to travel within the pterygopalatine canal along with the GP blood vessels. The opening of the GP foramen is a landmark for the administration of the GP block. The GP nerve can also be anesthetized with the AMSA block along with other maxillary nerve branches using a palatal technique.

The LP nerve serves as an afferent nerve for the soft palate and palatine tonsils. The LP nerve enters the LP foramen in the palatine bone near its junction with the sphenoid bone along with the LP blood vessels. The LP nerve then joins the GP nerve within the pterygopalatine canal. When administering the GP block some patients may become uncomfortable and may gag if the soft palate becomes inadvertently and harmlessly anesthetized, which is possible given the nearness of the LP nerve and its foramen (see Chapter 12).

Nasopalatine Nerve

The NP nerve originates in the mucosa of the anterior hard palate, palatal to the maxillary central incisors (see Figs. 10.4 and 10.20). This nerve serves as an afferent nerve for the anterior hard palate and the associated palatal periodontium and gingiva of the maxillary anterior teeth bilaterally from maxillary canine to canine in the maxillary anterior sextant as well as the nasal septal tissue (see Table 10.4).

Both the right and left NP nerves enter the incisive canal by way of the incisive foramen, deep to the incisive papilla, thus exiting the oral cavity. The opening of the incisive foramen and its incisive papilla are both landmarks for the administration of the NP block that anesthetizes both the right and left NP nerves (see Chapter 12). The NP nerves can also be anesthetized with the AMSA block along with other maxillary nerve branches using a palatal technique.

The NP nerve then travels along the nasal septum. Communication also occurs with the GP nerve terminal fibers in the associated palatal periodontium and gingiva of the maxillary canine, which may complicate the use of local anesthesia in the region (see Chapter 12).

Mandibular Nerve

The third nerve division or V_3 of the trigeminal nerve is the mandibular nerve, which is the short main trunk formed by the merger of a

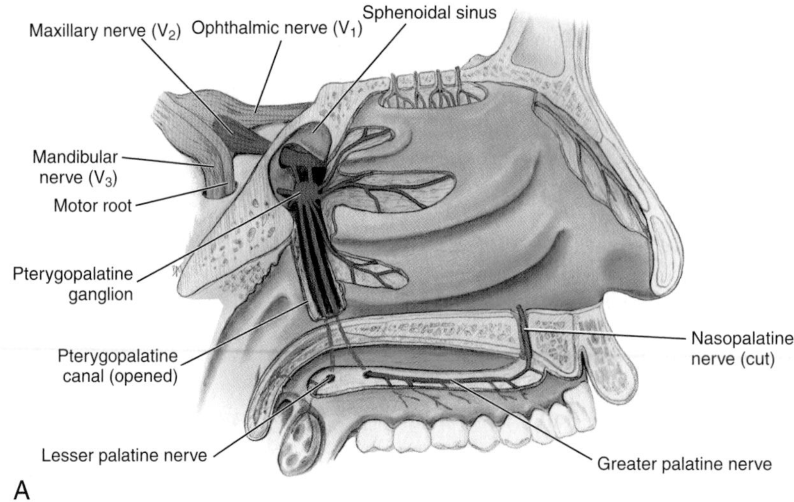

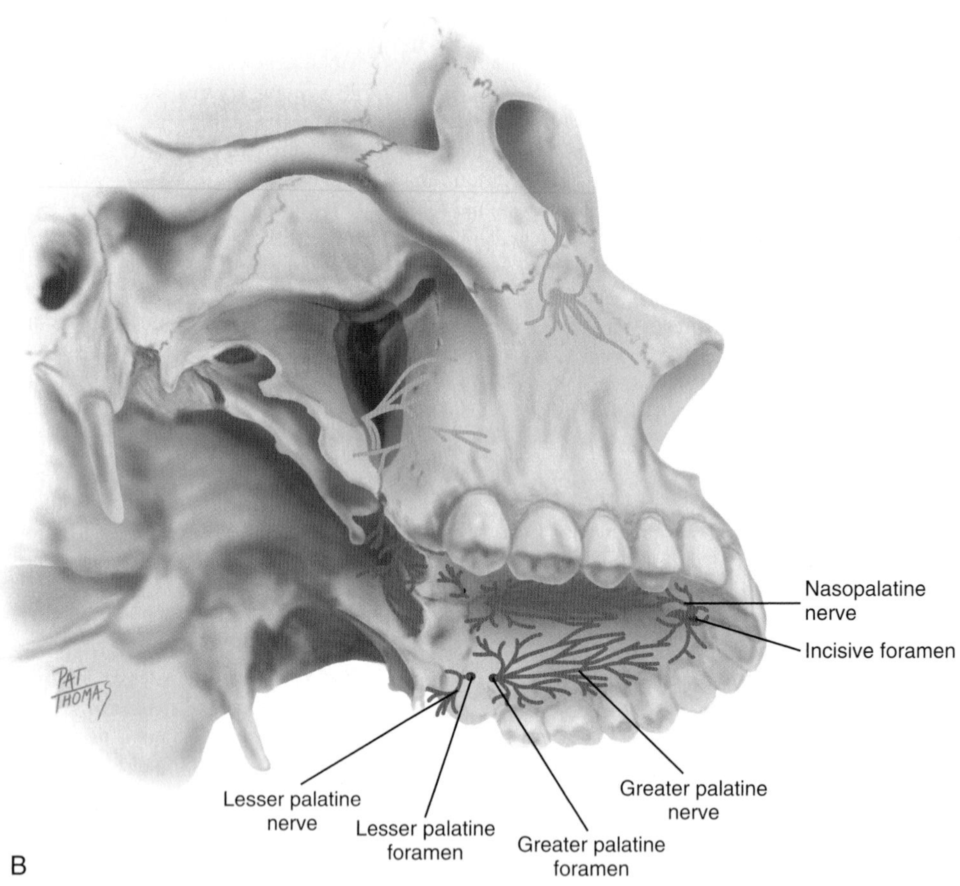

Fig. 10.20 Medial cutaway view of the lateral nasal wall and opened pterygopalatine canal highlighting the maxillary nerve (V_2) and its palatine branches, which include the greater, lesser, and nasopalatine nerves. Note that the nasal septum is removed, thus severing the nasopalatine nerve (A) and shown from an antero-lateral view of the skull and its hard palate (B). (From Fehrenbach MJ, Herring SW: *Illustrated anatomy of the head and neck,* ed 6, St Louis, 2021, Saunders/Elsevier.)

smaller anterior trunk and a larger posterior trunk within the infratemporal fossa before the nerve passes through the foramen ovale of the sphenoid bone to enter the skull (Figs. 10.21–10.23). The infratemporal fossa is inferior to the temporal fossa, which is located in the temporal region on each side of the face but superior to the pterygopalatine fossa. The mandibular nerve then joins with the ophthalmic and maxillary nerves to form the trigeminal ganglion of the trigeminal nerve. The mandibular nerve is the largest of the three divisions that form the trigeminal nerve. The mandibular nerve is also a mixed nerve with both afferent and efferent nerves; it contains the entire efferent part of the trigeminal nerve.

A few small branches come off the V_3 trunk or mandibular nerve before its separation into anterior and posterior trunks and include the meningeal branches, which are afferent nerves (see Chapter 2) for

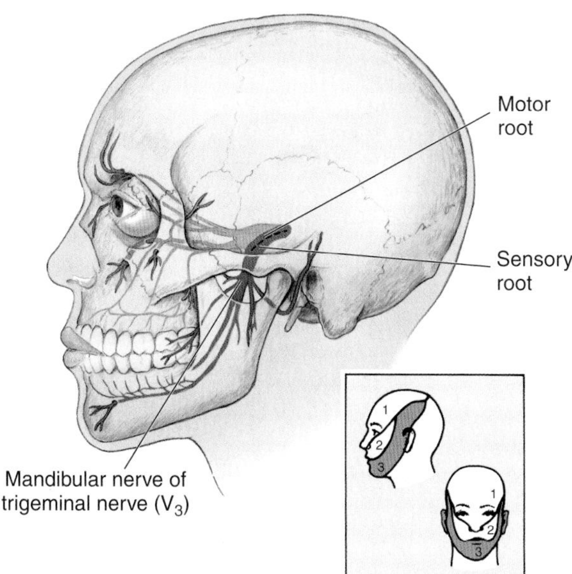

Fig. 10.21 Pathway of the mandibular nerve (V_3) of the trigeminal nerve is highlighted; note the innervation coverage for the mandibular nerve *(see inset).* (From Fehrenbach MJ, Herring SW: *Illustrated anatomy of the head and neck,* ed 6, St Louis, 2021, Saunders/Elsevier.)

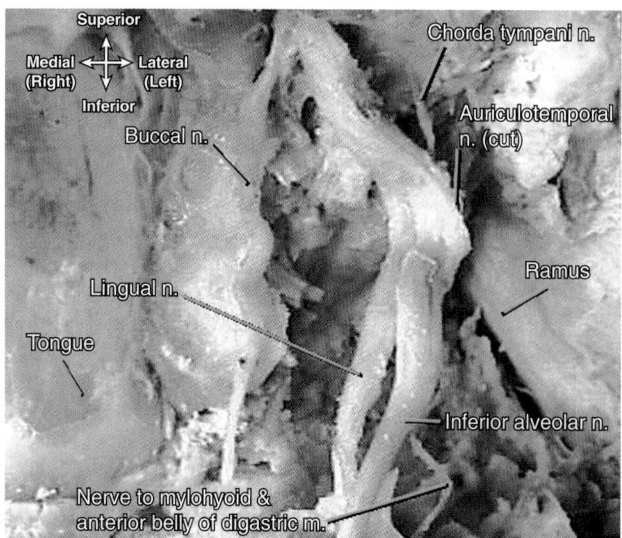

Fig. 10.22 Dissection of the mandibular nerve (V_3) of the trigeminal nerve. (From Fehrenbach MJ, Herring SW: *Illustrated anatomy of the head and neck,* ed 6, St Louis, 2021, Saunders/Elsevier.)

parts of the dura mater (see Fig. 10.26). In addition, there are muscular branches from the undivided mandibular nerve that serve as efferent nerves.

The anterior trunk of the mandibular nerve is formed by the merger of the (long) buccal nerve and additional muscular nerve branches (Fig. 10.24). The anterior trunk has both afferent and efferent nerves. The posterior trunk of the mandibular nerve is formed by the merger of the auriculotemporal, lingual, and IA nerves (see Fig. 10.14). The posterior trunk also has both afferent and efferent nerves.

Buccal Nerve

The buccal nerve (or long buccal nerve) serves as an afferent nerve for the skin of the cheek, buccal mucosa, and associated buccal periodontium and gingiva of the mandibular molars in one mandibular quadrant (see Table 10.4). The buccal nerve being discussed is located on the surface of the buccinator muscle (see Figs. 10.9, 10.10, 10.22–10.24). The buccal nerve then travels posteriorly in the cheek, deep to the masseter muscle. This buccal branch of the trigeminal nerve must not be confused with the buccal branch of the facial nerve, which is an efferent nerve that innervates the buccinator muscle and other muscles of facial expression.

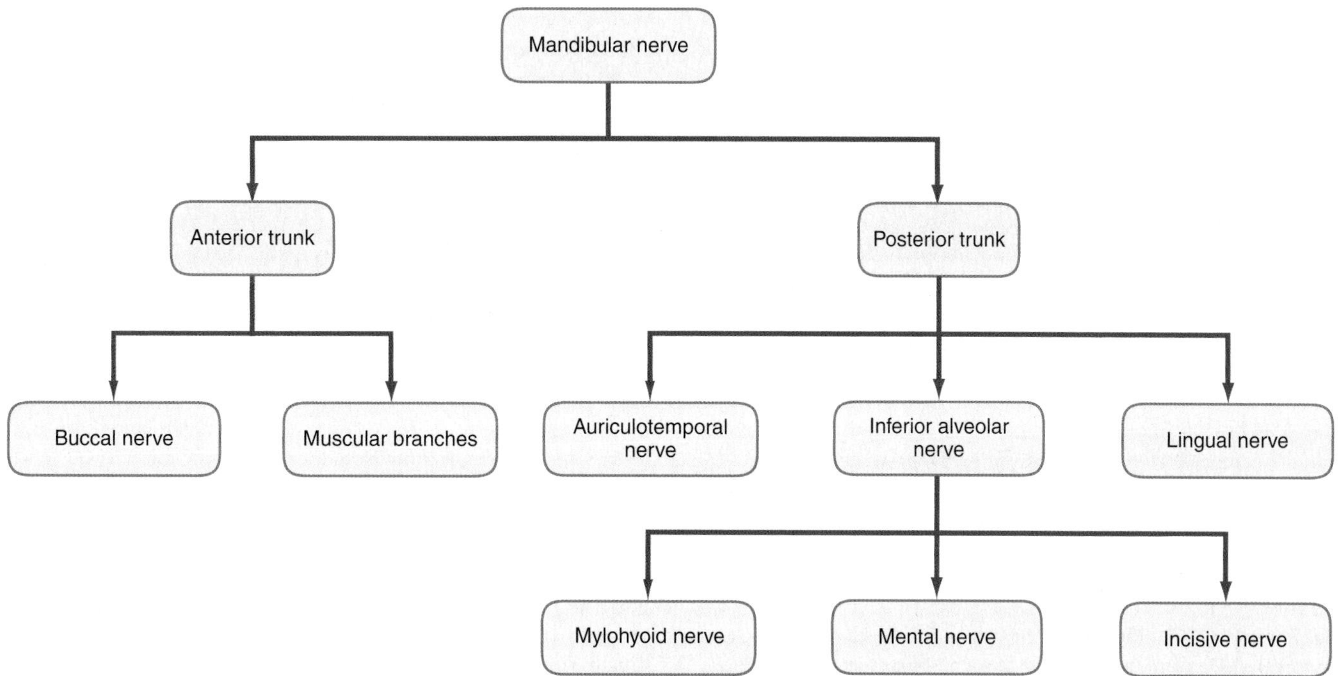

Fig. 10.23 Mandibular nerve (V_3) and its branches to the oral cavity. (From Fehrenbach MJ, Herring SW: *Illustrated anatomy of the head and neck,* ed 6, St Louis, 2021, Saunders/Elsevier.)

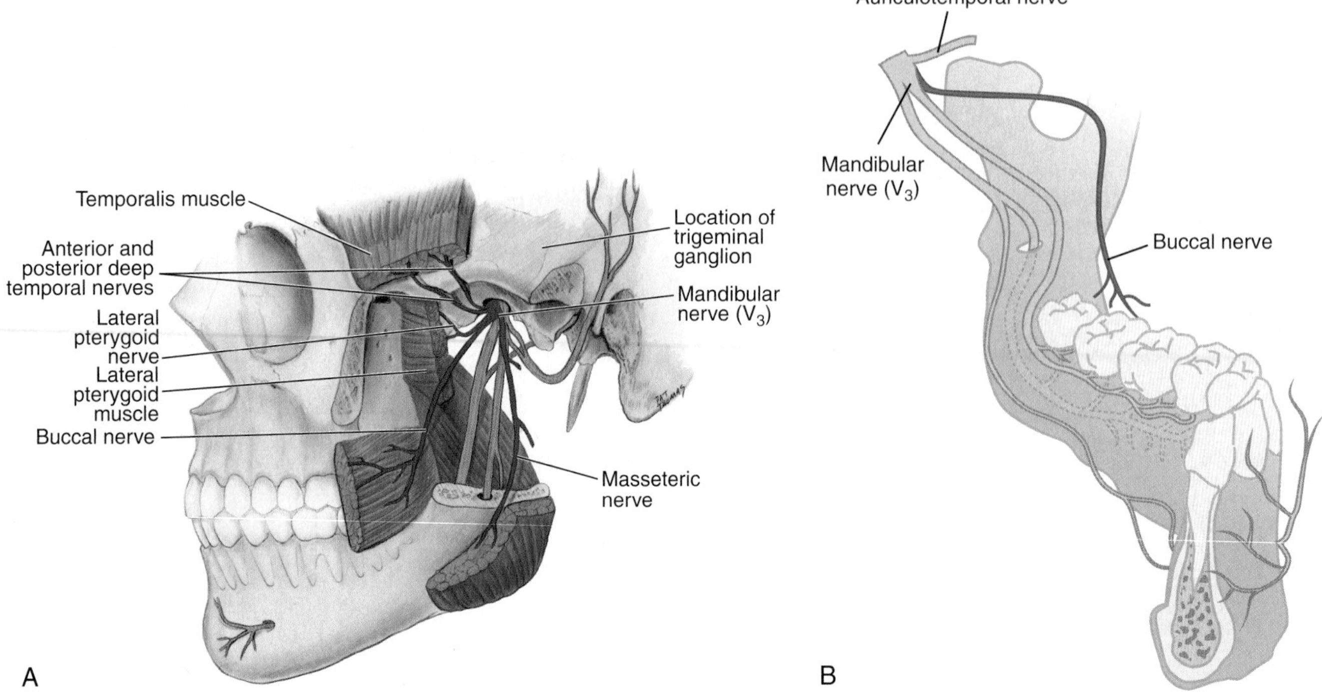

Fig. 10.24 Pathway of the anterior trunk of the mandibular nerve of the trigeminal nerve is highlighted from a lateral cutaway view (A) and from a medial cutaway view (B). (From Fehrenbach MJ, Herring SW: *Illustrated anatomy of the head and neck,* ed 6, St Louis, 2021, Saunders/Elsevier.)

The buccal nerve then crosses anteriorly on the anterior border of the mandibular ramus, distal and buccal to the most distal mandibular molar, and goes between the two heads of the lateral pterygoid muscle to join the anterior trunk of the V_3 or mandibular nerve. The anterior border of the mandibular ramus is a landmark for the administration of the buccal block (see Chapter 13). The buccal nerve is also anesthetized with both the G-G and V-A blocks, in most cases along with other branches of the mandibular nerve.

Muscular Branches and Auriculotemporal Nerve

Several muscular branches are part of the anterior trunk of V_3 or mandibular nerve (see Fig. 10.24). They begin from the motor root of the trigeminal nerve. The auriculotemporal nerve travels with the superficial temporal artery and vein and serves as an afferent nerve for the external ear, scalp, and TMJ (Figs. 10.25 and 10.26; see Figs. 10.22 and 10.23). The nerve also carries postganglionic parasympathetic nerve fibers to the parotid salivary gland. Important to note is that these parasympathetic fibers begin from the lesser petrosal branch of the glossopharyngeal or ninth cranial nerve, joining the auriculotemporal nerve only after relaying in the otic ganglion near the foramen ovale.

Communication of the auriculotemporal nerve with the facial nerve near the ear also occurs. The nerve courses deep to the lateral pterygoid muscle and neck of the mandible, then splits to encircle the middle meningeal artery and finally joins the posterior trunk of V_3 or mandibular nerve. The auriculotemporal nerve is anesthetized with the G-G block and also inadvertently in some cases with the IA block due to its nearness to the IA nerve (see Chapter 13).

Lingual Nerve

The lingual nerve is formed from afferent branches from the associated lingual periodontium and gingiva of mandibular teeth and from the body of the tongue. It first travels along the lateral surface of the tongue (Fig. 10.27; see Figs. 10.22, 10.23, 10.25, and 10.26). The lingual nerve then passes posteriorly, passing from the medial to the lateral side of the duct of the submandibular salivary gland by going inferior to the duct.

The lingual nerve communicates with the submandibular ganglion located superior to the deep lobe of the submandibular salivary gland (see Fig. 10.27). The submandibular ganglion is a part of the parasympathetic system (see Chapter 2). Parasympathetic efferent innervations for both the sublingual and submandibular salivary glands begin from the facial nerves (specifically, a branch of the facial nerve and the chorda tympani nerve) but travel along with the lingual nerve.

At the base of the tongue, the lingual nerve moves superiorly and runs between the medial pterygoid muscle and the mandible, anterior and slightly medial to the IA nerve. Thus the lingual nerve is also anesthetized when administering an IA block through localized diffusion of the local anesthetic agent due to its nearness to the IA nerve within the pterygomandibular space (see Chapter 13). In addition, both the G-G and V-A blocks can be used to anesthetize the lingual nerve along with other branches of the mandibular nerve.

Since the lingual nerve is only a short distance posterior and medial to the roots of the most distal mandibular molar and is covered only by a thin layer of oral mucosa, its location is sometimes visible clinically. Thus the lingual nerve can be endangered by dental procedures in this region such as the surgical extraction of mandibular third molars and possibly trauma from local anesthetic injections. Current research has implicated that paresthesia of the mandible after traumatic mandibular local anesthesia administration mainly involves the lingual nerve (see Chapters 13 and 16).

The lingual nerve then continues to travel superiorly to join the posterior trunk of the V_3 or mandibular nerve. Thus the lingual nerve serves as an afferent nerve for general sensation for the body of the tongue and floor of the mouth as well as the associated lingual periodontium and gingiva of the mandibular teeth to the midline in one mandibular quadrant (see Table 10.4).

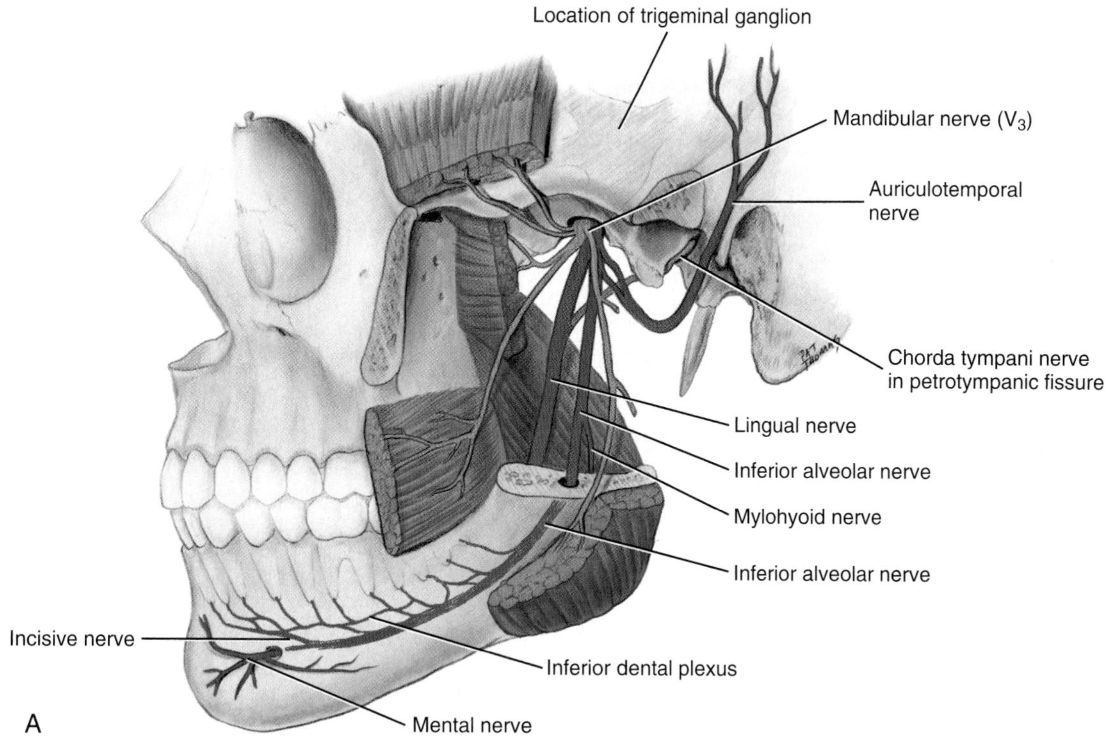

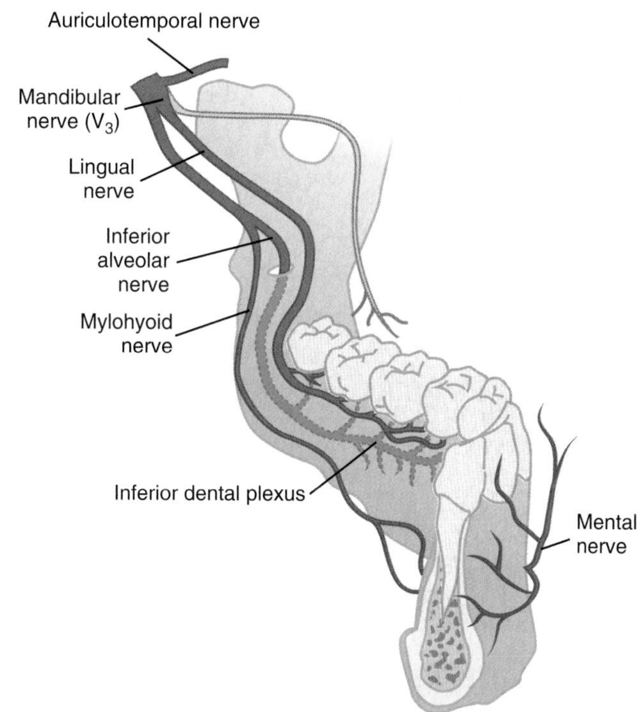

Fig. 10.25 Pathway of the posterior trunk of the mandibular nerve of the trigeminal nerve is highlighted from a lateral cutaway view (A) and from a medial cutaway view (B). (From Fehrenbach MJ, Herring SW: *Illustrated anatomy of the head and neck,* ed 6, St Louis, 2021, Saunders/Elsevier.)

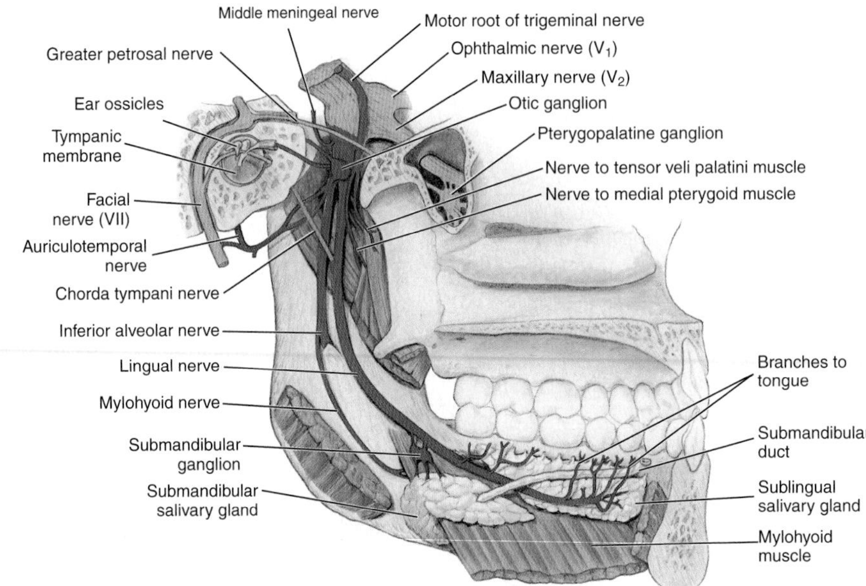

Fig. 10.26 Medial cutaway view of the mandible with the motor and sensory branches of the mandibular nerve is highlighted. (From Fehrenbach MJ, Herring SW: *Illustrated anatomy of the head and neck,* ed 6, St Louis, 2021, Saunders/Elsevier.)

Inferior Alveolar Nerve

The IA nerve is an afferent nerve formed from the merger of the mental nerve and incisive nerve (see Figs. 10.8–10.12, 10.22, 10.23, 10.25, and 10.27). The mental and incisive nerves are discussed later in this section.

After forming, the IA nerve continues to travel posteriorly through the mandibular canal along with the IA artery and vein. Then the IA nerve is joined by the dental branches as well as the interdental and interradicular branches from the surrounding periodontium to become part of the inferior dental plexus within mandibular arch.

The IA nerve then exits the mandible from the mandibular canal through the mandibular foramen where it is joined by the nearby mylohyoid nerve (discussed later). The mandibular foramen is an opening for the mandibular canal on the medial surface of the mandibular ramus. The mandibular foramen is located two-thirds to three-fourths the distance from the coronoid notch to the posterior border of the mandibular ramus and entirely within the pterygomandibular space (or pterygomandibular triangle, depending on the anatomy textbook source). Both the coronoid notch and pterygomandibular space are landmarks for the administration of the IA

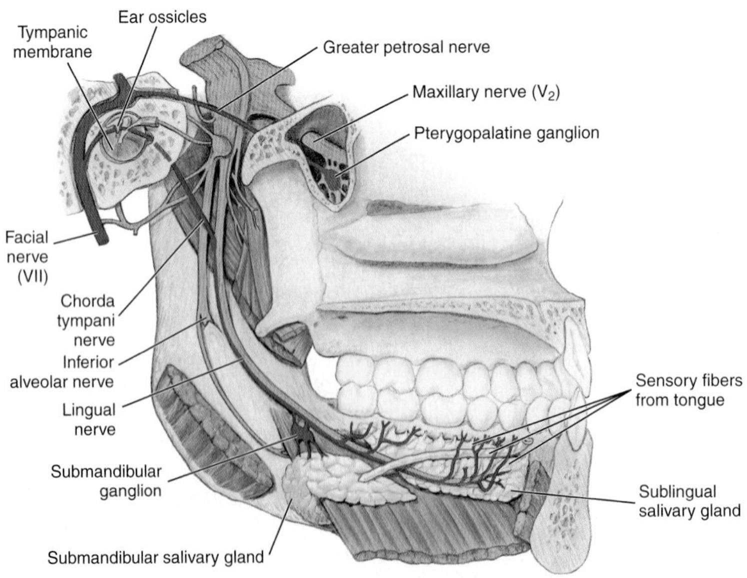

Fig. 10.27 Cutaway view of the pathway of the trunk of the facial nerve, greater petrosal nerve, and chorda tympani nerve is highlighted; note the relationship of the chorda tympani nerve with lingual nerve. (From Fehrenbach MJ, Herring SW: *Illustrated anatomy of the head and neck,* ed 6, St Louis, 2021, Saunders/Elsevier.)

block due to their relationship to the mandibular foramen (see Chapter 13).

The IA nerve then travels laterally to the medial pterygoid muscle, between the sphenomandibular ligament and mandibular ramus, posterior and slightly lateral to the lingual nerve. The sphenomandibular ligament can serve as a barrier during an incorrectly administered IA block that will only anesthetize the shallower lingual nerve (see Chapter 13). The IA nerve then joins the posterior trunk of the V_3 or mandibular nerve (see Figs. 10.25 and 10.26).

The IA nerve carries afferent innervations for the mandibular teeth and the associated facial periodontium and gingiva of mandibular anterior teeth and premolars as well as labial mucosa through its incisive and mental branches to the midline in one mandibular quadrant (see Table 10.4). The IA nerve and its branches along with the lingual nerve are anesthetized by the IA block within the pterygomandibular space (see Chapter 13). In addition, both the G-G and V-A blocks can be used to anesthetize the IA nerve along with other branches of the mandibular nerve at differing sites on the mandible.

In some cases there are two nerves present on the one side, creating bifid IA nerves. This situation can occur unilaterally or bilaterally and can be detected by the presence of a double mandibular canal upon radiographic assessment. Thus there can be more than one mandibular foramen, usually inferiorly located, either unilaterally or bilaterally along with the presence of bifid IA nerves. These variations must be kept in mind when administering local anesthesia for the mandibular teeth and associated tissue (see Chapter 13).

Mental Nerve

The mental nerve is composed of external branches that serve as afferent nerves for the chin, lower lip, and labial mucosa as well as the associated facial periodontium and gingiva of the mandibular anterior teeth and premolars to the midline in one mandibular quadrant (see Figs. 10.8–10.10, 10.23, and 10.25; see Table 10.4). The mental nerve then enters the mental foramen on the lateral surface of the mandible, usually inferior to the apices of the mandibular premolars. Palpation of the mental foramen before an administration of a local anesthetic agent will cause transient soreness to the area due to the presence of the nerve.

The opening of the mental foramen is a landmark for the administration of the mental block (see Chapter 13). The incisive block can also be administered at the same site to achieve anesthesia of the deeper incisive nerve resulting from additional amount of local anesthetic agent. In addition, the IA, G-G, or V-A blocks can be used to anesthetize the mental nerve along with other branches of the mandibular nerve from other target injection sites.

After entering via the mental foramen and traveling a distance within the mandibular canal, the mental nerve merges with the incisive nerve to form the IA nerve within the mandibular canal but before the IA nerve exits by way of the mandibular foramen.

Incisive Nerve

The incisive nerve is an afferent nerve composed of dental branches from the mandibular anterior teeth and premolars that originate in the pulp, exit the teeth through the apical foramina, and join with interdental branches from the surrounding periodontium to be part of the inferior dental plexus within the mandibular arch (see Figs. 10.8–10.10, 10.23, and 10.25). The incisive nerve serves as an afferent nerve for the mandibular anterior teeth and premolars and associated facial periodontium and gingiva to the midline in one mandibular quadrant (see Table 10.4).

The incisive nerve either begins as nerve endings within the mandibular anterior teeth or adjacent bone and soft tissue. The incisive nerve travels within the mandibular incisive canal, which is an anterior continuation of the mandibular canal that runs bilaterally between the mental foramina. The incisive nerve then merges with the mental nerve, just posterior to the mental foramen. The incisive nerve either terminates as nerve endings within the mandibular anterior teeth or adjacent lingual cortical bone and soft tissue.

The incisive nerve is anesthetized by the incisive block; it has the same landmark as the mental block, which is the opening of the mental foramen (see Chapter 13). The incisive nerve will go on next to merge with the IA nerve within the mandibular canal before the IA nerve exits by way of the mandibular foramen.

Crossover-innervation from the contralateral incisive nerve can also occur, which is an important consideration when administering local anesthesia for the mandibular anterior teeth and premolars and associated tissue (see Chapter 13). In addition, the incisive nerve can be anesthetized by way of the IA, G-G, or V-A blocks along with other branches of the mandibular nerve from other target injections.

Mylohyoid Nerve

After the IA nerve exits the mandibular foramen, a small branch occurs, the mylohyoid nerve (see Figs. 10.22, 10.25, and 10.26). This nerve pierces the sphenomandibular ligament and runs inferiorly and anteriorly in the mylohyoid groove and then onto the inferior surface of the mylohyoid muscle. The mylohyoid nerve serves as an efferent nerve to both the mylohyoid muscle and anterior belly of the digastric muscle (the posterior belly of the digastric muscle is innervated by a branch from the facial nerve) (see Table 10.4).

However, the mylohyoid nerve may in some cases also serve as an afferent nerve for the mandibular first molar (see Chapter 2), which needs to be considered when there is lack of clinical effectiveness of the IA block (see Chapter 13). If there is a concern, the mylohyoid nerve can be additionally anesthetized by giving a supraperiosteal injection for the tooth at the medial border of the mandible in the lingual soft tissue for the tooth (see Fig. 13.11 in Chapter 13) or possibly a periodontal ligament injection directly into the periodontium of the tooth (see Table 13.15, Figure AA in Chapter 13). The mylohyoid nerve is also anesthetized by either the G-G or V-A blocks along with other branches of the mandibular nerve.

FACIAL NERVE

The dental hygienist must also have an understanding of the seventh cranial (VII) or facial nerve and its importance when administering local anesthetics. The facial nerve carries both efferent and afferent nerves (see Chapter 2). The facial nerve emerges from the brain and enters the internal acoustic meatus within the temporal bone. Within the temporal bone, the nerve gives off a small efferent branch to the muscle in the middle ear and two larger branches, the greater petrosal and chorda tympani nerves, both of which carry parasympathetic fibers (see Figs. 10.26 and 10.27).

The main trunk of the facial nerve emerges from the skull through the stylomastoid foramen of the temporal bone and gives off two branches, the posterior auricular nerve and a branch to the posterior belly of the digastric and stylohyoid muscles (Fig. 10.28; see also Fig. 15.3 in Chapter 15). The facial nerve then passes into the parotid salivary gland and divides into numerous branches to supply the muscles of facial expression, but it does not innervate the parotid salivary gland itself (discussed next). Avoiding anesthesia of the facial nerve at this location within the parotid salivary gland is important when administering an IA or V-A block because it may result in transient facial paralysis if administered incorrectly (see Chapters 13 and 16).

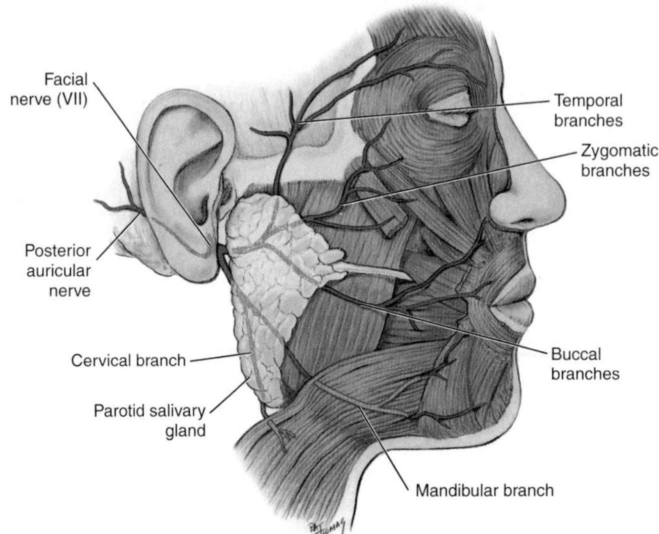

Fig. 10.28 Lateral view of the pathway of the branches of the facial nerve to the face as well as the muscles of facial expression is highlighted; note that the facial nerve is within the parotid salivary gland during its course. (From Fehrenbach MJ, Herring SW: *Illustrated anatomy of the head and neck,* ed 6, St Louis, 2021, Saunders/Elsevier.)

VASCULAR AND GLANDULAR STRUCTURES

The dental hygienist must also know the location of certain adjacent soft tissue structures to the orofacial nerves, such as major blood vessels and associated glandular tissue, to avoid inadvertently injecting these structures when administering local anesthesia. If these soft tissue structures are accidentally compromised, complications may occur (see Chapter 16). Blood vessels may be traumatized from being pierced by the needle and may result in hematomas.

In addition, if aspiration is not performed, an injection of agent directly into the vascular system might occur. Thus to avoid this complication, aspiration must always be attempted before administration of the local anesthetic agent into the oral cavity (see Chapter 11). The facial nerve within the parotid salivary gland may also be traumatized by the needle, which could result in transient facial paralysis. Infections may also be spread to deeper tissue by needle tract contamination.

However, the dental hygienist should use the hemostatic control properties of certain components of the local anesthetic agent to reduce the bleeding from smaller blood vessels in the region to be instrumented in order to provide better visibility and root coverage, especially within furcations and root concavities (see Chapter 4).

The vascular system of the head and neck, as is the case in the rest of the body, consists of an arterial blood supply, a capillary network, and venous drainage. A large network of blood vessels is a vascular plexus. The head and neck area contains certain important venous plexuses. Blood vessels also may communicate with each other by an anastomosis (plural, anastomoses), a connecting channel among the vessels.

An artery is a component of the vascular system that begins from the heart, carrying blood away from it. Each artery starts as a large vessel and branches into smaller vessels, each one a smaller artery or an arteriole. Each arteriole branches into even smaller vessels until it becomes a network of capillaries. Each capillary is smaller than an arteriole and can supply blood to a large tissue area only because there are so many of them.

A vein is another component of the vascular system. A vein, unlike an artery, travels to the heart and carries blood. After each smaller vein or venule drains the capillaries of the tissue area, the venules coalesce to become larger veins. Veins have a much larger diameter and are more numerous than arteries. Veins anastomose freely and have a greater variability in location in comparison with arteries. It is a common misconception that the veins of the head do not contain one-way valves like other veins of the vascular system. In fact, most veins in the face, but not all, have valves.

There are also different kinds of venous networks found in the body. *Superficial veins* are found immediately deep to the skin. *Deep veins* usually accompany larger arteries in a more protected location within the tissue. Venous sinuses are blood-filled spaces between the two layers of tissue. All these venous networks are connected by anastomoses.

Relating the structures supplied and the area's blood vessels is an important way of understanding the location of the various blood vessels and their relationship to the areas involved with the administration of local anesthesia. Remember that, unlike innervation supplied by the nerves to the muscles, which is a one-to-one relationship, blood supply is regional in coverage. Arteries supply the structures in their vicinity, and veins receive blood from the nearby structures. Associated salivary glandular tissue in the related regions will be noted during the overall discussion of the vascular system.

External Carotid Artery Orofacial Branches

The external carotid artery supplies the extracranial tissue of the head and neck, including the oral cavity (Figs. 10.29 and 10.30 and Table 10.5). The external carotid artery begins at the superior border of the thyroid cartilage at the termination of the common carotid artery and the carotid sheath. The external carotid artery travels superiorly in a more medial position in relationship to the internal carotid artery after arising from the common carotid artery. This chapter will only deal with the orofacial branches of the external carotid artery, which include the lingual artery and maxillary artery (see Table 10.5).

Lingual Artery

The lingual artery branches off the external carotid artery at the level of the hyoid bone (see Fig. 10.29). However, the artery does not accompany the corresponding nerve throughout its course. Instead the lingual artery travels anteriorly from the ventral surface to the apex of the tongue by way of its inferior surface to supply the tongue, tonsils, and

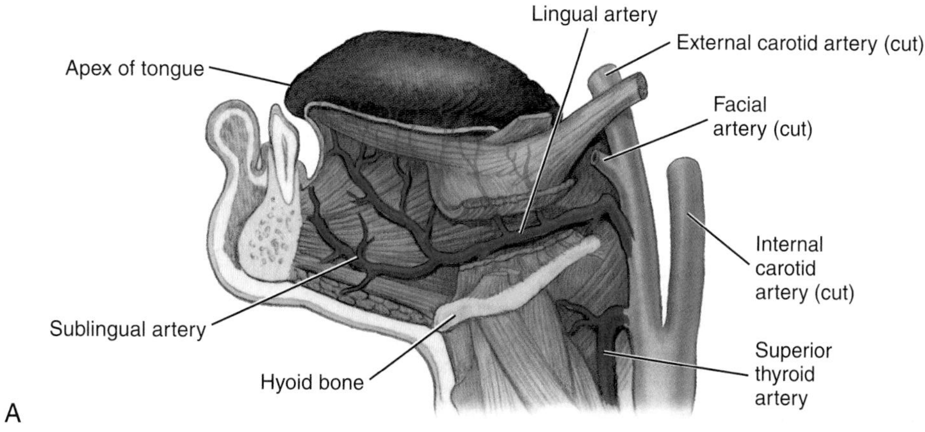

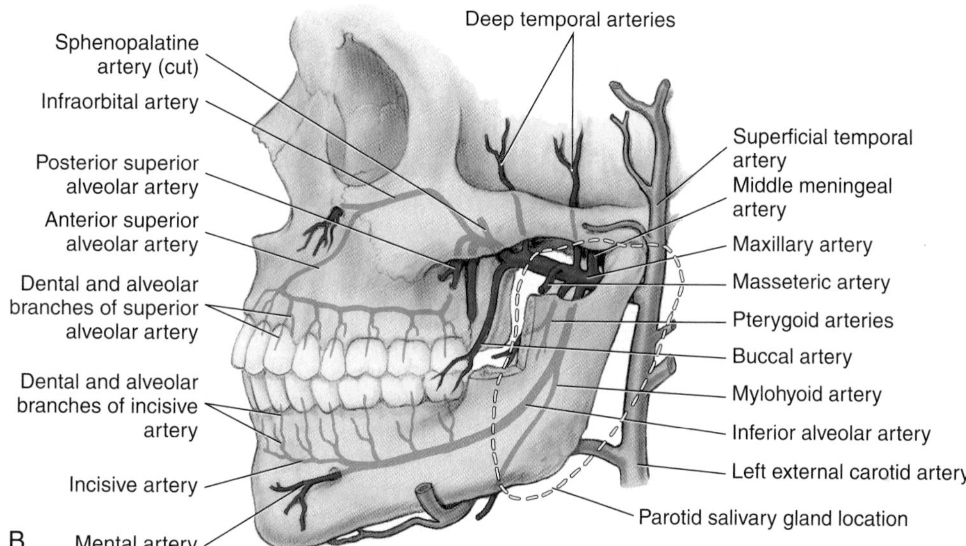

Fig. 10.29 Lateral views of the pathway of the external carotid artery with its major orofacial branches. Lingual artery with its sublingual artery is highlighted (A). Maxillary artery is highlighted except those branches to the nasal cavity and palate (see Fig. 10.30). Noted also is the location of the parotid salivary gland *(dashed lines)* (B). (From Fehrenbach MJ, Herring SW: *Illustrated anatomy of the head and neck,* ed 6, St Louis, 2021, Saunders/Elsevier.)

soft palate by way of the dorsal lingual arteries and deep lingual artery and other branches.

The sublingual artery also branches off the lingual artery to supply the mylohyoid muscle, suprahyoid muscles, sublingual salivary gland, and oral mucosa of the floor of the mouth as well as the lingual periodontium and gingiva of the mandibular teeth in most cases. However in a lesser number of cases, the mandibular lingual tissue is supplied along with or instead by the submental artery from the facial artery, another branch of the external carotid artery.

Maxillary Artery

The maxillary artery also branches off the external carotid artery but is inferior to the TMJ and turns anteromedially to the neck of the mandibular condyle to travel deep to the structures of the face (see Fig. 10.29). There it courses between the muscles of mastication and ascends toward and enters the pterygopalatine fossa.

The IA artery branches off the maxillary artery within the infratemporal fossa (see Fig. 10.29). The IA artery turns inferiorly to enter the mandibular foramen and then the mandibular canal along with the IA nerve and vein. The IA block also has a high percentage of positive aspiration with administration due to the nearness of the IA blood vessels to the IA nerve exiting the mandibular foramen, which is the target area for the block (see Chapter 13).

The mylohyoid artery branches off the IA artery before the main artery enters the mandibular canal by way of the mandibular foramen (see Fig. 10.29). The mylohyoid artery travels with the mylohyoid nerve in the mylohyoid groove on the medial surface of the mandible and supplies both the floor of the mouth and the mylohyoid muscle.

Within the mandibular canal, the IA artery gives off the dental and alveolar branches (see Fig. 10.29). The dental branches of the IA artery supply the pulp of the mandibular posterior teeth by way of each tooth's apical foramen. The alveolar branches of the IA artery supply the associated buccal periodontium and gingiva of the mandibular posterior teeth. The IA artery then branches into two arteries within the mandibular canal, the mental and incisive arteries.

The mental artery branches off the IA artery and enters the mandibular canal by way of the mental foramen along with the mental nerve (see Fig. 10.29). The mental foramen is located on the lateral surface of the mandible, usually inferior to the apices of the mandibular premolars. After the mental artery exits the canal, the artery

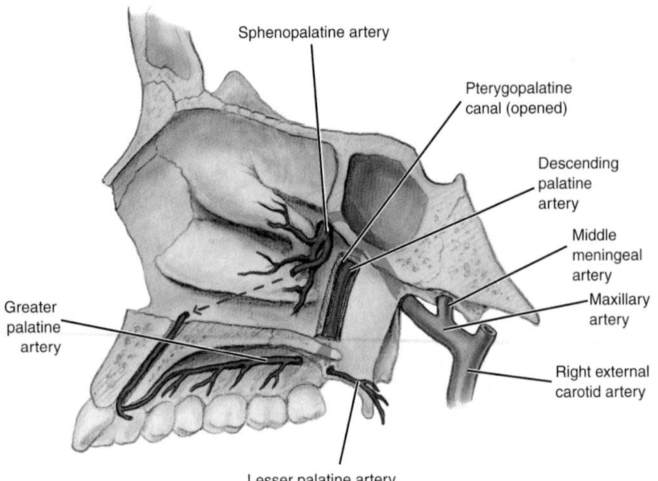

Fig. 10.30 Lateral cutaway view of the pathways of the greater palatine artery, lesser palatine artery, and sphenopalatine artery branching off the maxillary artery are highlighted. (From Fehrenbach MJ, Herring SW: *Illustrated anatomy of the head and neck,* ed 6, St Louis, 2021, Saunders/Elsevier.)

supplies the tissue of the chin and anastomoses with the inferior labial artery from the facial artery.

The incisive artery branches off the IA artery and remains within the mandibular canal along with the incisive nerve where it divides into dental and alveolar branches (see Fig. 10.29). The dental branches of the incisive artery supply the pulp of the mandibular anterior teeth by way of each tooth's apical foramen. The alveolar branches of the incisive artery supply the associated labial periodontium and gingiva of the mandibular anterior teeth and anastomose with the alveolar branches of the incisive artery on the other side.

In addition, both the mental and incisive blocks have a high percentage of positive aspiration with administration due to the nearness of both the mental artery and incisive artery to the mental and incisive nerves within the mental foramen, respectively, which is the target area for both blocks (see Chapter 13).

The maxillary artery also has orofacial branches that are located near the muscle they supply (see Fig. 10.29 and Table 10.5). These arteries all accompany branches of the mandibular nerve of the fifth cranial or trigeminal nerve. The deep temporal arteries supply both the anterior and posterior parts of the temporalis muscle. The pterygoid arteries supply the lateral and medial pterygoid muscles. The masseteric artery supplies the masseter muscle. The buccal artery passes to the buccal mucosa to supply the buccinator muscle and other soft tissues of the cheek.

Just after the maxillary artery leaves the infratemporal fossa and enters the pterygopalatine fossa, it gives off the PSA artery (see Fig. 10.29). Branches of the PSA artery enter the PSA foramina along with the PSA nerve on the outer posterior surface of the maxilla, where it gives off dental branches and alveolar branches. The PSA block has a high percentage of positive aspiration with administration due to the nearness of the PSA artery as well as the PSA vein to the PSA nerve as they all travel through the PSA foramina, which is the target area for the block (see Chapter 12).

The dental branches of the PSA artery supply the pulp of the maxillary posterior teeth by way of each tooth's apical foramen. The alveolar branches of the PSA artery supply the associated buccal periodontium and gingiva of the maxillary posterior teeth. Some branches also supply the mucous membranes of the maxillary sinus. The PSA artery also anastomoses with the ASA artery.

TABLE 10.5 Orofacial Branches of External Carotid Artery

Major Orofacial Branches	Further Orofacial Branches	Orofacial Structures Supplied
LINGUAL ARTERY		
Dorsal lingual and deep lingual		Tongue and tonsils
Sublingual		Mylohyoid muscle, suprahyoid muscles, sublingual salivary gland, and oral mucosa of the floor of the mouth as well as lingual periodontium and gingiva of mandibular teeth (possibly along with or alone by facial artery submental branch)
MAXILLARY ARTERY OROFACIAL BRANCHES		
Inferior alveolar arteries	Dental and alveolar branches, mylohyoid, mental, and incisive	Mandibular teeth with facial periodontium and gingiva, floor of the mouth, and mental region
Deep temporal(s)	Anterior and posterior	Temporalis muscle
Pterygoid(s)		Lateral and medial pterygoid muscles
Masseteric		Masseter muscle
Buccal		Buccinator muscle and buccal region
Posterior superior alveolar	Dental and alveolar branches	Maxillary posterior teeth with buccal periodontium and gingiva, maxillary sinus
Infraorbital	Orbital and terminal branches, anterior superior alveolar with dental and alveolar branches, and middle superior alveolar artery, if present	Maxillary anterior teeth with labial periodontium and gingiva as well as maxillary premolars with buccal periodontium and gingiva if latter artery is present, orbital region, and associated facial regions
Descending palatine	Greater palatine and lesser palatine(s)	Posterior hard palate and soft palate, and palatal periodontium and gingiva of maxillary posterior teeth by way of greater palatine
Sphenopalatine	Nasopalatine, posterior lateral nasal, and septal branches	Anterior hard palate and nasal cavity, and palatal periodontium and gingiva of maxillary anterior teeth by way of nasopalatine; nasal region and nasal cavity by others

After traversing the infratemporal fossa, the maxillary artery then enters the pterygopalatine fossa. Inferior and deep to the eye, the IO artery also branches in the pterygopalatine fossa but may share a common trunk with the PSA artery. The IO artery then enters the orbit through the inferior orbital fissure. While in the orbit, the IO artery travels in the IO canal. Within the IO canal, the IO artery provides orbital branches to the orbit and gives off the ASA artery that travels nearby to the ASA nerve.

Thus the ASA artery branches off the IO artery and gives off dental and alveolar branches (see Fig. 10.29). The dental branches of the ASA artery supply the pulp of the maxillary anterior teeth by way of each tooth's apical foramen. The alveolar branches of the ASA artery supply the associated labial periodontium and gingiva of the maxillary anterior teeth. The ASA artery also anastomoses with the PSA artery.

An MSA artery can be present and supplies the associated buccal periodontium and gingiva of the maxillary premolars. When present, the MSA artery branches from the IO artery within the IO canal and runs inferiorly along the lateral wall of the maxillary sinus toward the region of the maxillary canine and lateral incisors and anastomoses with the both ASA and PSA arteries.

After giving off these branches in the IO canal, the IO artery emerges onto the face from the IO foramen on the outer surface of the maxilla along with the IO nerve (see Fig. 10.29). The opening of the IO foramen is a landmark for the IO block (see Chapter 12). The artery's terminal branches supply parts of the face inferior to the orbit and anastomose with the facial artery.

Also in the pterygopalatine fossa, the maxillary artery gives off the descending palatine artery. This artery travels to the palate through the pterygopalatine canal and then terminates in both the GP artery and LP artery, which then travel along with the GP and LP nerves to exit by way of the GP and LP foramina to supply the posterior hard palate with the palatal periodontium and gingiva of the maxillary posterior teeth and soft palate, respectively (see Fig. 10.30). The GP foramen is a landmark for the GP block (see Chapter 12).

The maxillary artery ends by becoming the sphenopalatine artery, which supplies the nasal cavity. The sphenopalatine artery gives off the posterior lateral nasal branches and septal branches, including a NP branch that accompanies the NP nerve through the incisive foramen on the maxillae to supply the anterior hard palate with the palatal periodontium and gingiva of the maxillary anterior teeth. The incisive foramen is a landmark for the NP block (see Chapter 12).

Pterygoid Plexus of Veins

The pterygoid plexus of veins is a collection of small anastomosing vessels located around the lateral pterygoid muscle and surrounding the maxillary artery on each side of the face within the infratemporal fossa (Figs. 10.31 and 10.32). This vascular plexus anastomoses with both the facial and retromandibular veins. The pterygoid plexus of veins protects the maxillary artery from being compressed during mastication. By either filling or emptying, the pterygoid plexus of veins can accommodate changes in volume of the infratemporal fossa that occur when the mandible moves.

The pterygoid plexus of veins drains the veins from the deep parts of the face and then drains into the maxillary vein (see Fig. 10.32). The middle meningeal vein also drains the blood from the dura mater of the meninges of the brain into the pterygoid plexus of veins.

The pterygoid plexus of veins also drains the PSA vein, which is formed by the merging of its dental and alveolar branches. The dental branches of the PSA vein drain the pulp of the maxillary teeth by way of each tooth's apical foramen. The alveolar branches of the PSA vein drain the associated periodontium and gingiva of the maxillary teeth.

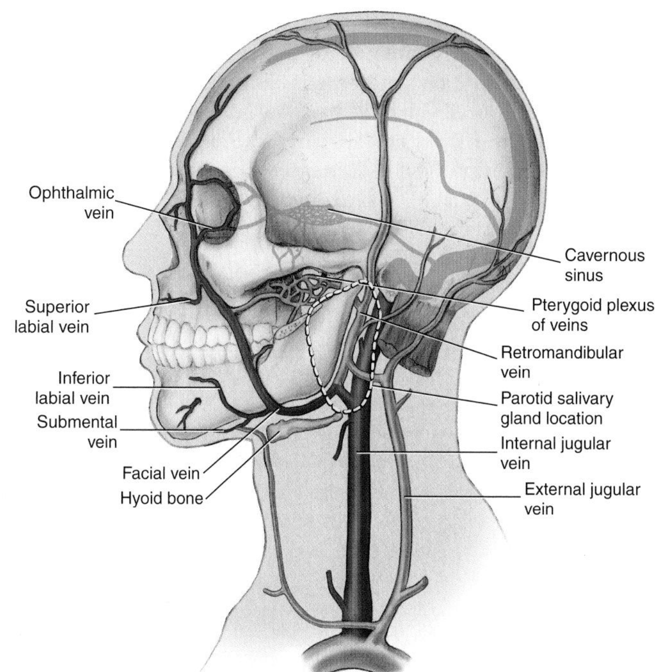

Fig. 10.31 Lateral view of the pathways of the retromandibular vein and external jugular vein to the orofacial region are highlighted including the anterior jugular vein. (From Fehrenbach MJ, Herring SW: *Illustrated anatomy of the head and neck,* ed 6, St Louis, 2021, Saunders/Elsevier.)

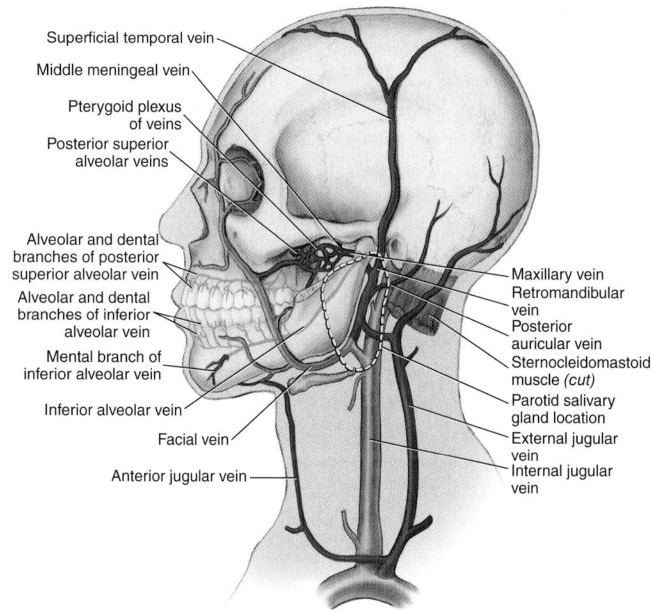

Fig. 10.32 Lateral view of the pathways of the internal jugular view and facial vein to the orofacial region are highlighted as well as the location of the cavernous sinus. (From Fehrenbach MJ, Herring SW: *Illustrated anatomy of the head and neck,* ed 6, St Louis, 2021, Saunders/Elsevier.)

The IA vein forms from the merging of its dental branches, alveolar branches, and mental branches in the mandible, where they also drain into the pterygoid plexus of veins. The dental branches of the IA vein drain the pulp of the teeth by way of each tooth's apical foramen. The alveolar branches of the IA vein drain the associated periodontium and gingiva of the mandibular teeth.

Some parts of the pterygoid plexus of veins are near the maxillary tuberosity, reflecting the drainage of dental tissue into the vascular plexus. Due to its location there is a possibility of piercing the pterygoid plexus of veins or nearby maxillary artery when a PSA block is administered incorrectly with the needle overinserted (see Chapter 12). When the pterygoid plexus of veins or even the nearby maxillary artery is pierced, as in this situation, a small amount of the blood escapes and enters the tissue, causing tissue tenderness, swelling, and the discoloration of a hematoma or bruise (see Fig. 16.2 in Chapter 16).

A spread of infection along the needle tract deep into the tissue can also occur when the PSA block is incorrectly administered with a contaminated needle. This may involve a serious spread of infection into the pterygoid plexus of veins and then on to the cavernous sinus, a venous sinus deep within the skull (see Fig. 10.32). Each cavernous sinus is located on the lateral surfaces of the body of the sphenoid bone. This may result in cavernous venous thrombosis (see Chapter 16).

Maxillary Vein

The maxillary vein begins within the infratemporal fossa by collecting blood from the pterygoid plexus of veins while accompanying the maxillary artery (see Fig. 10.32). Through the pterygoid plexus of veins, the maxillary vein receives the middle meningeal, PSA, IA veins as well as other veins such as those from the nasal cavity and palate, which are served by the maxillary artery. The maxillary vein then drains into the retromandibular vein, which forms part of the external jugular vein.

DENTAL HYGIENE CONSIDERATIONS

- Both the maxillary and mandibular dental arches have a dental plexus within either superior or inferior plexus, respectively, which is a network of nerves.
- Crossover-innervation occurs when there is overlap of terminal nerve fibers from the contralateral side of either dental arch, which then can affect the maxillary and mandibular anterior teeth and complicate anesthesia in both the maxillary and mandibular anterior sextants.
- The alveolar process of the maxillary teeth is less dense and more porous than the alveolar process of similar mandibular teeth, which allows a greater incidence of clinically effective local anesthesia for the maxillary arch when the local anesthetic agent is administered as a supraperiosteal injection or local infiltration than would occur with similar teeth on the mandibular arch.
- The canine eminence and apex of the maxillary canine are landmarks for the administration of the anterior superior alveolar (ASA) block that anesthetizes the ASA nerve.
- The middle superior alveolar (MSA) nerve is only present in approximately 28% of the population, and, when present, it is anesthetized by the MSA block. The landmark for the MSA block is the apex of the maxillary second premolar.
- The posterior superior alveolar (PSA) foramina and maxillary tuberosity are landmarks for the administration of the PSA block that anesthetizes the PSA nerve. The pterygoid plexus of veins or maxillary artery near the maxillary tuberosity may be pierced during the PSA block if administered incorrectly, causing a hematoma.
- The infraorbital (IO) foramen is a landmark for the administration of the IO block that anesthetizes the IO nerve and it is located approximately 10 mm inferior to the midpoint of the IO rim, and it is in a linear relationship on the ipsilateral side of the face with the more superior supraorbital notch of supraorbital rim as well as the pupil of the eye and corner of the mouth. When the IO nerve is anesthetized, both the ASA and MSA nerves are also anesthetized.
- The incisive foramen carries both branches of the right and left nasopalatine (NP) nerves and is the landmark along with its overlying incisive papilla for the administration of the NP block that anesthetizes both NP nerves.
- The greater palatine (GP) foramen is a landmark for the administration of the GP block that anesthetizes the GP nerve.
- Communication also occurs between the GP nerve and NP nerve terminal fibers, which may complicate the use of local anesthesia in the region.
- The median palatine raphe located on the hard palate is a landmark for the administration of the anterior middle superior alveolar (AMSA) block that anesthetizes the ASA, MSA, GP, and NP nerves as well as the GP block that anesthetizes the GP nerve.
- The alveolar process of the mandibular anterior teeth is less dense and more porous than the alveolar process of the mandibular posterior teeth. This allows a supraperiosteal injection or local infiltration of the mandibular anterior teeth by a local anesthetic agent to have greater incidence of clinically effective local anesthesia than the mandibular posterior teeth but less clinically effective overall than all the maxillary teeth.
- The mental foramen, which is located on the lateral surface of the mandible inferior to the apices of the mandibular premolars, is a landmark for the administration for both the mental and incisive blocks that anesthetize the mental and incisive nerves, respectively.
- The medial surface of the mandibular ramus is also a landmark for the administration of the inferior alveolar (IA) block as well as the Vazirani-Akinosi (V-A) mandibular block.
- The IA nerve and blood vessels as well as the lingual nerve are within the pterygomandibular space that has the overlying pterygotemporal depression, with both being landmarks for the IA block and V-A mandibular block.
- The coronoid notch and the mandibular foramen are landmarks for the administration of the IA block that anesthetizes the IA nerve. The mandibular foramen on the medial surface of the mandible is located two-thirds to three-fourths the distance from the coronoid notch to the posterior border of the mandibular ramus.
- In rare cases, a patient may have a bifid IA nerve, in which a second mandibular foramen may be present that needs to be considered.
- The mylohyoid nerve in some cases may also serve as an afferent nerve for the mandibular first molar and needs to be considered when there is lack of clinical effectiveness of the IA block.
- The seventh cranial or facial nerve may be inadvertently anesthetized during the IA block if administered incorrectly causing transient facial paralysis since the nerve travels through the parotid salivary gland.
- The anterior border of the mandibular ramus is a landmark for the administration of the buccal block that anesthetizes the (long) buccal nerve.
- The anteromedial border of the mandibular condylar neck is a landmark for the administration of the Gow-Gates (G-G) mandibular block.
- The IA, lingual, mental, incisive nerves and for the most part the buccal nerve as well as the mylohyoid and auriculotemporal nerves are anesthetized with the G-G block.
- The IA, lingual, mental, incisive nerves and for the most part the buccal nerve as well as the mylohyoid nerve are anesthetized with the V-A mandibular block.
- The location of major blood vessels and glandular tissue of the orofacial region must be known to avoid inadvertently injecting these structures when administering local anesthesia.
- The external carotid artery supplies the oral cavity by its orofacial arteries: the lingual and maxillary arteries.
- The IA, mental, incisive, and PSA blocks all have a high percentage of positive aspiration due to the nearness of the associated blood vessels to the target nerve.
- A spread of infection along the needle tract deep into the tissue can also occur when the PSA block is incorrectly administered with a contaminated needle; this may involve a serious spread of infection into the pterygoid plexus of veins or maxillary artery and then on to the cavernous sinus.

CHAPTER REVIEW QUESTIONS

1. Which of the following BEST describes the reason for greater incidence of clinically effective local anesthesia for the maxillary teeth when the local anesthetic agent is administered as a supraperiosteal injection than would occur with similar teeth on the mandibular arch?
   A. More porous alveolar process
   B. Denser alveolar process
   C. Presence of adjacent nerve canals
   D. Increased pulpal lymphatic channels
2. Which foramen carries branches of BOTH the right and left nasopalatine nerves?
   A. Greater palatine foramen
   B. Lesser palatine foramen
   C. Incisive foramen
   D. Infraorbital foramen
3. Which of the following is a landmark for the administration of the posterior superior alveolar local anesthetic block?
   A. Incisive foramen
   B. Maxillary tuberosity
   C. Palatine process
   D. Retromolar pad
4. Which of the following is a landmark for the administration of the anterior middle superior alveolar local anesthetic block?
   A. Incisive foramen
   B. Greater palatine foramen
   C. Median palatine raphe
   D. Lesser palatine foramen
5. Which of the following skull bones is the ONLY freely movable bone of the skull?
   A. Maxilla
   B. Zygomatic bone
   C. Palatal bone
   D. Mandible
6. The mental foramen is USUALLY located inferior to the apices of the mandibular
   A. first and second premolars
   B. first and second molars
   C. first premolar and canine
   D. central and lateral incisors
7. For which of the following mandibular teeth is a supraperiosteal local anesthetic injection MOST effective?
   A. Anterior teeth
   B. Premolars
   C. Molars
   D. Premolars and molars
8. Which of the following is a landmark for the administration of the inferior alveolar local anesthetic block?
   A. Mental foramen
   B. Coronoid notch
   C. Mandibular notch
   D. Incisive foramen
9. Which of the following is a landmark for the administration of the Gow-Gates mandibular local anesthetic block?
   A. Coronoid notch
   B. Mental foramen
   C. Condylar neck
   D. Mandibular canal
10. A patient may have a bifid inferior alveolar nerve. A second mandibular canal can be detected on radiographs.
   A. Both statements are correct.
   B. Both statements are NOT correct.
   C. The first statement is correct; the second statement is NOT correct.
   D. The first statement is NOT correct; the second statement is correct.
11. Which of the following nerves is present in ONLY approximately 28% of the population?
   A. Anterior superior alveolar
   B. Middle superior alveolar
   C. Posterior superior alveolar
   D. Infraorbital
12. Which of the following statements BEST describes the (long) buccal nerve?
   A. Efferent nerve for the facial gingiva of the mandibular anterior teeth
   B. Afferent nerve for the facial gingiva of the mandibular anterior teeth
   C. Efferent nerve for the buccal gingiva of the mandibular molars
   D. Afferent nerve for the buccal gingiva of the mandibular molars
13. Which of the following is the nerve division of the trigeminal nerve that does NOT innervate the teeth?
   A. Ophthalmic
   B. Maxillary
   C. Mandibular
   D. Facial
14. The zygomatic nerve is a branch of which of the following nerves?
   A. Ophthalmic
   B. Maxillary
   C. Mandibular
   D. Facial
15. Which nerve when anesthetized also anesthetizes BOTH the anterior and middle superior alveolar nerves?
   A. Posterior superior alveolar
   B. Inferior alveolar
   C. Incisive
   D. Infraorbital
16. Which of the following is considered the largest nerve division of the trigeminal nerve?
   A. Ophthalmic
   B. Maxillary
   C. Mandibular
   D. Facial
17. Which of the following nerves is formed from afferent branches from the body of the tongue?
   A. Inferior alveolar
   B. Lingual
   C. Mental
   D. Incisive
18. Which of the following nerves may ALSO innervate the mandibular first molar in some cases?
   A. Mylohyoid
   B. Mental
   C. Incisive
   D. Auriculotemporal

19. The mental nerve serves as an afferent nerve for the
    - **A.** labial mucosa of the mandibular anterior teeth
    - **B.** lingual gingiva of the mandibular anterior teeth
    - **C.** buccal mucosa of the mandibular posterior teeth
    - **D.** lingual gingiva of the mandibular posterior teeth

20. Which of the following local anesthetic blocks when administered INCORRECTLY may pierce the pterygoid plexus of veins causing a hematoma?
    - **A.** Anterior superior alveolar block
    - **B.** Middle superior alveolar block
    - **C.** Infraorbital block
    - **D.** Posterior superior alveolar block

11

Basic Injection Techniques

Demetra Daskalos Logothetis, RDH, MS

LEARNING OBJECTIVES

1. Describe the four anesthetic administration techniques.
2. List the steps to providing a successful injection, describe the importance of each, and discuss various rapport strategies to reduce stress in the patient.
3. Discuss basic injection techniques for computer-controlled local anesthetic delivery.

ADMINISTRATION TECHNIQUES

When choosing the appropriate administration technique, the dental hygienist must consider the area to be treated, the duration of anesthesia needed, and the comfort needs of the patient. Local anesthesia administration techniques are divided into four major categories: surface anesthesia, local infiltration, supraperiosteal injection (field block), and nerve block (Fig. 11.1).

Surface Anesthesia

Surface anesthesia is used when topical anesthetics are applied to the surface by gels, creams, or sprays to block the free nerve endings supplying the mucosal surfaces. The effect is short lasting and limited to the direct area of contact. Topical anesthetics are used as a preinjection technique to obtund the pain associated with needle insertion.

Local Infiltration

Local infiltration techniques are used when soft tissue anesthesia is needed in a limited area. The anesthesia is deposited close to the smaller terminal nerve endings, providing pain relief only in the area of anesthetic diffusion. Dental hygienists can use this technique during nonsurgical periodontal therapy when anesthesia is needed only in the immediate area of injection and for bleeding control provided by the vasoconstrictor.[1,2] The term local infiltration is frequently used incorrectly in dentistry to describe an injection where local anesthetic is deposited above the root of the tooth being treated. The correct term for this procedure is *supraperiosteal injection,* which is a field block and is described in the following paragraph.

Supraperiosteal Injection (Field Block)

A supraperiosteal injection, or a field block, is a form of regional anesthesia deposited near large terminal nerve branches. Anesthesia usually involves pulpal and soft tissue anesthesia of a single tooth in the maxilla (by depositing the anesthetic agent above the apex of the tooth to be anesthetized) except in the area of the anterior superior alveolar (ASA) block and middle superior alveolar (MSA) block, where anesthesia is achieved on more than one tooth using this technique (see Chapter 12). Supraperiosteal injections are most effective in the maxillary arch due to the porous nature of the bone, allowing the anesthetic to easily diffuse through the bone to the nerve. However, this technique can be used on the mandibular laterals and incisors and is an excellent injection technique when crossover anesthesia is needed (see Chapters 10, 12, and 13). In dentistry, supraperiosteal injections are often referred to incorrectly as infiltration injections (discussed above).

Nerve Block

Nerve block anesthesia refers to the injection of local anesthetic in the vicinity of a major nerve trunk to anesthetize the nerve's area of innervations, usually at a greater distance from the area of treatment. This technique offers an advantage over the other techniques by providing profound pulpal and soft tissue anesthesia over a larger area. The disadvantage is that arteries and veins accompany major nerve trunks, and the potential for piercing the artery or vein with this technique is greatly enhanced.[1] Examples of nerve blocks are the inferior alveolar (IA), posterior superior alveolar (PSA), anterior superior alveolar (ASA), middle superior alveolar (MSA), mental/incisive (MI), and infraorbital (IO) blocks.

STEPS TO PROVIDING A SUCCESSFUL INJECTION

The administration of local anesthetics will become routine to the experienced dental hygienist, but it is often a very stressful experience for the patient. For many patients, the fear and anticipation of pain from receiving a "shot" could produce an emergency situation.[3-5] Vasodepressor syncope is the most common medical emergency observed in the dental office, and it is most frequently linked to the administration of local anesthesia (see Chapter 17).[3-5]

Dental hygienists must be cognizant not to allow the administration of local anesthetics to become routine. Providing effective communication and psychological support is essential to build patient confidence and to reduce the risk of an emergency situation. Using the following steps (see also Table 11.1), the dental hygienist can provide appropriate pain control during and after the treatment in a safe, effective, and comfortable manner for the patient.

Step 1: Preanesthetic Patient Assessment and Consultation

The patient assessment should be conducted as described in Chapter 7, and vital signs should be obtained and recorded. Appropriate medical

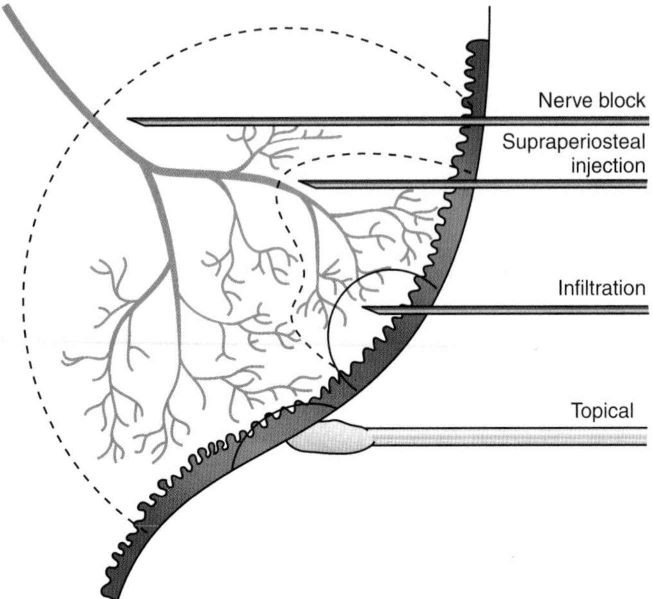

Fig. 11.1 Administration techniques used for anesthesia. Dashed lines and solid lines represent the areas of anesthesia produced by regional (nerve block, supraperiosteal injection) and local (infiltration, topical application) anesthetic techniques, respectively.

and dental consultations should be completed before administration of local anesthetics.

Determining Patient Anxiety

In addition to the physical and psychological evaluation of a patient to determine dental anxiety as described in Chapter 7, a Visual Analog Scale (VAS) is a tool used to help a person rate the intensity of certain sensations and feelings such as pain and anxiety. For example, the VAS for pain is a straight line with one end meaning no pain and the other end meaning the worst pain imaginable (see Fig. 1.2 in Chapter 1). A patient marks a point on the line that matches the amount of pain he or she feels. Though in dentistry "pain" is the most frequently existent feeling, dental patients have a lot more to share with the clinician that must be expressed by the patient in some concrete number.

The VAS is an effective tool for expressing or analyzing patients' feelings quantitatively, before and after seeking any kind of dental treatment. This concrete base can become the effective communication tool among the clinicians, as well as between the clinicians and the patients. In addition to rating pain, the simple VAS has proved to be a useful and valid measure of pretreatment anxiety (see Fig. 11.2). Most dental anxiety is influenced by the uncertainty of the impending dental procedures—specifically local anesthetic injections, past experience, and a patient's personality and coping style. Anxiety is an unpleasant emotion and may cause patients to avoid a planned treatment. The VAS may be a useful tool to measure pretreatment anxiety and certain

TABLE 11.1 Summary of Steps to Providing a Successful Injection

Step 1	Preanesthetic patient assessment and consultation • Conduct a patient assessment including vital signs and medical and dental consultations as necessary. • Determine patient anxiety. • Select an anesthetic based on the patient's medical history, duration of treatment, postoperative pain control, volume of anesthetic needed for the procedure, need for hemostasis, and possibility of self-mutilation. • Determine maximum recommended dose based on the anesthetic selected.
Step 2	Confirm care plan • Develop in collaboration with the patient and confirm with the patient before treatment.
Step 3	Informed consent • Discuss benefits and risks to treatment. • Discuss risks involved in not receiving treatment. • Review informed consent with the patient and have him or her sign. In the case of a minor, have parent or guardian sign.
Step 4	Determine injection(s) based on the areas needing to be anesthetized, the presence of infection, and the need for hemostasis.
Step 5	Prepare equipment as described in Chapter 9.
Step 6	Check the anesthetic equipment. • Bevel orientation if indicated. • Proper anesthetic flow. • Engaged harpoon. • Personal protective equipment is in place for the clinician and protective eyewear for the patient.
Step 7	Position patient in a supine position.
Step 8	Tissue preparation and patient communication • Apply topical antiseptic or have the patient rinse with chlorhexidine (optional). • Apply topical anesthetic for 1–2 minutes (this is a good time to visualize and practice the needle angulations, as well as a time to provide supportive communication to the patient).
Step 9	Dry tissue and visualize or palpate the penetration site to determine any needle access problems.
Step 10	Establish a fulcrum while holding the syringe palm up, large window up for the greatest stability of the syringe and visibility of the local anesthetic cartridge.
Step 11	Make the tissue taut to assist with visibility of the injection site and ease of tissue penetration with the needle.
Step 12	Keep the syringe out of the patient's sight to help prevent any unnecessary anxiety for the patient, and always know the location of the uncovered needle at all times.
Step 13	Gently insert the needle and watch for signs of discomfort and slowly move toward the target while communicating to the patient in a positive manner.

TABLE 11.1 Summary of Steps to Providing a Successful Injection (*Cont.*)

Step 14	Aspirate to prevent the possibility of an intravascular injection. If a clear bubble comes into the cartridge, the aspiration is negative. If blood enters the cartridge, the aspiration is positive and the needle should be redirected (little blood), or remove the needle from the mouth and change the cartridge and needle (blood fills the cartridge). If the harpoon becomes disengaged during aspiration, remove the needle from the tissue and safely cap. Remove the needle from the syringe and reengage the harpoon. Attach the needle back onto the syringe and repeat the injection.
Step 15	Slowly deposit the anesthetic at a rate of 1 mL of solution per minute or approximately 2 minutes for an entire cartridge.
Step 16	After completion of the injection, slowly withdraw the needle from the tissue and safely cap the needle using the one-handed scoop technique.
Step 17	Observe the patient to monitor any signs of a reaction to the anesthetic or from the procedure.
Step 18	Document the procedure.

patient characteristics that might serve to warn the dental professional about the potential presence of increased preprocedure anxiety. The use of a VAS might allow detection of patients with high anxiety, encouraging appropriate steps to ameliorate this anxiety.

Selection of Anesthetic

The selection of the anesthetic should be based on the patient's medical history, taking into consideration many additional factors:

- *The physical status of the patient:* The choice of local anesthetic agent and vasoconstrictor must be based on the patient's physical status and the medications the patient is taking. Absolute and relative contraindications should be carefully evaluated, and an anesthetic agent with the least adverse effects according to the patient's physical status should be selected.
- *Duration of treatment and postoperative pain control:* Duration of effect in pulpal and soft tissue varies for each agent, and consideration should be made as to whether profound pulpal anesthesia is indicated. For nonsurgical periodontal therapy in shallow pockets with soft tissue sensitivity but no root sensitivity, a short-acting anesthetic such as 3% mepivacaine may be appropriate. For half-mouth nonsurgical periodontal therapy with deep pockets and heavy deposits, a longer-acting anesthetic may be appropriate.
- *Volume of anesthetic:* Profound pulpal anesthesia necessary for restorative procedures, extractions, and nonsurgical periodontal therapy with heavy deposits, for example, is essential and will require more anesthetic volume than less invasive procedures.
- *Need for hemostasis:* Limited visibility decreases the efficiency in providing thorough deposit removal. If heavy bleeding is anticipated, a vasoconstrictor should be selected to constrict the blood vessels for greater visibility. Caution should be taken when using epinephrine 1:50,000 in patients with significant cardiovascular disease. For excessive bleeding, an intraseptal injection is recommended with epinephrine 1:50,000 in small amounts directly into the area of bleeding for greatest visibility and hemostatic control (see Chapters 12 and 13).

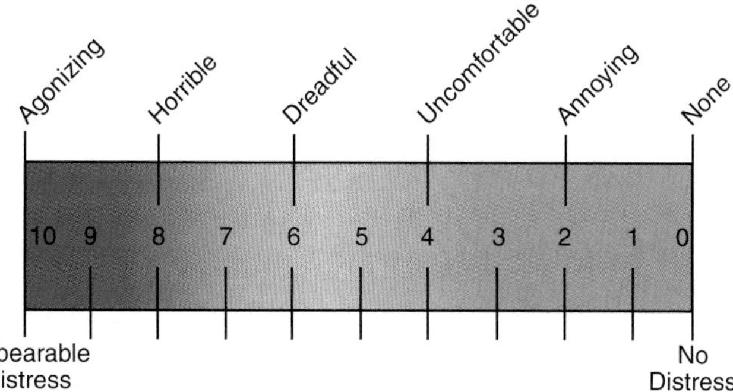

Fig. 11.2 Visual Analog Scale to determine the patient's anxiety level.

- *Possibility of self-mutilation:* Small children and patients with special needs are more prone to bite themselves while numb, causing self-mutilation. Longer-acting anesthetics should be avoided.
- *Determining maximum recommended dose:* The patient's maximum recommended dose (MRD) should be calculated based on the selected anesthetic and the patient's medical history and documented in the patient's chart (see Chapters 7 and 8).

Step 2: Confirm Care Plan

The care plan should be developed by the dental hygienist in collaboration with the patient and confirmed before treatment. If the dental hygiene care plan involves nonsurgical periodontal therapy with anesthesia, the dental hygienist should carefully determine the extent of periodontal involvement and how much of the treatment can be realistically accomplished in one visit. Local anesthesia should only be administered in the areas of treatment that can be completed in one visit. Overestimating the treatment and administering more anesthesia than necessary should be avoided.

Depending on the time available for treatment and the extent of periodontal involvement, the dental hygienist should design a care plan by dividing the mouth into sextants, quadrants, or half mouth for treatment. Figs. 11.3 to 11.5 illustrate examples of nonsurgical periodontal therapy with anesthesia care plan designs. With advanced periodontal disease and heavy deposits, the dental hygienist may only realistically be able to complete a few teeth in a single visit. The dental hygienist should then divide the mouth into sextants rather than quadrants for treatment (see Fig. 11.3). If either sextant or quadrant dental hygiene treatment is planned on the maxillary arch (see Figs. 11.3 and 11.4A–B), the PSA block is given before any of the other maxillary facial injections, as well as any maxillary palatal injections, to allow the necessary time for the larger molars to become completely anesthetized, with instrumentation proceeding in the same manner. After the PSA block, the MSA and then the ASA blocks (or IO block instead) is then given (in that order). For patients with initial to moderate periodontal disease, the dental hygienist may complete one to two quadrants during a single visit. When two quadrants (half mouth) are treated in a single visit, it is recommended to treat upper and lower quadrants on either the right or left side of the patient's face (Fig. 11.5A–B). The dental hygienist should avoid administering local anesthetics to both the mandibular right and left quadrants during a single treatment to prevent the inability of the patient to control his or her mandible. Administering bilateral inferior alveolar blocks also increases the possibility of the patient causing self-mutilation of their soft tissue (see Chapter 16). If half-mouth treatment is planned, the inferior alveolar and buccal blocks are given first, then the maxillary facial, and then palatal injections follow in order as described earlier, with instrumentation proceeding first on the maxillary arch. This allows time for the entire mandibular arch to become completely anesthetized. When designing the dental hygiene care plan, the dental

Sextant Treatment Plan

Sextant #2/appointment #2

ASA	Bilateral anterior superior alveolar block
NP	Nasopalatine block

Injections should be given in the order listed with instrumentation beginning on the facial anterior teeth

Sextant #1/appointment #1

PSA	Right posterior superior alveolar block
MSA	Right middle superior alveolar block
GP	Right greater palatine block

Injections should be given in the order listed with instrumentation beginning on the buccal posterior teeth

Sextant #3/appointment #3

PSA	Left posterior superior alveolar block
MSA	Left middle superior alveolar block
GP	Left greater palatine block

Injections should be given in the order listed with instrumentation beginning on the buccal posterior teeth

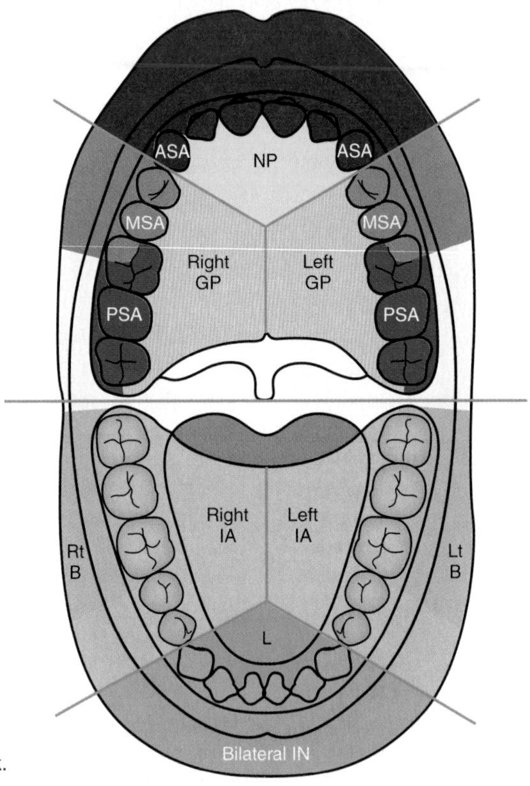

Sextant #6/appointment #6

IA	Right inferior alveolar block
B	Right buccal block

Injections should be given in the order listed with instrumentation beginning on the buccal posterior teeth

Note: The lingual nerve will be anesthetized through diffusion of the local anesthetic agent from the IA block. A separate lingual injection is not necessary.

Sextant #4/appointment #4

IA	Left inferior alveolar block
B	Left buccal block

Injections should be given in the order listed with instrumentation beginning on the buccal posterior teeth

Note: The lingual nerve will be anesthetized through diffusion of the local anesthetic agent from the IA block. A separate lingual injection is not necessary.

Sextant #5/appointment #5

IN	Bilateral incisive block
L	Lingual supraperiosteal injections

Injections should be given in the order listed with instrumentation beginning on the facial anterior teeth

Note: Since the IA block will not be administered for this sextant, lingual supraperiosteal injections will be needed to anesthetize the lingual tissue.

Fig. 11.3 Example of a dental hygiene care plan utilizing sextant nonsurgical periodontal therapy with anesthesia. The mouth is divided into six sextants for six appointments. (Modified from Fehrenbach MJ, Herring SW: *Illustrated anatomy of the head and neck,* ed 6, St Louis, 2021, Saunders/Elsevier.)

hygienist must consider the amount of anesthetic needed to complete the procedure (always staying within the patient's MRD).

Step 3: Informed Consent

The benefits and risks associated with all treatment including the administration of local anesthetics should be discussed, as should the risks involved in not receiving treatment. The dental hygienist should discuss with the patient the type of anesthetic that will be used and the injection procedure. The patient should be advised of the temporary numbing feeling associated with the administration of the drug and the anticipated duration of anesthesia. After the care plan discussion, informed consent to treatment should be given by the patient. In the

Quadrant Treatment Plan: Option 1

Quadrant #1/appointment #1

PSA	Right posterior superior alveolar block
MSA	Right middle superior alveolar block
ASA	Right anterior superior alveolar block
GP	Right greater palatine block
NP	Nasopalatine

Injections should be given in the order listed with instrumentation beginning on the buccal posterior teeth
Note: Can substitute IO block for MSA and ASA blocks (see Fig. 11.4B)

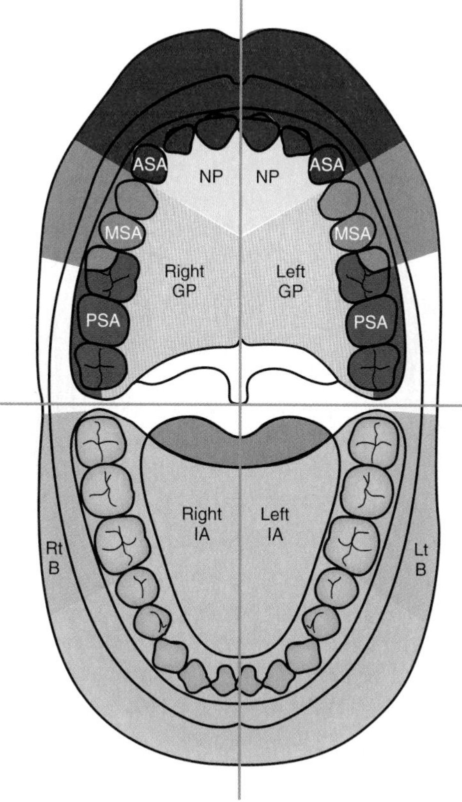

Quadrant #2/appointment #2

PSA	Left posterior superior alveolar block
MSA	Left middle superior alveolar block
ASA	Left anterior superior alveolar block
GP	Left greater palatine block
NP	Nasopalatine

Injections should be given in the order listed with instrumentation beginning on the buccal posterior teeth
Note: Can substitute IO block for MSA and ASA blocks (see Fig. 11.4B)

Quadrant #4/appointment #4

IA	Right inferior alveolar block
B	Right buccal block

Injections should be given in the order listed with instrumentation beginning on the buccal posterior teeth

Note: The lingual nerve will be anesthetized through diffusion of the local anesthetic agent from the IA block. A separate lingual injection is not necessary.

Quadrant #3/appointment #3

IA	Left inferior alveolar block
B	Left buccal block

Injections should be given in the order listed with instrumentation beginning on the buccal posterior teeth

Note: The lingual nerve will be anesthetized through diffusion of the local anesthetic agent from the IA block. A separate lingual injection is not necessary.

A

Quadrant Treatment Plan: Option 2

Quadrant #1/appointment #1

PSA	Right posterior superior alveolar block
IO	Right infraorbital block
GP	Right greater palatine block
NP	Nasopalatine

Injections should be given in the order listed with instrumentation beginning on the buccal posterior teeth
Note: Can substitute MSA and ASA blocks for IO block (see Fig. 11.4A)

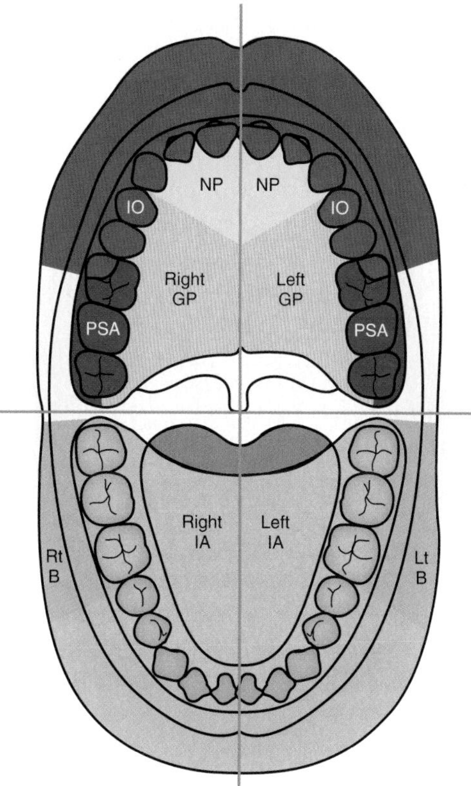

Quadrant #2/appointment #2

PSA	Left posterior superior alveolar block
IO	Left infraorbital block
GP	Left greater palatine block
NP	Nasopalatine

Injections should be given in the order listed with instrumentation beginning on the buccal posterior teeth
Note: Can substitute MSA and ASA blocks for IO block (see Fig. 11.4A)

Quadrant #4/appointment #4

IA	Right inferior alveolar block
B	Right buccal block

Injections should be given in the order listed with instrumentation beginning on the buccal posterior teeth

Note: The lingual nerve will be anesthetized through diffusion of the local anesthetic agent from the IA block. A separate lingual injection is not necessary.

Quadrant #3/appointment #3

IA	Left inferior alveolar block
B	Left buccal block

Injections should be given in the order listed with instrumentation beginning on the buccal posterior teeth

Note: The lingual nerve will be anesthetized through diffusion of the local anesthetic agent from the IA block. A separate lingual injection is not necessary.

B

Fig. 11.4 Two examples of dental hygiene care plans utilizing quadrant nonsurgical periodontal therapy with anesthesia. (A) Quadrant option 1: The mouth is divided into four quadrants for four appointments, administering the anterior superior alveolar (ASA) and the middle superior alveolar (MSA) blocks instead of the infraorbital (IO) block. (B) Quadrant option 2: The mouth is divided into four quadrants for four appointments, administering the IO block instead of the ASA and the MSA blocks. (Modified from Fehrenbach MJ, Herring SW: *Illustrated anatomy of the head and neck,* ed 6, St Louis, 2021, Saunders/Elsevier.)

Half-mouth Treatment Plan: Option 1

Half mouth #1/appointment #1

IA	Right inferior alveolar block
B	Right buccal block
PSA	Right posterior superior alveolar block
MSA	Right middle superior alveolar block
ASA	Right anterior superior alveolar block
GP	Right greater palatine block
NP	Nasopalatine block

Injections should be given in the order listed with instrumentation beginning on the buccal posterior teeth of the maxillary quadrant
Note: Can substitute IO block for MSA and ASA blocks (see Fig. 11.5B)

Note: The lingual nerve will be anesthetized through diffusion of the local anesthetic agent from the IA block. A separate lingual injection is not necessary.

Half mouth #2/appointment #2

IA	Left inferior alveolar block
B	Left buccal block
PSA	Left posterior superior alveolar block
MSA	Left middle superior alveolar block
ASA	Left anterior superior alveolar block
GP	Left greater palatine block
NP	Nasopalatine block

Injections should be given in the order listed with instrumentation beginning on the buccal posterior teeth of the maxillary quadrant
Note: Can substitute IO block for MSA and ASA blocks (see Fig. 11.5B)

Note: The lingual nerve will be anesthetized through diffusion of the local anesthetic agent from the IA block. A separate lingual injection is not necessary.

A

Half-mouth Treatment Plan: Option 2

Half mouth #1/appointment #1

IA	Right inferior alveolar block
B	Right buccal block
PSA	Right posterior superior alveolar block
IO	Right infraorbital block
GP	Right greater palatine block
NP	Nasopalatine block

Injections should be given in the order listed with instrumentation beginning on the buccal posterior teeth of the maxillary quadrant
Note: Can substitute MSA and ASA blocks for IO block (see Fig. 11.5A)

Note: The lingual nerve will be anesthetized through diffusion of the local anesthetic agent from the IA block. A separate lingual injection is not necessary.

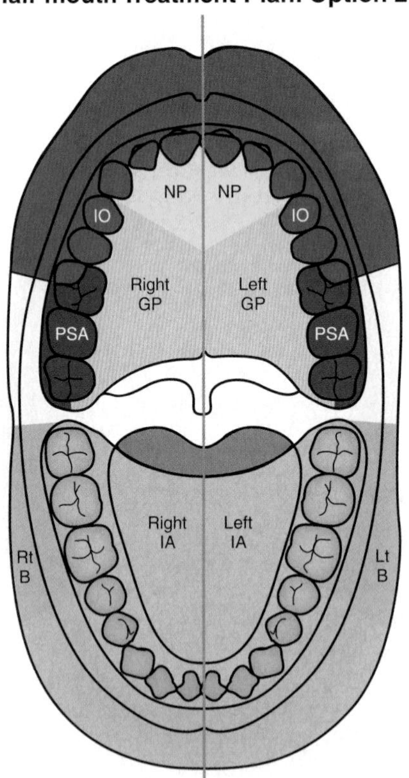

Half mouth #2/appointment #2

IA	Left inferior alveolar block
B	Left buccal block
PSA	Left posterior superior alveolar block
IO	Left infraorbital block
GP	Left greater palatine block
NP	Nasopalatine block

Injections should be given in the order listed with instrumentation beginning on the buccal posterior teeth of the maxillary quadrant
Note: Can substitute MSA and ASA blocks for IO block (see Fig. 11.5A)

Note: The lingual nerve will be anesthetized through diffusion of the local anesthetic agent from the IA block. A separate lingual injection is not necessary.

B

Fig. 11.5 Two examples of dental hygiene care plans utilizing half-mouth nonsurgical periodontal therapy with anesthesia. (A) Half-mouth option 1: The mouth is divided in half (maxillary/mandibular) for treatment of two quadrants in one appointment, administering the anterior superior alveolar (ASA) and the middle superior alveolar (MSA) blocks instead of the infraorbital (IO) block. (B) Half-mouth option 2: The mouth is divided in half (maxillary/mandibular) for treatment of two quadrants in one appointment, administering the IO block instead of the ASA and the MSA blocks. (Modified from Fehrenbach MJ, Herring SW: *Illustrated anatomy of the head and neck,* ed 6, St Louis, 2021, Saunders/Elsevier.)

1. I consent to the recommended procedure or treatment ______________________
   ____
   to be completed by Dr./Ms. ______________.
2. The procedure(s) or treatment(s) have been described to me.
3. I have been informed of the purpose of the procedure or treatment.
4. I have been informed of the alternatives to the procedure or treatment.
5. I understand that the following risk(s) may result from the procedure or treatment:
   ____
   ____
   ______________________.
6. I understand that the following risk(s) may occur if the procedure or treatment is not completed:
   ____
   ____
   ____
   ______________________.
7. I do—do not—consent to the administration of anesthetic.
   a. I understand that the following risks are involved in administering anesthesia:
   ____
   ____
   ____
   ______________________.
   b. The following alternatives to anesthesia were described: ______________
   ____
   ______________________.

All my questions have been satisfactorily answered.

Signature: ______________________
Date

Representative: ______________________
Date

Signature of Witness: ______________________
Date

Fig. 11.6 Example of informed consent. (From Bowen DM, Pieren JA: *Darby and Walsh: dental hygiene theory and practice,* ed 5, St Louis, 2020, Elsevier.)

case of a minor, the informed consent must be given by the parent or guardian. Fig. 11.6 is a sample informed consent form that includes the consent to the administration of anesthetics. The written agreement of the care plan becomes a legal contract between the patient and the dental hygienist.[2]

Step 4: Selection of Injection

After the care plan has been determined, the dental hygienist should determine the appropriate injections for complete pulpal and/or soft tissue anesthesia. There are many factors to take into consideration for injection selection:

- *Areas needing to be anesthetized:* For maximum patient comfort, the dental hygienist should select injections to completely anesthetize the areas needed with minimal tissue penetrations, such as choosing nerve blocks rather than supraperiosteal injections for larger treatment areas. In addition, the dental hygienist should take into consideration the density of the bone in the area of treatment and the selection of injection technique. Supraperiosteal injections are much more effective on the maxilla because the bone is callous. The mandible requires nerve blocks because the cortical plate is thick. The mandibular anterior teeth are more conducive to supraperiosteal injections but to a lesser degree than the maxilla.
- *Presence of infection:* Infection in the area of anesthetic administration will decrease the effectiveness of the anesthetic. The acidic nature of the anesthetic deposited into acidic tissue from the infection decreases the ability of the anesthetic to readily dissociate for nerve penetration (see Chapter 3). It is recommended that nerve blocks be administered away from the infected area.
- *Hemostasis:* If hemostasis is needed in the area for greater visibility, an intraseptal injection is recommended with a high-level vasoconstrictor directly into the papilla. Epinephrine 1:50,000 produces the greatest hemostatic control (see Chapters 4, 12, and 13).

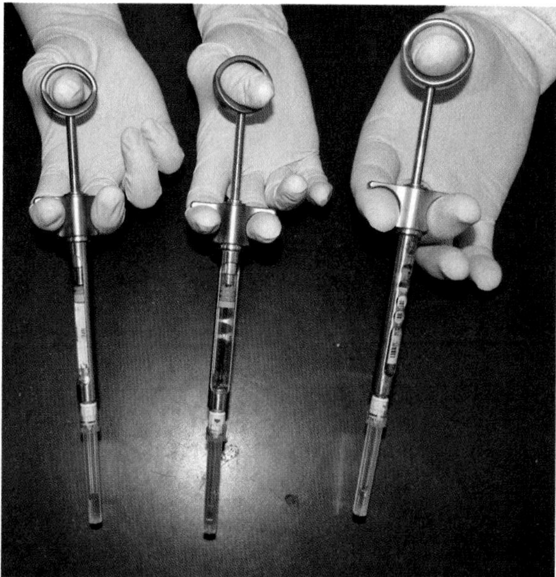

Fig. 11.7 Syringe selection depending on the hand size of the dental hygienist. Small (blue) Septodont syringe should only be used for very small hands, medium (silver) Septodont syringe is typically used for average hand size, and large (gold) Septodont syringe is used for larger hands. An important factor to consider in selecting a syringe is the ability to pull back on the thumb ring in an easy manner to achieve an aspiration.

Step 5: Preparation of Equipment

The preparation of equipment should be completed as described in Chapter 9. The appropriate selection of a syringe is important, taking into consideration the hand size of the dental hygienist and the hygienist's ability to properly conduct the aspiration test (Fig. 11.7). The bulkiness of the anesthetic syringe and the length of dental anesthetic needles can be frightening to the patient; therefore they should be covered or placed out of the patient's sight (Fig. 11.8). The equipment may be set up before the patient's arrival if the care plan and selection of appropriate anesthetic has already been determined at a previous appointment. However, any recent changes in the patient's medical history may require a modification in anesthetic selection.

Step 6: Check the Anesthetic Equipment

Before administration of the local anesthetic, the dental hygienist should check the needle bevel orientation for planned injections in close proximity to the periosteum. The bevel should be oriented toward the bone (see Fig. 9.27 in Chapter 9). For these injections, the

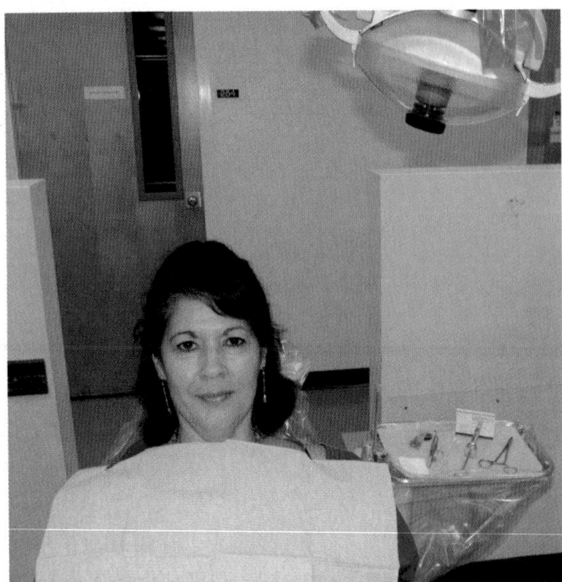

Fig. 11.8 Equipment placed out of patient's sight.

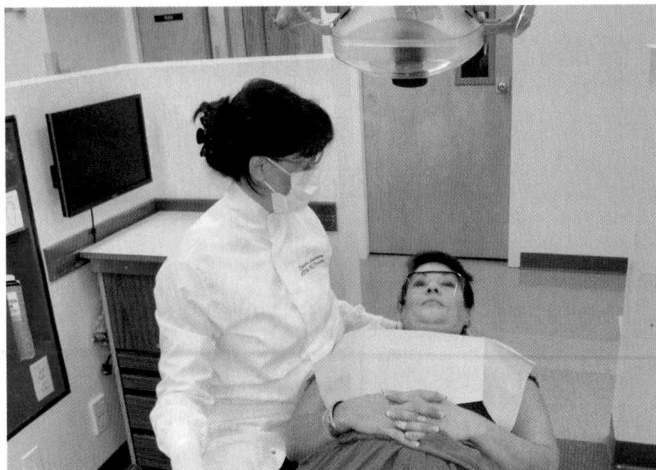

Fig. 11.9 Proper supine positioning.

bevel indicator (see Fig. 9.28 in Chapter 9) should be turned opposite the large window. This will ensure that when the dental hygienist is holding the syringe palm up with the large window facing him or her, the bevel will be toward the bone when the injection is commenced. Although the bevel of the needle does not affect success rates of the injection, it will provide added comfort to the patient and less trauma to the periosteum if the bone is contacted.

It is recommended to expel a few drops of anesthetic to ensure free flow of the solution. The dental hygienist should confirm that the harpoon is fully secured into the rubber stopper by gently pulling back on the thumb ring. The syringe is then ready for use. The dental hygienist should confirm that all protective equipment is in place, including recapping devices and personal protective equipment for the clinician and protective eyewear for the patient. Protective patient eyewear is critical for all dental hygiene procedures, especially during the administration of local anesthesia, as even a drop of local anesthetic inadvertently entering the patient's eye, or the needle being accidentally dropped near or into the eye, could cause severe or permanent damage.[6]

Step 7: Patient Position

Supine positioning (head and heart parallel to the floor, Fig. 11.9) with the patient's feet slightly elevated is the most effective position to administer anesthesia. Because supine positioning is the recommended position to treat vasodepressor syncope, this decreases the risk of a patient fainting before, during, or after the administration of the anesthetic.[3,4] The dental hygienist should ask the patient to turn his or her head appropriately for the greatest visibility of the penetration site.

Step 8: Tissue Preparation and Patient Communication

A topical antiseptic (Betadine or Merthiolate) may be applied to the tissue to reduce the possibility of septic material entering the soft tissue.[3] This step is optional, and before application the patient must be screened for a possible allergy to iodine. The tissue should be dried with a 2 × 2 gauze square (Fig. 11.10A), and the antiseptic should be applied to the area of needle insertion with a cotton-tipped applicator (see Fig. 11.10B). A chlorhexidine prerinse can also be used instead of Betadine to lower intraoral bacterial counts. This is also useful for nonsurgical periodontal therapy when using an ultrasonic scaler to reduce microbial counts.

A topical anesthetic should be applied after the topical antiseptic; this should be applied only to the area of needle insertion (see Fig. 11.10C). Topical anesthetics are commonly used before needle insertion to provide soft tissue anesthesia of the terminal nerve endings; these are most effective when applied according to manufacturer recommendations and are typically indicated for 1 to 2 minutes. Topical anesthetics do not contain vasoconstrictors and are absorbed rapidly when applied to the mucous membranes. Because of the rapid absorption and higher concentrations of surface applications, caution should be taken to avoid toxic reactions (see Chapter 6). While applying the topical anesthetic, the dental hygienist may use the cotton-tipped applicator to visualize and practice the angulations necessary for the injection (see Fig. 11.10D).

During application of the topical anesthetic, it is also a good time for supportive communication with the patient to help alleviate his or her fears. Communicating in a positive manner will enhance the patient's trust in the clinician and demonstrate the clinician's desire to provide a pain-free injection. For example, the dental hygienist might say: "I am applying a topical anesthetic for 2 minutes to numb the surface of the tissue, which will provide a more comfortable experience for you, and then I will make sure to administer the anesthetic slowly, which will provide additional comfort." (Do not use negative words, such as *pain, shot,* or *hurt;* see Chapter 18 for more information on effective communication before the administration of local anesthetics.)

Step 9: Dry Tissue and Visualize or Palpate the Penetration Site

After the application of topical anesthetic, redry the injection site to remove any excess topical anesthetic and to provide a dry area for effective visualization of the injection site. Palpate appropriate areas to determine any needle access problems associated with exostosis and to determine the insertion point (such as with the IA block).

Step 10: Establish a Fulcrum

Pick up the prepared syringe, palm up, making sure the large window is facing up in clear view. See Fig. 11.11 for correct hand positioning. The syringe should never be passed over the patient's face. The anesthetic syringe is large and can be cumbersome, so syringe stabilization is necessary. Selection of an appropriate fulcrum is determined by the clinician's finger length, personal preference, and physical abilities. A firm hand rest is essential to providing safe, comfortable injections. Of particular importance to a firm hand rest is ensuring syringe stability necessary for proper aspiration with limited needle movement. A fulcrum must always be used, and as with dental hygiene instrumentation,

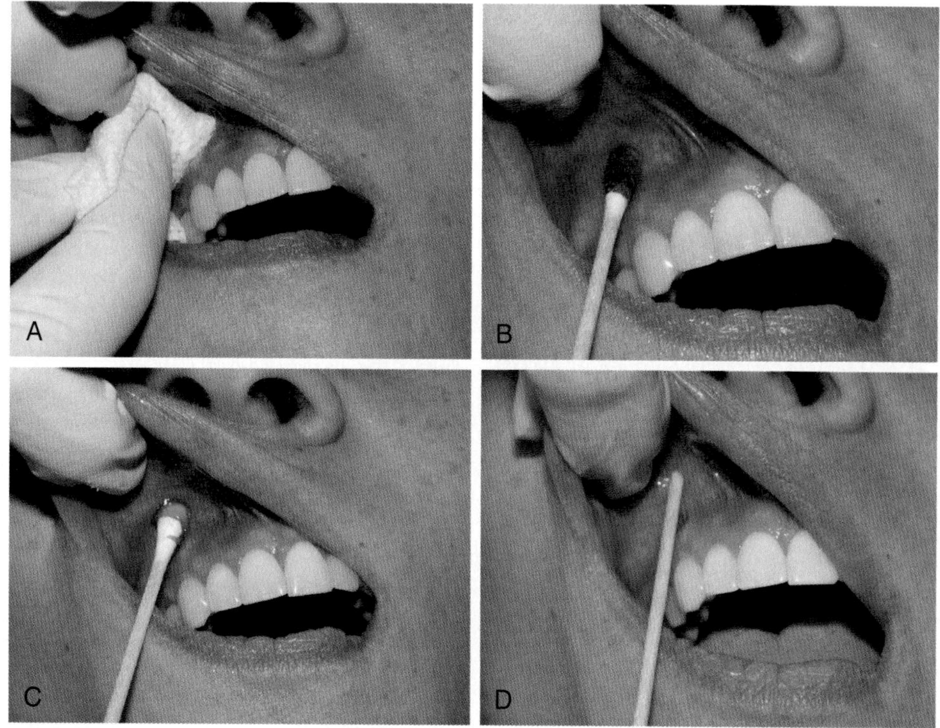

Fig. 11.10 (A) Drying of the tissue. (B) Applying topical antiseptic. (C) Applying topical anesthetic. (D) Using cotton-tipped applicator to visualize and practice injection angulations before needle insertion.

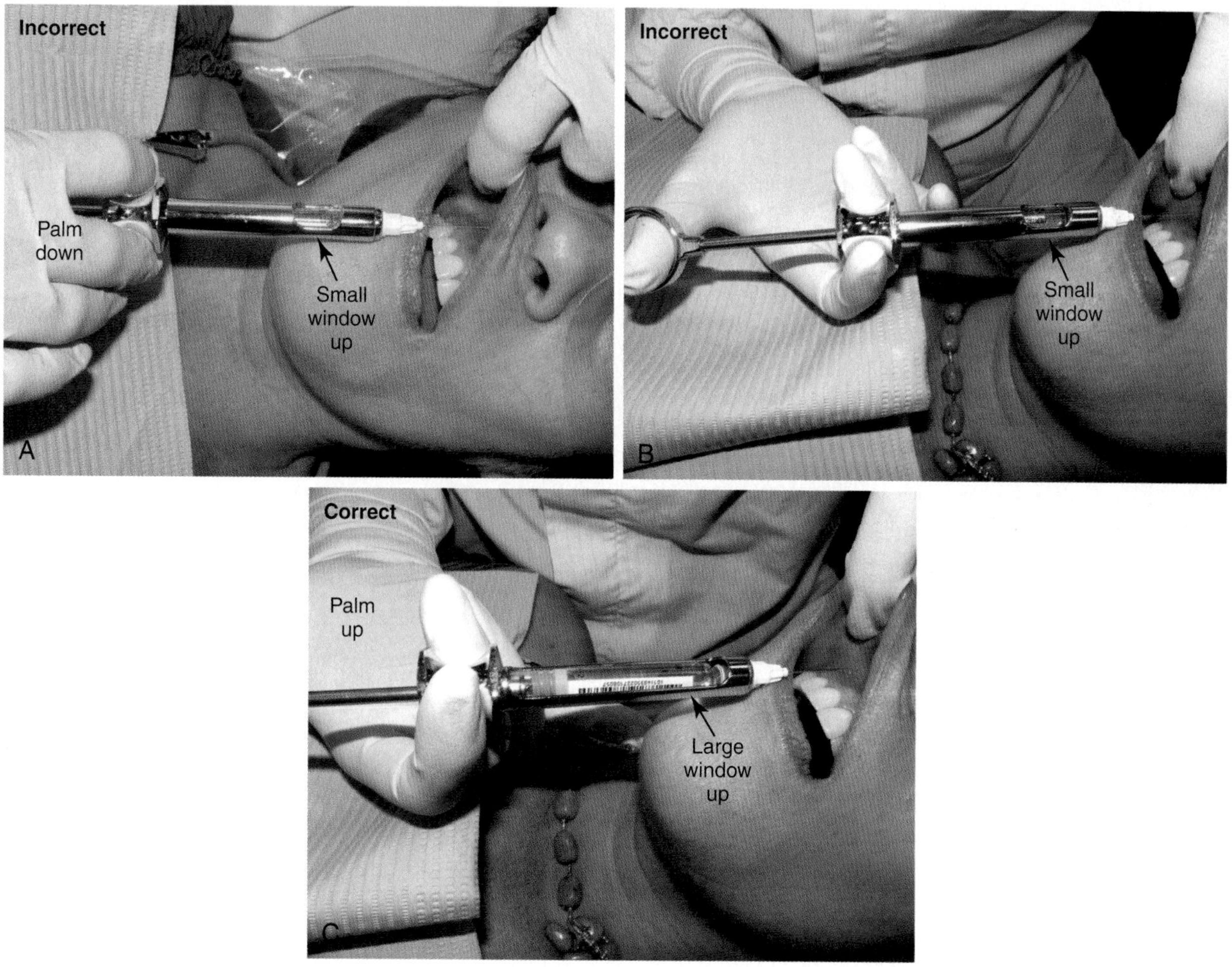

Fig. 11.11 (A) Palm down, large window down (incorrect). (B) Palm up, large window down (incorrect). (C) Palm up, large window up (correct).

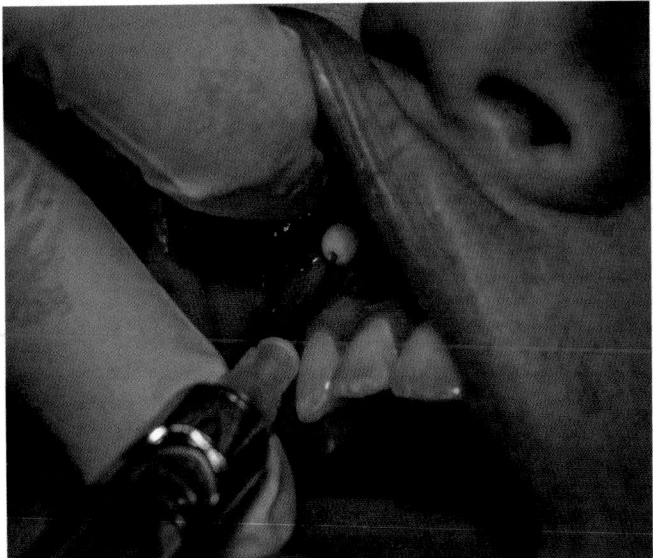

Fig. 11.12 Utilization of a syringe set up with a training needle for students to practice needle angulation and stable fulcrums prior to administering their first injections.

secure extraoral fulcrums are acceptable. The dental hygienist should never use the patient's arm to rest the syringe-holding arm. Any sudden movement of the patient's arm may cause injury to the patient or dental hygienist. Dental hygienists with small hands may not be able to achieve appropriate stabilization using only the fingers of their dominant hand. If firm finger placement cannot be achieved, the dental hygienist may maintain stability through arm-to-body support. For student dental hygienists or practicing dental hygienists administering their first local anesthetic injections on a fellow classmate, some degree of nervousness and shaking of the hands is to be expected. Syringe stabilization using firm fulcrums will help alleviate the shaking. Students are encouraged to practice maintaining correct needle angulation and a solid fulcrum using the syringe with a capped needle or a training needle (see Fig. 11.12 and Chapter 9) before administering the injection. Fig. 11.13 illustrates successful fulcrums; additional fulcrums are demonstrated for each injection technique in Chapters 12 and 13.

Step 11: Make Tissue Taut

Retracting the tissue taut at the penetration site (Fig. 11.14A) will assist the dental hygienist with visibility of the injection site and allow easier, less traumatic needle insertion. A 2 × 2 piece of sterile gauze may be used if the tissue is slippery (see Fig. 11.14B).

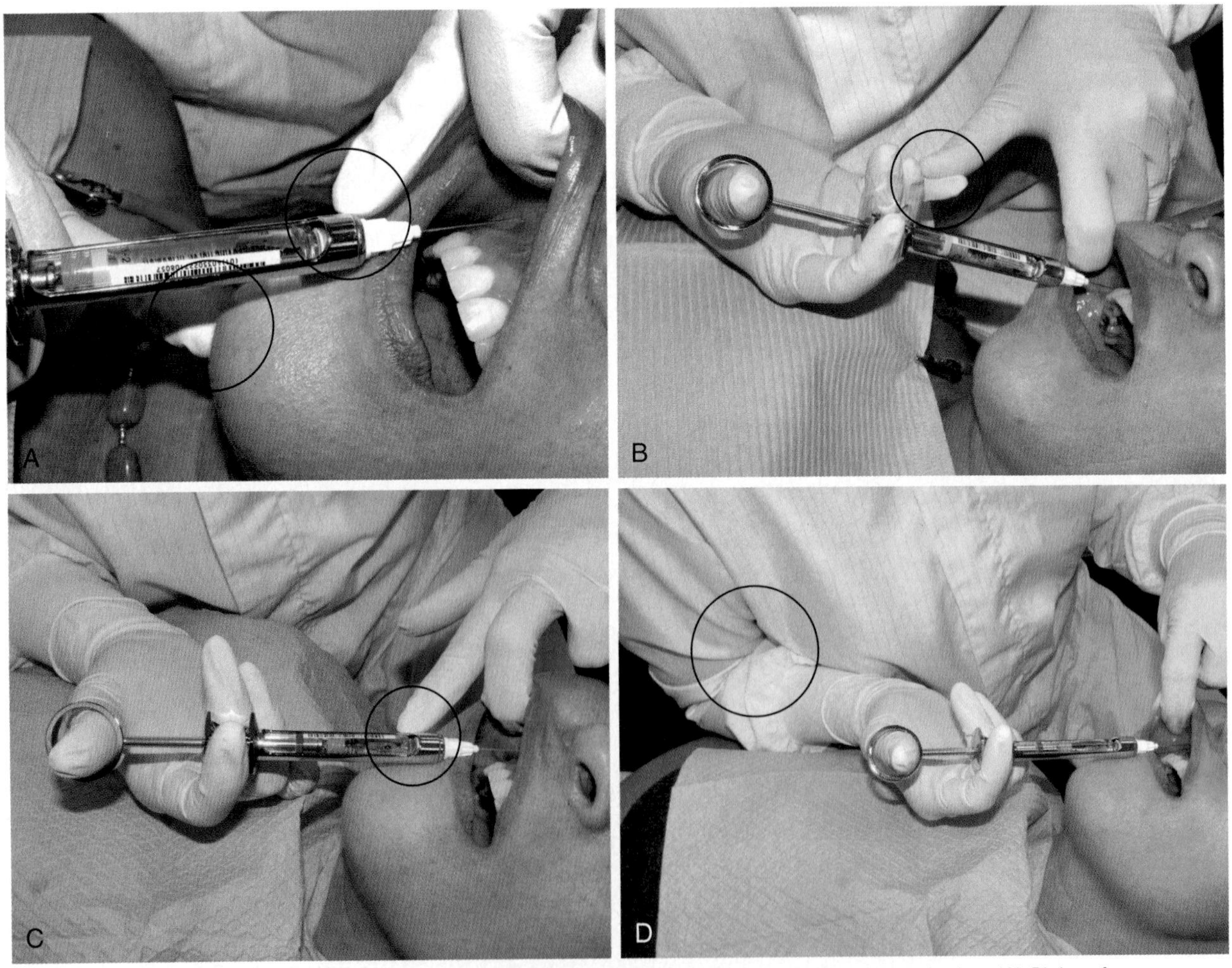

Fig. 11.13 Example of an appropriate fulcrum during the administration of local anesthetics. (A) Pinky of dominant hand resting on patient's chin; index finger of nondominant hand supporting the syringe barrel. (B) Double-handed fulcrum. (C) Index finger of nondominant hand supporting the syringe barrel. (D) Arm to body fulcrum.

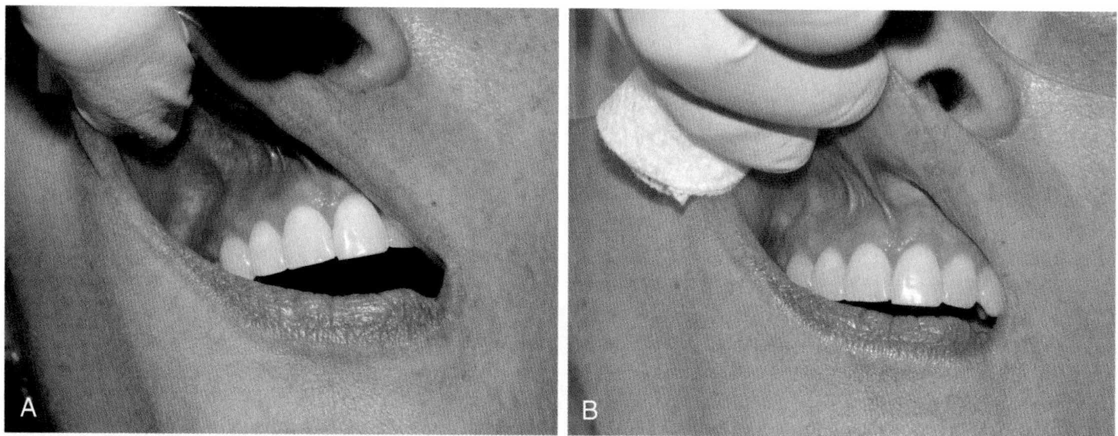

Fig. 11.14 (A) Pulling the tissue taut; no sterile gauze used. (B) Pulling the tissue taut, using sterile gauze for slippery tissue.

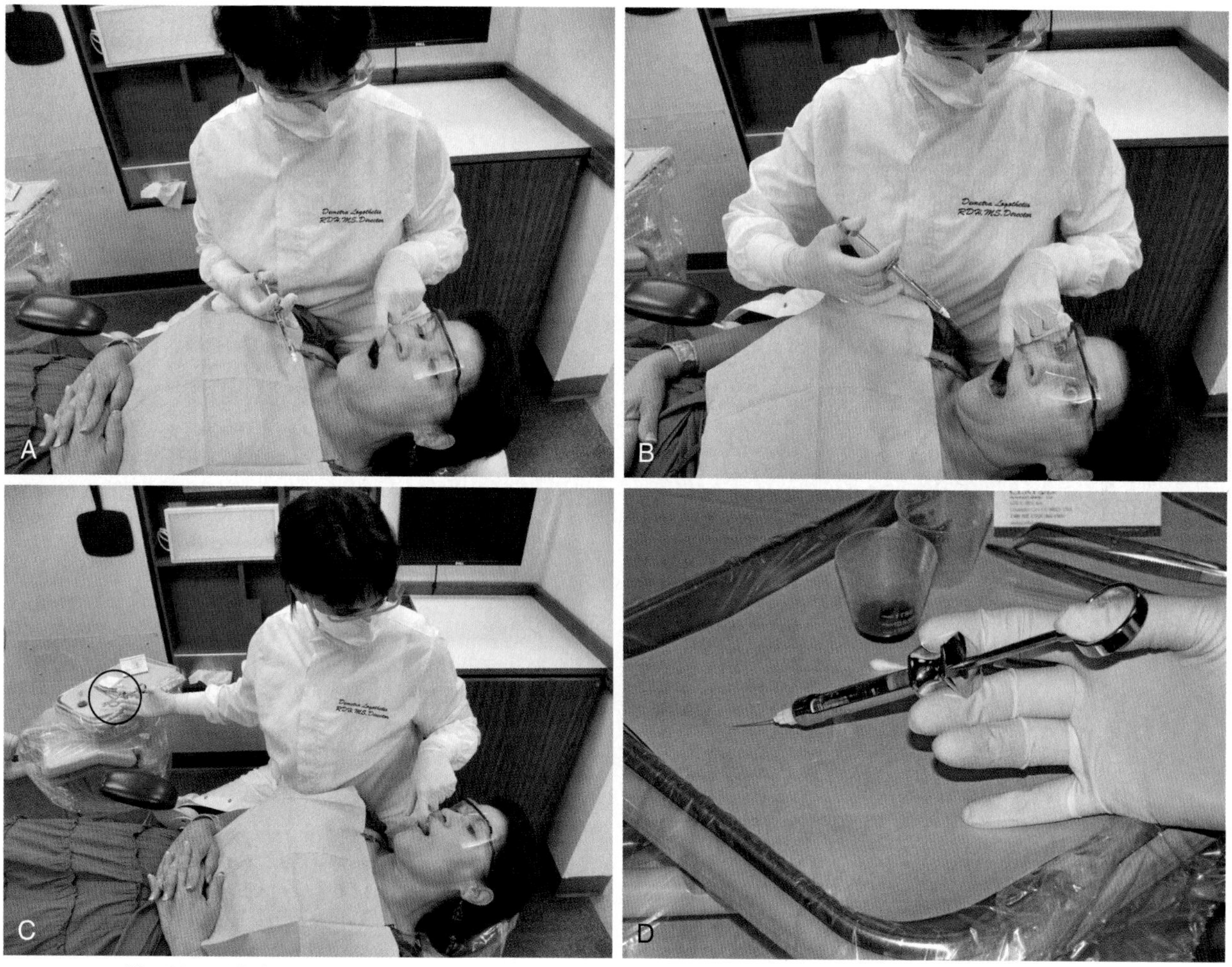

Fig. 11.15 (A) Correct: keeping syringe out of patient's sight (keep syringe low out of patient's direct line of vision without contaminating the needle). (B) Incorrect: syringe in direct line of patient's sight, producing fear. (C) Incorrect: dental hygienist not paying attention to the location of the uncovered needle, causing accidental contamination of the needle from a nonsterile surface. (D) Close-up view of dental hygienist's hand demonstrating needle contamination from a nonsterile surface.

Step 12: Keep Syringe out of the Patient's Sight

Keeping the syringe out of the patient's sight will help prevent any unnecessary anxiety for the patient (Fig. 11.15A). The sight of the dental needle and the large anesthetic syringe could provoke excess anxiety, leading to a possible medical emergency (see Fig. 11.15B). It is important, however, that the dental hygienist knows the exact location of the uncovered needle at all times. This can prevent accidental needlestick exposure to the clinician or touching the needle to a nonsterile surface outside of the patient's mouth before the injection and thus contaminating the needle (see Fig. 11.15C–D). If the needle is accidentally contaminated, discard the needle in the sharps container, and attach a new sterile needle to the syringe prior to injection.

Step 13: Gently Insert the Needle, Watch, Communicate

Techniques of distraction, such as shaking the lip and pulling the soft tissue over the needle, are often used at this point. Devices have been designed to produce vibration as the injection is being administered. Two examples are DentalVibe (BING Innovations LLC, Boca Raton, FL; Fig. 11.16) and Vibraject (Newport Coast, CA; Fig. 11.17). Distractor techniques, however, are not needed and may actually cause pain from the needle movement in the tissue, and the clinician needs to maintain sight of the needle tip at all times. A recent study compared pediatric patients' pain during needle insertion and injection during the administration of the inferior alveolar block injected by either a traditional syringe or the DentalVibe Injection Comfort System. Results demonstrated that there was no statistically significant difference for pain evaluation during needle insertion and injection for each technique. However, a negative correlation was found on the Face, Legg, Cry, Consolability Scale between age and pain scores during injection after using the DentalVibe.[7] Proper injection techniques, as described in this chapter, such as the application of topical anesthetic, keeping the tissue taut, using an effective fulcrum, and injecting slowly, will produce comfortable injections.

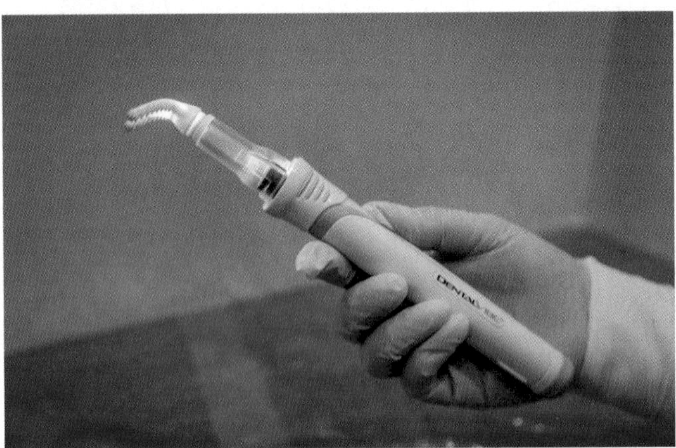

Fig. 11.16 DentalVibe unit.

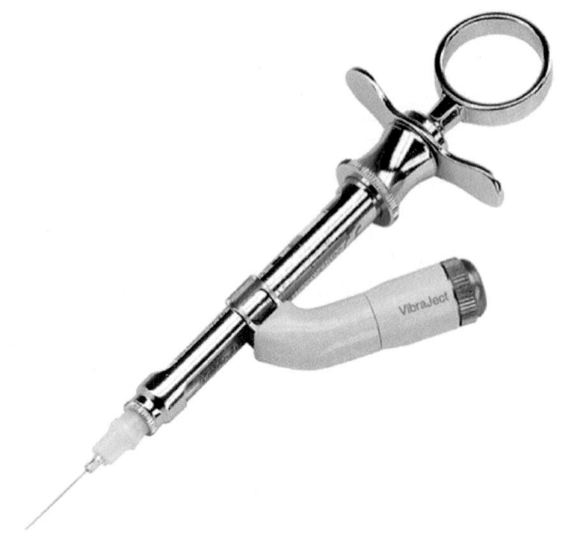

Fig. 11.17 VibraJect. (From Malameds: *Handbook of local anesthesia*, ed 7, St Louis, 2020, Elsevier.)

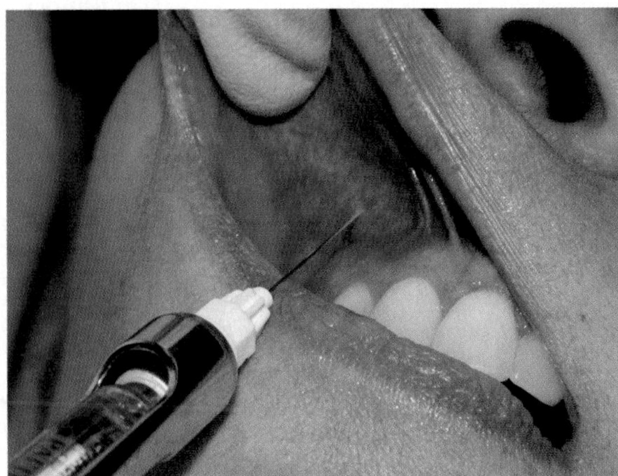

Fig. 11.18 Needle insertion; bevel is covered.

Gently insert the needle until the bevel is covered, keeping the tissue taut (Fig. 11.18). This is the needle insertion point or injection site. Watch for signs of discomfort or distress. Slowly move toward the target while communicating to the patient in a positive manner. A few drops of anesthetic will be unconsciously deposited ahead of the needle due to the gentle contact by the clinician's thumb on the inner surface of the thumb ring. Proceed slowly, using appropriate angulations, to the depth of needle insertion, which is the target location or deposit location of the anesthetic.

Step 14: Aspiration

To prevent the possibility of an intravascular injection, an aspiration test should be conducted before any anesthetic agent is deposited. This is one of the most important steps to reduce the incidence of injecting anesthetic agent directly into a blood vessel. Once the target location is reached, aspirate by pulling back on the thumb ring (only about 1–2 mm for standard syringes) to change the pressure in the cartridge from positive to negative (Fig. 11.19A). Care should be taken not to allow the thumb ring to slip down to the bottom of the thumb, making it difficult to achieve the full range of backward motion needed for a successful aspiration (see Fig. 11.19B). For self-aspirating syringes, this is accomplished by applying positive pressure to either the thumb ring or thumb disk and releasing it to create the negative pressure (Fig. 11.20). The needle should not move with either type of syringe. Beginners, especially those who do not have a firm fulcrum, have a tendency to overexaggerate the pulling back motion of the thumb ring, which pulls the needle away from the proper depth of penetration.

After the initial successful negative aspiration, the dental hygienist should rotate the barrel of the syringe about 45 degrees and aspirate a second time. This is called aspirating on two planes. This ensures that the needle is not located within a blood vessel and possibly abutting the blood vessel wall drawing the lining of the blood vessel over the lumen of the needle during the aspiration test, providing a false-negative aspiration (Fig. 11.21). This slight rotation will reposition the bevel away from the wall of a blood vessel, allowing blood to enter the cartridge during the second aspiration test. When injecting near highly vascular areas, such as near the pterygoid venous plexus with the PSA block, the dental hygienist should aspirate several times during the injection to ensure that any movement of the needle has not placed it within the blood vessel.

Any blood entering the cartridge is considered a positive aspiration. A clear air bubble, or no return after definite movement backward of

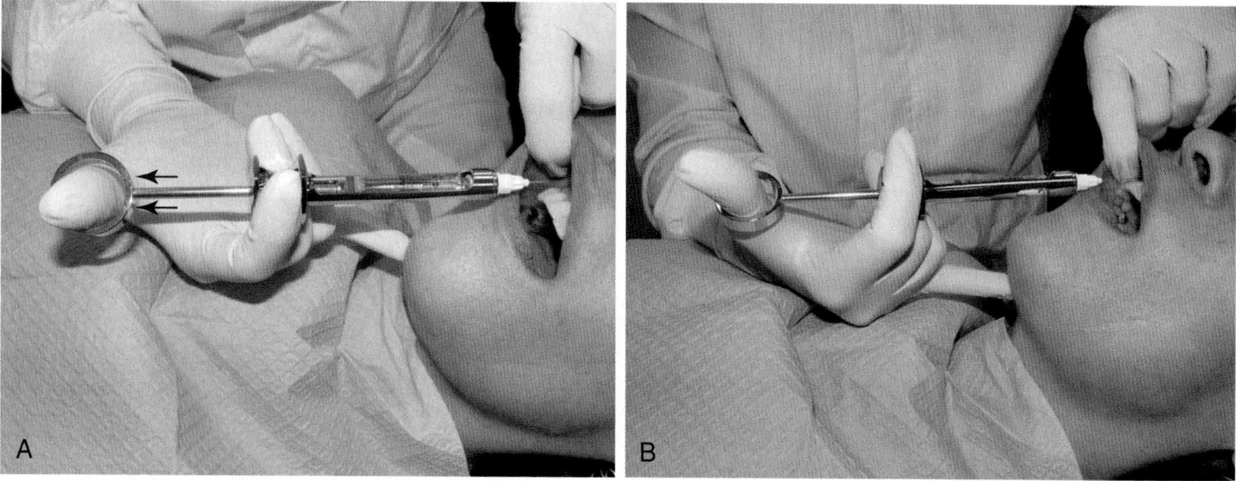

Fig. 11.19 Aspiration using a standard syringe. (A) Pulling back on the thumb ring for standard syringe with thumb ring in correct location for full range of backward motion. (B) Thumb ring not in proper location, restricting full range of backward motion.

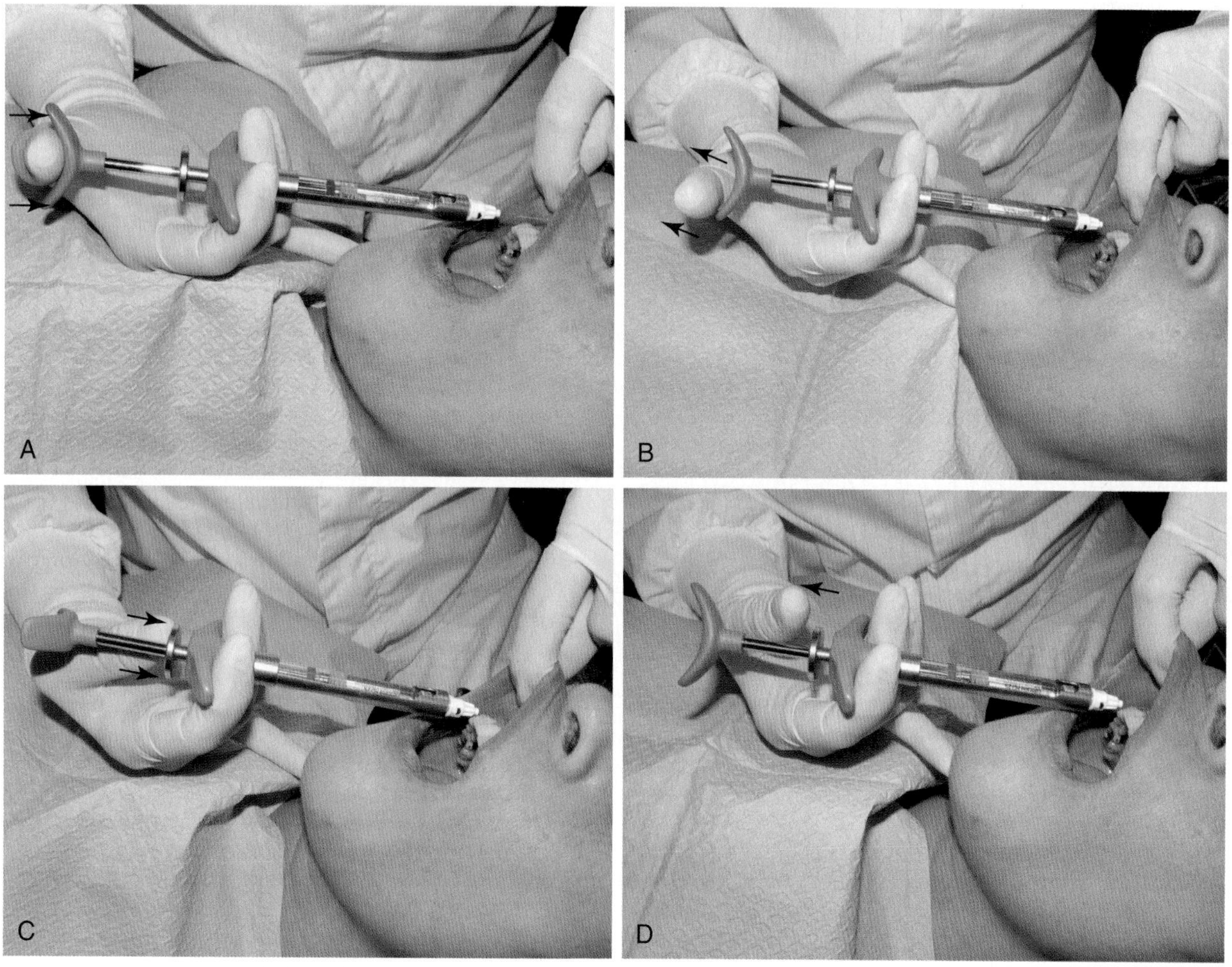

Fig. 11.20 Aspiration using a self-aspirating syringe. (A) Applying positive pressure to thumb ring for self-aspirating syringe. (B) Releasing positive pressure from thumb ring to create negative pressure. (C) Applying positive pressure to thumb disk for self-aspirating syringe. (D) Releasing positive pressure from thumb disk to create negative pressure.

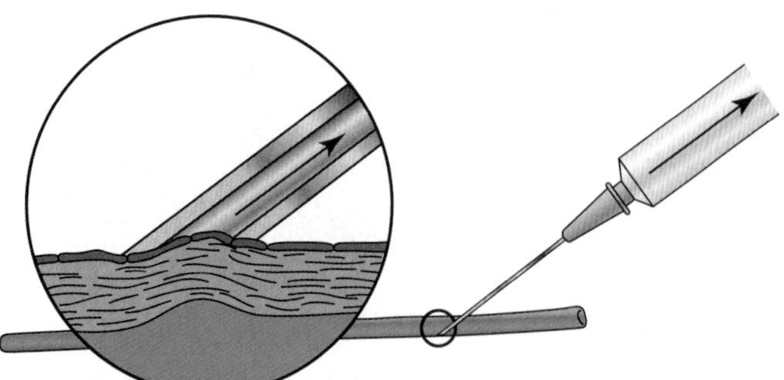

Fig. 11.21 Negative pressure during aspiration pulls the vessel wall against the bevel of the needle, giving a false-negative result.

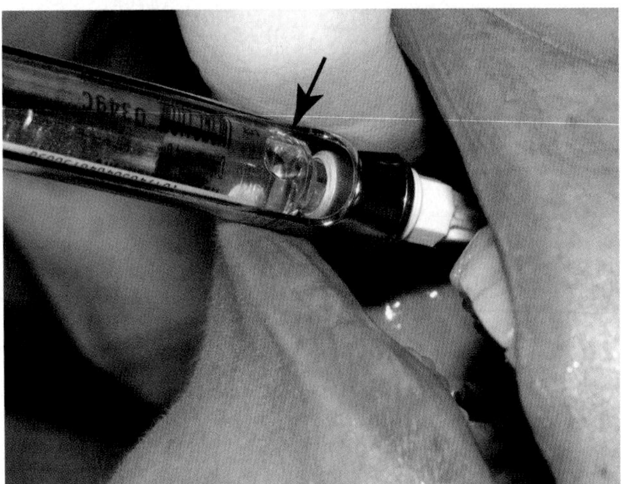

Fig. 11.22 Negative aspiration produces a clear bubble.

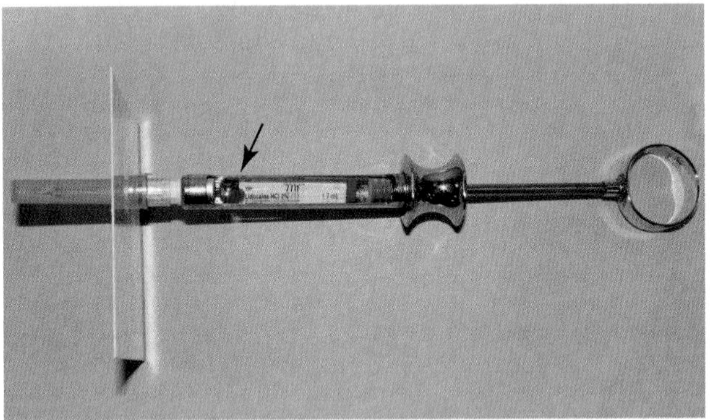

Fig. 11.23 Positive aspiration with little blood entering the cartridge; redirection and reaspiration is possible.

the rubber stopper, is a negative aspiration (Fig. 11.22). If a positive aspiration is observed, the dental hygienist is required to address the situation immediately. If only a small amount of blood has entered the cartridge and does not obstruct the view of successive aspirations, the dental hygienist can slightly reposition the needle a few millimeters, and the aspiration can be reattempted. If the second aspiration is negative, the anesthetic can be delivered (Fig. 11.23). If blood fills and clouds the cartridge or a second aspiration cannot be clearly seen after redirection, it is necessary to remove the syringe from the tissue, change the cartridge and needle, and redo the procedure (Fig. 11.24).

If repeated positive aspirations are observed at the same injection site, it may be necessary for the dental hygienist to consider postponing

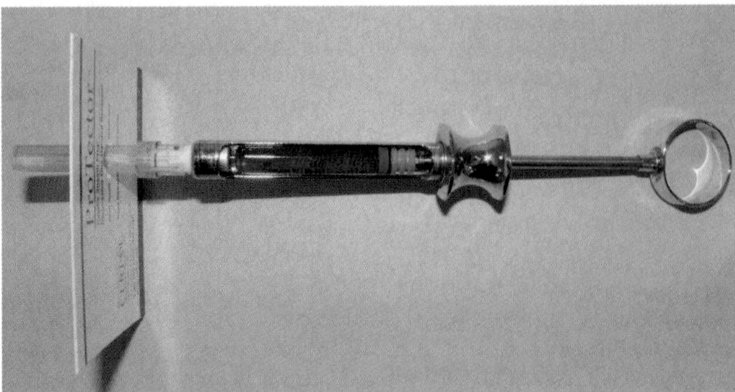

Fig. 11.24 Positive aspiration filling the cartridge; it is necessary to remove the syringe, change the cartridge and needle, and redo the procedure.

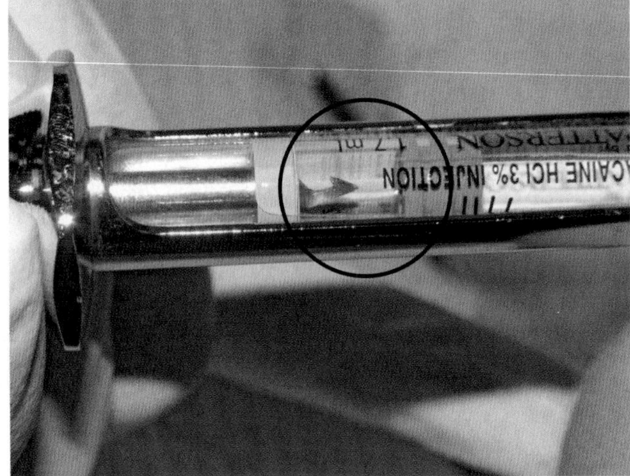

Fig. 11.25 Disengagement of the harpoon during aspiration: The dental hygienist must remove the needle from the tissue, reengage the harpoon, and redo the procedure.

treatment or treating a different section of the mouth, if possible. Repeated penetrations in the same area can cause bleeding at the target location and increased risk of hematoma, trismus, postoperative pain, and infection. Effective patient communication and education regarding these concepts is an important component to the delivery of local anesthetics so that the patient is aware that best practices are maintained at all times.[2]

Disengagement of the harpoon from the rubber stopper can occur when the dental hygienist is attempting aspiration (Fig. 11.25). This is usually caused by a dull harpoon or improper engagement during setup. If the harpoon disengages, the dental hygienist cannot ensure that a negative aspiration has occurred; the syringe must be removed, the harpoon must be reembedded into the rubber stopper, and the procedure must be redone. The best practice to reembed the needle into the rubber stopper is to recap the needle (using the one-handed scoop technique), remove the needle from the syringe, and apply pressure to the thumb ring. If the dental hygienist attempts to reembed the harpoon into the rubber stopper with the needle still on, anesthetic solution will be expressed without the harpoon adequately embedding into the rubber stopper.

Step 15: Slowly Deposit the Local Anesthetic Agent

Once the dental hygienist has reached the target location and has successfully aspirated on two planes, the anesthetic should be deposited slowly by gently and evenly pressing on the thumb ring. Slowly

BOX 11.1 Recommended Method to Ensure Slow Deposit of Solution

After negative aspiration on two planes → deposit slowly ¼ cartridge of solution → reaspirate (negative) → continue to deposit another ¼ solution → reaspirate (negative) → continue to deposit another ¼ solution to complete the procedure.

This process will take approximately 2 minutes, ensuring the slow flow of solution and aspirating throughout the procedure in case of needle movement.

depositing the anesthetic agent is a very important safety factor for two reasons: it reduces the risk of overdose even if the anesthetic is accidentally administered intravascularly, and it prevents the tearing of tissue.[3] In addition, it improves patient comfort. The anesthetic should be deposited at a rate of 1 mL of solution per minute.[2] Local anesthetic cartridges contain 1.8 mL of solution, so an entire cartridge would be deposited in approximately 2 minutes for most injections. It is important to continue communicating with the patient while administering the anesthetic. The dental hygienist should inform the patient why the anesthetic is being deposited slowly, for example: "I am depositing the anesthetic slowly to improve comfort." See Box 11.1 for a recommended method for slow deposition of anesthetic while implementing the safety of reaspiration.

Step 16: Slowly Withdraw the Syringe and Safely Cap the Needle

After completion of the injection, slowly withdraw the needle from the tissue. The procedure is not completed until the needle is safely capped. Once the needle leaves the tissue, it is contaminated with blood, tissue, and saliva and must be covered with its protective shield before anything else is done. This prevents inadvertent operator needle puncture. Because dental procedures require multiple injections, it is impractical to change the needle after each injection, disposing of it immediately in the sharps container after the injection as is required in other medical professions. It is therefore recommended that the needle be capped using at least the basic Centers for Disease Control and Prevention (CDC)-recommended one-handed scoop method (Fig. 11.26; see Chapter 9 and Appendices 11.1 and 11.2). Safer needle recapping devices or fabricated methods are available to help the dental hygienist secure the needle shield, allowing for easy, safe capping of a contaminated needle (see Fig. 11.27).

Step 17: Observe the Patient for Possible Reaction to Anesthetic

After the safe covering of the contaminated needle, the dental hygienist should observe the patient to monitor any signs of a reaction to the

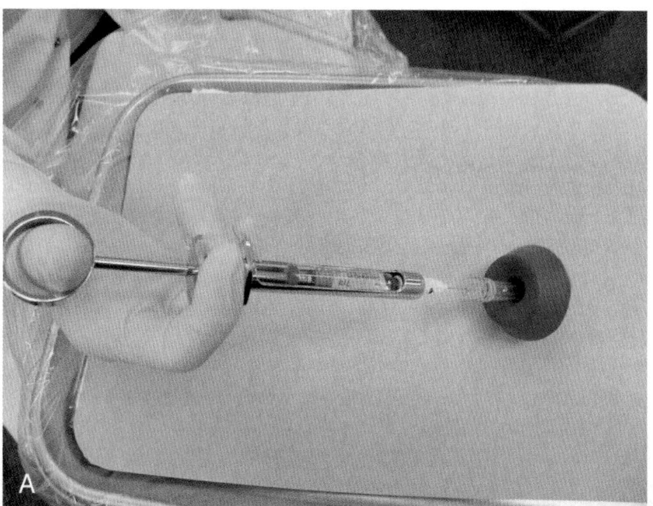

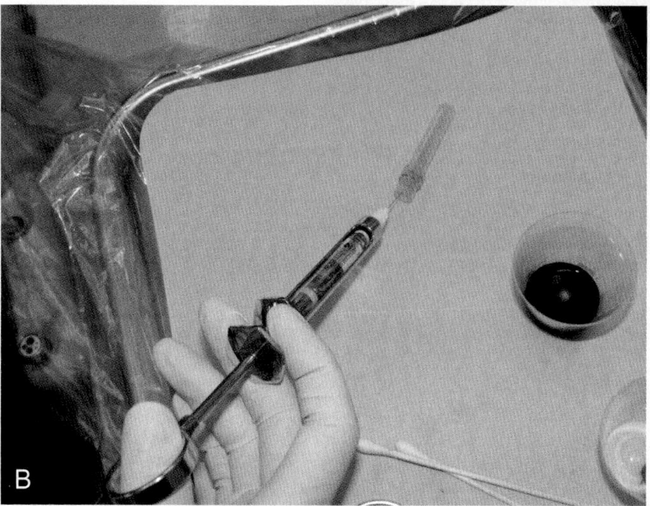

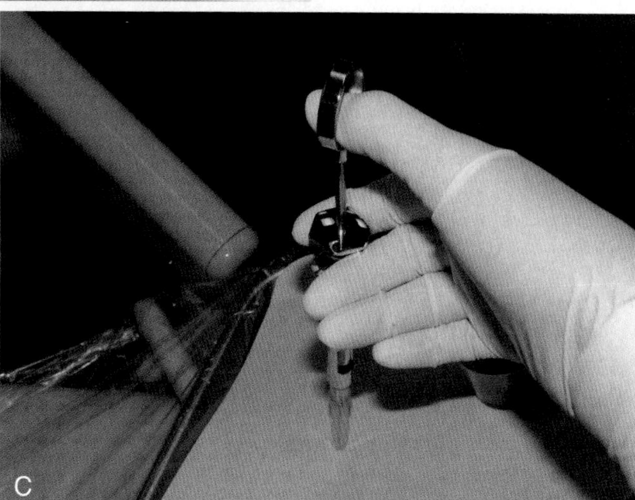

Fig. 11.26 Needle capping procedures. (A) One-handed scoop method with recapping device. (B) Basic one-handed scoop method without recapping device. (C) Securing the cap one-handed without a recapping device.

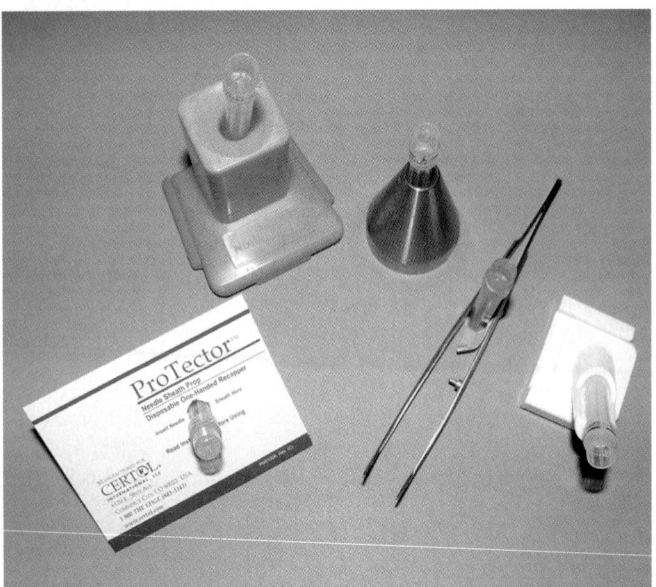

Fig. 11.27 Recapping devices are the preferred method to safely cap needles.

anesthetic or from the procedure. Most reactions, or dental emergencies associated with the administration of an anesthetic, occur within 5 minutes after the procedure.[5] Therefore the dental hygienist should remain in the room while the anesthetic blood levels increase and observe the patient for possible signs of an adverse reaction. If no adverse reactions are demonstrated, the dental hygienist should evaluate the effectiveness of the anesthetic, which should take approximately 3 to 10 minutes depending on the dissociation constant (pK_a) of the selected anesthetic (see Chapter 3) and the injection technique.

Step 18: Document Procedure

After the procedure, document the injection in the patient's permanent record. This should include (1) the date of drug administration; (2) the drug used and concentration; (3) the vasoconstrictor used, if any, and dilution; (4) the amount of drug and vasoconstrictor administered in milligrams (because dental cartridges are unique to the dental profession, recording the amount of drug administered in milligrams is more universally understood, and if medical assistance is needed during an emergency, the paramedics will understand milligrams and not cartridges); (5) the gauge and type of needle; (6) the injections administered; (7) the time of administration; and (8) any patient reactions and treatment. The time the drug was administered is important for long procedures when additional anesthetic might be needed, especially when a patient has received an anesthetic agent close to the MRD. By noting the time, the dental hygienist may be able to administer more anesthetic once the half-life of the drug is considered. See Table 11.2 for examples of patient documentation.

BASIC INJECTION TECHNIQUES FOR COMPUTER-CONTROLLED LOCAL ANESTHETIC DELIVERY

As discussed in Chapter 9, the computer-controlled local anesthetic delivery (C-CLAD) can be used effectively for both maxillary and mandibular anesthesia. See Fig. 11.28 for the Wand STA system faceplate legend. The C-CLAD is beneficial for increasing patient comfort for all local anesthetic injections and particularly during palatal and PDL injections where the tissue compliance is lower.

Steps to Achieving a Successful Supraperiosteal Injection Using the Wand STA System

1. Set the Wand STA system on the normal mode (Fig. 11.28F), which allows the Wand STA unit to function with two distinct flow rates: the slow-flow and rapid-flow rates. For this injection, the slow-flow rate should be used.
2. Turn the aspiration button on (Fig. 11.28G).
3. After the application of topical anesthetic, insert the 1-inch needle in the first layer of tissue at the injection site as described in Chapter 12 for supraperiosteal injections.

TABLE 11.2 Examples of Treatment Notes After the Administration of 1.6 Cartridges of Lidocaine 2% 1:100,000 Epinephrine

EXAMPLE 1
No complications following the administration of local anesthesia.

Date	Treatment	Signature
1/12/21	Medical history reviewed, no significant findings. BP 120/85, P 65, R 14. Patient consented to treatment with local anesthesia. 5% lidocaine topical, 57.6 mg of lidocaine 2% 1:100,000 epinephrine (0.028 mg) was administered for the Rt. IA, B blocks using 25-gauge long needle at 9:00 a.m.; no patient reaction or complications.	D Logothetis

EXAMPLE 2
Local anesthetic complication following the administration of local anesthesia.

Date	Treatment	Signature
1/12/21	Medical history reviewed, no significant findings. BP 120/85, P 65, R 14. Patient consented to treatment with local anesthesia. 5% lidocaine topical, 57.6 mg of lidocaine 2% 1:100,000 epinephrine (0.028 mg) was administered for the Rt. IA, B blocks using 25-gauge long needle at 9:00 a.m. Hematoma developed immediately after the Rt. IA block. Applied pressure and ice to the area and instructed the patient to continue with ice today and apply warm packs tomorrow. Patient requested treatment be postponed. Released patient after no further swelling developed. Further home care instructions were given to the patient.	D Logothetis
1/12/21	Follow-up phone call at 5 p.m. Patient is doing much better, swelling has decreased. No further complications. Informed patient to call if any problems arise. Scheduled patient for follow-up appointment.	D Logothetis

B, Buccal; *BP*, blood pressure; *IA*, inferior alveolar; *P*, pulse; *R*, respiration.

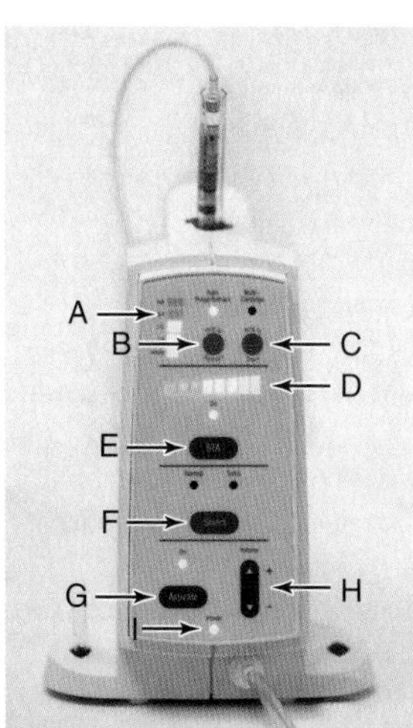

Fig. 11.28 Wand STA system faceplate legend.

4. Begin the slow-flow rate by lightly pressing on the foot pedal. After three audible beeps, the Wand STA unit will announce "cruise control." Upon hearing the "cruise control" announcement, remove foot from the foot pedal to continue the slow-flow rate on cruise control. Continue inserting the needle until the deposit location is reached.
5. Aspirate to make sure the needle is not in a blood vessel by depressing and releasing the foot pedal once.
6. If the aspiration is negative, continue to administer the anesthetic at the slow-flow rate to administer as much anesthetic as indicated under traditional syringe techniques (see Chapters 12 and 13).
7. Once the recommended amount of anesthetic is administered, depress and release the foot pedal, wait for three beeps, and slowly back the needle out of the tissue. This will prevent anesthetic spray back into the patient's mouth.
8. Safely recap the needle using the one-handed scoop technique.

Steps to Achieving a Successful Inferior Alveolar Block Using the Wand STA

1. Set the Wand STA system on the normal mode (Fig. 11.28F), which allows the Wand STA unit to function with two distinct flow rates: the slow-flow and rapid-flow rates. For this injection, both the slow-flow and rapid-flow rates can be used.
2. Turn the aspiration button on (Fig. 11.28G).
3. After the application of topical anesthetic, insert a 25- or 27-gauge long needle into the first layer of tissue at the injection site as described in Chapter 13 for the inferior alveolar block.
4. Begin the slow-flow rate by lightly pressing on the foot pedal. After three audible beeps, the Wand STA unit will announce "cruise control." Upon hearing the "cruise control" announcement, remove foot from the foot pedal to continue the slow-flow rate on cruise control.
5. Using the bidirectional technique (rotating the needle at a full 180° back and forth to prevent needle deflection), continue to insert the needle slowly with the anesthetic flowing at the slow-flow rate until the deposit location is reached.
6. Once the needle has reached the deposit location, aspirate to make sure the needle tip is not in a blood vessel by depressing and releasing the foot pedal once.
7. If the aspiration is negative, continue to administer the anesthetic at the slow-flow rate until one-quarter of the cartridge has been administered, and then, if desired, fully depress the foot pedal to go to rapid-flow rate to administer as much anesthetic as indicated under the traditional syringe technique (see Chapter 13). Aspirate again by depressing and releasing the foot pedal after every quarter of the cartridge.
8. Once the recommended amount of anesthetic is administered, depress and release the foot pedal, count three beeps, and slowly back the needle out of the tissue. This will prevent anesthetic spray back into the patient's mouth.
9. Safely recap the needle using the one-handed scoop technique.

Steps to Achieving a Successful Anterior Middle Superior Alveolar Block Using the Wand STA

1. Keep the Wand STA system on the STA mode (Fig. 11.28E).
2. Locate the injection site, which is between the free gingival margin and the midpalatal suture, bisecting the premolars as described in Chapter 12 for the anterior middle superior alveolar (AMSA) block.
3. Using the prepuncture technique to increase patient comfort, place the bevel of the ½-inch needle on the injection site with the needle at about a 45° angle and apply pressure to the back of the needle and tissue with a cotton-tipped applicator (Fig. 11.29). Depress the foot pedal lightly to start the slow-flow rate. After three audible beeps, the system will announce "cruise control." Continue to administer the anesthetic without penetrating the tissue at the slow-flow rate for about 8 to 10 seconds.
4. Slowly rotate the needle to pierce the tissue. This prepuncture technique numbs up the palatal tissue.
5. After a pause of 5 to 6 seconds, with the anesthetic flowing at the slow-flow rate, continue to rotate the needle with a back and forth motion toward the palatal tissue for another 1 to 2 mm before pausing.
6. Every 4 to 5 seconds, slowly advance the needle about 1 mm (creating an anesthetic pathway) until you reach the deposit location: the palatal bone. Maintain the needle bevel toward the bone. You will notice distinct blanching on the palatal tissue as an effect of the vasoconstrictor.
7. Once the desired amount of anesthetic is administered, depress and release the foot pedal, listen for three audible beeps, and slowly back the needle out of the tissue. This will prevent anesthetic spray back into the patient's mouth.
8. Safely recap the needle using the one-handed scoop technique.

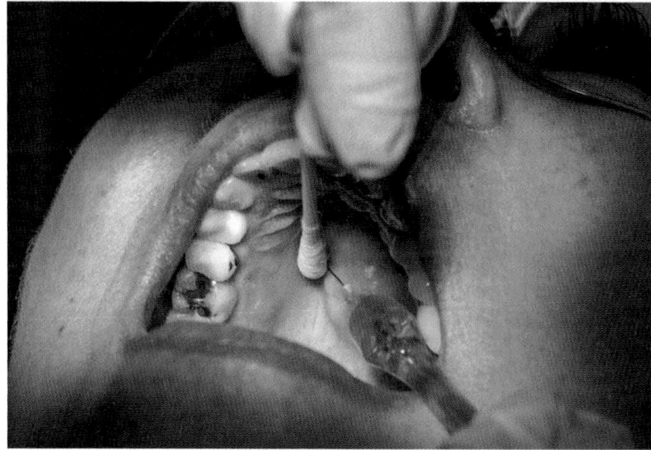

Fig. 11.29 Demonstration of prepuncture technique: Place the bevel of the needle on the injection site. Apply pressure to the back of the needle and tissue with a cotton-tipped applicator, and administer the anesthetic at the slow-flow rate when using the Wand STA system for about 8 to 10 seconds. The prepuncture technique can be used for all palatal injections.

DENTAL HYGIENE CONSIDERATIONS

- Dental hygienists should never allow the administration of local anesthetics to become routine. Dental hygienists should always take great care in the preanesthetic assessment, drug selection, and drug delivery.
- Vasodepressor syncope is the most common medical emergency observed in the dental office, and it is most frequently associated with the administration of local anesthesia.
- If two quadrants are to be completed in a single visit, anesthesia should be administered to upper and lower quadrants on the same side of the patient's face, administering the mandibular anesthesia first.
- Profound pulpal anesthesia necessary for restorative procedures, nonsurgical periodontal therapy with heavy deposits, and extractions require more anesthetic volume than less invasive procedures.
- Nerve block anesthesia provides profound anesthesia over a larger area with fewer injections needed.
- Good patient communication before and during the injection will help alleviate the patient's fears.
- Keeping the syringe and needle out of the patient's range of vision may prevent unnecessary anxiety.
- The dental hygienist must know the exact location of the uncovered needle at all times to prevent needlestick exposure, or accidentally touching the needle to a nonsterile surface outside of the patient's mouth before the injection and thus contaminating the needle.
- If the needle is accidentally contaminated before the injection, discard the needle in the sharps container, and attach a new sterile needle prior to injection.
- A firm fulcrum allows the dental hygienist to properly control the anesthetic syringe and provides ease of aspiration and a safer, more comfortable injection.
- Arteries and veins accompany major nerve trunks, and there is a greater potential for piercing an artery or vein during nerve blocks. Therefore proper technique and aspiration prior to injection is essential.
- The dental hygienist should aspirate on two planes before depositing anesthetic to ensure that the needle is not abutting the blood vessel wall, providing a false-negative aspiration.
- If the blood of a positive aspiration does not completely fill the cartridge, the dental hygienist can slightly reposition the needle and attempt a second aspiration.
- If repeated positive aspirations are observed at the same injection site, it may be necessary for the dental hygienist to consider postponing treatment or selecting a different sextant or quadrant to treat.
- If the harpoon disengages after an aspiration, the dental hygienist must remove the needle from the tissue and the harpoon must be reembedded into the rubber stopper. The procedure will need to be redone.
- To provide safe and comfortable injections, the dental hygienist should administer the anesthetic agent slowly at a rate of 1.8 mL over approximately 2 minutes for most injections.
- The dental hygienist should always cap the contaminated needle using the one-handed scoop method and using a needle shield prop.
- The dental hygienist should observe the patient for possible adverse reactions to the anesthetic and should never leave the patient unattended after providing anesthesia.

CASE STUDY 11.1 The Patient Is Feeling Anxious After Administration of a Local Anesthetic

A 130-lb patient is in the office for a routine class I amalgam on tooth #19. The patient's medical history reveals that she is nervous about the dental appointment, has a history of hypertension, and is taking Lopressor. The dental hygienist calculates the patient's maximum recommended dose (MRD) and determines that the patient can have 2.2 cartridges of 2% lidocaine 1:100,000 epinephrine. The dental hygienist begins the administration of the inferior alveolar block. Once the needle is at the injection site, the dental hygienist aspirates and hears a popping noise, which startles the patient. The dental hygienist is concerned about the patient's nervousness and quickly injects the cartridge of anesthetic. Shortly after the completion of the injection, the patient is experiencing increased heart rate and blood pressure and a throbbing headache. The dental hygienist leaves the patient in a supine position to make her more comfortable.

Critical Thinking Questions

- Why can the patient only receive 2.2 cartridges of the selected anesthetic?
- What postinjection reaction is the patient experiencing?
- What is the likely cause of the reaction?
- What could the dental hygienist have done to prevent the reaction?
- How should the dental hygienist properly treat the reaction?

CHAPTER REVIEW QUESTIONS

1. Surface anesthesia can be achieved by all of the following EXCEPT one. Which one is the EXCEPTION?
   A. Gels
   B. Creams
   C. Sprays
   D. Injections
2. When soft tissue anesthesia is needed in a limited area, it is best to perform a:
   A. Supraperiosteal
   B. Local infiltration
   C. Nerve block
   D. Surface anesthesia
3. The dental hygienist will provide nonsurgical periodontal therapy of teeth #18 to #24. Which injection administration technique should the dental hygienist use?
   A. Supraperiosteal
   B. Local infiltration
   C. Nerve block
   D. Surface anesthesia

4. If the dental hygienist wants to anesthetize tooth #12, which injection administration technique should the clinician use?
   A. Supraperiosteal
   B. Local infiltration
   C. Nerve block
   D. Surface anesthesia
5. When half-mouth periodontal treatment with anesthesia is required, it is best to begin with which injection?
   A. Posterior superior alveolar
   B. Inferior alveolar
   C. Anterior superior alveolar
   D. Middle superior alveolar
6. What is the most common medical emergency observed in the dental office?
   A. Cardiac arrest
   B. Vasodepressor syncope
   C. Seizures
   D. Respiratory failure
7. During the preanesthetic assessment, what are appropriate clinical considerations?
   A. Vital signs
   B. Length of appointment
   C. Anticipated postoperative pain control
   D. All are important considerations
8. When checking the armamentarium, why is it important to expel a few drops of the anesthetic agent?
   A. To decrease the amount of anesthetic that would be administered to the patient
   B. To ensure the harpoon is fully engaged into the rubber stopper
   C. To ensure the rubber stopper is not sticky
   D. To ensure a free flow of anesthetic through the needle
9. What is the recommended patient position when administering anesthesia?
   A. Supine
   B. Semisupine
   C. Upright
   D. Head below heart level
10. The dental hygienist should aspirate on two planes before depositing anesthetic. After a positive aspiration, the dental hygienist must always change the cartridge and redo the procedure.
    A. Both statements are correct.
    B. Both statements are NOT correct.
    C. The first statement is correct; the second statement is NOT correct.
    D. The first statement is NOT correct; the second statement is correct.
11. Topical anesthetic should be applied after the application of a topical antiseptic. Topical antiseptic can be used to decrease infection.
    A. Both statements are correct.
    B. Both statements are NOT correct.
    C. The first statement is correct; the second statement is NOT correct.
    D. The first statement is NOT correct; the second statement is correct.
12. After the patient has consented to treatment, when is a good time to communicate with the patient to alleviate fears of needle injection?
    A. After the procedure is over so as to not distract the clinician from the procedure
    B. When preparing the equipment
    C. When inserting the needle
    D. When preparing the tissue for injection
13. All of the following are the benefits of establishing a fulcrum during the administration of a local anesthetic EXCEPT one. Which one is the EXCEPTION?
    A. To ensure safe, comfortable injections
    B. To ensure proper aspiration without needle movement
    C. To provide more stability
    D. To clearly see a positive aspiration
14. Pulling the tissue taut before needle insertion helps all of the following EXCEPT one. Which one is the EXCEPTION?
    A. Visibility
    B. Ease of needle insertion
    C. Ease of needle penetration through the tissue
    D. Burning sensation felt by the patient
15. What is the main goal of aspirating on two planes?
    A. To determine whether the bevel of the needle is abutting against a blood vessel providing a false-negative aspiration on the first aspiration test
    B. To determine definite backward movement of the rubber stopper
    C. To determine whether disengagement of the harpoon occurred
    D. To provide the clinician a second chance to see if a clear bubble entered the cartridge
16. What is the minimum number of times a clinician should aspirate before administering the anesthetic solution?
    A. One
    B. Two
    C. Zero, only during nerve blocks
    D. Four
17. All of the following are benefits to depositing anesthetic agent slowly EXCEPT one. Which one is the EXCEPTION?
    A. Improves patient comfort
    B. Reduces risk of overdose
    C. Insures effective aspiration
    D. Prevents tearing of tissue
18. After removing the needle, what is the immediate next step?
    A. Rinsing the patient's mouth
    B. Documenting the procedure
    C. Recapping the needle
    D. Monitoring the patient for reactions
19. When do most reactions or dental emergencies associated with the administration of local anesthetics happen?
    A. Before the procedure
    B. When the patient gets home
    C. Within 5 minutes of the procedure
    D. Within 1 hour of the procedure
20. After the local anesthetic procedure, what information is important to document?
    A. Anesthetic used and amount in cartridges
    B. Anesthetic used and amount in milligrams
    C. Vasoconstrictor used and amount in cartridges
    D. Vasoconstrictor used and amount in milligrams
    E. B and C only
    F. B and D only

REFERENCES

1. Jastak T, Yagiela J, Donaldson D. *Local anesthesia of the oral cavity.* St Louis: Saunders; 1995.
2. Bowen DM, Pieren JA. *Darby and Walsh dental hygiene: theory and practice.* ed 5. St. Louis: Elsevier; 2020.
3. Malamed S. *Handbook of local anesthesia.* ed 7. St Louis: Elsevier; 2020.
4. Malamed SF. *Medical emergencies in the dental office.* ed 7. St Louis: Mosby; 2015.
5. Matsuura H. Analysis of systemic complications and deaths during dental treatment in Japan. *Anesth Prog.* 1989;36:219–228.
6. Kelsch N. Jenn's vision: A true lesson in best practices. Dentistry IQ. http://www.dentistryiq.com/articles/2014/08/jenn-s-vision-a-true-lesson-in-best-practices.html.
7. Elbay M, Şermet Elbay Ü, Yıldırım S, Uğurluel C, Kaya C, Baydemir C. Comparison of injection pain caused by the DentalVibe Injection System versus a traditional syringe for inferior alveolar nerve block anaesthesia in paediatric patients. *Eur J Paediatr Dent.* Jun 2015;16(2):8–123.

APPENDIX 11.1: SHARPS MANAGEMENT: CENTERS FOR DISEASE CONTROL AND PREVENTION GUIDELINES FOR INFECTION CONTROL IN THE DENTAL HEALTH CARE SETTING

Exposure Prevention Facts

Preventing occupational exposures in dentistry can significantly preclude the transmission of hepatitis B (HBV), hepatitis C (HCV), and human immunodeficiency virus (HIV) to dental health care personnel (DHCP).

Occupational exposures occur through percutaneous injury (e.g., a needlestick or cut with a sharp object), and through contact between potentially infectious blood, tissues, body fluids, and mucous membranes of the eye, nose, mouth, or nonintact skin.

The incidence of occupational exposures is not reduced for the experienced clinician.

Occupational exposures in dentistry are preventable when standard precautions are consistently used and devices engineered to alleviate sharps injuries are employed.

Standard Precautions

Engineering controls incorporate safer designs of instruments to reduce the exposures to blood and other potentially infectious material (OPIM) from sharp instruments and needles. These include self-sheathing anesthetic needles to reduce percutaneous injuries.

Needles are a substantial source of percutaneous injury in dental practice, and engineering of safe devices and work-practice controls for needle handling are paramount. The 2001 Occupational Safety and Health Administration (OSHA) bloodborne pathogens standards as mandated by the Needlestick Safety and Prevention Act of 2000 emphasizes the need for employers to consider available safer needle devices and to involve clinicians (e.g., dentists, hygienists, and dental assistants) in identifying and choosing such devices.

Safety controls for needles and other sharps are mandatory, which include placing used disposable syringes and needles, scalpel blades, and other sharp items in appropriate puncture-resistant containers located as close as feasible to the area of use.

Contaminated needles should never be recapped or otherwise manipulated by using both hands or directed toward any part of the body.

A one-handed scoop technique, a recapping device designed for holding the needle cap to facilitate one-handed recapping, or an engineered sharps injury protection device (e.g., needles with resheathing mechanisms) should be employed for recapping needles between uses and before disposal.

DHCP should never bend or break needles before disposal because this practice requires unnecessary manipulation and a greater chance for needlestick injury.

To prevent injuries, the DHCP should safely recap contaminated needles using the one-handed scoop technique before attempting to remove needles from nondisposable aspirating syringes. For procedures involving multiple injections with a single needle, the practitioner should recap the needle between injections by using a one-handed scoop technique or use a device with a needle-resheathing mechanism.

Avoid passing a syringe with an unsheathed needle between clinicians to avoid risk for injury.

Strategic Steps for Needlestick Prevention Programs

Form a sharps injury prevention team that includes workers to (1) develop, implement, and evaluate a plan to reduce needlestick injuries and (2) evaluate needle devices with safety features.

Identify priorities based on assessments of how needlestick injuries are occurring, patterns of device use in the institution, and local and national data on injury and disease transmission trends. Give the highest priority to needle devices with safety features that will have the greatest effect on preventing occupational infection.

When selecting a safer device, identify its intended scope of use in the dental care facility and any special technique or design factors that will influence its safety, efficiency, and user acceptability. Seek published, Internet, or other sources of data on the safety and overall performance of the device.

Conduct a product evaluation, making sure that the participants represent the scope of eventual product users. The following steps will contribute to a successful product evaluation:

- Train DHCP in the correct use of the new device.
- Establish clear criteria and measures to evaluate the device (safety feature evaluation forms are available).
- Conduct onsite follow-up to obtain informal feedback, identify problems, and provide additional guidance.
- Monitor the use of a new device after it is implemented to determine the need for additional training, solicit informal feedback on health care worker experience with the device (e.g., using a suggestion box), and identify possible adverse effects of the device on patient care.

Additional information for developing a safety program and for identifying and evaluating safer dental devices is available at https://www.cdc.gov/OralHealth/infectioncontrol/forms.htm and https://www.cdc.gov/niosh/topics/bbp (state legislation on needlestick safety).

APPENDIX 11.2: SAFE AND UNSAFE NEEDLE RECAPPING TECHNIQUES

Exposures to bloodborne pathogens can happen by getting stuck with a contaminated needle or getting cut by a sharp instrument that has blood on it. Job-related needlesticks can lead to serious or potentially fatal infections from bloodborne pathogens such as hepatitis B virus (HBV), hepatitis C virus (HCV), or human immunodeficiency virus (HIV). Even when a serious infection is not transmitted, the emotional effect of a needlestick injury can be severe and long-lasting. It is essential that dental health care providers consistently employ safe needle handling, recapping, and disposal of contaminated needles based upon the Centers for Disease Control and Prevention (CDC) and Occupational Safety and Health Administration (OSHA) guidelines for infection control in the dental health care setting. A one-handed scoop technique is crucial to safe and effective needle recapping in the dental setting. The use of recapping devices with the one-handed scoop method provides safer engineering controls for recapping procedures. The following examples demonstrate "safe" and "unsafe" needle recapping techniques.

"Safe" one-handed scoop method using weighted needle cap holder.

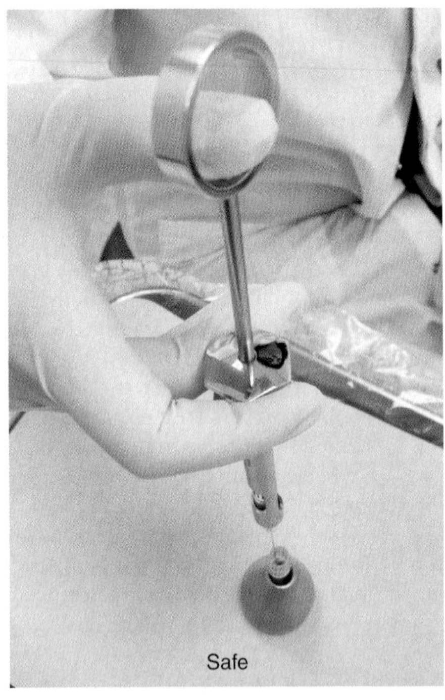

"Safe" basic one-handed scoop method without recapping device.

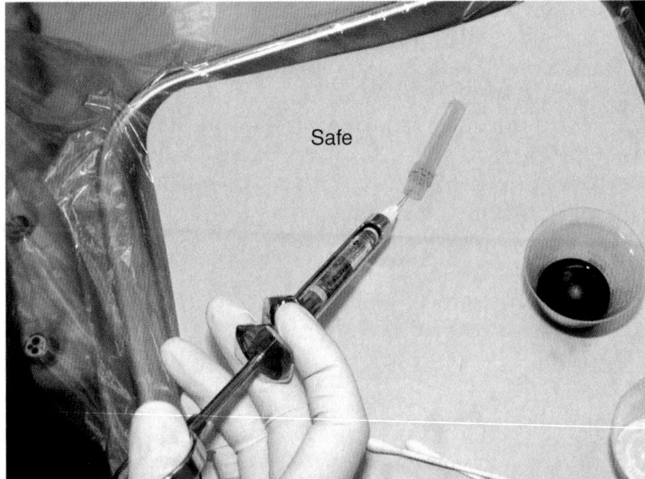

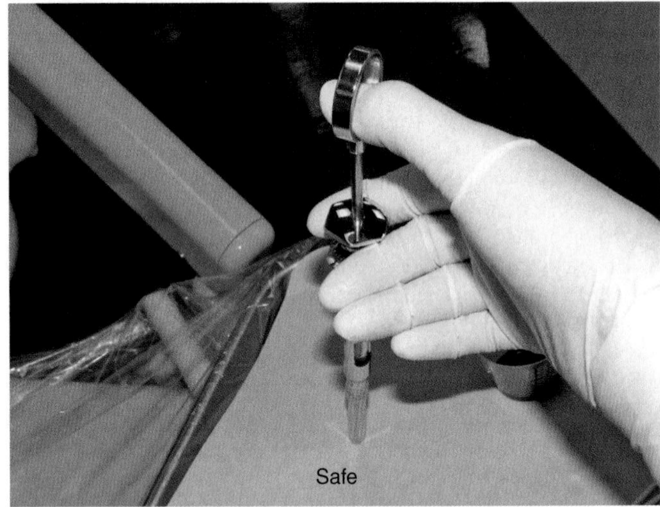

"Safe" one-handed scoop method using plastic recapping devices.

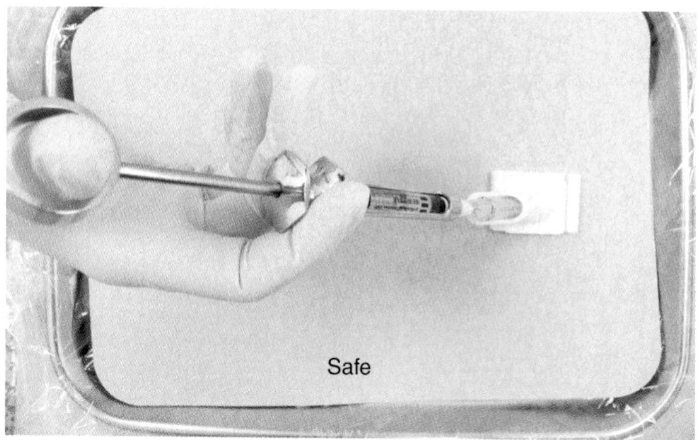

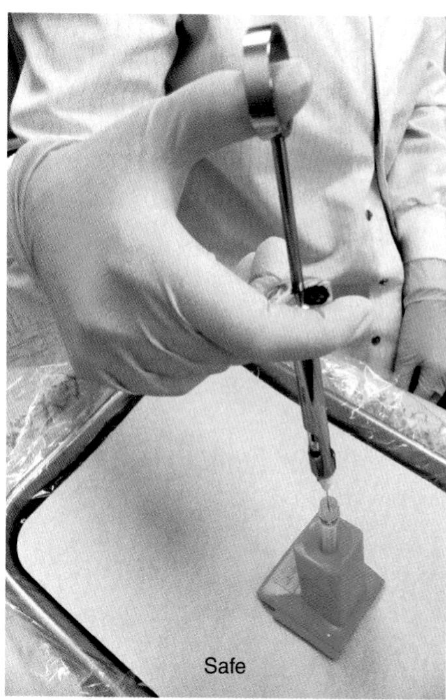

"Unsafe" two-handed technique holding the needle cap should never be performed.

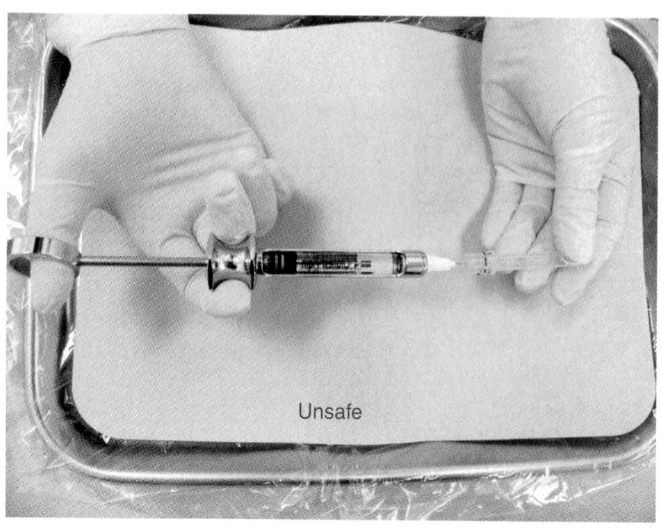

"Unsafe" two-handed techniques holding the rubber recapping device should never be performed.

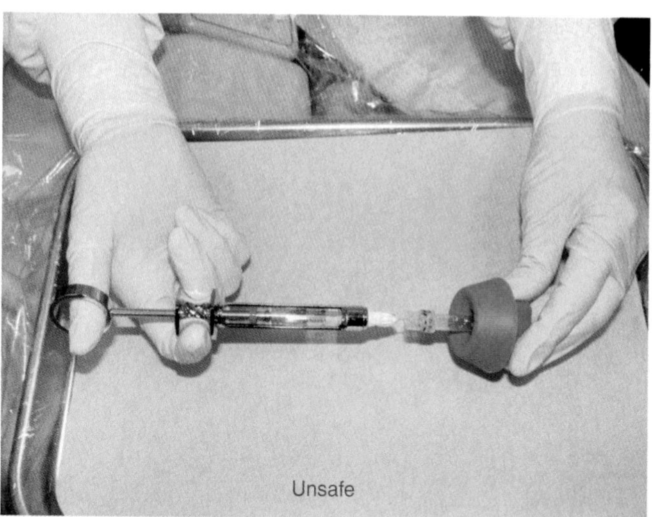

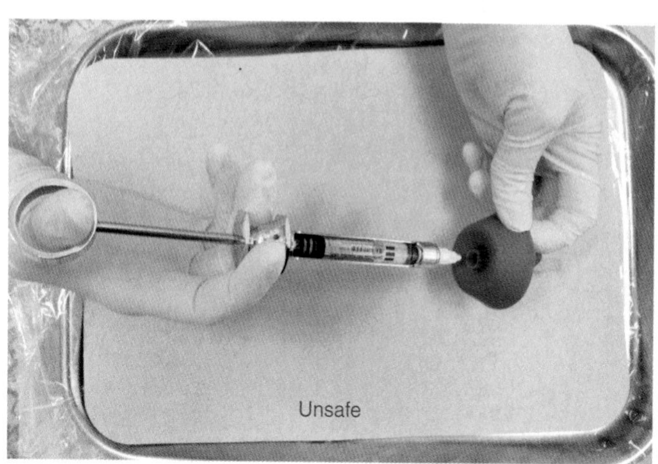

"Safe" one-handed technique using assisted rubber recapping device.

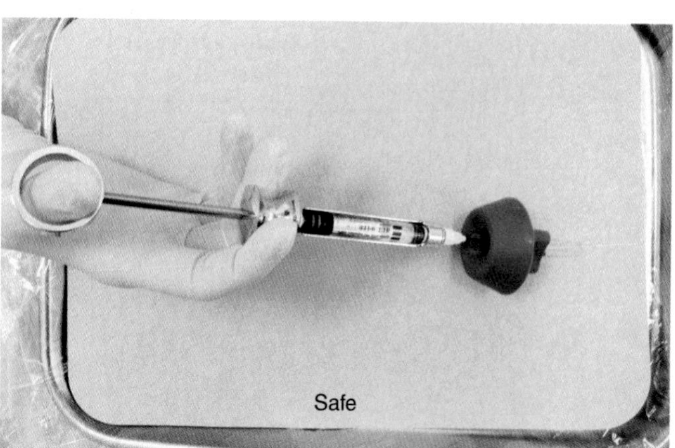

"Unsafe" two-handed technique utilizing the needle sheath prop. Note that it is unsafe to hold the card at the corner, as well as in the back of the card, as the needle can easily penetrate the card and injure the clinician and should never be used in this manner.

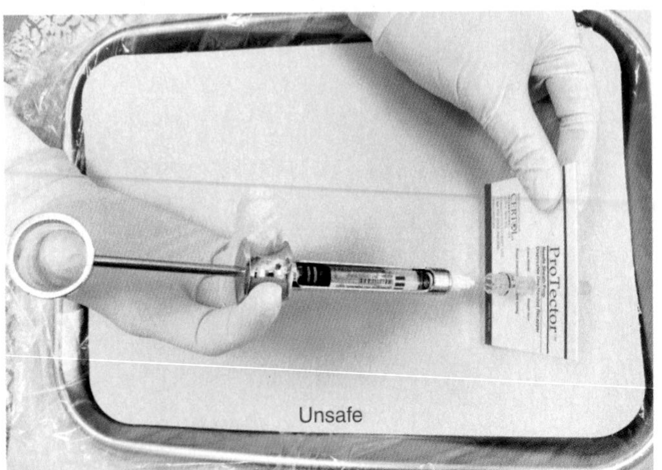

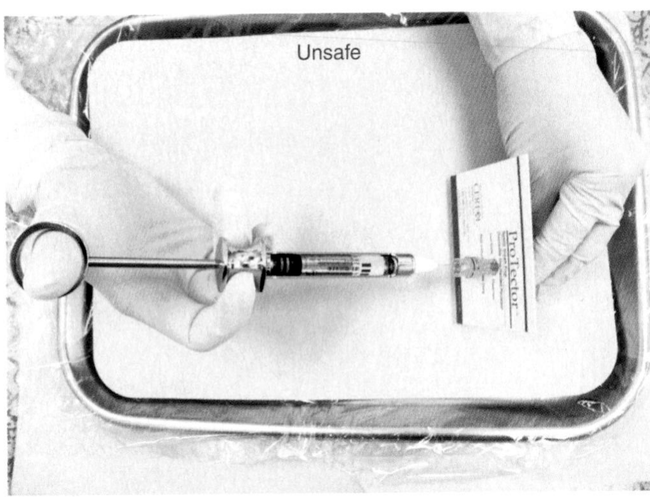

"Safe" one-handed scoop technique with a needle sheath prop to aid in covering and securing the contaminated needle. This device is disposable after use and is the preferred recapping device.

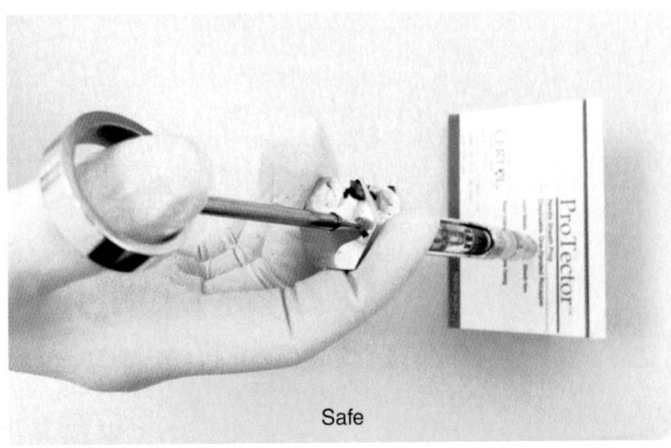

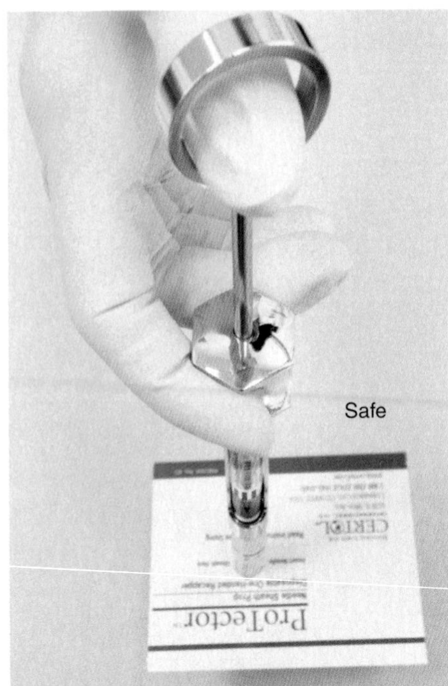

"Safe" one-handed shielding of safety syringe.

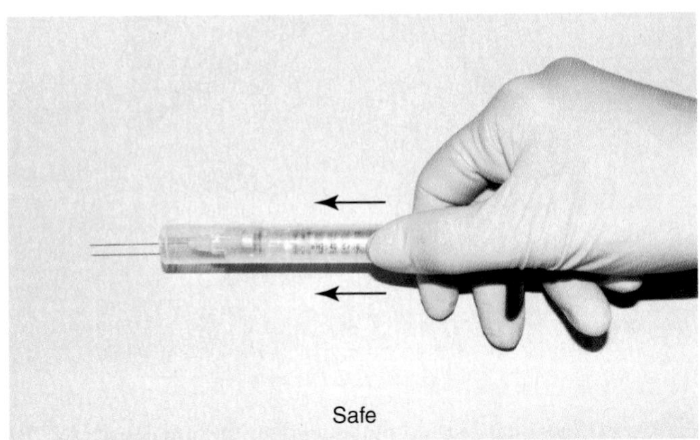

12

Maxillary Anesthesia

Margaret Fehrenbach, RDH, MS and Demetra Daskalos Logothetis, RDH, MS

LEARNING OBJECTIVES

1. Discuss the importance of understanding the anatomy of the maxillary nerve and its branches when it comes to the utilization of local anesthesia within the maxillary arch.
2. Discuss the clinical effectiveness of maxillary nerve blocks in relationship to anatomy and compare them to similar mandibular nerve blocks.
3. Concerning the three supplementals that can be administered within the maxillary arch as well as the mandibular arch, including the supraperiosteal, intraseptal, and periodontal ligament injections:
   - List and describe the supplemental injections.
   - Identify the target location of each.
   - Demonstrate the correct placement of the local anesthetic for each injection within the maxillary arch on a skull, peer, and patient.
4. Concerning the four maxillary facial nerve blocks, including the posterior superior alveolar, middle superior alveolar, anterior superior alveolar, and infraorbital blocks:
   - List and describe the various types of maxillary facial nerve blocks.
   - Identify the correct tissue inserted into by the local anesthetic needle for each maxillary facial injection.
   - Identify the target location for the maxillary facial nerve blocks and demonstrate correct administration of local anesthesia during dental hygiene clinical practice.
   - Discuss the indications of clinically effective injections as well as possible complications.
5. Concerning the three palatal nerve blocks, including the greater palatine, nasopalatine, and anterior middle superior alveolar blocks:
   - List and describe the various types of palatal nerve blocks.
   - Identify the correct tissue inserted into by the local anesthetic needle for each palatal injection.
   - Identify the target location for the palatal nerve blocks and demonstrate correct administration of local anesthesia during dental hygiene clinical practice.
   - Discuss the indications of clinically effective injections as well as possible complications.
6. Discuss common technique errors associated with maxillary injections.

INTRODUCTION TO MAXILLARY ANESTHESIA

The dental hygienist must understand how the maxillary nerve of the fifth cranial or trigeminal nerve and its branches can be anesthetized in various ways for patient pain management with clinically effective hemostatic control depending on the extent of procedure anticipated and the structures requiring local anesthesia (see Table 10.4 in Chapter 10).[1] In addition, the dental hygienist must also understand that administering maxillary anesthesia has its own considerations compared to administering mandibular anesthesia.[2]

First, most local anesthesia of the maxilla is more clinically effective than that of the mandible because the facial cortical plate of the maxillae is less dense and more porous than that of the mandible over similar teeth; anesthesia from the palatal surface is also possible (see Chapters 10 and 13).[1,2] This decrease in density of the maxillae compared to the mandible can be demonstrated with a panoramic radiograph (see Figs. 10.2 and 10.8 in Chapter 10).

Second, there is less anatomic variation of both the maxillae and palatine bones as well as the associated nerves with respect to local anesthetic landmarks than there is in similar mandibular structures, making the maxillary injections more routine and usually without the need for troubleshooting if there is lack of clinical effectiveness of anesthetic administered (see Chapter 10).[1,2] However, this does not mean that maxillary injections do not have any complications that can occur (see later discussion and related tables).[3] But unlike mandibular arch anesthesia, the entire maxillary arch can usually undergo anesthesia within one appointment without serious complications.

MAXILLARY SUPPLEMENTAL INJECTIONS

There are three supplemental injections that can be administered within the maxillary arch as well as the mandibular arch (see Chapter 13). The maxillary supplemental injections all have a high level of clinical effectiveness when administered correctly.[3] The supplemental injections have an associated visual analog scale (VAS) ranging from 0 to 6 when using the correct technique by the clinician (see Chapter 1).[4] The higher-end range is due to two of these injections entering into the cancellous bone of the alveolar process and not always being administered following a nerve block. However, the administration of all of these injections is of a short duration. The **supraperiosteal injection** is recommended when pulpal anesthesia is needed on a single tooth or when anesthesia of the associated periodontium and gingiva is needed in a localized area.

The next two injections are *intraosseous injections* since the agent is deposited into the alveolar process that supports the teeth. The **intraseptal injection** is recommended when there is a need for additional hemostatic control with the interdental periodontium and gingiva

PROCEDURE BOX 12.1 Supraperiosteal Injection Procedure

Step 1 Assume the correct clinician position depending on area anesthetized.

Step 2 Ask the supine patient to open and then retract the patient's lip pulling the tissue taut using the thumb and index finger of the nondominant hand (one inside and one outside); sterile gauze may be used to help retract slippery tissue.

Step 3 Prepare the alveolar mucosa within the height (or depth) of the mucobuccal fold or lingual tissue of the intended dental arch superior (or inferior) to the apex (or apices) of the selected tooth (as discussed in Chapter 11) and palpate the injection site or needle insertion point to confirm that only soft tissue is injected (see Table 12.1, Fig. A2).

Step 4 Using a 27-gauge short needle in the syringe of the dominant hand, orient the bevel of the needle away from the large window of the syringe to confirm bevel orientation toward the bone.

Step 5 Establish a fulcrum (see Table 12.1, Fig. B for fulcrum recommendations).

Step 6 Place the syringe parallel with the long axis of the tooth with the large window facing the clinician.

Step 7 Insert the needle within the height (or depth) of the mucobuccal fold or lingual tissue of the intended dental arch, parallel to the long axis of the tooth; the needle depth may vary but is approximately 3 to 5 mm, or until the bevel is superior (or inferior) to the apex (or apices) of the tooth (see Table 12.1, Fig. C). There should be no bony contact upon insertion.

Step 8 Aspirate within two planes.

Step 9 If negative aspiration, slowly deposit approximately 0.6 mL of agent (one-third of cartridge) over approximately 20 seconds; if the tissue balloons, the clinician is injecting too rapidly.

Step 10 Carefully withdraw the syringe and immediately recap the needle using the one-handed scoop method utilizing a needle sheath prop (see Chapter 11).

Step 11 Wait approximately 3 to 5 minutes until anesthesia takes effect before starting treatment.

between adjacent teeth. The periodontal ligament (PDL) injection is recommended when pulpal anesthesia as well as anesthesia of the associated periodontium and gingiva is indicated on a single tooth.

If there is any pulpal anesthesia for these supplemental injections present, such as that obtained for the supraperiosteal or PDL injections, it is achieved through anesthesia of each tooth's dental branches as they extend into the pulp by way of each apical foramen from the dental plexus.[1] Both the hard and soft tissue of the associated periodontium and gingiva are anesthetized by way of the interdental and interradicular branches for each tooth.

Maxillary Supraperiosteal Injection

A supplemental injection, the supraperiosteal injection, commonly incorrectly referred to as *local infiltration,* is recommended for pulpal anesthesia in one tooth or when anesthesia of the associated facial or lingual periodontium and gingiva is needed in a localized area (Table 12.1, Figs. A–C, and Procedure Box 12.1).[5] The supraperiosteal injection can be administered on any tooth of either dental arch. The supraperiosteal injection is administered by depositing the anesthetic agent either superior for the maxillary arch or inferior for the mandibular arch to the apex (or apices) of the tooth to be anesthetized. For mandibular supraperiosteal injection, see Chapter 13. In the case of the maxilla with its less dense and more porous bone, the anesthetic agent readily diffuses through its thinner facial cortical plate to anesthetize the terminal fibers of the superior dental plexus (see Chapter 10).[1,2]

The supraperiosteal injection is especially useful for dental hygiene care during limited nonsurgical periodontal therapy when the anesthetic is used in combination with a vasoconstrictor to provide anesthesia and hemostasis in a smaller circumscribed area, such as during maintenance or recare appointments.[6] However, because the anesthetic is deposited in close proximity to the area of treatment, any severe inflammation or infection in the area may inhibit achieving profound anesthesia.[1,3] In this situation, it is recommended to instead administer the anesthetic agent at a distance from the involved site using a nerve block where healthier tissue is located, thus allowing for more profound anesthesia (see Chapters 3 and 11).

Finally, supraperiosteal injections are also not recommended when several teeth within the quadrant need to be anesthetized. Using supraperiosteal injections for nonsurgical periodontal therapy of several teeth within the quadrant would require several supraperiosteal injections and thus larger volumes of anesthetic agent to achieve anesthesia of the entire quadrant as well as increased patient discomfort with an increased number of injection sites.[3,6] Therefore using nerve block anesthesia techniques would be a more appropriate choice for this situation (see Figs. 11.3–11.5 in Chapter 11).[7]

Target Area and Injection Site for Supraperiosteal Injection

The target area or deposit location for the supraperiosteal injection of either dental arch is superior (or inferior) to the apex (or apices) of the selected tooth (see Table 12.1, Fig. A1). Because the root lengths of teeth vary, the depth of needle insertion will vary. For the maxillary arch, the clinician should review the average root lengths of the maxillary teeth to help make this adjustment of needle depth more accurate (Table 12.2).[8,9] A review of the average root length for mandibular teeth will be needed for the mandibular arch when administering similar supraperiosteal injections (see Table 13.14 in Chapter 13).

The injection site or needle insertion point for the supraperiosteal injection is usually within the height (or depth) of the mucobuccal fold or lingual tissue of the intended dental arch with the needle inserted superior (or inferior) to the apex (or apices) of the tooth to be anesthetized (see Table 12.1, Fig. A2). The bevel orientation of the needle should be toward the alveolar process and the needle should be inserted parallel to the long axis of the tooth. The needle is advanced until the tip is superior (or inferior) to the apex (or apices) for the deposit location of the selected tooth, without contacting bone in order to reduce trauma, and then the injection is administered (see Table 12.1, Fig. C).

For injections involving facial anesthesia, the agent is administered within the height (or depth) of the mucobuccal fold and thus within the soft tissue of the redder superior alveolar mucosa, avoiding the firmer and pinker inferior attached gingiva with its underlying bone of the alveolar process (Fig. 12.1).[9] For both facial and lingual injections, the cotton-tipped applicator is used to locate this general target area by gently palpating the injection site or needle insertion point to confirm soft tissue entry before the needle is inserted as well as providing topical anesthesia. It is important to advise the patient that a slight prick of the needle may be felt before proceeding.

To increase patient comfort during supplemental injections, the needle should not be moved within the tissue, nor should the patient's upper lip be shaken, which was mistakenly recommended in the past.[10] In this so-called "distractor" technique, the clinician used the retraction finger or thumb to shake the patient's upper lip to distract the patient during the injection; however, this movement may increase discomfort when the needle bevel is moved and the anesthetic agent may not be actually administered at the target area.[11] Instead, to reduce patient discomfort, topical anesthetic should be used initially and the local anesthetic agent should be deposited slowly (see Chapter 11).[10] Access issues can also occur with supraperiosteal injections similar to that with maxillary facial nerve blocks (discussed later).

TABLE 12.1 Supraperiosteal Injection Review

Indications	Procedures on selected tooth and facial or lingual periodontium and gingiva
Nerves anesthetized	Terminal branches of dental plexus of selected tooth
Teeth anesthetized	Selected tooth
Other structures anesthetized	Facial or lingual periodontium and gingiva of anesthetized tooth
Administration technique	See Procedure Box 12.1
Needle gauge and length	27-gauge short
Target area/Deposit location Fig. A = Example: Supraperiosteal injection of maxillary central incisor	Superior (or inferior) to apex (or apices) of selected tooth
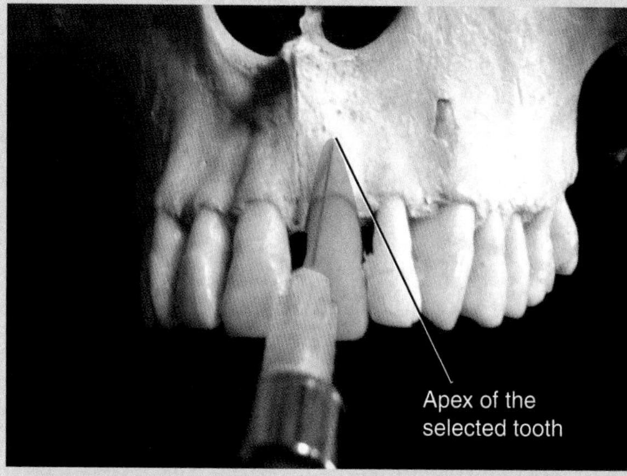 *1,* Example: Target area and distribution of anesthesia of supraperiosteal injection of maxillary central incisor (Courtesy Margaret J. Fehrenbach, RDH)	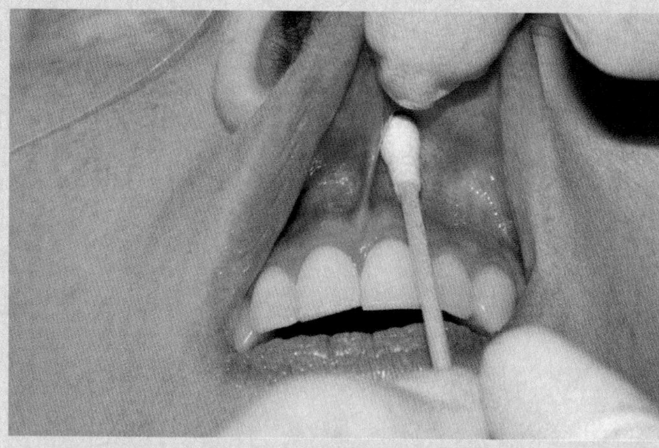 *2,* Example: Palpation within height of maxillary mucobuccal fold superior to apex of maxillary central incisor to confirm soft tissue deposition.
Clinician position	Varies with different teeth; clinician should be positioned for greatest visibility
Syringe stabilization with fulcrums Fig. B = Example: Supraperiosteal injection of maxillary central incisor	Varies with different teeth; clinician should use fulcrums with greatest support
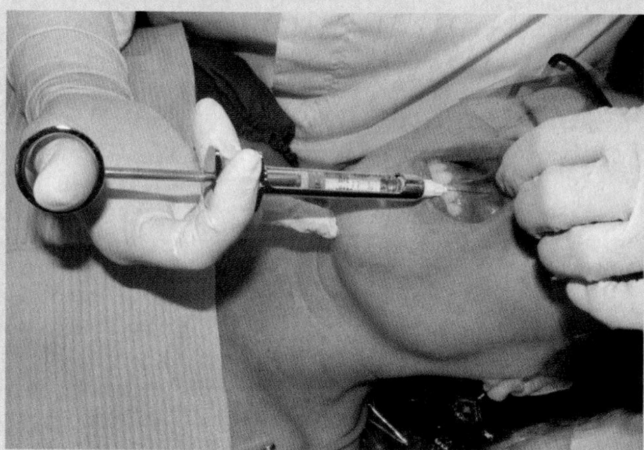 *1,* Example: Rest pinky finger of dominant hand on patient's chin	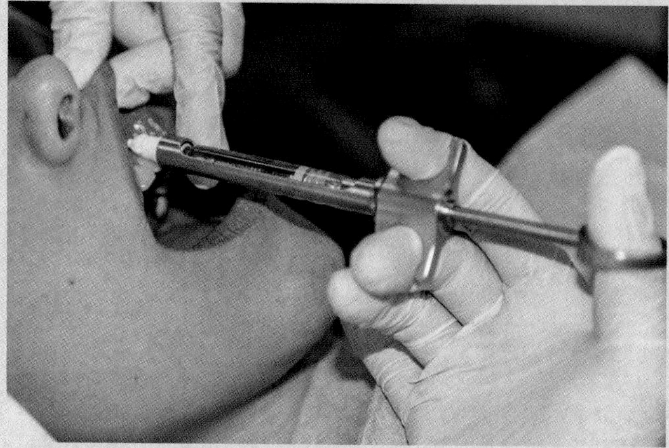 *2,* Example: Use index finger of retraction hand to gently support syringe barrel
Landmarks	Selected tooth Mucobuccal fold or lingual tissue of dental arch
Injection site/Needle insertion point	Superior (or inferior) to apex (or apices) of selected tooth within height (or depth) of mucobuccal fold or lingual tissue of dental arch (see Fig. A2)

(Continued)

TABLE 12.1 Supraperiosteal Injection Review (*Cont.*)

Depth of needle insertion Fig. C = Example: Supraperiosteal injection of maxillary central incisor	Varies based on location of apex (or apices) at approximately 3 to 5 mm (see Table 12.2 and Table 13.14 in Chapter 13)
Amount of anesthetic agent	Approximately 0.6 mL or one-third of cartridge
Length of time to deposit	Approximately 20 seconds

TABLE 12.2 Maxillary Teeth Average Root(s) Length(s)

Tooth	Average Root(s) Length(s) (mm)
Central incisor	13.0
Lateral incisor	13.0
Canine	17.0
First premolar	14.0
Second premolar	14.0
First molar	12.0 (buccal) 13.0 (lingual)
Second molar	11.0 (buccal) 12.0 (lingual)
Third molar	11.0

All data from Nelson S: *Wheeler's dental anatomy, physiology, and occlusion*, ed 9, St Louis, 2009, Saunders/Elsevier; in Fehrenbach MJ, Popowics T: *Illustrated dental embryology, histology, and anatomy*, ed 5, St Louis, 2020, Saunders/Elsevier.

Indications of Clinically Effective Supraperiosteal Injection and Possible Complications

Indications of a clinically effective supraperiosteal injection include numbness of any associated soft tissue and absence of discomfort during dental procedures. However, the patient may feel pain if the needle makes bony contact with the maxilla (or mandible); in this case, the needle should be withdrawn and reinserted farther away (or lateral) from the bone (Table 12.3).[10]

Inadequate anesthesia may result when agent is deposited directly over the apex (or apices) of the tooth or when an increased amount of dense facial cortical bone covers the apex (or apices); this situation is noted in children, near the maxillary central incisors where the apex (or apices) of the tooth lies beneath the nasal cavity as well as most of the mandibular arch (see Chapter 14).[3] Positive aspiration occurs in less than approximately 1% of cases; thus overinsertion with subsequent complications of hematoma is rare with supraperiosteal injections.[3]

Maxillary Intraseptal Injection

A supplemental intraosseous injection, the intraseptal injection, is used when there is a need for additional hemostatic control with the interdental periodontium and gingiva between adjacent teeth (Table 12.4, Figs. D–F, and Procedure Box 12.2). Thus a less diluted but smaller amount of vasoconstrictor can be used with the agent of choice, such as 2% lidocaine 1:50,000 epinephrine, in this localized area that requires additional hemostatic control (see Chapter 4).[3] The intraseptal injection is usually administered after the nerve block when used in conjunction with nonsurgical periodontal therapy for the region to allow for less discomfort of the needle entering the bone as well as having the usual dilution of vasoconstrictor (such as 1:100,000 epinephrine) already present to stem any gingival bleeding from the intraosseous injection.[6] Thus this injection is administered in an area that has an increased amount of blood vessels where the influence of the added less diluted vasoconstrictor can work. The clinician will find it useful for clinically effective hemostasis during nonsurgical periodontal therapy or when preparing the patient for periodontal surgical procedures by the periodontist.[7,12]

If the injection is administered without the nerve block, it can also provide short duration of anesthesia and hemostasis control of the associated facial or lingual periodontium and gingiva of two adjacent teeth without causing collateral numbness of the tongue or lower lip.[3]

The intraseptal injection can be used in either dental arch. Usually for the maxillary arch, the maxillary posterior sextant is a focus for this injection, but it is also useful for the maxillary anterior sextant if there has been advanced periodontal disease. Clinicians also find the injection useful if they feel the need for an additional injection on the labial interdental gingiva between the maxillary central incisors before a nasopalatine block on the palate for a highly sensitive patient.[3] For further discussion of the intraseptal injection and its use on the mandibular arch, see Chapter 13.

Target Area and Injection Site for Intraseptal Injection

The target area or deposit location is the terminal nerve endings within the bone marrow of the interdental septum or bone of the alveolar process associated with the associated periodontium and gingiva of two or more adjacent teeth (see Table 12.4, Fig. D).

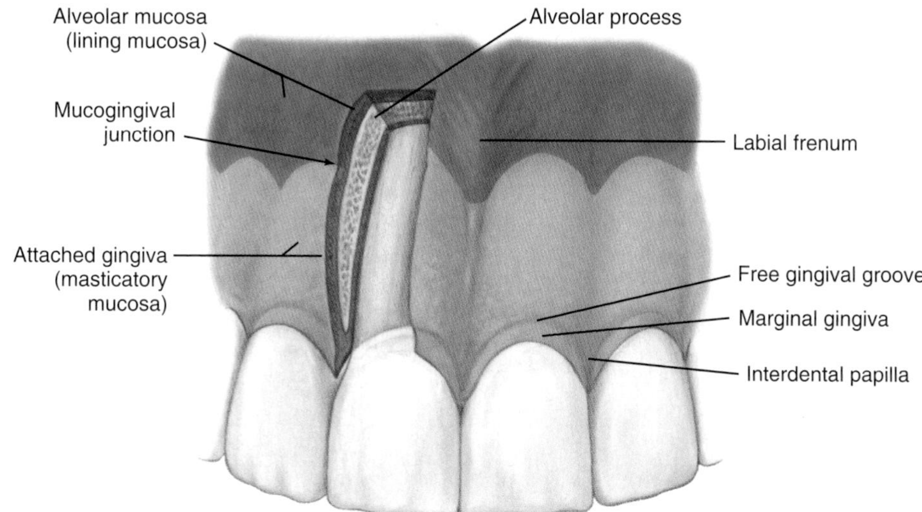

Fig. 12.1 For maxillary facial nerve blocks, as well as maxillary supraperiosteal injections, the needle is inserted within the height of the maxillary mucobuccal fold and thus within the softer and redder superiorly located alveolar mucosa, avoiding the firmer and pinker inferiorly located attached gingiva with its underlying bony alveolar process. Note that for certain mandibular nerve blocks, such as the mental block and incisive block as well as mandibular supraperiosteal injections, a similar method is used within the depth of the mandibular mucobuccal fold again within the softer and redder inferiorly located alveolar mucosa, avoiding the firmer and pinker superiorly located attached gingiva with its underlying bony alveolar process (see Chapter 13). (From Fehrenbach MJ, Popowics T: *Illustrated dental embryology, histology, and anatomy,* ed 5, St Louis, 2020, Saunders/Elsevier.)

TABLE 12.3 Supraperiosteal Injection Complications

Complication	Technique Adjustment
Pain on insertion with needle against periosteum	Withdraw needle and reinsert farther away (or lateral) from periosteum
Pain during injection from injecting too rapidly	Due to acidic anesthetic agent, care should be taken to inject slowly to not exceed recommended deposit time
Possibly inadequate anesthesia from injecting into area of infection and also risking needle tract infection	Instead administer appropriate nerve block (see Tables 12.6–12.18)
Possibly inadequate anesthesia from dense bone covering apex (or apices)	Instead administer appropriate nerve block (see Tables 12.6–12.18)

The injection site or needle insertion point is the center of the interdental papilla of the interdental gingiva, between the selected adjacent teeth (see Table 12.4, Fig. F). More specifically, the insertion is into the interdental papilla at approximately 2 mm from the tip and equidistant from the selected adjacent teeth on the dental arch. There is no need to use topical anesthesia on the attached gingival surface since the injection is a deeper intraosseous injection that is given within the alveolar process.[3] Stabilize the syringe and angle the needle correctly with the bevel toward the apex (apices) of the teeth. The needle and syringe should be at 45° to the long axes of the teeth and at 90° to the attached gingiva.

Slowly inject a few drops of agent as the needle enters the attached gingiva to increase patient comfort, advancing the needle until contacting the bone. Applying pressure, push the needle slightly deeper at approximately 1 to 2 mm into the cancellous bone of the interdental septum or bone and then administer the anesthetic. Use of a computer-controlled local anesthesia delivery device with short or extra-short needles (see Chapter 9) may be warranted with this injection since it slowly delivers the anesthetic agent, but standard or specialized syringes may also be used, usually with short or extra-short needles.[3]

Indications of Clinically Effective Intraseptal Injection and Possible Complications

If the injection is going to be clinically effective, there will be significant resistance to the deposition of the agent, at least with a standard syringe. Blanching of the tissue of the attached gingival surface will immediately be noted as the agent enters the tissue. Intravascular injection is extremely unlikely to occur so aspiration is not necessary.[3]

If the agent is not retained in the tissue upon administration, it is due to shallowness of the injection depth. To correct this, advance the needle farther into the interdental septum or bone and readminister.[3] Without the extensive soft tissue anesthesia, noted with other injections, especially most nerve blocks, patients may be concerned that they are not adequately anesthetized if given alone. The clinician will need to reassure patients that indeed the localized region is anesthetized. The advantages and disadvantages of an intraseptal injection are listed in Table 12.5.

Maxillary Periodontal Ligament Injection

A supplemental intraosseous injection, the PDL injection is used when pulpal anesthesia as well as anesthesia of the associated periodontium and gingiva is indicated on a single tooth mainly in the mandibular arch; the injection can also be used within the maxillary arch but is rarely used for the superior dental arch.[3] For more detailed discussion of the injection, including use on the mandibular arch, as well as advantages and disadvantages for the PDL injection, see Chapter 13.

TABLE 12.4 Intraseptal Injection Review

Indications	Two selected adjacent teeth usually already anesthetized by nerve block but requiring additional hemostatic control, using a less diluted vasoconstrictor such as epinephrine 1:50.000, with interdental periodontium and gingiva
Nerves anesthetized	Terminal endings within interdental septum or bone associated with periodontium and gingiva of two selected adjacent teeth unless already anesthetized by regional nerve block
Teeth anesthetized	None directly from injection; selected teeth are usually already anesthetized by nerve block
Other structures anesthetized	Associated facial or lingual periodontium and gingiva unless already anesthetized by nerve block
Administration technique	See Procedure Box 12.2
Needle gauge and length	27-gauge extra-short or short for standard or specialized syringe; also 30-gauge extra-short or short with computer-controlled local anesthetic delivery device
Target area/Deposit location 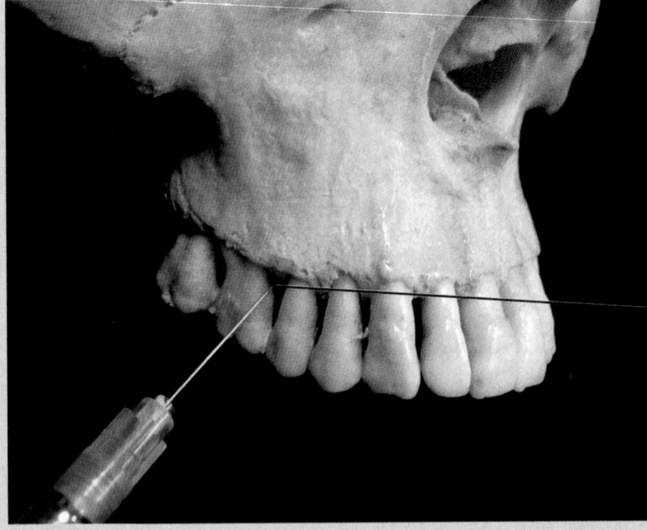 Fig. D = Example: Target area and distribution for buccal intraseptal injection between maxillary second premolar and first molar (Courtesy Margaret J. Fehrenbach, RDH.)	Interdental septum or bone of alveolar process between two selected adjacent teeth
Clinician position	Varies with different teeth; clinician should be positioned for greatest visibility
Syringe stabilization with fulcrums Fig. E = Example: Syringe stabilization with fulcrums for intraseptal injection 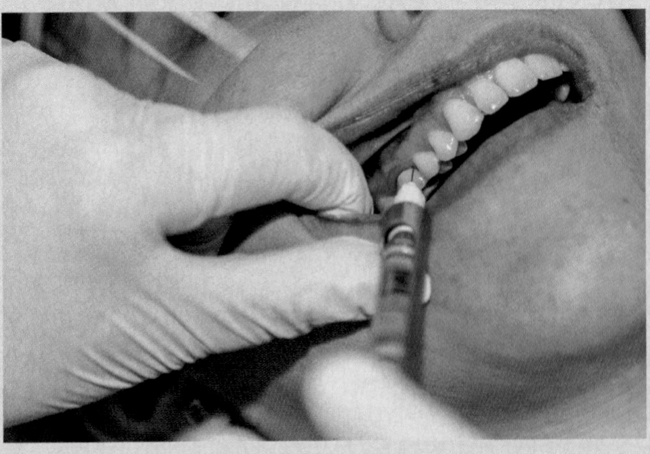	Against patient's teeth, lips, or face
Landmarks	Selected teeth Interdental papilla between selected adjacent teeth

TABLE 12.4 Intraseptal Injection Review (*Cont.*)

Injection site/Needle insertion point 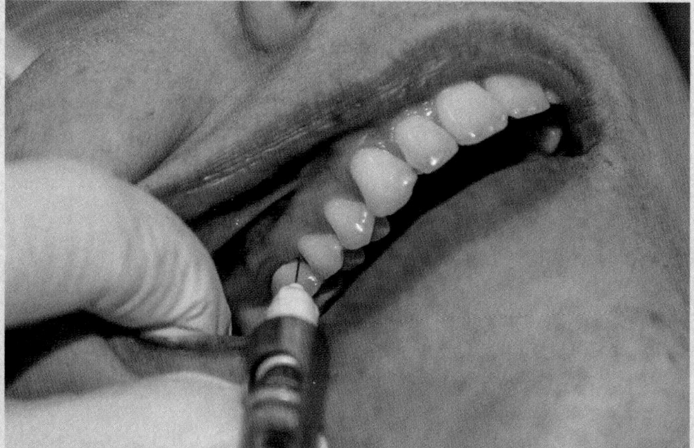 Fig. F = Example: Injection site for buccal intraseptal injection between maxillary second premolar and first molar	Center of interdental papilla at approximately 2 mm from tip and equidistant from selected adjacent teeth on dental arch
Depth of needle insertion	Approximately 1 to 2 mm into interdental septum or bone after bony contact (see Fig. F)
Amount of anesthetic agent	Approximately 0.2 to 0.4 mL or one to two stopper widths of anesthetic with standard or computer-controlled local anesthesia delivery device; one or two squeezes for specialized syringe
Length of time to deposit	Approximately 20 seconds

PROCEDURE BOX 12.2 Intraseptal Injection Procedure

Step 1 After administering the nerve block for region of the selected adjacent teeth continue to assume the correct clinician position depending on region anesthetized.

Step 2 Ask the supine patient to open and then retract the patient's lip pulling the tissue taut using the thumb and index finger of the nondominant hand (one inside and one outside); sterile gauze may be used to help retract slippery tissue.

Step 3 Prepare the center of the interdental papilla between the selected adjacent teeth (as discussed in Chapter 11).

Step 4 Assemble the standard or specialized syringe with a 27-gauge extra-short or short needle or use a computer-controlled delivery device with a 30-gauge extra-short or short needle after careful consideration of the situation. Using the syringe or handpiece in the dominant hand, orient the bevel of the needle toward the alveolar process.

Step 5 Clinician and patient positions as well as fulcrums vary from tooth to tooth.

Step 6 Stabilize the syringe or handpiece and angle the needle at 45° to the long axes of the teeth and at 90° to the attached gingiva, with the bevel toward the apices of the teeth (see Table 12.4, Fig. E).

Step 7 Insert the needle in the center of the interdental papilla of the selected adjacent teeth at approximately 2 mm from the tip and equidistant from the adjacent teeth on the arch (see Table 12.4, Fig. F). Slowly inject a few drops of agent as the needle enters the attached gingiva, advancing the needle until contacting the bone. Applying pressure, push the needle slightly deeper at 1 to 2 mm into the cancellous bone of the interdental septum or bone.

Step 8 Deposit approximately 0.2 to 0.4 mL of agent or one to two stoppers with standard or computer-controlled local anesthesia delivery device; one or two squeezes for the specialized syringe. There will be significant resistance to the deposition of the agent at least with the standard syringe. Blanching of the attached gingival surface will immediately be noted as the agent enters the tissue.

Step 9 Carefully withdraw the syringe or handpiece and immediately recap the needle using the one-hand scoop method utilizing a needle sheath prop (see Chapter 11).

Step 10 Rinse the patient's mouth. Inspect the region and stem any remaining bleeding with pressure using sterile gauze. Onset of action is immediate and treatment may commence.

MAXILLARY FACIAL NERVE BLOCKS

Maxillary facial nerve blocks anesthetizing various maxillary nerve branches have a high level of clinical effectiveness when administered correctly as they anesthetize both the pulp and various regions of the associated periodontium and gingiva (Fig. 12.2).[1,2] The maxillary facial injections have an associated VAS ranging from 0 to 2 using the correct technique by the clinician (see Chapter 1).[4] To achieve this level of patient comfort, there is usually avoidance of bony contact of the overlying sensitive periosteum of the maxilla with the needle during the injection except at the final deposition point of the infraorbital block.[10]

The target area or deposit location for the maxillary facial nerve blocks is superior to the apex (or apices) of the target tooth. Because the root lengths of teeth vary, the depth of needle insertion will vary. For the maxillary arch, the clinician should review the average root

TABLE 12.5 Advantages and Disadvantages of Intraseptal Injection

Advantages	Disadvantages
• Minimal volume needed of both the anesthetic and vasoconstrictor (1:50,000 dilution), which decreases the risk of systemic toxicity while providing profound hemostasis, an important consideration for patients with significant cardiovascular disease • Minimizes bleeding in localized area of treatment • Alternative or supplemental method when other options are ineffective or can be considered • Immediate (<30 seconds) onset of action • Postoperative complications such as paresthesia are unlikely since lingual nerve is not anesthetized in most cases • Absence of lip or tongue numbness that is particularly beneficial to children and special needs patients so as to decrease risk of self-inflicted trauma; also lessens postinjection discomfort	• Contraindicated in areas with localized infection or severe inflammation such as with advanced periodontal disease, severe caries, or endodontic lesion* • Multiple injections may be needed • Needle placement may be difficult without experience and with certain crowded dentitions or if patient has reduced interdental septum or bone • Anesthetic agent may leak into patient's mouth, especially without adequate levels of interdental septum or bone

*Most common reason cited for lack of clinical effectiveness of intraseptal injection.

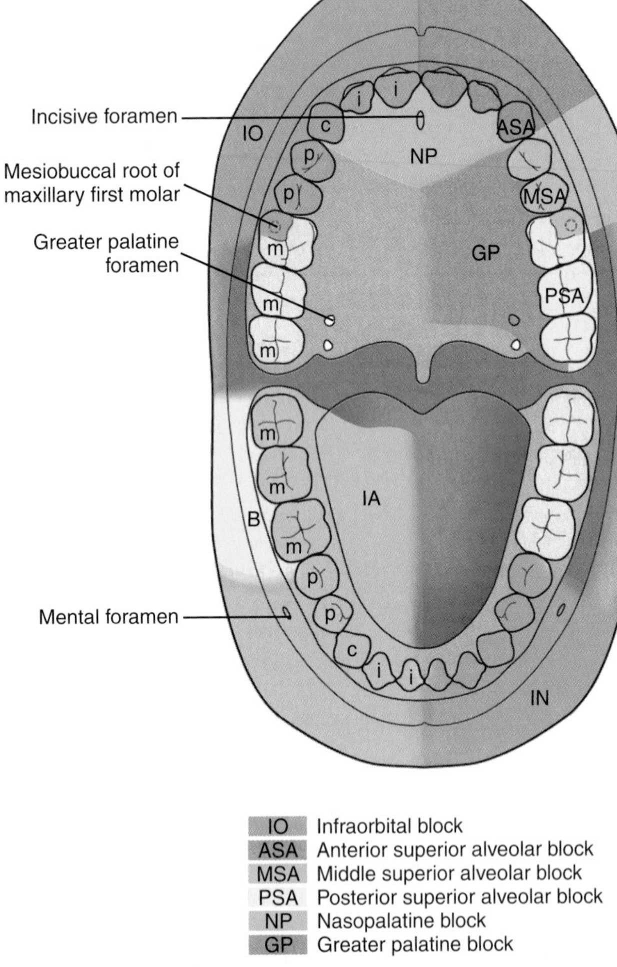

Fig. 12.2 Local anesthetic nerve blocks of the maxillary arch with the related structures anesthetized. Note that the anterior middle superior alveolar block is not included; see associated figures for more clarification of this nerve block. Note that the borders of each injection shown are approximate and that substantial overlap exists between nerves that can affect clinical anesthesia effectiveness. (From Fehrenbach MJ, Herring SW: *Illustrated anatomy of the head and neck,* ed 6, St Louis, 2021, Saunders/Elsevier.)

lengths of the maxillary teeth to help make this adjustment of needle depth more accurate (see Table 12.2).[8,9]

In all cases, the agent is administered within the height of the maxillary mucobuccal fold within the soft tissue of the redder superior alveolar mucosa, avoiding the firmer and pinker inferior attached gingiva with its underlying bone of the alveolar process (see Fig. 12.1).[9] To locate this general target area, the cotton-tipped applicator is used to gently palpate the injection site or needle insertion point to confirm soft tissue entry before the needle is inserted as well as providing topical anesthesia. It is important to advise the patient that a slight prick of the needle may be felt before proceeding.

To increase patient comfort during maxillary facial injections, the needle should not be moved within the tissue, nor should the patient's upper lip be shaken as previously discussed. Instead, to reduce patient discomfort, topical anesthesia is used initially and the local anesthetic agent should be deposited slowly (see Chapter 11).

The pulpal anesthesia for the maxillary facial injections is achieved through anesthesia of each tooth's dental branches as they extend into the pulp by way of each apical foramen from the superior dental plexus.[1,2] Both the hard and soft tissue of the associated periodontium and gingiva are anesthetized by way of the interdental and interradicular branches for each tooth (Table 12.6).

The **posterior superior alveolar (PSA) block** is a nerve block that is recommended for anesthesia of the maxillary molars and associated buccal periodontium and gingiva within one maxillary quadrant. The **middle superior alveolar (MSA) block** is a nerve block that is recommended for anesthesia of the maxillary premolars and associated buccal periodontium and gingiva within one maxillary quadrant. The **anterior superior alveolar (ASA) block** is a nerve block that is recommended for anesthesia of the maxillary anterior teeth and associated labial periodontium and gingiva to the midline within one maxillary quadrant. The **infraorbital (IO) block** is a nerve block that is recommended for anesthesia of the maxillary anterior teeth and premolars and associated facial periodontium and gingiva within one maxillary quadrant since it anesthetizes both regions covered by the MSA and ASA blocks.

If quadrant dental hygiene treatment is planned within the maxillary arch, the PSA block is administered before any of the other maxillary facial injections as well as any palatal injections to allow the necessary time for the larger maxillary molars to undergo pulpal anesthesia (see Chapter 11 and Fig. 11.4A–B). After the PSA block, the MSA and then ASA blocks (or IO block instead) are then administered in that order, and palatal injections follow for the maxillary quadrant. Instrumentation by the clinician proceeds in the same order as anesthesia.

TABLE 12.6 Nerve Blocks for Maxillary Teeth and Associated Structures

Maxillary Tooth and Structures	ASA Block	MSA Block	PSA Block	IO Block	NP Block	GP Block	AMSA Block
Central Incisor							
Pulp with labial periodontium and gingiva	X			X			X
Palatal periodontium and gingiva					X		X
Lateral Incisor							
Pulp with labial periodontium and gingiva	X			X			X
Palatal periodontium and gingiva					X		X
Canine							
Pulp with labial periodontium and gingiva	X			X			X
Palatal periodontium and gingiva					X		X
First Premolar							
Pulp with buccal periodontium and gingiva		X		X			X
Palatal periodontium and gingiva						X	X
Second Premolar							
Pulp with buccal periodontium and gingiva		X		X			X
Palatal periodontium and gingiva						X	X
First Molar							
Pulp with buccal periodontium and gingiva			X				
Palatal periodontium and gingiva						X	X
Second Molar							
Pulp with buccal periodontium and gingiva			X				
Palatal periodontium and gingiva						X	X
Third Molar							
Pulp with buccal periodontium and gingiva			X				
Palatal periodontium and gingiva						X	X

*Anesthesia for anatomic variants such as absence of middle superior alveolar nerve and resultant variance of mesiobuccal root of maxillary first molar is not included.
AMSA, Anterior middle superior alveolar; *ASA,* anterior superior alveolar; *GP,* greater palatine; *IO,* infraorbital; *MSA,* middle superior alveolar; *NP,* nasopalatine; *PSA,* posterior superior alveolar.
From Fehrenbach MJ, Herring SW: *Illustrated anatomy of the head and neck,* ed 6, St Louis, 2021, Saunders/Elsevier.

If half-mouth treatment is planned, both the inferior alveolar and buccal blocks are administered first (see Chapter 13), then the maxillary facial and palatal injections follow in that order. However, instrumentation initially begins first on the maxillary quadrant; this allows time for the entire mandibular quadrant to become anesthetized. See Fig. 11.5A–B in Chapter 11 for examples of nonsurgical periodontal therapy care plans using local anesthesia.

Local anesthesia should be administered only in the areas of treatment that can be completed in one visit. Overestimating the treatment to be completed on patients with heavy deposits and thus administering larger amount of agent than necessary should be avoided. Thus planning dental hygiene treatment must include local anesthesia as part of the overall treatment plan.[6]

In some cases, there can be access difficulties for the clinician on the approach of the needle to the target site. The patient may have the variation of exostoses present on the facial surface of the maxillary arch, especially within the maxillary posterior sextants, forcing the clinician to work around these bony growths to maintain proper angulation of the needle, keeping the needle parallel to the long axis of the target tooth (Fig. 12.3A).[13] Similarly, a bulky facial alveolar process of the maxilla may hinder ideal angulation of the needle; increasing retraction and moving the needle injection site or needle insertion point more superior usually helps the clinician adapt to this anatomic variation (Fig. 12.3B). Palpating the injection site or needle insertion point with a cotton-tipped applicator before the injection helps determine these needle access problems.[10]

Posterior Superior Alveolar Block

The PSA block in most cases anesthetizes the PSA nerve and thus the maxillary molars and associated buccal periodontium and gingiva within one maxillary quadrant if the MSA nerve is not present, which occurs in approximately 72% of cases (Table 12.7, Figs. G–K and Procedure Box 12.3).[1,3] However, in some cases the mesiobuccal root of the maxillary first molar is not innervated by the PSA nerve, but rather by the MSA nerve when present, which occurs in approximately 28% of cases. Therefore a second injection to anesthetize the MSA nerve by the MSA block is recommended after the administration of the PSA block (see next section, Middle Superior Alveolar Block) to

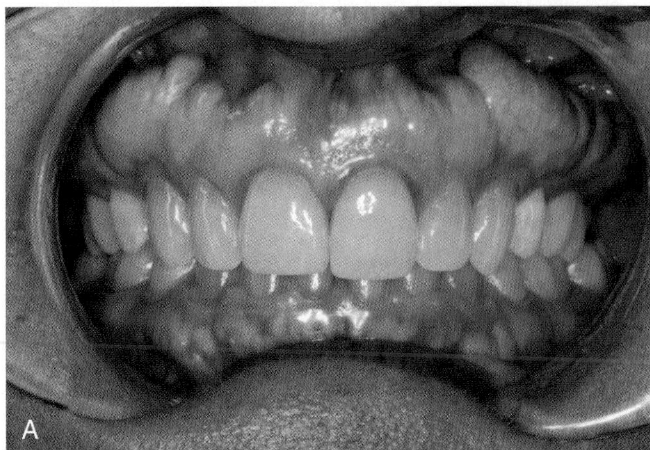

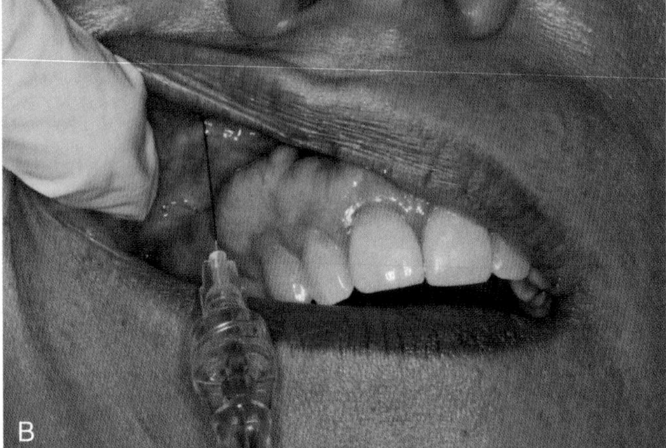

Fig. 12.3 (A) Exostoses present on the facial surface of the maxillary arch. (B) Clinician will need to work around the bony growth to maintain proper angulation of the needle by moving the needle injection site to a more superior location and still keeping the needle parallel to the long axis of the tooth. (Courtesy Sandra Arill, CRDH, Jackie Podboy-Navarro, CRDH, and Alina Guasch, CRDH.)

confirm pulpal anesthesia of all the roots of the maxillary first molar, even during maintenance or recare appointments since exact innervation coverage of the patient is unknown.[6]

In most cases the PSA block is used during quadrant or half-mouth nonsurgical periodontal therapy, but the dental hygienist should consider using this injection also during maintenance or recare appointments since in many cases the maxillary molars, especially unilaterally, are the first teeth involved in periodontal disease.[7] In addition, with many patients now retaining their maxillary third molars, this injection when done correctly can confirm the pulpal anesthesia of the potentially elusive third molars, unlike only using a supraperiosteal injection near the more accessible maxillary second molar.[1] If anesthesia of the associated palatal periodontium and gingiva of the maxillary posterior teeth is desired, the greater palatine block also may be necessary; this is an important consideration with any palatal molar furcation and root concavity involvement.[1,7,9]

Target Area and Injection Site for Posterior Superior Alveolar Block

The target area or deposit location for the PSA block is the PSA nerve branches entering the PSA foramina on the infratemporal surface of the maxilla (see Table 12.7, Fig. G). However, intraoral surface landmarks are also used to confirm nearness to the target area. Thus the PSA foramina are posterosuperior on the maxillary tuberosity as well as superior to the apices of the maxillary second molar.

The presently recommended depth of needle insertion is approximately 16 mm or three-fourths of a short needle. This depth for needle insertion should not vary much from patient to patient with an average skull size.[3] However, this average depth for the average-sized skull could be too deep for patients with smaller than average skull size, increasing the risk for hematoma (discussed later). In contrast, using the average depth of needle insertion in a patient with a larger than average skull size may not provide adequate anesthesia and a long needle may need to be used.[3] However, to decrease the risk for hematoma, a 27-gauge short needle is recommended except for patients with a large skull.[3]

Since student dental hygienists may be tested on clinical and written board examinations using this presently more commonly recommended method, it will be the method specifically described in detail in Table 12.7, Figs. G–K and Procedure 12.3.

However, a newer and more conservative needle insertion technique that is being used by clinicians may be considered. This conservative technique has known clinical effectiveness with initial research to reduce possible complications (discussed later) as the region being anesthetized allows for less depth due to allowance for tissue diffusion.[1,11] This conservative technique also includes avoidance of a long needle but significantly also going to less depth within the height of the mucobuccal fold of the maxillary arch at only approximately 5 to 6 mm or one-fourth of the short needle.[12] Initial studies were completed and now even more extensive recent studies are showing that this conservative technique is just as empirically effective in the clinic as the other more risky protocol since the space fills easily with the agent.[12]

To achieve visibility of the intraoral surface landmarks for maximum clinical effectiveness, ask the patient to partially open and to slide the mandible toward the injection side, opening the area for greater visibility. Many clinicians first palpate posterior to the zygomatic arch and then the alveolar mucosa is retracted vertically, approximately 10 mm posterior to the zygomatic arch so that the posterior part of the maxillary tuberosity is exposed. This is accomplished by pulling the tissue taut using the index finger for intraoral retraction and thumb for extraoral retraction on the dominant side (and vice versa on nondominant side) for visibility and to help with a fulcrum. If horizontal retraction is incorrectly used instead, the overlying upper lip will prevent needle access using the correct angulation.[10] If these small initial steps are done correctly, a concavity in the maxillary mucobuccal fold distal to the maxillary tuberosity will be present allowing for easier access to the target site.

Resting the finger on the posterior surface of the zygomatic arch when retracting can make the clinician feel more confident.[10] Some clinicians suggest a distraction to the insertion to the needle by gently pressing downward on the skin surface slightly posterior to the zygomatic arch during retraction. In addition, a slight pinching of the lip while it is being held open also adds to the distraction.

The injection site or needle insertion point for the PSA block is within the height of the maxillary mucobuccal fold superior to the apices of the maxillary second molar, as well as posterior to the zygomatic arch (Figs. 12.4 and 12.5; see Table 12.7, Fig. J). The needle is inserted within the height of the maxillary mucobuccal fold and advanced in a direction superior to the tooth apices without contacting the bone of the maxilla in order to reduce trauma and then the injection is administered (see Table 12.7, Fig. K). Thus the clinician "enters over the second and administers over the third".

It is important to make sure that the needle will be superior to the apices of the maxillary second molar before entering the tissue, especially on the nondominant side where visualization may be difficult.

TABLE 12.7 Posterior Superior Alveolar Block Review

Indications	Procedures on maxillary molars within one maxillary quadrant; will need to administer ASA and MSA blocks as well as GP and NP blocks to complete maxillary quadrant anesthesia; will need to administer GP block to complete maxillary posterior sextant anesthesia
Nerves anesthetized	PSA nerve
Teeth anesthetized	Maxillary molars in approximately 72% of cases; however, mesiobuccal root of maxillary first molar is not anesthetized in approximately 28% of cases due to presence of MSA nerve
Other structures anesthetized	Buccal periodontium and gingiva of anesthetized teeth
Administration technique	See Procedure 12.3
Needle gauge and length	25- or 27-gauge short
Target area/Deposit location	PSA foramina on infratemporal surface of maxilla and posterosuperior on maxillary tuberosity

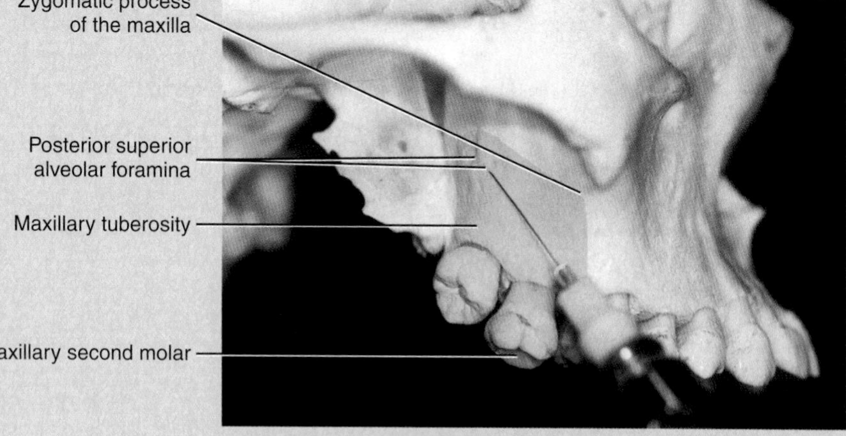

Fig. G = Target area and distribution of anesthesia for PSA block (From Fehrenbach MJ, Herring SW: *Illustrated anatomy of the head and neck,* ed 6, St Louis, 2021, Saunders/Elsevier)

Fig. H = Clinician position of right-handed clinician for PSA block

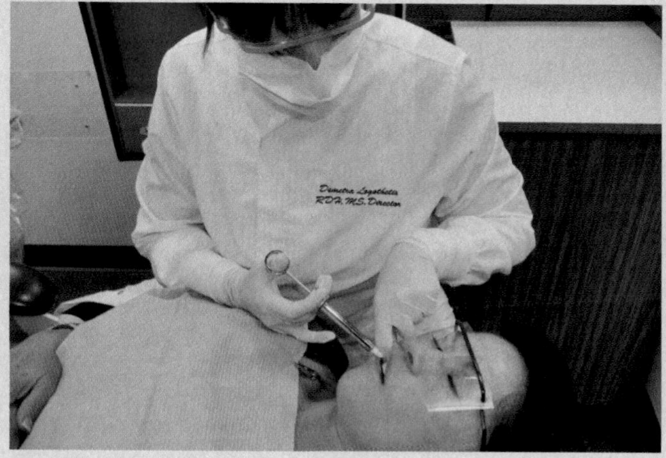

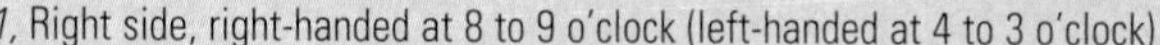

1, Right side, right-handed at 8 to 9 o'clock (left-handed at 4 to 3 o'clock)

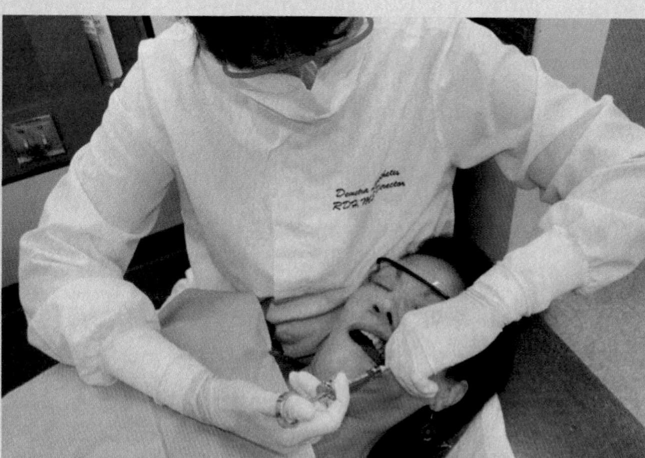

2, Left side, right-handed at 10 o'clock (left-handed at 2 o'clock)

(*Continued*)

TABLE 12.7 Posterior Superior Alveolar Block Review (*Cont.*)

Fig. I = Syringe stabilization with fulcrums for PSA block

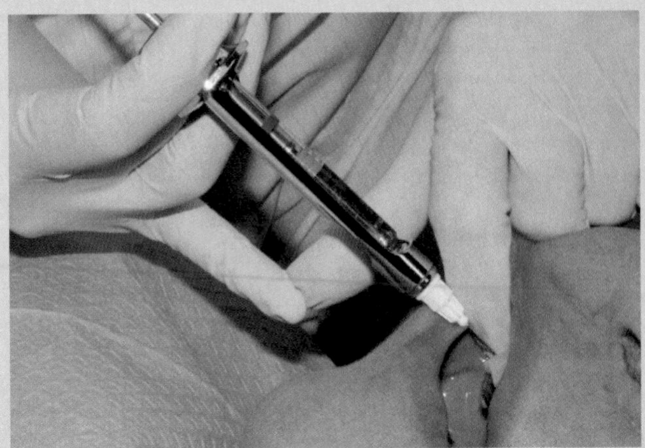

1, Double finger support

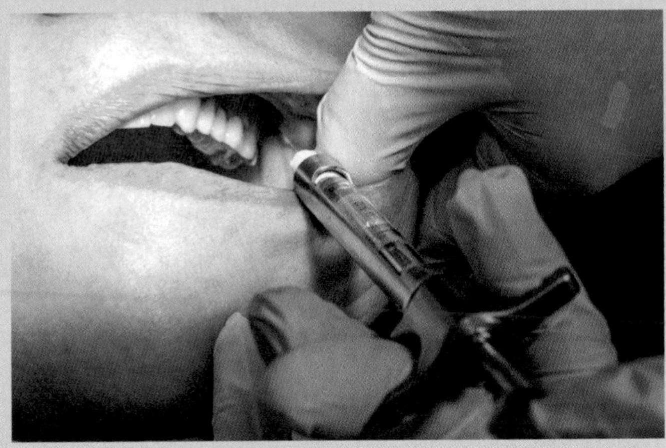

2, Rest syringe barrel on index finger or thumb of retraction hand for left side and if possible use pinky finger of dominant hand to rest on chin

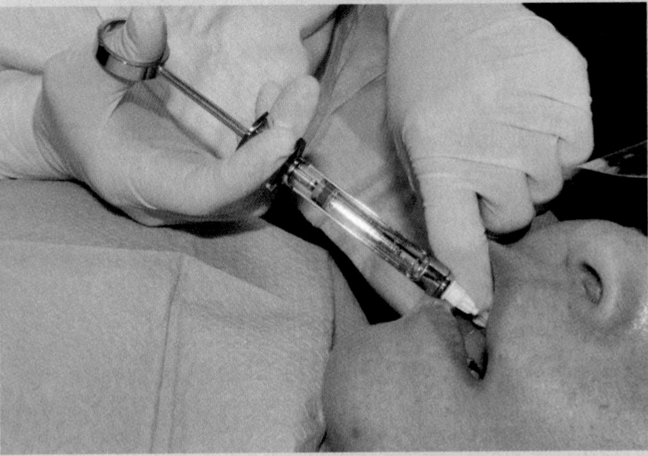

3, Syringe barrel resting on index finger of retraction hand for right side and if possible use pinky finger of dominant hand to rest on chin

Landmarks	Maxillary tuberosity Posterior superior alveolar foramina Maxillary mucobuccal fold Maxillary second molar Zygomatic arch Maxillary occlusal plane
Injection site/Needle insertion point 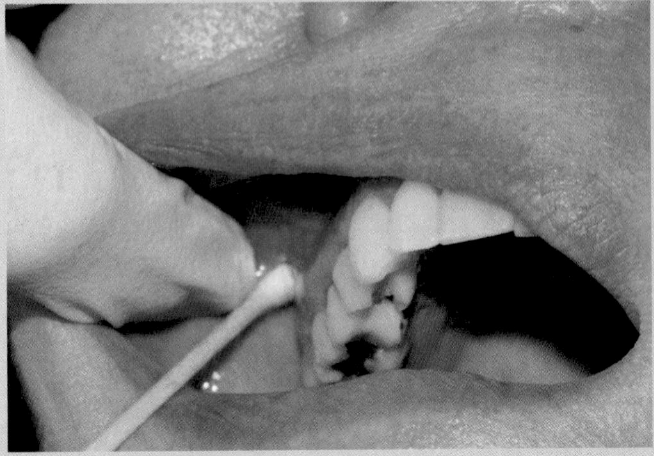 Fig. J = Injection site for PSA block	Within height of maxillary mucobuccal fold superior to apices of maxillary second molar, posterior to maxilla arch and with correct angulations to maxillary occlusal plane and long axis of tooth

TABLE 12.7 Posterior Superior Alveolar Block Review (*Cont.*)

Depth of needle insertion 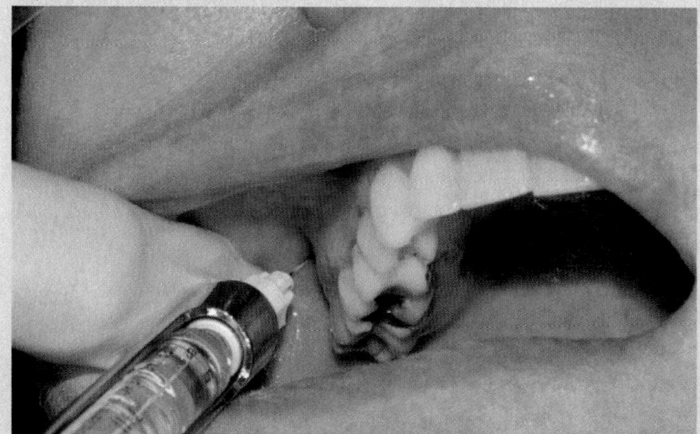 Fig. K = Needle insertion for PSA block (when not using conservative technique)	Approximately 16 mm or three-fourths of short needle (when not using conservative technique)
Amount of anesthetic agent	Approximately 0.9 to 1.8 mL or one-half to one cartridge
Length of time to deposit	Approximately 60 to 90 seconds

ASA, anterior superior alveolar; *GP,* greater palatine; *MSA*, middle superior alveolar; *NP,* nasopalatine; *PSA*, posterior superior alveolar.

PROCEDURE BOX 12.3 Posterior Superior Alveolar Block Procedure

Step 1 Assume the correct clinician position for right side, right-handed at 8 to 9 o'clock (left-handed at 4–3 o'clock); left side, right-handed at 10 o'clock (left-handed at 2 o'clock; see Table 12.7, Fig. H).

Step 2 Ask the supine patient to partially open and to slide the mandible toward the injection side, opening the area for greater visibility. Retract the cheek vertically and not horizontally, pulling the tissue taut using the index finger for intraoral retraction and thumb for extraoral retraction on the dominant side (and vice versa on nondominant side) for visibility and to help with a fulcrum. Sterile gauze may be used to help retract slippery tissue.

Step 3 Prepare the alveolar mucosa within the height of the maxillary mucobuccal fold superior to the apices of the maxillary second molar (as discussed in Chapter 11) and palpate the injection site or needle insertion point to confirm that only soft tissue is injected (see Table 12.7, Fig. J).

Step 4 Using a 25- or 27-gauge short needle in the syringe of the dominant hand orient the bevel of the needle away from the large window of the syringe to confirm the bevel orientation is toward the bone.

Step 5 Establish a fulcrum by resting the syringe on the index finger or thumb that is retracting the cheek to confirm that the syringe is backward at 45° to the long axis of the tooth, while the finger rests posterior to the zygomatic arch while retracting (see Table 12.7, Fig. I for fulcrum recommendations). The syringe should be extended from the ipsilateral corner of the mouth, possibly pressing downward on the lower lip to maintain the angulations.

Step 6 Insert the needle within the height of the maxillary mucobuccal fold superior to the apices of the maxillary second molar and gently advance the needle in an upward, inward, and backward direction at 45° in each direction until desired depth of the needle is achieved at 16 mm or three-fourths of the short needle for most situations (unless using the conservative technique) (Table 12.7, Fig. K). Angulation may need adjusting once the syringe is in the mouth but before tissue is entered; do not move the needle in the tissue to establish correct angulation. There should be no bony contact upon insertion.

Step 7 Aspirate within three planes due to the high vascularity in the area of anesthetic deposition and to confirm that the bevel of the needle is not abutted against the interior of a blood vessel providing a false aspiration. To accomplish this, first aspirate as usual at the depth of insertion. If aspiration is negative, rotate the syringe barrel gently toward the clinician and reaspirate; if aspiration is negative, rotate the syringe barrel gently back to the original position and aspirate again.

Step 8 If a negative aspiration is achieved after each of three aspirations, slowly deposit approximately 0.9 to 1.8 mL of agent (one-half to one cartridge) over approximately 60 to 90 seconds and aspirate in the same plane after each fourth of the cartridge is administered.

Step 9 Carefully withdraw the syringe, possibly stepping it up near the final removal movements to avoid nicking the lower lip with the tip of the needle and immediately recap the needle using the one-handed scoop method utilizing a needle sheath prop (see Chapter 11).

Step 10 Wait approximately 3 to 5 minutes until anesthesia takes effect before starting treatment.

Otherwise, not all of the three maxillary molars or their associated tissue will be effectively anesthetized if the anesthetic agent is incorrectly administered superior to the apices of the maxillary first molar.

In addition, the correct needle and syringe barrel angulation to the injection site or needle insertion point must be maintained throughout the injection using three different orientations but only one insertion movement. This angulation should be superiorly (or upward) at 45° to the maxillary occlusal plane and medially (or inward) at 45° to the midsagittal plane. The angulation also needs to be posteriorly (or backward) at 45° to the long axis of the maxillary second molar and conforming to the contour of the maxillary tuberosity.[1,3]

To accomplish this injection in these three planes within one pass, the syringe barrel should be extended from the ipsilateral corner of the mouth, possibly pressing downward on the lower lip to maintain the angulations (Fig. 12.6). This possibly complex orientation, along with all the discussed injections, can be practiced using a long cotton-tipped applicator or a training needle set up on the syringe (see Chapters 9 and 11) to palpate the insertion site and to visualize the needle and

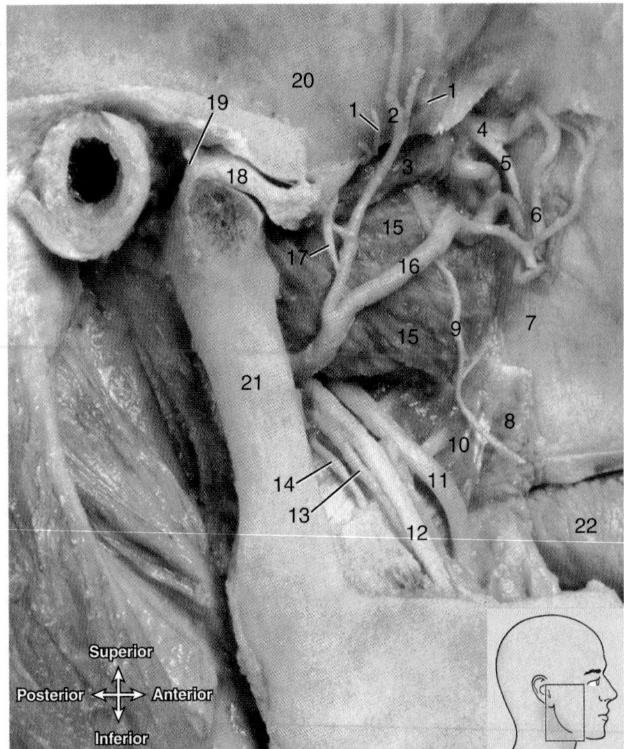

Fig. 12.4 Dissection of the right infratemporal fossa to show the injection site or needle insertion point for the posterior superior alveolar block (*inset:* note removal of the lateral pterygoid muscle, zygomatic arch, and part of the mandible). The inferior alveolar block injection site or needle insertion point is also shown and is discussed in Chapter 13. *1,* Deep temporal nerve; *2,* Deep temporal artery; *3,* Lateral pterygoid muscle; *4,* Maxillary nerve; *5,* Posterior superior alveolar nerve; *6,* Posterior superior alveolar artery; *7,* Infratemporal surface of maxilla; *8,* Buccinator muscle; *9,* Buccal nerve; *10,* Medial pterygoid muscle; *11,* Lingual nerve; *12,* Inferior alveolar nerve; *13,* Inferior alveolar artery; *14,* Mylohyoid nerve; *15,* Lateral pterygoid muscle; *16,* Maxillary artery; *17,* Masseteric nerve; *18,* Joint disc of the temporomandibular joint with mandibular condyle; *19,* Joint capsule; *20,* Temporal bone; *21,* Mandibular ramus; *22,* Tongue. (From Logan BM, Reynold PA, Hutching RT: *McMinn's color atlas of head and neck anatomy,* ed 4, London, 2010, Mosby. In Fehrenbach MJ, Herring SW: *Illustrated anatomy of the head and neck,* ed 6, St Louis, 2021, Saunders/Elsevier.)

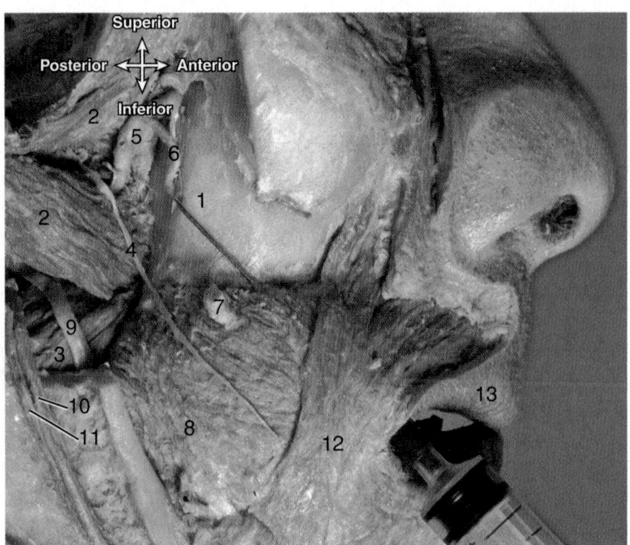

Fig. 12.5 Dissection showing the needle at the injection site or needle insertion point for a posterior superior alveolar block. *1,* Posterior surface of maxilla; *2,* Lateral pterygoid muscle; *3,* Medial pterygoid muscle; *4,* Buccal nerve; *5,* Maxillary artery; *6,* Posterior superior alveolar nerve and vessels; *7,* Parotid salivary duct; *8,* Buccinator muscle; *9,* Lingual nerve; *10,* Inferior alveolar nerve; *11,* Inferior alveolar artery; *12,* Corner of lip; *13,* Upper lip. (From Logan BM, Reynold PA, Hutching RT: *McMinn's color atlas of head and neck anatomy,* ed 4, London, 2010, Mosby. In Fehrenbach MJ, Herring SW: *Illustrated anatomy of the head and neck,* ed 6, St Louis, 2021, Saunders/Elsevier.)

barrel angulations.[1,10] Many clinicians note that if retraction is done correctly for the PSA block, the intraoral retracting finger points to the injection site. Other say that having the maxillary occlusal plane at 45° to the floor helps with overall orientation.

When attempting the nondominant side for the PSA block, the correct angulation of the needle and syringe barrel may be harder again to ascertain from across the patient's face; however, the needle should follow the same pathway as the nondominant arm, always toward the surface of the maxilla and the clinician's body.

With the PSA block there should be no bending of the needle shank in order to accomplish the necessary needle and syringe barrel angulations as discussed.[3] The needle can break when bent and there is little control over the needle direction, needle angulation, and needle bevel. Nor should any change in direction of the needle within the tissue to obtain correct angulation be performed as this may cause trauma since the correct angulations should be established before entering the soft tissue.[10,11]

Since the PSA block is usually administered first before other needed injections in the maxillary quadrant (discussed earlier), the PSA block is an effective way to introduce the patient to less discomfort with local anesthesia as performed by a competent clinician (see Chapter 11). These lower levels of discomfort come from the fact that the injection does not contact bone and the relatively large area of soft tissue into which the local anesthetic agent is deposited. In addition, it does not involve any nerve "shock."[1,3] This early introduction will go a long way toward relaxing the patient for further injections to complete either within the maxillary quadrant or with half-mouth anesthesia.[10]

Indications of Clinically Effective Posterior Superior Alveolar Block and Possible Complications

Usually there are no overt indications of a clinically effective PSA block. Thus the patient frequently has difficulty determining the extent of anesthesia because the lip or the tongue does not feel numb as occurs with the more commonly used inferior alveolar block or mandibular block.[1] Instead, the patient will state that the teeth in the area feel dull when gently tapped and there will be an absence of discomfort during dental procedures. It may be necessary to inform the patient of this situation before starting the procedure so as to reduce fears that the local anesthetic agent has not worked.

Inadvertent and harmless anesthesia of branches of the mandibular nerve may also occur with a PSA block because these branches may be located at a more superior level and thus lateral to the PSA nerve in some cases.[1,11] This injection may result in subsequent levels of mandibular lingual anesthesia and numbness of the lower lip in some patients; thus it is important to try to avoid depositing lateral to the PSA nerve.

As discussed, the maxilla should not be contacted at any time during the PSA injection. If bone is contacted immediately after the needle is inserted into the soft tissue, the medial angle of the syringe barrel toward the maxillary occlusal plane is too great at more than 45°. Instead, the syringe barrel needs to be closer to the maxillary occlusal plane thus reducing the medial angle to less than 45°. The clinician

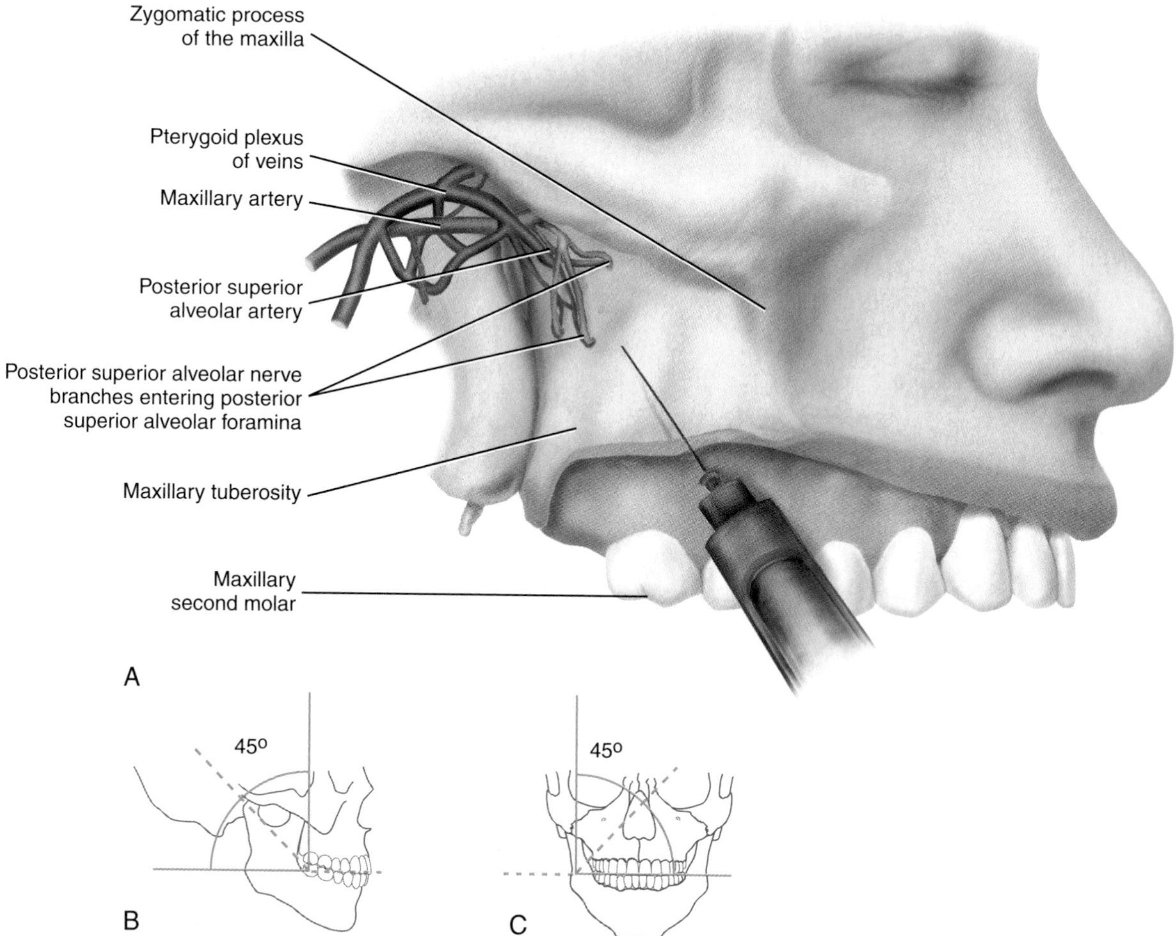

Fig. 12.6 (A) Correct insertion of the needle during a posterior superior alveolar block is superior to the apices of the maxillary second molar without contacting the maxilla. If the needle is overinserted, it can pierce the pterygoid plexus of the veins and maxillary artery, which may lead to complications such as a hematoma. (B) To prevent this complication, the needle and syringe barrel angulation should be superiorly *(or upward)* at 45° to the maxillary occlusal plane. (C) Additionally the needle and syringe barrel angulation needs to be medially *(or inward)* at 45° to the midsagittal plane as well as posteriorly *(or backward)* at 45° to the long axis of the maxillary second molar. (From Fehrenbach MJ, Herring SW: *Illustrated anatomy of the head and neck,* ed 6, St Louis, 2021, Saunders/Elsevier.)

needs to remove the syringe and reinsert the needle to reduce any further trauma to the tissue to perform this alternative needle insertion.

Positive aspiration is approximately 3.1%; it is the third highest rate of all the block injections due to the nearness of the PSA blood vessels.[1,3,11] Thus clinicians recommend aspiration several times within different planes before administration to reduce risk and to further reaspirate if there is any movement of the needle within the tissue. In addition, clinicians believe that the PSA block should not be used in children due to its inherent risks and have found clinical effectiveness with using supraperiosteal injections instead for the maxillary posterior sextant (see Chapter 14).

Complications can occur if the needle is advanced too deep into the tissue as when using a long needle instead of a recommended short one during a PSA block (Table 12.8; see Figs. 12.5 and 12.6).[3] The needle may pierce the deeper pterygoid plexus of veins and the maxillary artery if overinserted, possibly damaging these blood vessels within the infratemporal fossa (see Chapter 10).[1] This results in a bluish-reddish extraoral swelling of hemorrhaging blood that may form an extraoral hematoma in the tissue covering the infratemporal fossa on the affected side of the face a few minutes after the injection. The lesion progresses over time inferiorly and anteriorly toward the lower anterior region of the cheek (see Chapter 16).

This temporary hematoma can be overwhelming to both the patient and to the clinician. In addition, unlike other blocks, there is no easily accessible intraoral area for the PSA block to which pressure can be applied to stop the hemorrhage. And even though this is a basic risk of local anesthetic injections, care must be taken to avoid this situation.[3] Aspiration should always be attempted before all injections as outlined before administration in order to avoid injection into blood vessels and damaging them (see Chapter 11).

In addition, if the needle is contaminated, there may be a spread of needle tract infection from the infratemporal space to the even deeper cavernous sinus (see Chapter 16).[1,14,15] The clinician should always assess the infection level of the patient before proceeding with dental care and use strict standard infection control at all times during the procedure (see Chapter 11).

Middle Superior Alveolar Block

The MSA block anesthetizes the maxillary premolars and the mesiobuccal root of the maxillary first molar as well as the associated buccal

TABLE 12.8 Posterior Superior Alveolar Block Complications

Complication	Technique Adjustment/ Recommendation
Bone is contacted because the angle of needle is too great since the syringe barrel toward midline at more than 45°	Withdraw syringe and reinsert needle closer to maxillary occlusal plane and thus reducing angle to less than 45°
Hematoma caused by overinsertion of needle that pierces and damages the pterygoid plexus of veins and/or maxillary artery	Use more conservative technique in future with only short needle by only advancing to one-fourth of short needle or 5 to 6 mm and/or modify depth of needle for children and small adults; avoid use in children if possible (see Chapter 14); use extraoral pressure over hematoma in region with sterile gauze square and reassure patient
Mandibular anesthesia from branches of mandibular division of trigeminal nerve located lateral to PSA nerve	Avoid depositing lateral to PSA nerve

PSA, Posterior superior alveolar.

periodontium and gingiva within one maxillary quadrant if the MSA nerve is present to be anesthetized, which occurs in approximately 28% of cases (Table 12.9, Figs. L–P and Procedure Box 12.4). When the MSA nerve is absent as occurs in approximately 72% of cases, the region is instead innervated by both the PSA and the ASA nerves as part of the superior dental plexus, but mainly by the ASA nerve.[1,3,11] Thus to confirm complete anesthesia to the entire maxillary quadrant, most clinicians administer this block even though the MSA nerve may not be present or when only instrumenting the maxillary premolars.[3]

Using this block will confirm complete patient comfort when the dental hygienist is instrumenting the maxillary first premolar with its mesial root depression that is prone to heavier deposits.[9] If anesthesia of the associated palatal periodontium and gingiva of the maxillary premolars is necessary, the greater palatine block may also be indicated.

Target Area and Injection Site for Middle Superior Alveolar Block

The target area or deposit location for the MSA block is the MSA nerve, if present, as part of the superior dental plexus that is located superior to the apex of the maxillary second premolar (Fig. 12.7; see Table 12.9, Fig. L). Thus the injection site or needle insertion point is within the height of the maxillary mucobuccal fold superior to the apex of the maxillary second premolar (see Table 12.9, Fig. O).

Some clinicians suggest a distraction to the insertion to the needle by gently pressing downward on the skin surface slightly anterior to

TABLE 12.9 Middle Superior Alveolar Block Review

Indications	Procedures on maxillary premolars within one maxillary quadrant
Nerves anesthetized	MSA nerve when present in approximately 28% of cases; mainly ASA nerve as well as PSA nerve when MSA nerve is absent in approximately 72% of cases
Teeth anesthetized	Maxillary premolars and mesiobuccal root of maxillary first molar
Other structures anesthetized	Buccal periodontium and gingiva of anesthetized teeth as well as buccal mucosa and upper lip
Administration technique	See Procedure Box 12.4
Needle gauge and length	27-gauge short
Target area/Deposit location	Superior to apex of maxillary second premolar

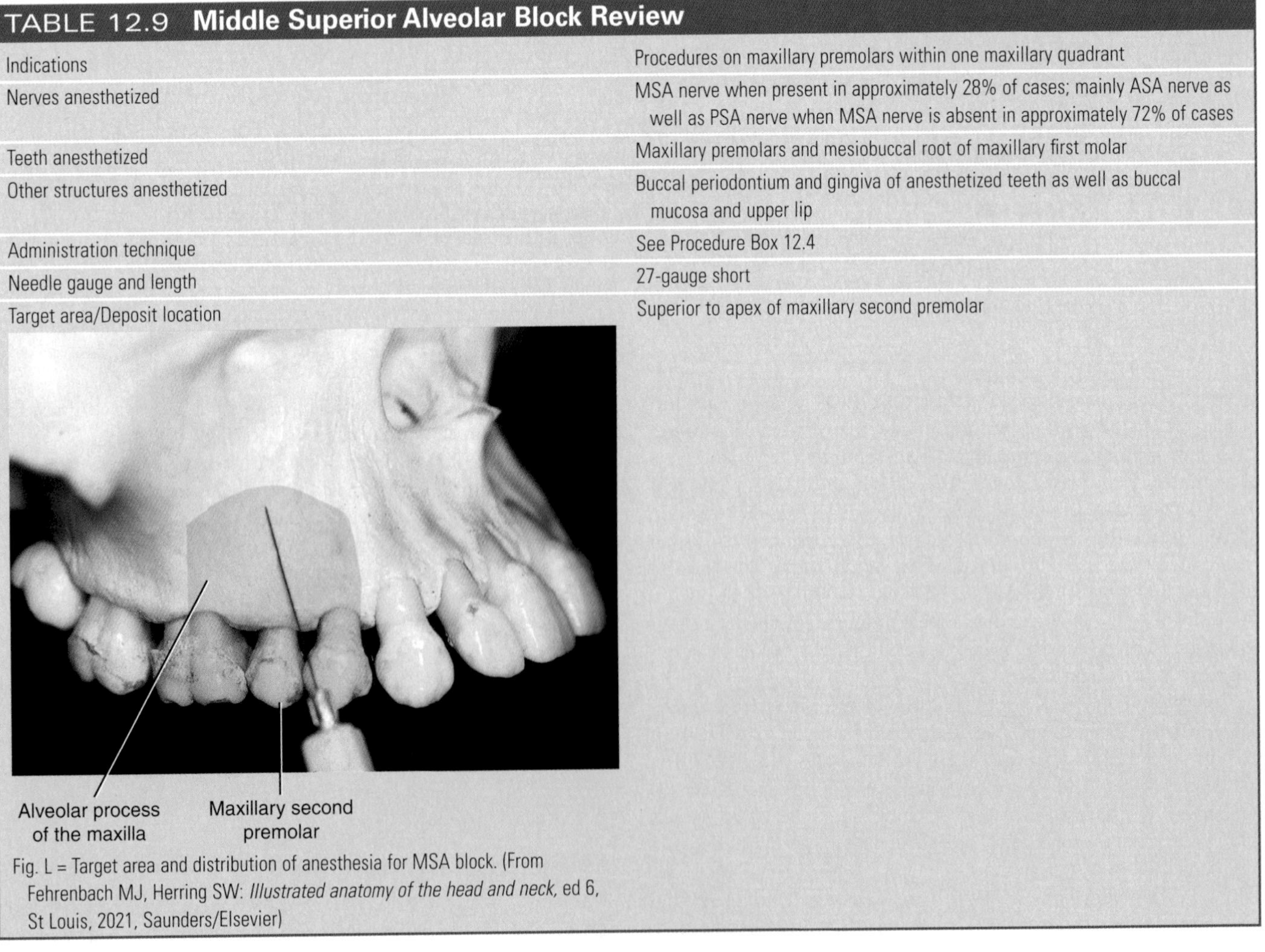

Fig. L = Target area and distribution of anesthesia for MSA block. (From Fehrenbach MJ, Herring SW: *Illustrated anatomy of the head and neck*, ed 6, St Louis, 2021, Saunders/Elsevier)

TABLE 12.9 Middle Superior Alveolar Block Review (*Cont.*)

Fig. M = Clinician position of right-handed clinician for MSA block (same as for ASA block or IO block)

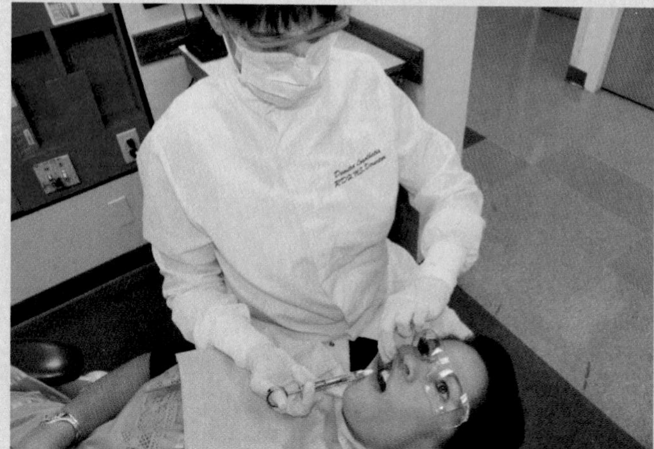

1, Right side, right-handed at 8 o'clock (left-handed at 4 o'clock)

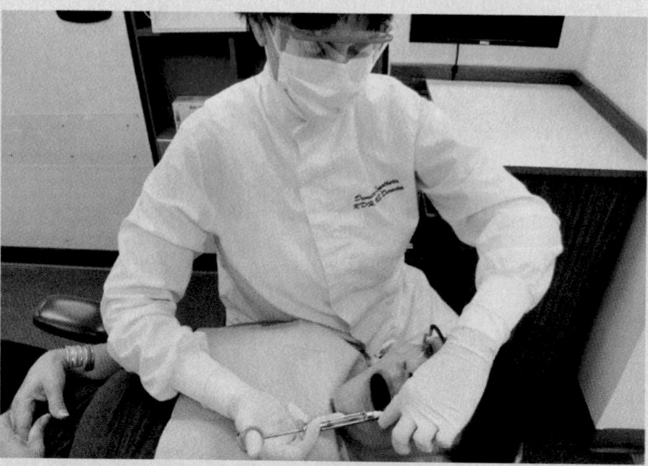

2, Left side, right-handed at 9 o'clock (left-handed at 3 o'clock)

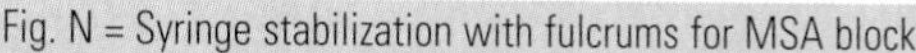

Fig. N = Syringe stabilization with fulcrums for MSA block

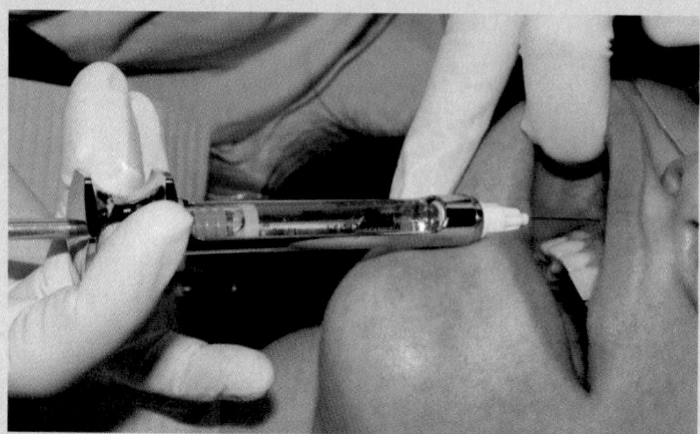

1, Support syringe barrel with finger from retraction hand

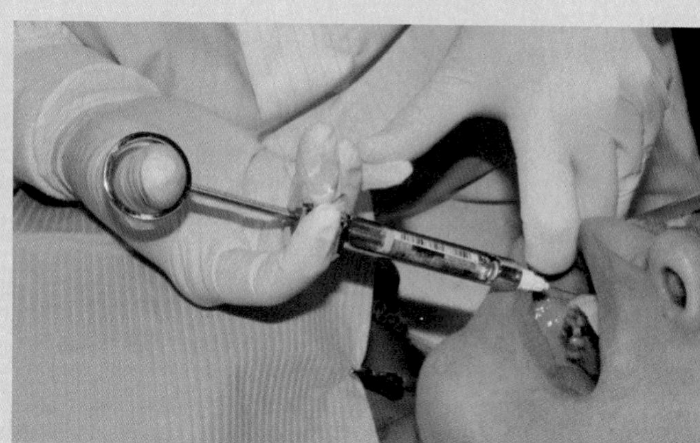

2, Double finger support

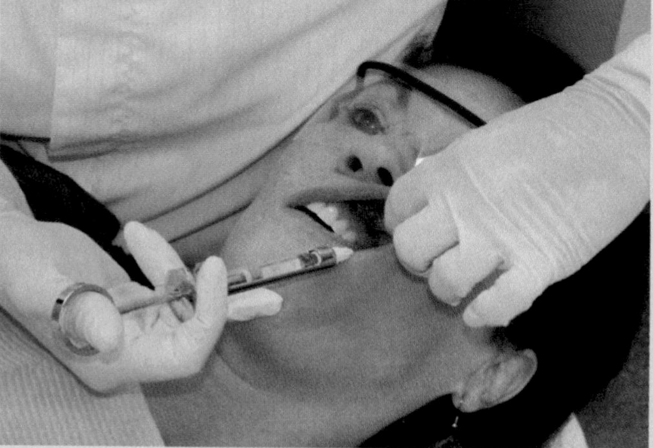

3, Rest pinky finger of dominant hand on patient's chin

(*Continued*)

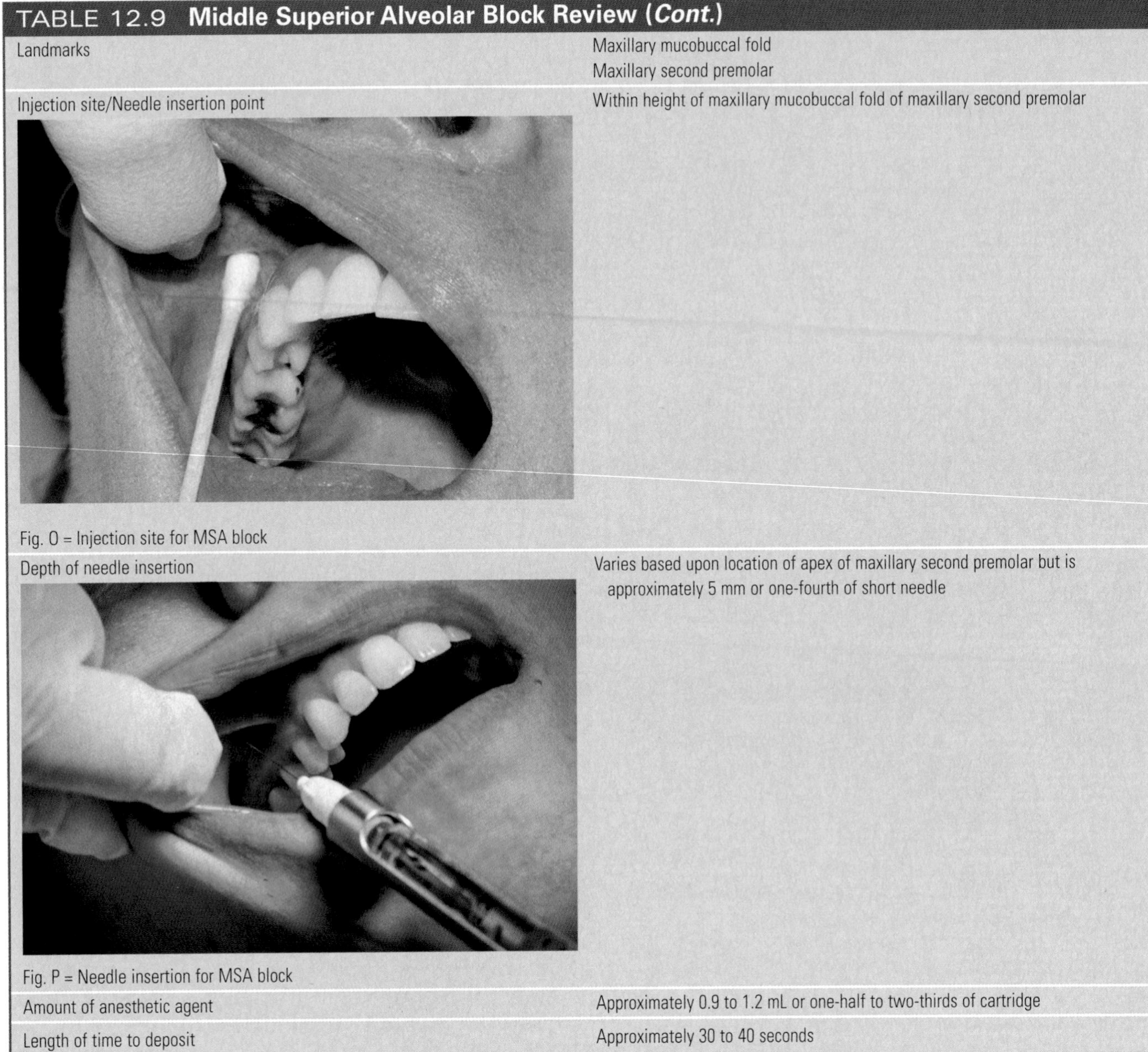

TABLE 12.9 Middle Superior Alveolar Block Review (*Cont.*)	
Landmarks	Maxillary mucobuccal fold Maxillary second premolar
Injection site/Needle insertion point Fig. O = Injection site for MSA block	Within height of maxillary mucobuccal fold of maxillary second premolar
Depth of needle insertion Fig. P = Needle insertion for MSA block	Varies based upon location of apex of maxillary second premolar but is approximately 5 mm or one-fourth of short needle
Amount of anesthetic agent	Approximately 0.9 to 1.2 mL or one-half to two-thirds of cartridge
Length of time to deposit	Approximately 30 to 40 seconds

ASA, Anterior superior alveolar; *IO*, infraorbital; *MSA*, middle superior alveolar.

the zygomatic arch during retraction. In addition, a slight pinching of the lip while it is being held open also adds to the distraction.

The needle is then angled at approximately 10° off an imaginary line drawn parallel to the long axis of the maxillary second premolar and following the contour of the maxilla. The needle is inserted within the height of the maxillary mucobuccal fold and advanced until its tip is located superior to the apex of the maxillary second premolar without contacting the maxilla in order to reduce trauma, and then the injection is administered (see Table 12.9, Fig. P).

As previously noted, because the root length varies, the depth of needle insertion superior to the apex of the maxillary second premolar will vary. For the MSA block, the clinician should review the average root length of the maxillary second premolar to help make this adjustment of needle depth more accurate to achieve a clinically effective injection (see Table 12.2).[8]

If one of the maxillary premolars has been extracted during orthodontic therapy, thereby moving the still present premolar from the original place within the dental arch, the target area can initially be estimated by administering the injection equidistant from the maxillary tuberosity to the midline within the maxillary arch to provide the most clinically effective anesthetic coverage to the region.[9,16]

Finally, adjusting the upper lip by pulling it more anteriorly helps to avoid having the needle go through any large buccal frena. If not able to avoid these tissue variations, administer the injection slightly posterior rather than anterior to the recommended site for more complete coverage of these intended posterior teeth and their associated tissue.[10]

Indications of Clinically Effective Middle Superior Alveolar Block and Possible Complications

Indications of a clinically effective MSA block include harmless tingling and numbness of the upper lip and absence of discomfort during dental procedures. Positive aspiration less than approximately 3.1%; thus overinsertion with complications such as a hematoma is rare with the MSA block (Table 12.10).[3]

PROCEDURE BOX 12.4 Middle Superior Alveolar Block Procedure

Step 1 Assume the correct clinician position for right side, right-handed at 8 o'clock (left-handed at 4 o'clock); left side, right-handed at 9 o'clock (left-handed at 3 o'clock; see Table 12.9, Fig. M).

Step 2 Ask the supine patient to open and then retract the upper lip, pulling the tissue taut; sterile gauze may be used to help retract slippery tissue. Pull the upper lip more anteriorly to avoid having to go through any large frena if present.

Step 3 Prepare the alveolar mucosa within the height of the maxillary mucobuccal fold superior to the apex of the maxillary second premolar (see Chapter 11) and palpate the injection site or needle insertion point to confirm only soft tissue is injected (see Table 12.9, Fig. O).

Step 4 Using a 27-gauge short needle in the syringe of the dominant hand, orient the bevel of the needle away from the large window of the syringe to confirm the bevel orientation is toward the bone.

Step 5 Establish a fulcrum (see Table 12.9, Fig. N for fulcrum recommendations).

Step 6 Place the syringe parallel with the long axis of the tooth with the large window facing the clinician.

Step 7 Insert the needle within the height of the maxillary mucobuccal fold superior to the apex of the maxillary second premolar; the needle depth may vary based on the location of the apex of the maxillary second premolar but is approximately 5 mm or one-fourth of a short needle or until the bevel is slightly superior to the apex of the tooth (see Table 12.9, Fig. P). There should be no bony contact upon insertion.

Step 8 Aspirate within two planes.

Step 9 If a negative aspiration is achieved slowly deposit approximately 0.9 to 1.2 mL of agent (one-half to two-thirds of cartridge) over approximately 30 to 40 seconds; if the tissue balloons, injection is too rapid.

Step 10 Carefully withdraw the syringe and immediately recap the needle using the one-handed scoop method utilizing a needle sheath prop (see Chapter 11).

Step 11 Wait approximately 3 to 5 minutes until anesthesia takes effect before starting treatment.

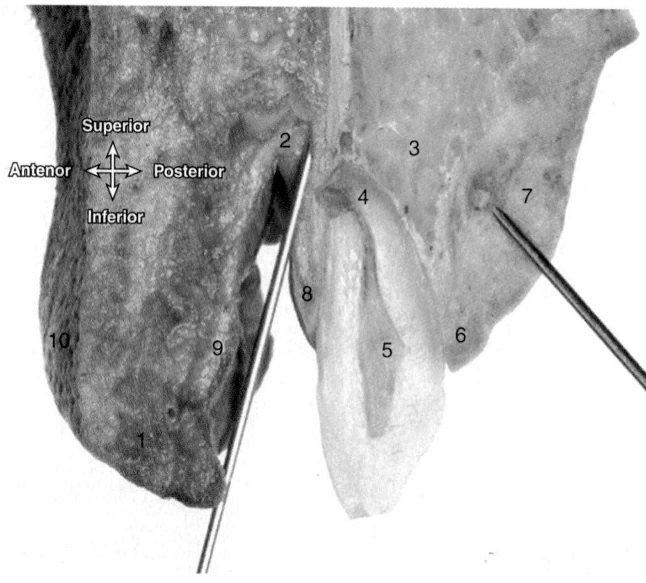

Fig. 12.7 Dissection of the maxilla through the permanent maxillary first premolar with one needle *(to left)* at the injection site or needle insertion point for middle superior alveolar block and the other needle *(to right)* at the injection site or needle insertion point for the anterior middle superior alveolar block. *1,* Upper lip; *2,* Height of maxillary mucobuccal fold; *3,* Alveolar process of maxilla; *4,* Apex of tooth; *5,* Pulp cavity; *6,* Palatal gingival margin; *7,* Mucoperiosteum of anterior hard palate; *8,* Buccal gingival margin; *9,* Labial mucosa; *10,* Buccal mucosa. (From Logan BM, Reynold PA, Hutching RT: *McMinn's color atlas of head and neck anatomy,* ed 4, London, 2010, Mosby. In Fehrenbach MJ, Herring SW: *Illustrated anatomy of the head and neck,* ed 6, St Louis, 2021, Saunders/Elsevier.)

TABLE 12.10 Middle Superior Alveolar Block Complications

Complication	Technique Adjustment
Presence of large buccal frenum (frena) at site of needle insertion	Insert needle more posterior to injection site and retract lip and buccal frenum (frena) more anteriorly to avoid going through large frenum (frena); however, avoid moving injection site too anterior and lose anesthetic coverage
Only one premolar present due to extraction for orthodontic therapy	Inject equidistant within maxillary arch to provide most clinically effective anesthetic coverage
Pain on insertion with needle against periosteum	Withdraw needle and reinsert farther away (or lateral) from periosteum
Pain during injection from injecting too rapidly	Due to acidic anesthetic agent, care should be taken to inject slowly so as to not exceed recommended deposit time
Inadequate anesthesia from injecting inferior to apex of maxillary second premolar	Increase depth of insertion upon reinsertion to confirm placement of agent superior to apex of maxillary second premolar
Possible inadequate anesthesia from dense bone covering apex (or apices)	Instead administer IO block (see Table 12.13)
Possible inadequate anesthesia from injecting into area of infection or risk of needle tract infection	Instead administer IO block (see Table 12.13)

IO, Infraorbital.

Anterior Superior Alveolar Block

The ASA block anesthetizes the ASA nerve and thus the maxillary anterior teeth and associated labial periodontium and gingiva to the midline within one maxillary quadrant. It is commonly used in conjunction with an MSA block instead of using an IO block alone to anesthetize these teeth (Table 12.11, Figs. Q–U, and Procedure Box 12.5). Communication occurs between the MSA nerve and both the ASA and PSA nerves as part of the superior dental plexus. Some clinicians consider the ASA block to be only a supraperiosteal injection but since it has a larger area of anesthesia and the local anesthetic agent is deposited near the larger nerve trunk of the ASA nerve, it can be considered a nerve block.[1,3]

In addition, in some cases there is overlap of the right and left ASA nerves and the tissue they innervate due to crossover-innervation; this may need to be taken into account when using local anesthesia in this area (see Chapter 10). Crossover-innervation is the overlap of terminal

TABLE 12.11 Anterior Superior Alveolar Block Review	
Indications	Procedures on maxillary anterior teeth within one maxillary quadrant; use also for crossover-innervation on contralateral quadrant following ASA block or IO block
Nerves anesthetized	ASA nerve
Teeth anesthetized	Maxillary anterior teeth
Other structures anesthetized	Labial periodontium and gingiva of anesthetized teeth as well as labial mucosa and upper lip
Administration technique	See Procedure Box 12.5
Needle gauge and length	27-gauge short
Target area/Deposit location	Superior to apex of maxillary canine
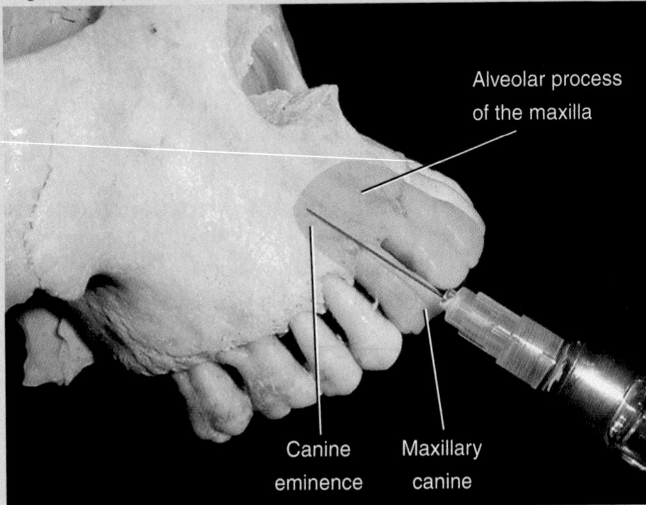 Fig. Q = Target area and distribution of anesthesia for ASA block (From Fehrenbach MJ, Herring SW: *Illustrated anatomy of the head and neck,* ed 6, St Louis, 2021, Saunders/Elsevier)	
Fig. R = Clinician position of right-handed clinician for ASA block (same as for MSA or IO blocks)	
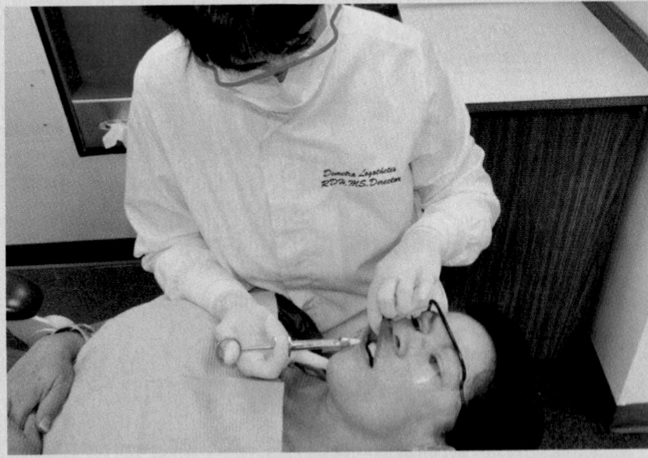 *1,* Right side, right-handed at 8 o'clock (left-handed at 4 o'clock)	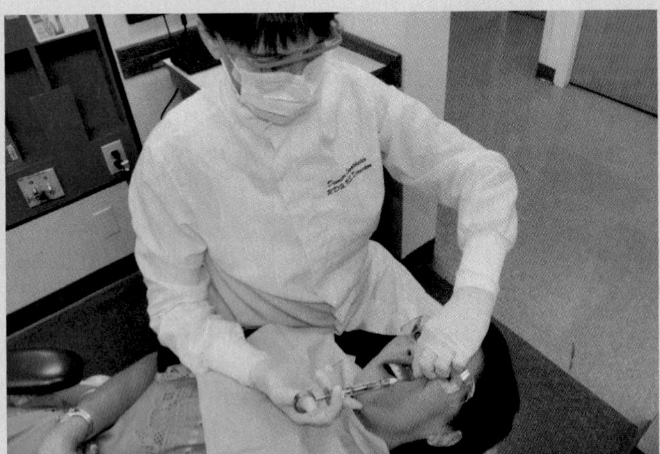 *2,* Left side, right-handed at 9 o'clock (left-handed at 3 o'clock)

TABLE 12.11 Anterior Superior Alveolar Block Review (*Cont.*)

Fig. S = Syringe stabilization with fulcrums for ASA block	
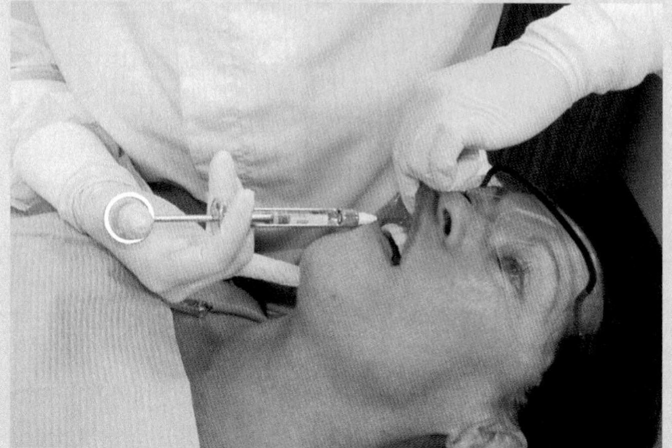 *1.* Rest pinky finger of dominant hand on patient's chin	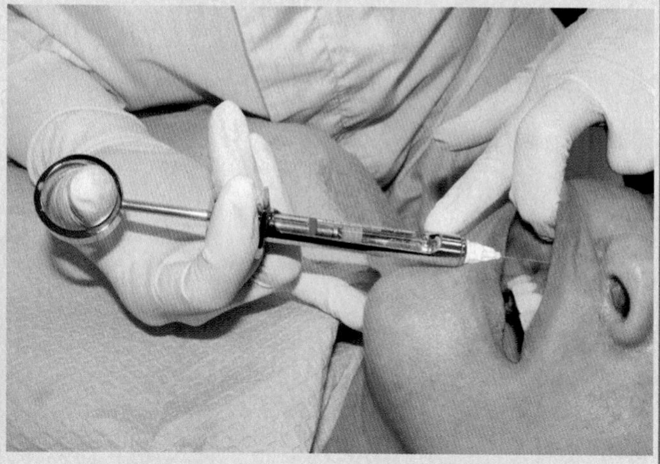 *2.* Support syringe barrel with finger from retraction hand
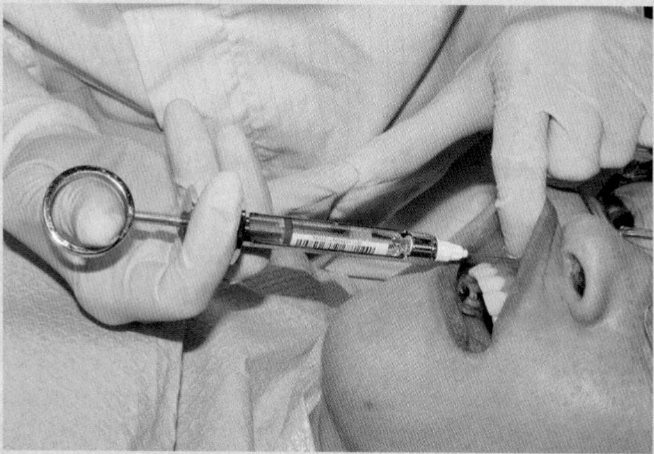 *3.* Double finger support	
Landmarks	Maxillary mucobuccal fold Maxillary canine Canine eminence
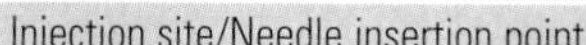 Injection site/Needle insertion point 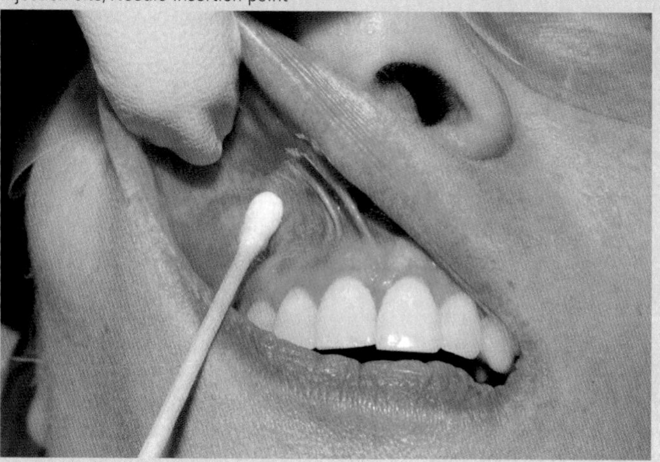 Fig. T = Injection site for ASA block	Within height of maxillary mucobuccal fold of maxillary canine and just medial to and parallel to canine eminence

(*Continued*)

TABLE 12.11 Anterior Superior Alveolar Block Review (*Cont.*)

Depth of needle insertion	Varies based on location of apex of maxillary canine but is approximately 5 to 6 mm
Fig. U = Needle insertion for ASA block	
Amount of anesthetic agent	Approximately 0.9 to 1.2 mL or one-half to two-thirds of cartridge
Length of time to deposit	Approximately 30 to 40 seconds

ASA, Anterior superior alveolar; *IO,* infraorbital; *MSA,* middle superior alveolar.

PROCEDURE BOX 12.5 Anterior Superior Alveolar Block Procedure

Step 1 Assume the correct clinician position for right side, right-handed at 8 o'clock (left-handed at 4 o'clock) or left side, right-handed at 9 o'clock (left-handed at 3 o'clock; see Table 12.11, Fig. R).

Step 2 Ask the supine patient to open and then retract the upper lip by pulling the tissue taut outward and then upward only at the tip using the index finger and thumb of the nondominant hand (one inside and one outside); sterile gauze can be wrapped around the tip to help retract slippery tissue.

Step 3 Prepare the alveolar mucosa within the height of the maxillary mucobuccal fold superior to the apex of the maxillary canine, just medial to and parallel with the canine eminence (see Chapter 11) and palpate the injection site or needle insertion point to confirm only soft tissue is injected (see Table 12.11, Fig. T).

Step 4 Using a 27-gauge short needle in the syringe, orient the bevel of the needle away from the large window of the syringe to confirm the bevel orientation is toward the bone.

Step 5 Establish a fulcrum (see Table 12.11, Fig. S for fulcrum recommendations).

Step 6 Place the syringe parallel with the long axis of the tooth with the large window facing the clinician.

Step 7 Insert the needle within the height of the maxillary mucobuccal fold at the apex of the maxillary canine, just medial to and parallel with the canine eminence and approximately 10° off an imaginary line drawn to the long axis of the tooth; the needle depth may vary based on the location of the apex of the maxillary canine, but it is approximately 5 to 6 mm or one-fourth of the needle or until the bevel is slightly superior to the apex of the tooth (see Table 12.11, Fig. U). There should be no bony contact upon insertion.

Step 8 Aspirate within two planes.

Step 9 If a negative aspiration is achieved, slowly deposit approximately 0.9 to 1.2 mL of agent (one-half to two-thirds of cartridge) over approximately 30 to 40 seconds; if the tissue balloons, injection is too rapid.

Step 10 Carefully withdraw the syringe and immediately recap the needle using the one-handed scoop method utilizing a needle sheath prop (see Chapter 11).

Step 11 Wait approximately 3 to 5 minutes until anesthesia takes effect before starting treatment.

nerve fibers from the contralateral side of the dental arch.[1,5] Thus additional bilateral injections of the ASA block or supraperiosteal injection over the contralateral maxillary central incisor may be indicated if the patient is still feeling discomfort during treatment. If anesthesia of the associated palatal periodontium and gingiva of the maxillary anterior teeth is necessary, the nasopalatine block may also be indicated.

Target Area and Injection Site for Anterior Superior Alveolar Block

The target area or deposit location for the ASA block is the ASA nerve superior to the apex of the maxillary canine (see Table 12.11, Fig. Q). The injection site or needle insertion point is within the height of maxillary mucobuccal fold, just medial to and parallel with canine eminence (see Table 12.11, Fig. T).

Retraction of the upper lip will be very important for the ASA block to achieve visibility as well as taut tissue for the needle to go through at the correct injection site and with less tissue trauma created.[10] If the clinician takes the tip of the lip directly over the tooth and then pulls it outward and then upward like pulling up a window blind instead of just pushing it up, then the height of the maxillary mucobuccal fold opens up for insertion. In addition, sterile gauze folded over the edge of the lip before retraction can help prevent slippage during administration, but do not allow the gauze to obstruct the view of the injection site.

Some clinicians suggest a distraction to the insertion to the needle by gently pressing downward on the skin surface near the nose during retraction. In addition, a slight pinching of the lip while it is being held open also adds to the distraction.

The needle is then angled at approximately 10° off an imaginary line drawn parallel to the long axis of the maxillary canine and following the contour of the maxilla. The needle is inserted within the height of the maxillary mucobuccal fold just mesial to the maxillary canine and advanced until its tip is superior to the apex of the maxillary canine without contacting the maxilla so as to reduce trauma, and then the injection is administered (see Table 12.11, Fig. U).

Since the root length varies, the depth of needle insertion related to the apex of the maxillary canine will vary.[9] For the ASA block, the clinician should review the average root length of the maxillary canine to help make this adjustment of needle depth more accurate to achieve a clinically effective injection (see Table 12.2).[8]

If the patient needs extensive nonsurgical periodontal therapy within the maxillary arch, the patient's treatment plan should use a sextant approach instead of quadrant, along with the additional administration of a nasopalatine block to confirm anesthesia of the associated palatal periodontium and gingiva of the teeth within the maxillary anterior sextant (see Fig. 11.3 in Chapter 11).[6]

TABLE 12.12 Anterior Superior Alveolar Block Complications

Complication	Technique Adjustment
Pain on insertion with needle against periosteum	Withdraw needle and reinsert farther away (or lateral) from periosteum
Pain during injection from injecting too rapidly	Due to acidic anesthetic agent, care should be taken to inject slowly to not exceed recommended deposit time
Inadequate anesthesia from injecting inferior to the apex of maxillary canine	Increase depth of insertion upon reinsertion to assure placement of agent just superior to apex of maxillary canine
Possibly inadequate anesthesia from crossover-innervation of contralateral ASA nerve	Additional bilateral ASA block or supraperiosteal injection over contralateral maxillary central incisor (see Tables 12.11 and 12.1)
Possibly inadequate anesthesia from dense bone covering apex	Instead administer IO block (see Table 12.13)
Possibly inadequate anesthesia from injecting into area of infection or risking needle tract infection	Instead administer IO block (see Table 12.13)

ASA, Anterior superior alveolar; *IO*, infraorbital.

Indications of Clinically Effective Anterior Superior Alveolar Block and Possible Complications

Indications of a clinically effective ASA block include harmless tingling and numbness of the upper lip and an absence of discomfort during dental procedures. Positive aspiration is less than approximately 1%; thus overinsertion with complications such as a hematoma is rare with the ASA block (Table 12.12).[3]

Infraorbital Block

The IO block anesthetizes the IO nerve as well as both the ASA and MSA nerves to cover the regions of both the MSA and ASA blocks with one injection. Thus the IO block anesthetizes the maxillary anterior teeth and premolars, as well as the associated facial periodontium and gingiva to the midline within one maxillary quadrant (Table 12.13, Figs. V–Y, and Procedure Box 12.6). Some clinicians believe that this block should be referred to as the *ASA block* to reflect the anesthetized tissue, but the more useful name comes from the IO nerve anesthetized.[1,11] The additional administration of the PSA block completes maxillary quadrant anesthesia.[9] However, if anesthesia of the associated palatal periodontium and gingiva of the maxillary anterior teeth and premolars is necessary, both the nasopalatine block and the greater palatine block may also be indicated; this is an important consideration with any root concavity involvement.

Branches of the IO nerve to the ipsilateral upper lip, side of the nose, and lower eyelid are also inadvertently anesthetized during the IO block (see Table 12.13, Fig. V2). In addition, in many cases the contralateral ASA nerve can involve crossover-innervation, so an additional supraperiosteal injection over the contralateral maxillary central incisor or bilateral injections of either the IO block or ASA block (depending on extent of procedures) may be indicated if the patient is still feeling discomfort during treatment.[1]

Target Area and Injection Site for Infraorbital Block

The target area or deposit location for the IO block is the IO nerve after entering the IO foramen (see Table 12.13, Fig. V). Within the IO foramen, both the ASA and MSA nerves move superiorly to join the IO nerve after it enters.

To locate the IO foramen, extraorally palpate the midpoint of the patient's IO rim and then move approximately 10 mm slightly inferior while applying pressure until the depression created by the IO foramen is felt, surrounded by smoother bone (Fig. 12.8).[2] Clinicians can palpate a "notch" or more correctly a depression in the midpoint of the IO rim created by the more vertical zygomaticomaxillary suture located

TABLE 12.13 Infraorbital Block Review

Indications	Procedures on maxillary anterior teeth and premolars within one maxillary quadrant or if other injections considered would not be as clinically effective due to dense bone or local infection such as supraperiosteal injection, MSA block, or ASA block
Nerves anesthetized	IO nerve ASA nerve MSA nerve Inferior palpebral nerve Lateral nasal nerve Superior labial nerve
Teeth anesthetized	Maxillary anterior teeth and premolars as well as mesiobuccal root of maxillary first molar in approximately 28% of cases

(*Continued*)

TABLE 12.13 Infraorbital Block Review (*Cont.*)

Other structures anesthetized	Facial periodontium and gingiva of anesthetized teeth; upper lip to midline; medial part of cheek; side of nose; lower eyelid
Administration technique	See Procedure Box 12.6
Needle gauge and length	27-gauge long or 27-gauge short for children (or small adults)
Target area/Deposit location Fig. V = Target area and distribution of anesthesia for IO block	IO foramen that is approximately 10 mm inferior to midpoint of IO rim with zygomaticomaxillary suture
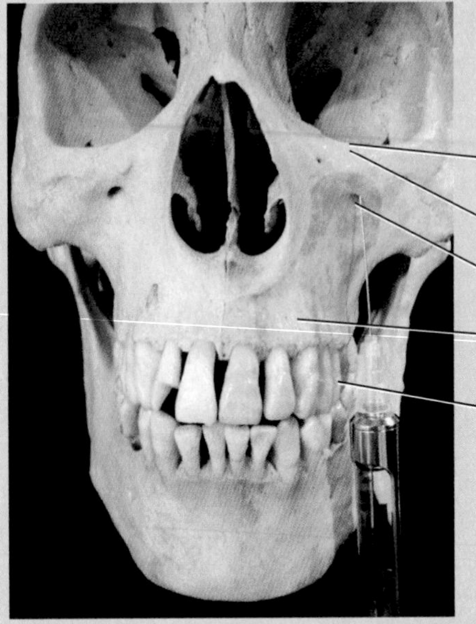 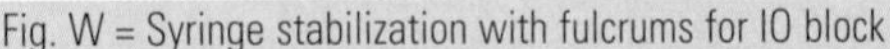	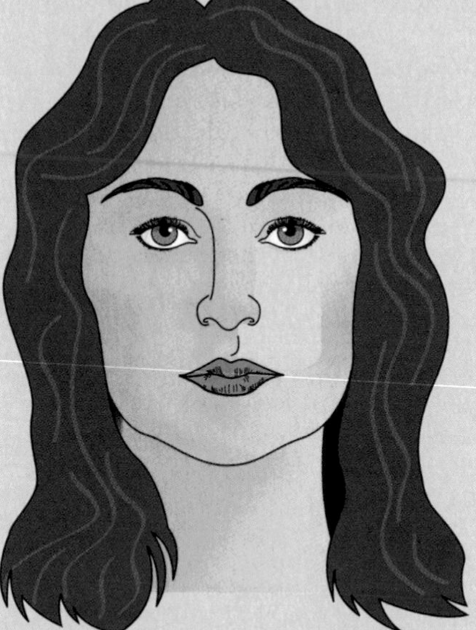
1, Distribution of anesthesia for IO block (From Fehrenbach MJ, Herring SW: *Illustrated anatomy of the head and neck,* ed 6, St Louis, 2021, Saunders/ Elsevier)	*2,* Facial view of extraoral distribution of IO block
Clinician position	Right side, right-handed at 8 o'clock (left-handed at 4 o'clock). Left side, right-handed at 9 o'clock (left-handed at 3 o'clock, same as MSA or ASA blocks; see Table 12.11, Fig. R)
Fig. W = Syringe stabilization with fulcrums for IO block	
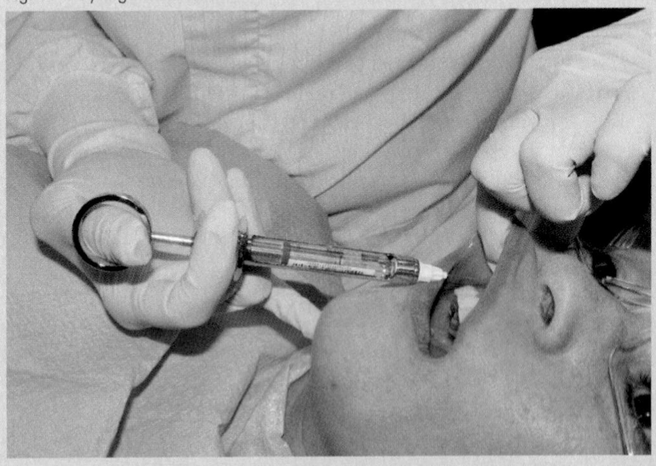	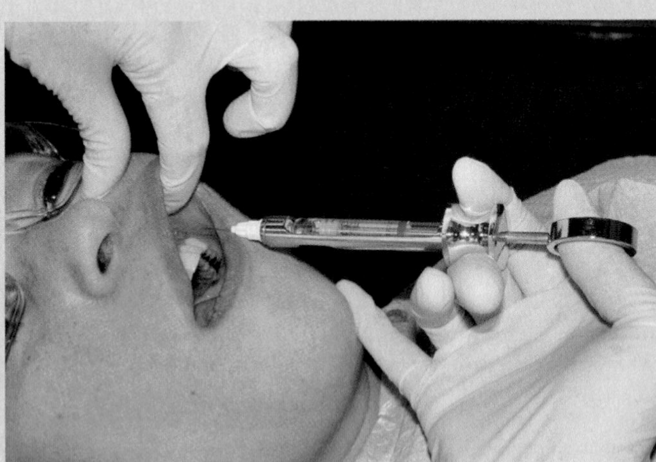
1, Pinky finger of dominant hand resting on patient's chin for right side	*2,* Pinky finger of dominant hand resting on patient's chin for left side

TABLE 12.13 Infraorbital Block Review (*Cont.*)

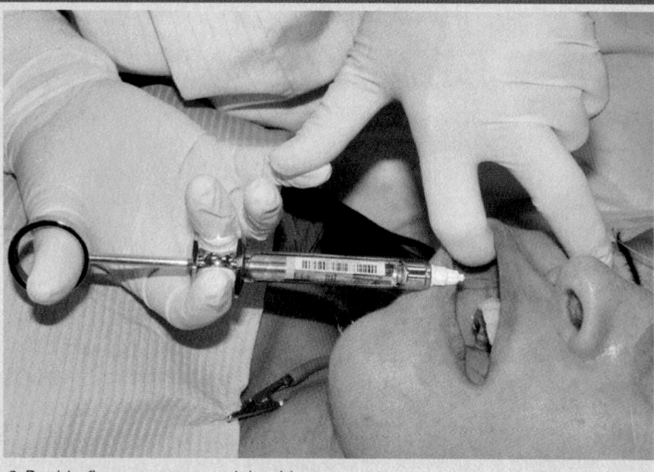

3, Double finger support on right side

Landmarks	*Extraoral:* IO rim Zygomaticomaxillary suture IO foramen *Intraoral:* Maxillary first premolar Maxillary mucobuccal fold
Injection site/Needle insertion point 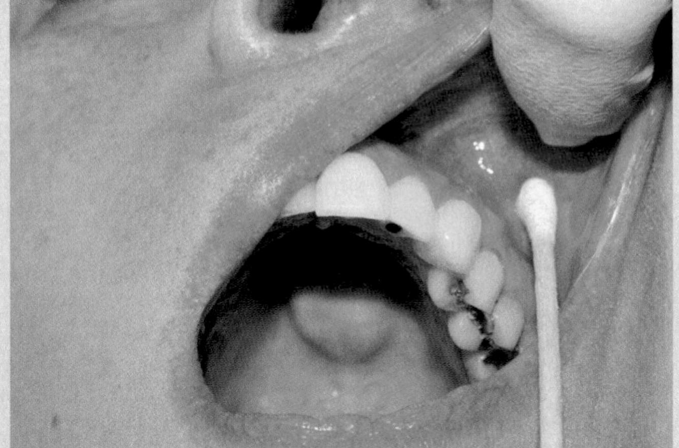 Fig. X = Injection site for IO block	Within height of maxillary mucobuccal fold superior to apices of maxillary first premolar
Depth of needle insertion Fig. Y = Needle insertion for IO block	Approximately 16 mm or one-half of long needle or three-fourths of short needle
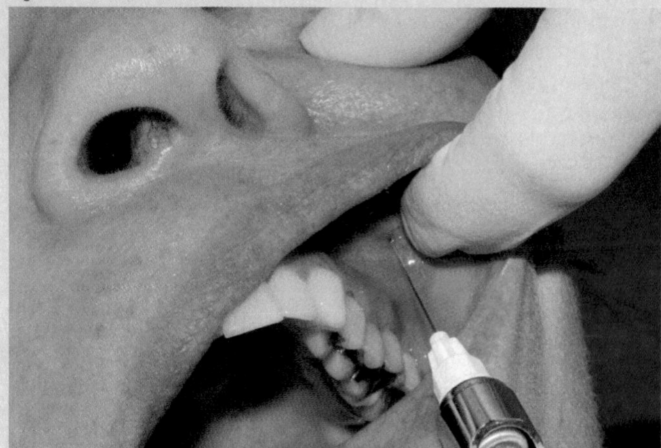 *1,* Needle insertion for IO block showing finger pressure over IO foramen	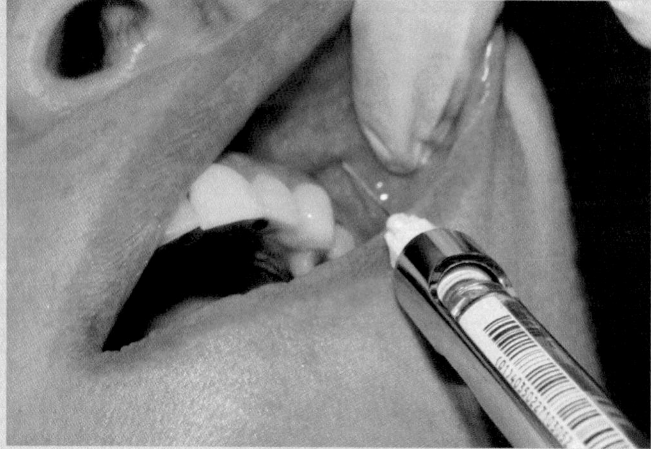 *2,* Needle depth for IO block approximately 16 mm or one-half of long needle
Amount of anesthetic agent	Approximately 0.9 to 1.2 mL or one-half to two-thirds of cartridge
Length of time to deposit	Approximately 30 to 40 seconds

ASA, Anterior superior alveolar; *IO,* infraorbital; *MSA,* middle superior alveolar.

PROCEDURE BOX 12.6 Infraorbital Block Procedure

Step 1 Assume the correct clinician position for right side, right-handed at 8 o'clock (left-handed at 4 o'clock); left side, right-handed at 9 o'clock (left-handed at 3 o'clock, same as middle superior alveolar [MSA] or anterior superior alveolar [ASA] blocks; see Table 12.11, Fig. R).

Step 2 Ask the supine patient to open and then retract the upper lip, pulling the tissue taut outward and then upward only at the tip with the index finger or thumb of the nondominant hand (one inside and one outside); sterile gauze may be wrapped around the tip to help retract slippery tissue.

Step 3 Prepare the alveolar mucosa within the height of the maxillary mucobuccal fold superior to the apices of the maxillary first premolar (see Chapter 11) and palpate the injection site or needle insertion point to confirm soft tissue is injected (see Table 12.13, Fig. X).

Step 4 Using a 27-gauge long needle or 27-gauge short for children (or small adults) in the syringe in the dominant hand, orient the bevel of the needle away from the large window of the syringe to confirm the bevel orientation is toward the bone.

Step 5 Locate the infraorbital foramen (see Figs. 12.8 and 12.9) by palpating extraorally for the midpoint of the infraorbital rim of the orbit and moving approximately 10 mm slightly inferior with the index finger or thumb of the nondominant hand; maintain finger pressure at the infraorbital foramen before, during, and after the injection. Advise patient that some discomfort might be felt with this slight pressure.

Step 6 Establish a fulcrum (see Table 12.13, Fig. W for fulcrum recommendations).

Step 7 Place the syringe parallel with the long axis of the maxillary first premolar orienting the needle in line with the infraorbital foramen using the finger over the foramen as a guide, with the large window facing the clinician (see Table 12.13, Fig. Y1).

Step 8 Insert the needle within the height of the maxillary mucobuccal fold superior to the apices and parallel to the long axis of the maxillary first premolar and approximately 16 mm or one-half of a long needle or three-fourths of a short needle, until the needle gently contacts bone at the superior rim of the infraorbital foramen (see Table 12.13, Fig. Y2).

Step 9 Aspirate within two planes.

Step 10 If negative aspiration is achieved, slowly deposit approximately 0.9 to 1.2 mL of agent (one-half to two-thirds of cartridge) over approximately 30 to 40 seconds. The clinician will be able to feel the agent being deposited beneath the finger over the infraorbital foramen.

Step 11 Carefully withdraw the syringe and immediately recap the needle using the one-handed scoop method utilizing a needle sheath prop (see Chapter 11).

Step 12 Maintain pressure and massage the agent into the infraorbital foramen for approximately 2 minutes after the injection.

Step 13 Wait approximately 3 to 5 minutes until anesthesia takes effect before starting treatment.

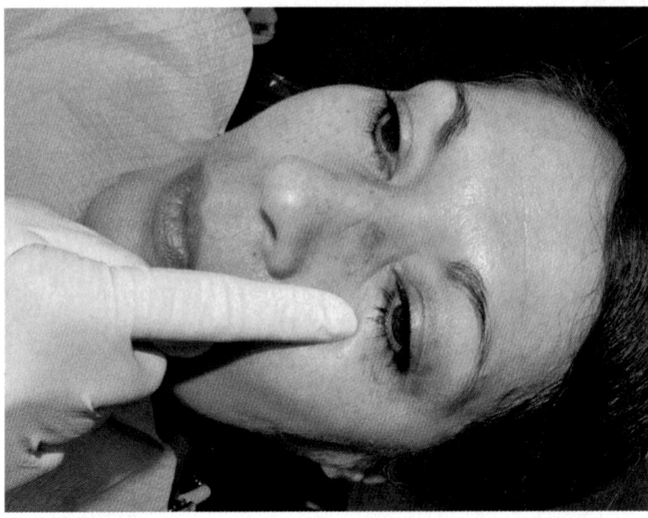

Fig. 12.8 Palpation of the depression created by the infraorbital foramen for the infraorbital block by palpating extraorally for the midpoint infraorbital rim of the orbit with the zygomaticomaxillary suture and moving approximately 10 mm slightly inferior.

between the maxilla (medial part) and the zygomatic bone (lateral part) that both form the IO rim (see Chapter 10).[1] The patient may feel soreness when pressure is applied to the IO foramen due to the presence of the nearby nerve. There is also a linear relationship on the ipsilateral side of the face with the ipsilateral supraorbital notch, pupil of the eye looking forward, midpoint of the IO rim with its zygomaticomaxillary suture, IO foramen, and corner of the mouth (Fig. 12.9).

The injection site or needle insertion point for the IO block is within the height of the maxillary mucobuccal fold superior to the apices of the maxillary first premolar (Table 12.13, Fig. X). A preinjection approximation of the depth of needle insertion for the IO block can be made by placing one finger on the IO foramen and the other finger on the proposed injection site or needle insertion point and then estimating the distance between the two fingers. The approximate depth of needle insertion for the IO block may vary, but usually it is one-half of a long needle and three-fourths of a short needle.

The approximate depth of needle insertion for the IO block may vary. In a patient with a higher or deeper maxillary mucobuccal fold or more superiorly located IO foramen, less tissue insertion will be required than in a patient with a much lower or shallower maxillary mucobuccal fold or more superior IO foramen.[1,2] In addition, retraction of the upper lip will be very important for the IO block to achieve visibility and a taut tissue as discussed earlier with the ASA block.[10]

The needle is inserted for the IO block within the height of the maxillary mucobuccal fold superior to the apices of the maxillary first premolar while keeping the finger of the other hand on the IO foramen during the injection to help keep the syringe toward the IO foramen (Table 12.13, Fig. Y1). The needle is advanced while keeping it parallel with the long axis of the tooth to avoid premature contact with the maxilla. The point of gentle contact of the needle with the maxilla should be at the superior rim of the IO foramen and then the injection is administered (Table 12.13, Fig. Y2).

Maintaining the needle in contact with the bone prevents overinsertion and possible puncture of the orbit, although that is a rare occurrence.[3] Once the needle is carefully withdrawn and capped, an important postinjection procedure is to maintain pressure and massage the agent into the IO foramen for approximately 2 minutes to enhance anesthetic agent diffusion.[3]

Indications of Clinically Effective Infraorbital Block and Possible Complications

Indications of a clinically effective IO block include harmless tingling and numbness of the ipsilateral upper lip, medial part of the cheek, side of the nose, and lower eyelid because there is inadvertent anesthesia of the branches of the IO nerve.[1] Additionally, there is numbness of the teeth and associated tissue along the distribution of the ASA and MSA nerves and absence of discomfort during dental procedures. Rarely, the complication of a hematoma may develop across the lower eyelid and the tissue between it and the IO foramen due to nearness of the area blood vessels (Table 12.14).[3]

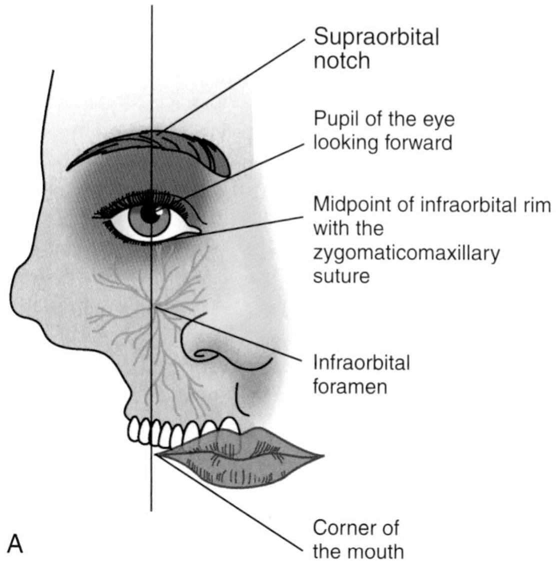

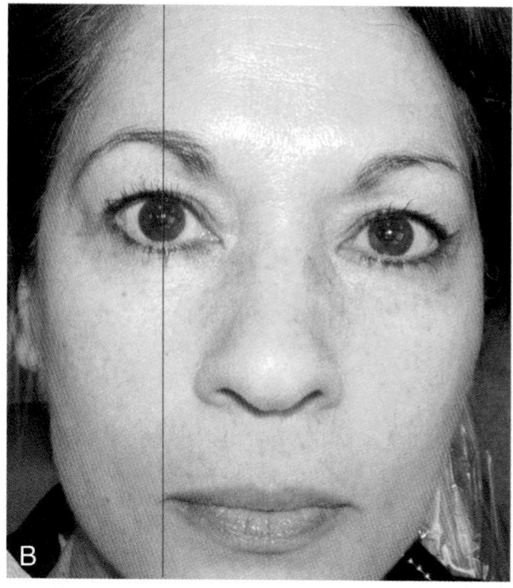

Fig. 12.9 (A) Linear relationship on the ipsilateral side of the face between the supraorbital notch, pupil of the eye looking forward, midpoint of the infraorbital rim with the zygomaticomaxillary suture, infraorbital foramen, and corner of the mouth. (B) Facial view of linear relationship that involves the infraorbital foramen.

TABLE 12.14 Infraorbital Block Complications

Complication	Technique Adjustment
Pain on insertion with needle against periosteum	Withdraw needle and reinsert farther away (or lateral) from periosteum
Inadequate anesthesia from needle contacting bone inferior to IO foramen	Direct needle toward finger over IO foramen to help line up needle with IO foramen, making sure to contact bone
Possibly inadequate anesthesia from crossover-innervation of contralateral ASA nerve	Additional contralateral ASA block (Table 12.11) or supraperiosteal injection over contralateral maxillary central incisor (Table 12.1)

ASA, Anterior superior alveolar; *IO,* infraorbital.

PALATAL NERVE BLOCKS

The palatal nerve blocks also anesthetize various branches of the maxillary nerve. However, all the palatal nerve blocks have a somewhat higher associated VAS range of 2 to 4, even when using correct technique by the clinician since there is bony contact, including initially the sensitive mucoperiosteum overlying maxilla and palatal bones; in contrast, most maxillary facial injections have a lower associated VAS range from 0 to 2 since they are administered through soft tissue and have no bony contact except for the IO block (see Chapter 1).[4,10]

However, there is no need to avoid the clinically effective palatal injections because of their somewhat greater level of discomfort; the clinician and the rest of the dental team should also be careful in their discussion of this type of injection in front of the patient.[10] The goal is overall pain management as well as clinically effective hemostatic control. This is especially needed during the longer appointment time needed for nonsurgical periodontal therapy when instrumenting exposed roots with dentinal hypersensitivity.[6,9]

Topical anesthetics have very limited action on keratinized tissue such as the hard palate (Chapter 11) but should be used for any additional comfort that they can provide.[9,10] However, because the overlying palatal tissue is dense and adheres firmly to the underlying bones of the palate, the use of pressure anesthesia with a cotton-tipped applicator before, during, and after the injection to blanch the tissue will reduce patient discomfort.[1,10] This pressure anesthesia of the tissue produces a dull ache that blocks pain impulses that comes from needle insertion and agent deposition. The greater palatine block may produce a slightly lower associated VAS range than the nasopalatine block since the tissue surrounding the greater palatine foramen is not as firmly adherent to the bone as those around the incisive foramen and therefore is better able to accommodate the volume of agent deposited.[4] This still does not preclude the use of the nasopalatine block since there may be greater deposits on the palatal surfaces of anterior teeth due to deeper periodontal pockets and exposure to food debris.

When using pressure anesthesia, it is important to advise patients that they may feel some slight discomfort from the gentle pressure and that there may still be an initial slight prick of the needle. It is also important to keep the cotton-tipped applicator firmly engaged with the hard palatal tissue surface; this also reassures the patient that the applicator, which feels like it is near the soft palate, will not be moving down the throat to be possibly choked on.

A cotton-tipped applicator is the best tool to use to accomplish pressure anesthesia because its padded roundness results in less damaging pressure than using the ends of metal instruments.[3,10] After topical anesthetic has been placed with the cotton-tipped applicator, a new cotton-tipped applicator without topical anesthesia should be used to confirm minimal slippage while still being able to bear down on the tissue with the pressure anesthesia during the injection.[10]

The use of the computer-controlled local anesthesia delivery device (see Chapter 9) is commonly used for the palatal injections since such a device regulates both the pressure and volume ratio of agent delivered, which is not readily attained with a standard syringe. Some clinicians use a bidirectional rotation needle insertion technique with the handpiece of the delivery device syringe instead of the usual linear insertion technique to allow the needle to more easily enter the firmer tissue of the hard palate.[3]

In addition, a prepuncture technique with the computer-controlled local anesthesia delivery device that acts as a type of topical anesthesia can also be used by placing the bevel of the needle toward the palatal tissue with a cotton-tipped applicator on top of the needle tip (see Chapter 11 and Fig. 11.29).[3] The clinician then applies light pressure on the cotton-tipped applicator to slightly puncture the tissue while administering a small amount of the agent from the delivery device without leakage. The cotton-tipped applicator is removed from on top of the needle, and the rest of the agent is then administered with less discomfort. There is no need for the pressure anesthesia from the cotton-tipped applicator at any time during the injection.

At all times, the needle will naturally withdraw from the mucoperiosteum when bony contact is made with the hard palate, so there is no need to withdraw farther upon bony contact and possibly miss the depth needed to reach the target area. As discussed previously, the use of a topical anesthetic or additional prepuncture technique as well as the slow deposition of the local anesthetic agent will also reduce patient discomfort.[10]

Since the palatal tissue adheres so tightly to the bone and the injection is quite shallow, the agent may leak out of the injection site or needle insertion point and run down the patient's throat. Quickly rinsing the patient's mouth immediately after safe capping of the needle will help reduce any bad taste of the agent (see Chapter 11). Although positive aspiration is less than approximately 1% for all palatal injections, because of the increased vascularity and density of the palatal tissue, the tissue may continue to slightly bleed even after the removal of the needle and rinsing. Pressure against the palatal tissue with folded sterile gauze, always avoiding contacting the nearby posteriorly located yellower soft palate, will stem the slight bleeding and prevent the patient (or clinician) from becoming alarmed.[3]

It may also be necessary to work around the variation of a midline palatal torus if present or a high-vaulted palate when giving the palatal injections; the clinician must try to maintain the perpendicular angle to the palatal tissue as much as possible during the injections to maintain the correct angulation (see Chapter 11 and Fig. BB2).[16]

Palatal anesthesia usually involves anesthesia of both the soft and hard tissue of the palate including the associated palatal periodontium and gingiva. However in most cases palatal anesthesia alone, with one exception, usually does not provide any pulpal anesthesia to the maxillary teeth nor anesthesia of the associated facial periodontium and gingiva.[1,2,11] Additional administration of maxillary facial injections would be needed for complete coverage of either a maxillary sextant or a maxillary quadrant when planning dental treatment.

The **greater palatine (GP) block** is a nerve block that is recommended for anesthesia of the associated palatal periodontium and gingiva for the maxillary posterior teeth within the maxillary posterior sextant. The **nasopalatine (NP) block** is a nerve block that is recommended for anesthesia of the associated palatal periodontium and gingiva for the maxillary anterior teeth bilaterally from maxillary canine to canine within the maxillary anterior sextant.

Separate from these palatal blocks that only provide anesthesia of the palatal soft tissue and not any pulpal anesthesia, is another block administered on the hard palate: the **anterior middle superior alveolar (AMSA) block**. The AMSA block is a palatal nerve block that also provides pulpal anesthesia. This block is recommended for anesthesia of maxillary teeth and their associated facial and lingual periodontium and gingiva to the midline within one maxillary quadrant, except for those structures innervated by the PSA nerve. Thus the maxillary molars and associated buccal periodontium and gingiva are not involved in the anesthesia provided by this block. However, if using the AMSA block, the PSA block is additionally administered first in most cases to complete maxillary quadrant anesthesia.

If quadrant dental hygiene treatment is planned within the maxillary arch, the GP block is administered after any maxillary facial nerve blocks but before the NP block, with instrumentation proceeding in the same manner to have complete anesthesia coverage (see Chapter 11). Because of its regional coverage of the palatal region, the GP block covers the molar and premolar sextant for nonsurgical periodontal therapy (see Fig. 11.3 in Chapter 11). The NP block and its use with sextants or even quadrants is discussed in detail later.

Greater Palatine Block

The GP block anesthetizes the GP nerve and thus the posterior hard palate and the associated palatal periodontium and gingiva of the ipsilateral maxillary posterior teeth within the maxillary posterior sextant (Table 12.15, Figs. Z–DD, and Procedure Box 12.7).

Because the GP block does not provide pulpal nor associated facial periodontium and gingiva anesthesia of the maxillary posterior teeth, the additional administration of the PSA and MSA blocks or the IO block may also be indicated, especially during nonsurgical periodontal therapy, because dentinal hypersensitivity is possible when instrumenting exposed root surfaces.[6,7,9]

In addition, anesthesia of the associated palatal periodontium and gingiva of the maxillary first premolar may prove inadequate because of overlapping nerve fibers from the anteriorly located NP nerve when instrumenting within the maxillary posterior sextant.[1] This lack of anesthesia may be corrected by additional administration of the NP block if the patient is still feeling discomfort, especially with the considerations of maxillary premolar root concavity involvement.[6,9]

Target Area and Injection Site for Greater Palatine Block

The target area or deposit location for the GP block is the GP nerve entering the GP foramen from its location in the deepest part of the interface between the mucoperiosteum and the bone of the posterior hard palate (see Table 12.15, Fig. Z).

The GP foramen is noted as a depression on the palatal surface, usually at the junction of the alveolar process of the maxilla and posterior hard palate, as well as superior to the apices of the maxillary

TABLE 12.15 Greater Palatine Block Review

Indications	Palatal procedures of maxillary premolars and molars within one maxillary posterior sextant
Nerves anesthetized	GP nerve
Teeth anesthetized	None
Other structures anesthetized	Posterior hard palate and palatal periodontium and gingiva of ipsilateral maxillary posterior teeth
Administration technique	See Procedure Box 12.7
Needle gauge and length	27-gauge extra-short or short with standard syringe or 30-gauge extra-short or short with computer-controlled local anesthetic delivery device

TABLE 12.15 Greater Palatine Block Review (*Cont.*)

Target area/Deposit location	GP foramen at junction of alveolar process of maxilla and hard palate as well as superior to apices of maxillary second or third molar and midway between median palatine raphe (suture) and palatal gingival margin of maxillary molar

Median palatine suture
Posterior hard palate
Alveolar process of the maxilla
Maxillary second molar
Greater palatine foramen
Horizontal plate of the palatine bone

Fig. Z = Target area and distribution of anesthesia for GP block (From Fehrenbach MJ, Herring SW: *Illustrated anatomy of the head and neck,* ed 6, St Louis, 2021, Saunders/Elsevier)

Fig. AA = Clinician position of right-handed clinician for GP block

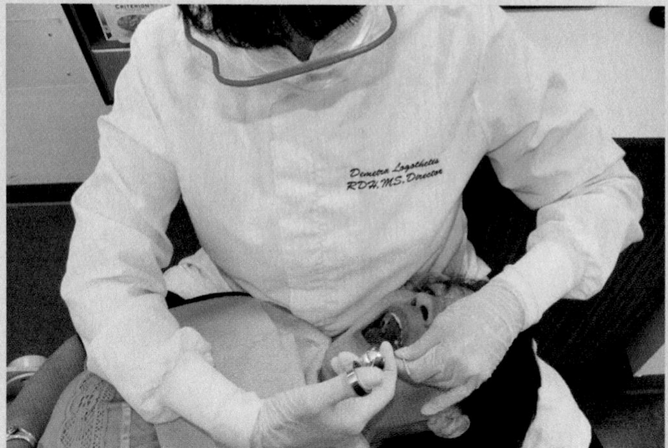

1, Right side, right-handed at 8 to 9 o'clock (left-handed at 4 to 3 o'clock)

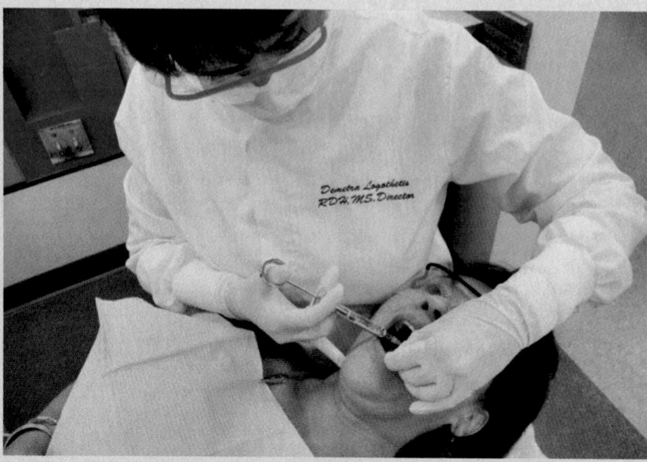

2, Left side, right-handed at 11 o'clock (left-handed at 1 o'clock)

Fig. BB = Syringe stabilization with fulcrums for GP block (same as AMSA block)

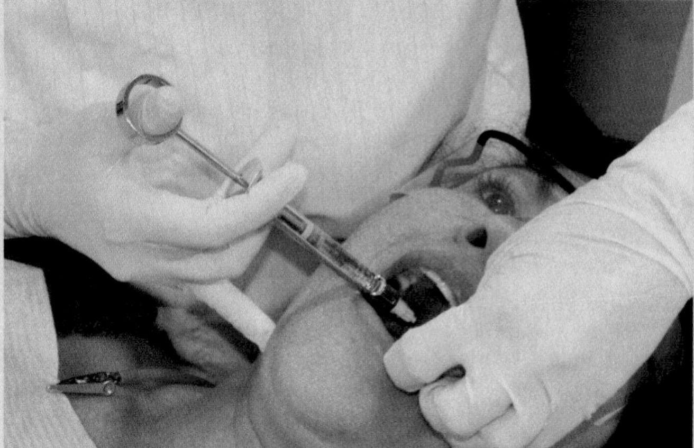

1, Pinky finger resting on patient's chin for left side

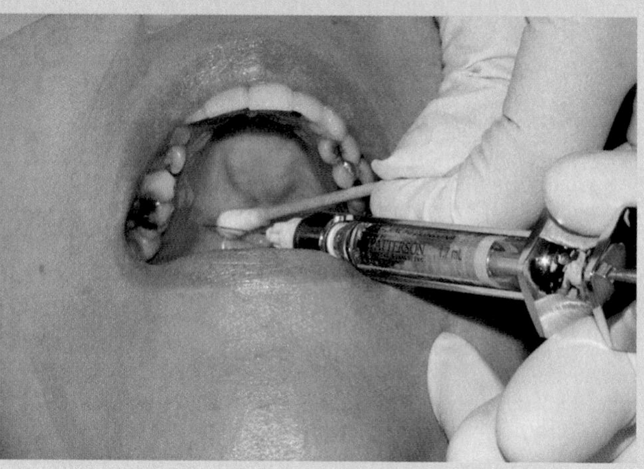

2, Syringe barrel resting on index finger of nondominant hand and pinky finger of dominant hand on chin for right side

(*Continued*)

TABLE 12.15 Greater Palatine Block Review (*Cont.*)

Landmarks	Maxillary second or third molar Junction of alveolar process of maxilla and posterior hard palate Median palatine raphe (suture) Palatal gingival margin GP foramen
Injection site/Needle insertion point 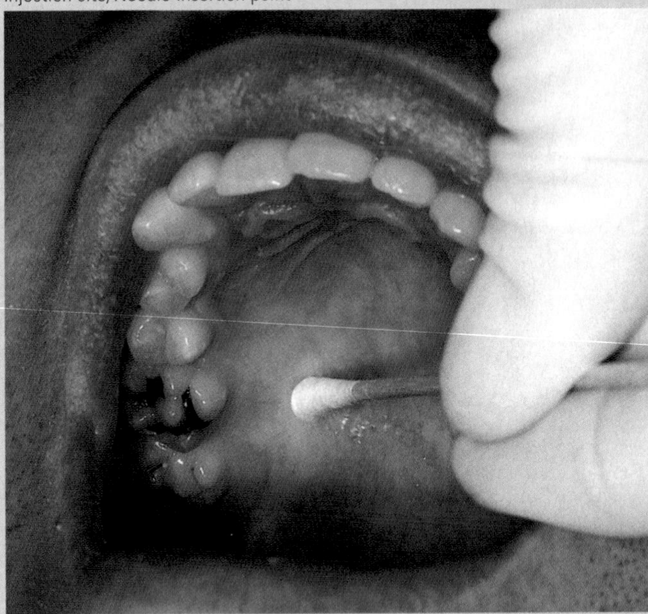 Fig. CC = Injection site for GP block (From Fehrenbach MJ, Herring SW: *Illustrated anatomy of the head and neck*, ed 6, St Louis, 2021, Saunders/Elsevier)	Palatal tissue 1 to 2 mm slightly anterior to greater palatine foramen
Depth of needle insertion Fig. DD = Needle insertion for GP block (From Fehrenbach MJ, Herring SW: *Illustrated anatomy of the head and neck*, ed 6, St Louis, 2021, Saunders/Elsevier) 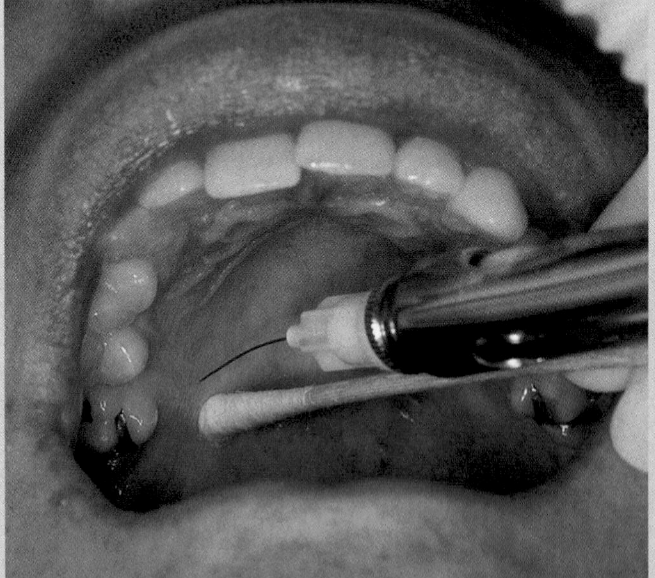 *1,* Without prepuncture technique: Cotton-tipped applicator is placed firmly on greater palatine foramen and needle is inserted slightly anterior to cotton-tipped applicator	Approximately 4 to 6 mm or until contact with palatine bone 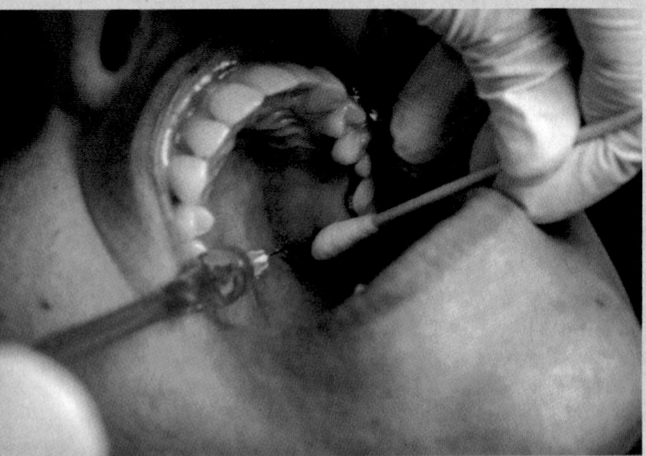 *2,* With prepuncture technique: Apply pressure on needle bevel and tissue with cotton-tipped applicator
Amount of anesthetic agent	Approximately 0.45 to 0.6 mL or one-fourth to one-third of cartridge until blanching of palatal tissue
Length of time to deposit	Minimum of 30 seconds

AMSA, Anterior middle superior alveolar; *GP,* greater palatine.

PROCEDURE BOX 12.7 Greater Palatine Block Procedure

Step 1 Assume the correct clinician position for right side, right-handed at 8 to 9 o'clock (left-handed at 4–3 o'clock); left side, right-handed at 11 o'clock (left-handed at 1 o'clock; see Table 12.15, Fig. AA).

Step 2 Ask the patient to open and extend the neck either to the right or left. Locate the greater palatine foramen by gently sliding a cotton-tipped applicator along the posterior hard palate surface, starting at the junction of the maxillary alveolar process and the posterior hard palate foramen near the maxillary first molar, and moving distally until the cotton-tipped applicator falls into the depression of the greater palatine foramen. Usually the foramen is located superior to the apices of either the maxillary second or third molar (see Table 12.15, Fig. CC). Be careful not to contact the more yellow-tinged soft palate with the applicator or else gagging may occur.

Step 3 Prepare the tissue 1 to 2 mm slightly anterior to the greater palatine foramen (see Chapter 11).

Step 4 Determine whether to use a 27-gauge extra-short or short needle with a standard syringe or 30-gauge extra-short or short needle with a computer-controlled local anesthetic delivery device. With the syringe or handpiece in the dominant hand, orient the bevel of the needle toward the posterior hard palate.

Step 5 Determine whether to use the prepuncture technique for surface pain control. *Without prepuncture technique:* Using a new cotton-tipped applicator in the nondominant hand, apply firm pressure with the applicator over the greater palatine foramen on the surface of the hard palate until tissue is blanched. Advise patient that he or she may feel some slight discomfort from the pressure.

Step 6 *For both techniques:* Establish a fulcrum (see Table 12.15, Fig. BB for fulcrum recommendations).

Step 7 *Without prepuncture technique:* Direct the syringe or handpiece from the contralateral side of the mouth at 90° to the posterior hard palate toward the cotton-tipped applicator, with the large window facing the clinician. *For prepuncture technique:* Place the bevel of the needle on the injection site without penetrating the tissue. Apply pressure to the back of the needle and tissue with a cotton-tipped applicator and slowly dispense anesthetic agent to produce a topical anesthetic effect. If using a computer-controlled local anesthetic delivery device, depress the foot pedal lightly to start the slow-flow rate. After three audible beeps the system will announce "cruise control"; continue to administer the anesthetic without penetrating the tissue at the slow-flow rate for about 8 to 10 seconds.

Step 8 *For both techniques:* Insert the needle approximately 4 to 6 mm, possibly using the bidirectional rotation needle insertion technique, at 1 to 2 mm slightly anterior to the greater palatine foramen until the palatine bone is gently contacted. *Without prepuncture technique:* Maintain pressure with the cotton-tipped applicator throughout the injection and a short time after the agent is deposited (see Table 12.15, Fig. DD1). *With prepuncture technique:* Continue to hold the cotton-tipped applicator over the needle tip with the bevel facing the tissue and continue to dispense a small amount of agent (see Table 12.15, Fig. DD2), then remove the applicator.

Step 9 *For both techniques:* Aspirate.

Step 10 *For both techniques:* If negative aspiration is achieved, slowly deposit approximately 0.45 to 0.6 mL of agent (one-fourth to one-third of cartridge) over a minimum of 30 seconds; tissue in area will blanch even further when the anesthetic is administered. *With prepuncture technique:* Inspect the tissue to make sure the agent is not overblanching it; slow it down or stop if excessive blanching of the palatal tissue occurs (see Table 12.16).

Step 11 *For both techniques:* Carefully withdraw the syringe or handpiece and immediately recap the needle using the one-handed scoop method, utilizing a needle sheath prop (see Chapter 11).

Step 12 *For both techniques:* Rinse the patient's mouth. Inspect the region and stem any remaining bleeding with pressure using sterile gauze. Be careful not to contact the soft palate. Wait approximately 3 to 5 minutes until anesthesia takes effect before starting treatment.

second molar (in children) or third molar (in adults), which is approximately 10 mm medial and directly superior to the palatal gingival margin (Fig. 12.10). Thus this depression can be palpated approximately midway between the median palatine raphe overlying the median palatine suture and the palatal gingival margin of the maxillary molar; this is where pressure anesthesia is applied for the injection.[1]

In patients who have a vaulted palate, the GP foramen appears closer to the dentition.[1] Conversely, in patients with a more shallow palate, the foramen appears closer to the midline. In patients lacking a visible depression for the GP foramen, the other surface landmarks are useful and palpation of the area may help with emphasizing the depression of the foramen.

The injection site or needle insertion point for the GP block is the palatal tissue approximately 1 to 2 mm slightly anterior to the GP foramen (see Table 12.15, Fig. CC). The needle is inserted into the previously blanched palatal tissue at a 90° to the posterior hard palate, with the needle bowing slightly (see Table 12.15, Fig. DD). The needle is advanced until the palatine bone is gently contacted and then the injection is administered.

Pressure anesthesia is performed utilizing a cotton-tipped applicator on nearby palatal tissue, before, during, and for a short time after the injection unless prepuncture technique with the computer-controlled local anesthesia delivery device is used with the GP block.[10]

There is no need to enter the GP canal when administering the injection.[3] Although such an entrance is not potentially hazardous, it

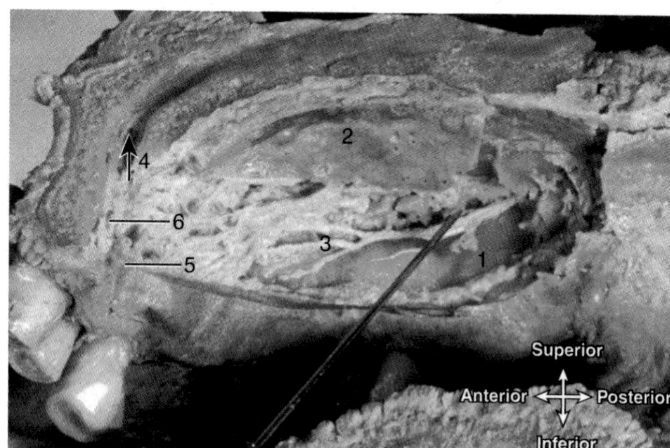

Fig. 12.10 Dissection of the hard palate showing a needle at the injection site or needle insertion point for the greater palatine block. Note the landmarks for the nasopalatine block are also shown. *1,* Greater palatine foramen; *2,* Mucoperiosteum of the hard palate; *3,* Greater palatine nerve traveling horizontally; *4,* Incisive canal *(with arrow), 5,* Incisive foramen; *6,* Nasopalatine nerve. (From Logan BM, Reynold PA, Hutching RT: *McMinn's color atlas of head and neck anatomy,* ed 4, London, 2010, Mosby. In Fehrenbach MJ, Herring SW: *Illustrated anatomy of the head and neck,* ed 6, St Louis, 2021, Saunders/Elsevier.)

is also not necessary for this block and it would be difficult with the angulation of the needle as recommended.

Indications of Clinically Effective Greater Palatine Block and Possible Complications

Indications of a clinically effective GP block are numbness in the posterior hard palate and absence of discomfort during dental procedures. Some patients may become uncomfortable and may gag if the soft palate is contacted or becomes inadvertently and harmlessly anesthetized, which is a distinct possibility given the nearness of the lesser palatine (LP) nerve and the LP foramen (Table 12.16; see Chapter 10).[1]

Nasopalatine Block

The NP block anesthetizes the anterior hard palate and the associated palatal periodontium and gingiva of the maxillary anterior teeth bilaterally from the maxillary right canine to the left canine within the maxillary anterior sextant (Table 12.17, Figs. EE–II, and Procedure Box 12.8). Both the right and the left NP nerves are anesthetized by this one block so only one injection is needed for both sides of the anterior hard palate.[1] The NP block is used when anesthesia of the associated palatal periodontium and gingiva is necessary for two or more maxillary anterior teeth. The injection is particularly useful on the more difficult nonsurgical periodontal therapy cases that are treated in sextants as well as in patients who have extensive palatal deposits as discussed or severe periodontal inflammation with heavy bleeding in the region (see Chapter 11).

In some cases, more than one injection may have been used by clinicians when administering the NP block, such as entering the labial interdental gingiva initially for a first injection and then following up with the second injection of the NP block from the palate with the thought of reducing soft tissue discomfort on the palate near the incisive papilla.[3] As discussed earlier, the intraseptal injection can be given on the labial interdental gingiva between the maxillary central incisors for a highly sensitive patient. However if administered correctly, one injection can usually be used comfortably for the average patient. In addition, creative dental hygiene treatment planning using sextants

TABLE 12.16 Greater Palatine Block Complications

Complication	Technique Adjustment
Inadequate anesthesia from injecting too far anterior to GP foramen	Direct needle more posteriorly toward GP foramen upon reinsertion
Inadequate anesthesia of maxillary first premolar due to overlapping from NP nerve	Additional NP block (see Table 12.17)
Inadvertently anesthetized LP nerve because its LP foramen is nearby; patient gags slightly due to soft palate anesthesia or contact	Reassure patient and have patient avoid swallowing any food or drink until anesthesia wears off and avoid contact with soft palate
Excessive blanching of palatal tissue that may lead to postoperative tissue ischemia and sloughing	Slowing or stopping delivery device to let agent dissipate as well as controlling overall amount used

GP, Greater palatine; *LP,* lesser palatine; *NP,* nasopalatine.

TABLE 12.17 Nasopalatine Block Review

Indications	Palatal procedures of maxillary anterior teeth from maxillary canine to canine within maxillary anterior sextant
Nerves anesthetized	NP nerve
Teeth anesthetized	None
Other structures anesthetized	Anterior hard palate and palatal periodontium and gingiva of maxillary anterior teeth bilaterally
Administration technique	See Procedure Box 12.8
Needle gauge and length	27-gauge extra-short or short with standard syringe or 30-gauge extra-short or short with computer-controlled local anesthetic delivery device
Target area/Deposit location	At incisive foramen on anterior hard palate of maxilla deep to incisive papilla and palatal to maxillary central incisors

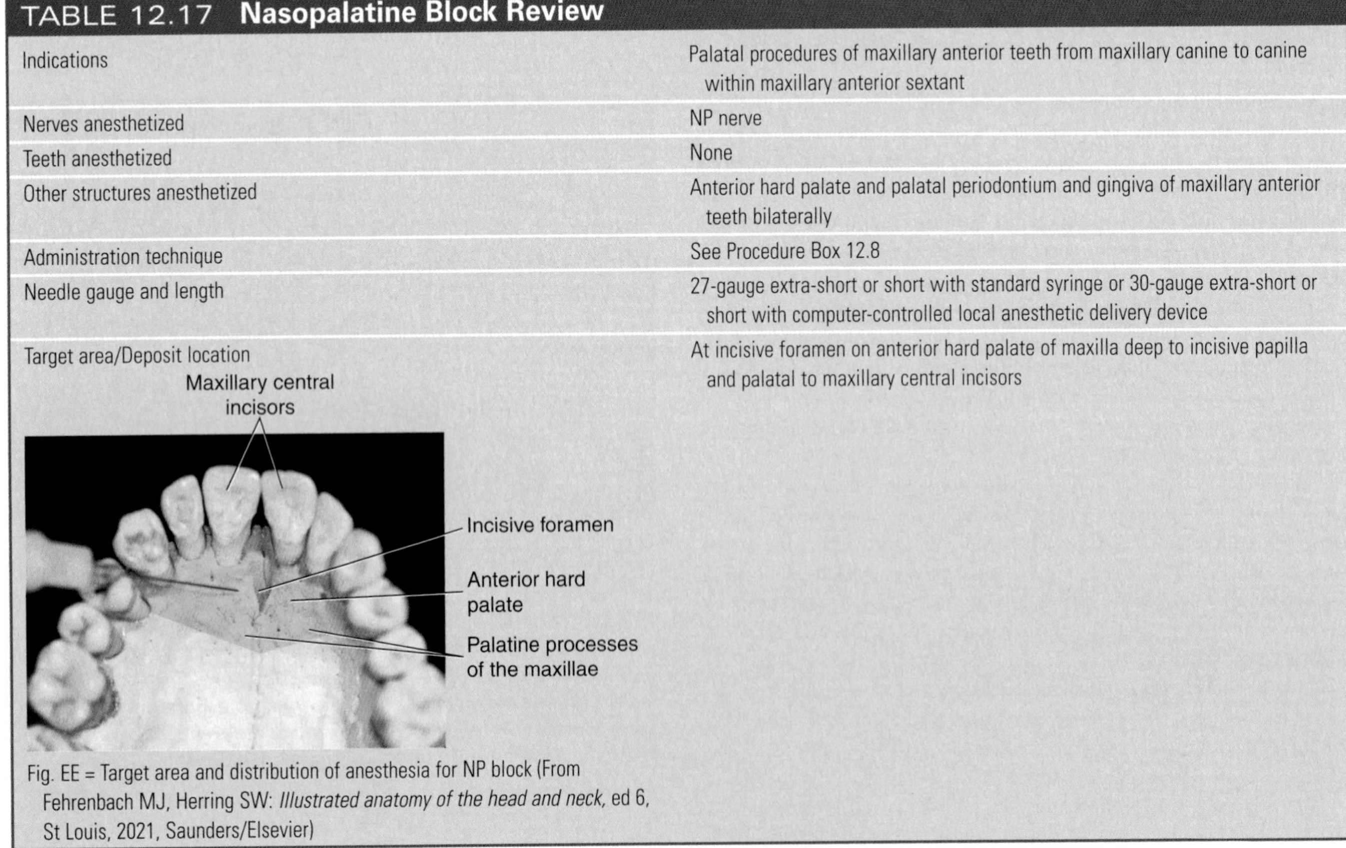

Fig. EE = Target area and distribution of anesthesia for NP block (From Fehrenbach MJ, Herring SW: *Illustrated anatomy of the head and neck,* ed 6, St Louis, 2021, Saunders/Elsevier)

TABLE 12.17 Nasopalatine Block Review (*Cont.*)

Clinician position 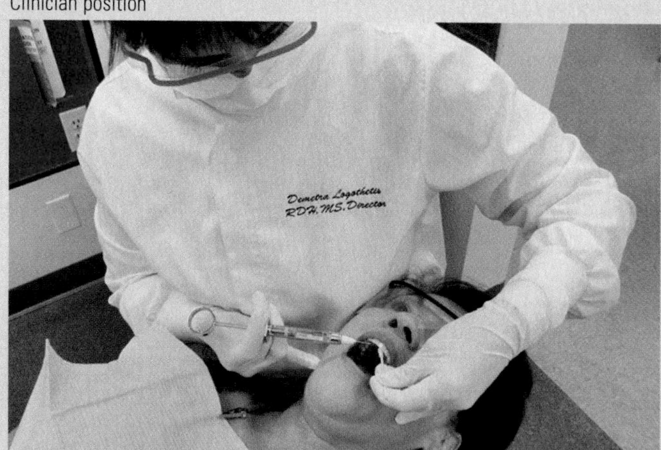 Fig. FF = Clinician position of right-handed clinician for NP block	Right-handed at 11 o'clock; left-handed at 1 o'clock
Syringe stabilization with fulcrums for NP block 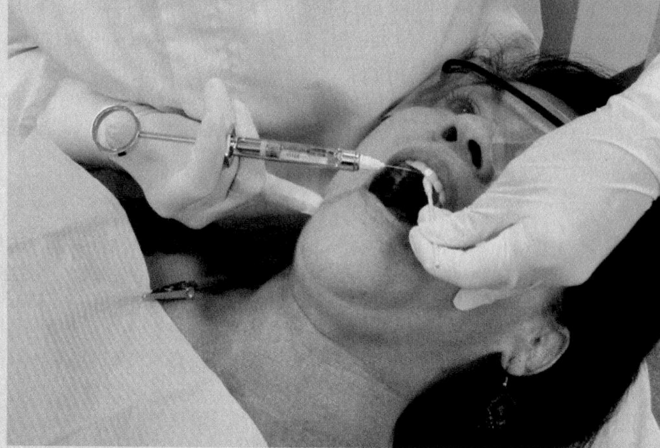 Fig. GG = Finger of dominant hand resting on patient's chin	
Landmarks	Maxillary central incisors Anterior hard palate of maxillae Incisive papilla Incisive foramen
Injection site/Needle insertion point 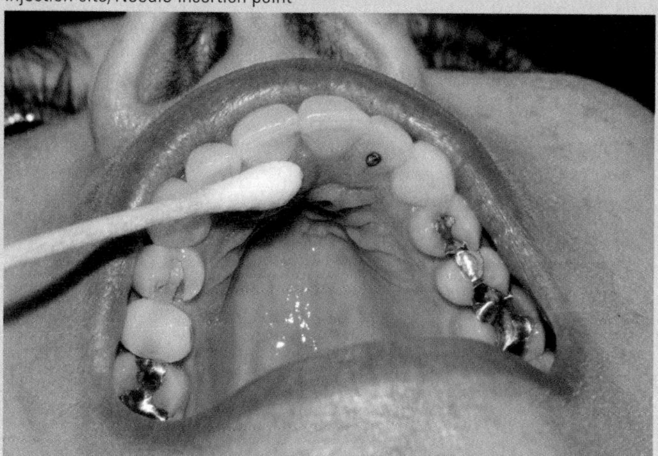 Fig. HH = Injection site for NP block	Palatal tissue lateral to incisive papilla and palatal to maxillary central incisors

(*Continued*)

TABLE 12.17 Nasopalatine Block Review (*Cont.*)

Depth of needle insertion Fig. II = Needle insertion for NP block	Approximately 4 to 5 mm or until gentle contact with maxilla
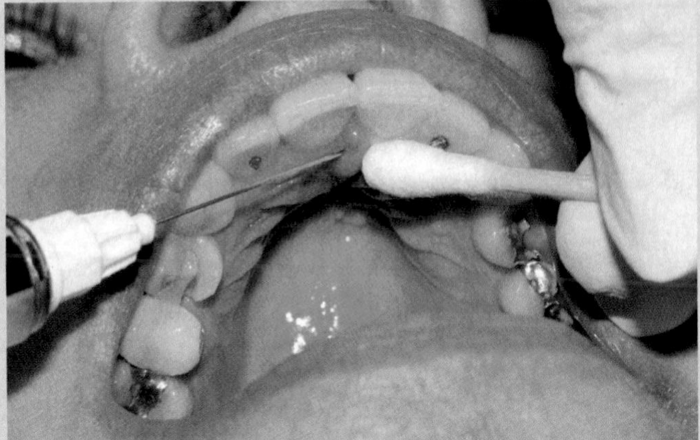 *1,* Without prepuncture technique: Cotton-tipped applicator is placed firmly on contralateral side of incisive papilla and needle is inserted on lateral side of incisive papilla toward clinician	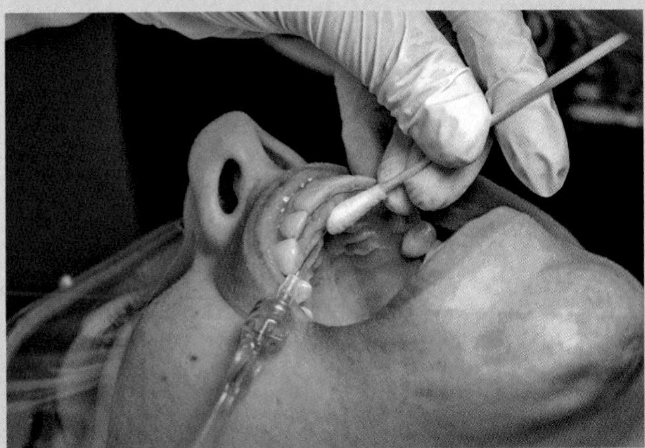 *2,* With prepuncture technique: Apply pressure on needle bevel and tissue with cotton-tipped applicator
Amount of anesthetic agent	Approximately 0.45 mL or one-fourth of cartridge until blanching of palatal tissue
Length of time to deposit	Minimum of 30 seconds

NP, Nasopalatine.

PROCEDURE BOX 12.8 Nasopalatine Block Procedure

Step 1 Assume the correct clinician position for right-handed at 11 o'clock; left-handed at 1 o'clock (see Table 12.17, Fig. FF).

Step 2 Ask the patient to open and extend the neck comfortably backward.

Step 3 Prepare the tissue on the lateral side of the incisive papilla toward the clinician (see Chapter 11 and see Table 12.17, Fig. HH).

Step 4 Determine whether to use a 27-gauge extra-short or short needle with a standard syringe or 30-gauge extra-short or short needle with a computer-controlled local anesthetic delivery device. With the syringe or handpiece in the dominant hand, orient the bevel of the needle toward the anterior hard palate.

Step 5 Determine whether using the prepuncture technique or not for surface pain control. *Without prepuncture technique:* Using a new cotton-tipped applicator in the nondominant hand, apply firm pressure with the applicator on the contralateral side of the incisive papilla until tissue is blanched. Maintain pressure with the cotton-tipped applicator throughout the injection as well as a short time after the agent is deposited. Advise patient that he or she may feel some slight discomfort from the pressure.

Step 6 *For both techniques:* Establish a fulcrum (see Table 12.17, Fig. GG).

Step 7 *Without prepuncture technique:* Direct the syringe or handpiece from the contralateral side of the mouth at 40° toward the lateral side of base of the incisive papilla with the large window facing the clinician. *For prepuncture technique:* Place the bevel of the needle on the injection site without penetrating the tissue. Apply pressure to the back of the needle and tissue with a cotton-tipped applicator and slowly dispense anesthetic agent to produce a topical anesthetic effect. If using a computer-controlled local anesthetic delivery device, depress the foot pedal lightly to start the slow-flow rate; after three audible beeps the system will announce "cruise control"; continue to administer the anesthetic without penetrating the tissue at the slow-flow rate for about 8 to 10 seconds.

Step 8 *For both techniques:* Insert the needle approximately 4 to 5 mm, possibly using the bidirectional rotation needle insertion technique, into the tissue on the lateral side of the incisive papilla toward the clinician until the bone of the maxilla is gently contacted. *Without prepuncture technique:* Maintain pressure with the cotton-tipped applicator throughout the injection and a short time after the agent is deposited (see Table 12.17, Fig. II1). *With prepuncture technique:* Continue to hold the cotton-tipped applicator over the needle tip with the bevel facing the tissue and continue to dispense a small amount of agent (see Table 12.17, Fig. II2) and then remove the applicator.

Step 9 *For both techniques:* Aspirate.

Step 10 *For both techniques:* If negative aspiration is achieved, slowly deposit approximately 0.45 mL of agent (one-fourth of cartridge) over a minimum of 30 seconds; tissue in area will blanch even further when the anesthetic is administered. *With prepuncture technique:* Inspect the tissue to make sure the agent is not overblanching it; slow it down or stop if excessive blanching of the palatal tissue occurs (see Table 12.18).

Step 11 *For both techniques:* Carefully withdraw the syringe or handpiece and immediately recap the needle using the one-handed scoop method utilizing a needle sheath prop (see Chapter 11).

Step 12 *For both techniques:* Rinse the patient's mouth. Inspect the region and stem any remaining bleeding with pressure using sterile gauze. Wait approximately 3 to 5 minutes until anesthesia takes effect before starting treatment.

and administering only one NP block may be helpful in these more sensitive patients with heavier deposits (see Fig. 11.3 in Chapter 11).

However, the NP block does not provide pulpal nor associated facial periodontal and gingiva anesthesia of the maxillary anterior teeth, so additional anesthesia such as the ASA block or the IO block may be indicated and is usually administered before this block. In addition, anesthesia of the associated palatal periodontium and gingiva of the maxillary canines may prove inadequate because of overlapping nerve fibers from the posteriorly located GP nerves.[1] This lack of anesthesia may be corrected by additional administration of the GP block if the patient is still feeling discomfort during treatment.

In addition, the target area on the anterior hard palate surrounding the incisive papilla is prone to previous trauma from food products, for example, hot coffee, tea, or pizza cheese or rough nacho chips, so care needs to be taken to work around any trauma that may be present.[16]

Target Area and Injection Site for Nasopalatine Block

The target area or deposit location for the NP block is both the right and left NP nerves entering the incisive foramen of the maxillae from the mucosa of the anterior hard palate, deep to the incisive papilla, and palatal to the maxillary central incisors (Fig. 12.11; see Table 12.17, Fig. EE). The incisive foramen is located at the midline between the articulating palatine processes of the maxillae of the anterior hard palate.

However, the injection site or needle insertion point is the palatal tissue lateral to the incisive papilla toward the clinician, which is usually located at the midline approximately 10 mm palatal to the maxillary central incisors in case there is no telltale bulge of the structure of the incisive papilla present (see Table 12.17, Fig. HH).[1] Never insert the needle directly into the incisive papilla because this can be extremely painful.[3]

Pressure anesthesia is performed utilizing a cotton-tipped applicator on palatal tissue on the contralateral side of the incisive papilla throughout, before, during, and for a short time after the injection

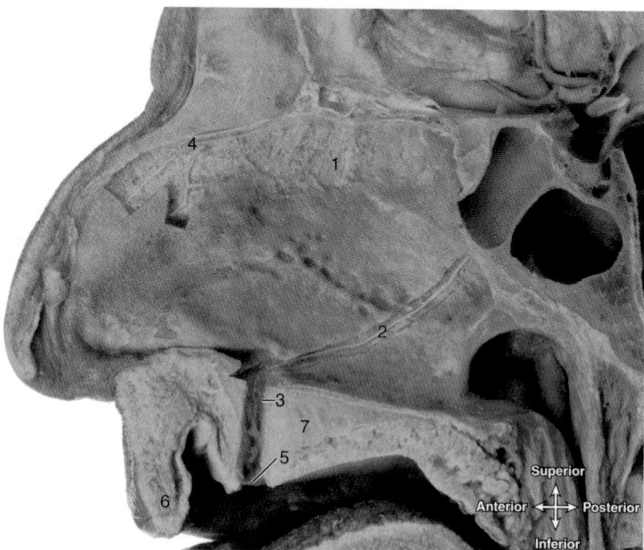

Fig. 12.11 Dissection of the left side of the nasal septum near the target area or deposit location for the nasopalatine block. *1,* Olfactory nerve; *2,* Nasopalatine nerve; *3,* Incisive canal; *4,* Anterior ethmoidal nerve; *5,* Incisive foramen; *6,* Upper lip; *7,* Anterior hard palate. (From Logan BM, Reynold PA, Hutching RT: *McMinn's color atlas of head and neck anatomy,* ed 4, London, 2010, Mosby. In Fehrenbach MJ, Herring SW: *Illustrated anatomy of the head and neck,* ed 6, St Louis, 2021, Saunders/Elsevier.)

unless prepuncture technique with the computer-controlled local anesthesia delivery device is used with the NP block (Chapter 11).[10]

The needle is inserted for this block into the previously blanched palatal tissue at 45° to the anterior hard palate (see Table 12.17, Fig. II). The needle is advanced into the tissue until the maxilla is gently contacted and then the injection is administered. There is no need to enter the incisive canal via the foramen for the NP block; in fact the needle cannot enter foramen with the recommended position of the needle.[3]

However, for another nerve block, the needle does enter deeper into the incisive canal using a similar needle insertion but with a different angulation.[3] With the expanding use of the computer-controlled local anesthesia delivery device, it was discovered that clinicians could also administer a nerve block to the entire maxillary anterior sextant, which has been named the palatal (approach) ASA (P-ASA) block, which allows for innervation of both the ASA block and the NP block regions. Thus the anterior branches of the ASA nerve as well as the NP nerve are anesthetized.[3,17]

As discussed, the P-ASA uses a similar initial tissue point of entry, the lateral aspect of the incisive papilla toward the clinician as the NP block, but differs in its final target since the needle is positioned within the incisive canal at a depth of approximately 6 to 10 mm[3] (Fig. 12.12). This results in anesthesia of the maxillary anterior teeth and associated labial periodontium and gingiva bilaterally as well as the additional anesthesia of the associated palatal periodontium and gingiva bilaterally, but without causing the usual collateral anesthesia of the upper lip and face.

The P-ASA block is a nerve block that can be used when performing cosmetic dentistry procedures because after the procedures are completed, the clinician can immediately and accurately assess the patient's smile line.[3] However, similar to the AMSA block that will be discussed next, clinicians may find that the longer deposit time of approximately 3 to 4 minutes and variable depth and duration of clinically effective anesthesia (especially with the maxillary canines) and lower level of clinically effective hemostatic control make its use compromised for nonsurgical periodontal therapy by the dental hygienist.[1,17] Potential also exists for postinjection pain, temporary numbness or paresthesia, and incisive papilla swelling or soreness.[1,17]

Indications of Clinically Effective Nasopalatine Block and Possible Complications

Indications of a clinically effective NP block include numbness in the anterior hard palate and absence of discomfort during dental procedures. Complications such as hematoma are extremely rare (Table 12.18).

Anterior Middle Superior Alveolar Block

The AMSA block anesthetizes a large area that is innervated by the ASA, MSA, GP, and NP nerves within the maxillary arch (Table 12.19, Figs. JJ–LL, and Procedure Box 12.9). Thus the single-site palatal injection of the AMSA block can anesthetize the maxillary anterior teeth and premolars as well as associated facial periodontium and gingiva of anesthetized teeth to the midline along with the mesiobuccal root of the maxillary first molar within one maxillary quadrant, hard palate with the associated palatal periodontium and gingiva of the ipsilateral maxillary posterior teeth and maxillary anterior teeth bilaterally.

This anesthesia is without the usual collateral anesthesia of the upper lip and face.[1,3] However, the ipsilateral maxillary molars may have anesthesia of the associated palatal periodontium and gingiva but do not have pulpal anesthesia nor anesthesia of the associated buccal periodontium and gingiva. Additional administration of the PSA block will add this necessary anesthesia coverage to complete maxillary quadrant anesthesia.[13]

This injection is commonly used when performing cosmetic dentistry because after the procedures are completed, the clinician can immediately and accurately assess the patient's smile line.[3,13] Studies show that this injection is best accomplished with a computer-controlled local anesthesia delivery device (see Chapter 9) because it regulates both the pressure and volume ratio of the agent delivered, which is not readily attained with a standard syringe.[1,3,13,18] In addition, more recent studies show that due to the extensive anatomy involved, this block may be variable in the depth and duration of clinically effective anesthesia and does not provide a high enough level of clinically effective hemostatic control.[1,13,19]

This then compromises the use of the AMSA block for nonsurgical periodontal therapy by the dental hygienist that usually needs a full depth and long duration of clinically effective anesthesia as well as clinically effective hemostatic control to complete the treatment.[1,13] Instead, reliance on the more clinically effective nerve blocks allows the

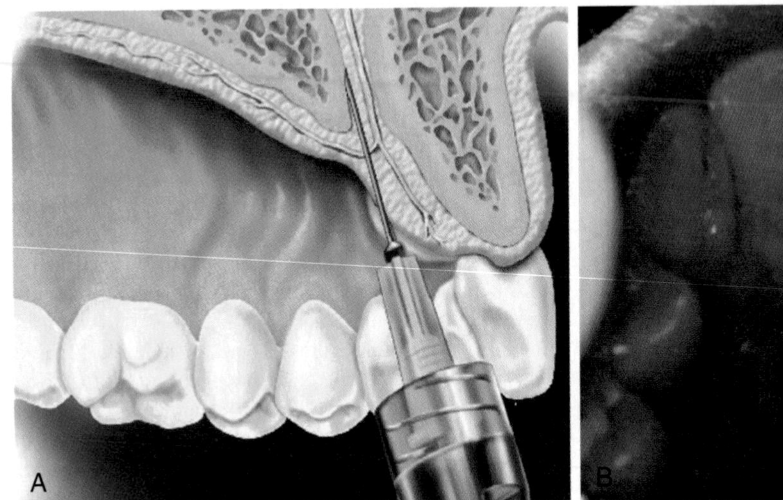

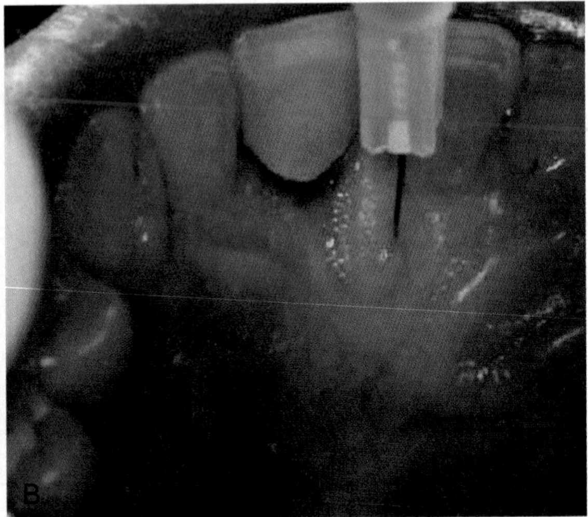

Fig. 12.12 (A) Syringe orientation of the palatal (approach)-anterior superior alveolar block demonstrating the needle positioned within the incisive foramen. (B) Needle insertion for the palatal (approach)-anterior superior alveolar block. (From Malamed S: *Handbook of local anesthesia*, ed 7, St Louis, 2018, Mosby/Elsevier.)

TABLE 12.18 Nasopalatine Block Complications

Complication	Technique Adjustment
Inadequate anesthesia of maxillary canine due to overlapping from GP nerve	Additional GP block (see Table 12.15)
Density of tissue and constricted area for anesthetic deposition may cause agent to appear around needle insertion site during administration	Inject slowly and rinse patient's mouth following safe capping of needle
Excessive blanching of palatal tissue that may lead to postoperative tissue ischemia and sloughing with delivery device	Slowing or stopping delivery device to let agent dissipate as well as controlling overall amount used

GP, Greater palatine.

TABLE 12.19 Anterior Middle Superior Alveolar Block Review

Indications	Procedures on maxillary anterior teeth and premolars within one maxillary quadrant; will need to administer PSA block to complete maxillary quadrant anesthesia
Nerves anesthetized	ASA nerve MSA nerve if present GP nerve NP nerve
Teeth anesthetized	Maxillary anterior teeth and premolars along with maxillary first molar mesiobuccal root within one maxillary quadrant
Other structures anesthetized	Facial periodontium and gingiva of anesthetized teeth to midline; hard palate and palatal periodontium and gingiva of ipsilateral maxillary posterior teeth and maxillary anterior teeth bilaterally; no regional soft tissue anesthesia of upper lip and face
Administration technique	See Procedure Box 12.9
Needle gauge and length	30-gauge extra-short or short with computer-controlled local anesthetic delivery device or 27-gauge extra-short or short with standard syringe

TABLE 12.19 Anterior Middle Superior Alveolar Block Review (*Cont.*)

Target area/Deposit location 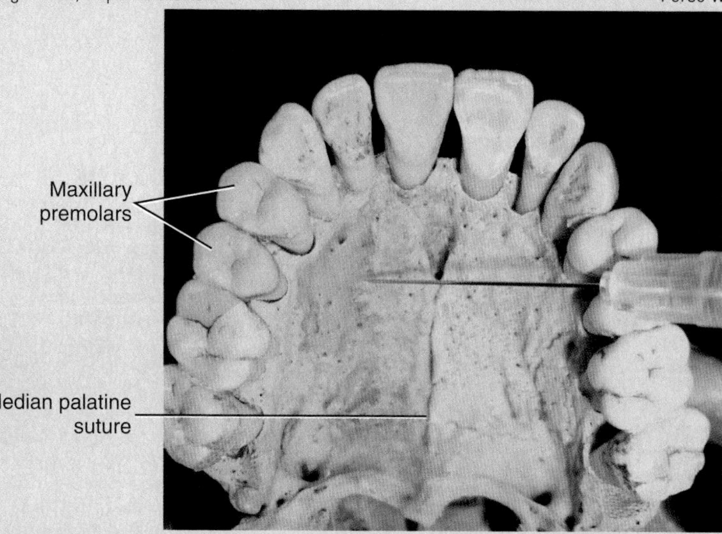 Fig. JJ = Target area and distribution of anesthesia for AMSA block (From Fehrenbach MJ, Herring SW: *Illustrated anatomy of the head and neck,* ed 6, St Louis, 2021, Saunders/Elsevier)	Pores within maxilla of hard palate
Clinician position	Same as GP block; right side, right-handed at 8 to 9 o'clock (left-handed at 4 to 3 o'clock). Left side, right-handed at 11 o'clock (left-handed at 1 o'clock). (See Table 12.15, Fig. AA.)
Syringe stabilization with fulcrums	Same as GP block; see Table 12.15, Fig. BB
Landmarks	Maxillary premolars Palatal gingival margin Median palatine raphe (suture)
Injection site/Needle insertion point 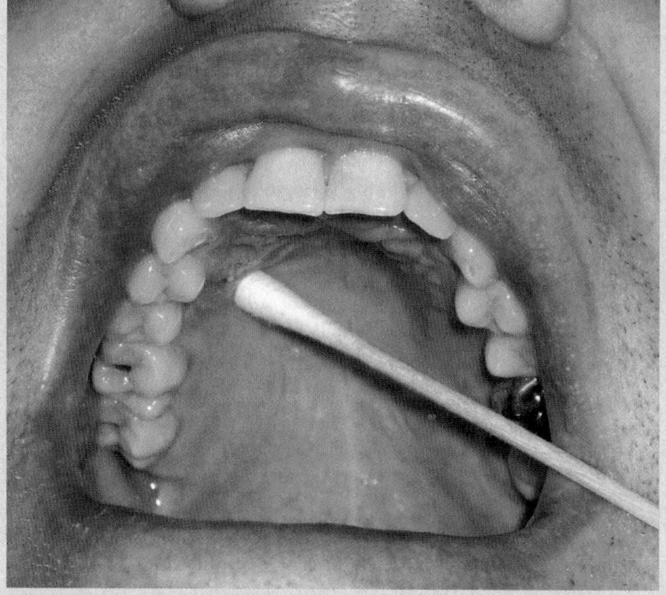 Fig. KK = Injection site for AMSA block (From Fehrenbach MJ, Herring SW: *Illustrated anatomy of the head and neck,* ed 6, St Louis, 2021, Saunders/Elsevier)	Area on hard palate superior to apices of maxillary premolars and midway between palatal gingival margin and median palatal raphe (suture)

(*Continued*)

TABLE 12.19 Anterior Middle Superior Alveolar Block Review (*Cont.*)

Depth of needle insertion Fig. LL = Needle insertion for AMSA block	Approximately 4 to 7 mm until gentle contact with bone of palate
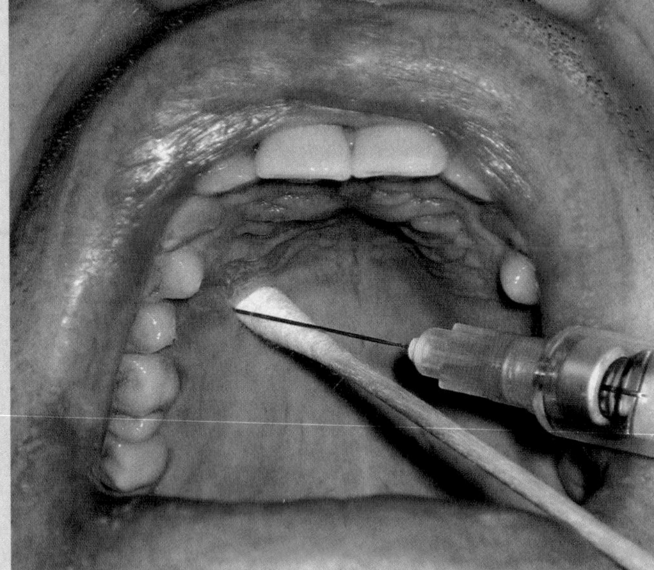 *1,* Without prepuncture technique: Maintain pressure with cotton-tipped applicator throughout injection and for short time after (From Fehrenbach MJ, Herring SW: *Illustrated anatomy of the head and neck,* ed 6, St Louis, 2021, Saunders/Elsevier)	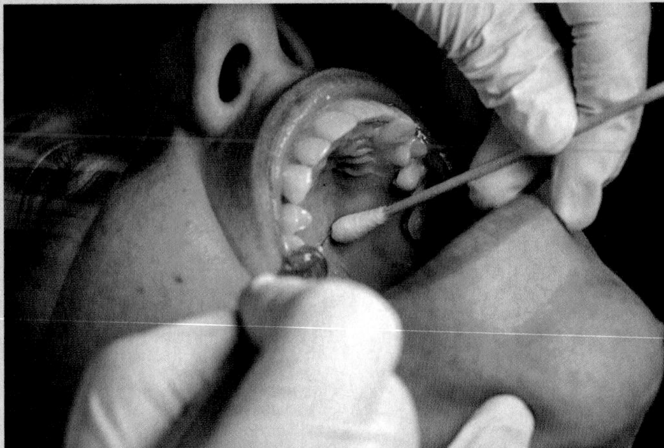 *2,* With prepuncture technique: Apply pressure on needle bevel and tissue with cotton-tipped applicator.
Amount of anesthetic agent	Approximately 1.4 to 1.8 mL until blanching of palatal tissue
Length of time to deposit	Approximately 0.5 mL per minute

AMSA, Anterior middle superior alveolar; *ASA,* anterior superior alveolar; *GP,* greater palatine; *MSA,* middle superior alveolar; *NP,* nasopalatine; *PSA,* posterior superior alveolar.

dental hygienist to treatment plan instrumentation in either maxillary sextants or maxillary quadrants with more confidence of both pain and hemostatic control.[1,13,18]

Target Area and Injection Site for Anterior Middle Superior Alveolar Block

The target area or deposit location for the AMSA block is the pores within the maxilla of the hard palate (see Table 12.19, Fig. JJ). As the agent diffuses through the pores, it has access from the anterior to middle part of the superior dental plexus, which then anesthetizes the teeth and associated facial and palatal periodontium and gingiva as discussed earlier (see Fig. 12.7).[1,13,20]

The injection site or needle insertion point for the AMSA block is on the hard palate superior to the apices of the maxillary premolars and midway between the palatal gingival margin and the median palatal raphe overlying the median palatine suture (see Table 12.19, Fig. KK). Orientation of the handpiece of the syringe from the computer-controlled local anesthesia delivery device should be from the contralateral premolars. The previously blanched tissue is approached with the needle at 45° to the hard palate until the maxilla is gently contacted and then the injection is administered (see Table 12.19, Fig. LL).

Indications of Clinically Effective Anterior Middle Superior Alveolar Block and Possible Complications

Indications of a clinically effective AMSA block include variable numbness of the large area that is usually innervated by the ASA, MSA, GP, and NP nerves. Blanching of the palatal tissue also remains present following the AMSA block due to the increased agent dispensed. However, if excessive, it may cause possibly painful postoperative tissue ischemia and sloughing (Table 12.20).[3] Thus if excessive blanching of the palatal tissue is beginning to be noted, slowing or stopping the delivery device for a few seconds to let the agent dissipate as well as controlling the overall amount of agent used, will diminish the chance of this postoperative event. Other complications are extremely rare.

COMMON TECHNIQUE ERRORS ASSOCIATED WITH MAXILLARY INJECTIONS

Most technique errors associated with maxillary injections are due to the angulation of the needle and syringe barrel and are usually associated with the maxillary facial injections. To confirm safe and effective pain control, the dental hygienist should follow all recommended injection technique guidelines addressed in this chapter. This section describes common technique errors associated with maxillary facial injections.

Common Errors With Supraperiosteal Injections, Anterior Superior Alveolar, or Middle Superior Alveolar Blocks

The most common technique error associated with supraperiosteal injections or ASA and MSA blocks is the angle of the needle and syringe barrel. The angle of the syringe barrel should be parallel to the

PROCEDURE BOX 12.9 Anterior Middle Superior Alveolar Block Procedure

Step 1 Assume the correct clinician position for right side, right-handed at 8 to 9 o'clock (left-handed at 4–3 o'clock); left side, right-handed at 11 o'clock (left-handed at 1 o'clock; see Table 12.15, Fig. AA).

Step 2 Ask the patient to open and extend the neck either to the right or left.

Step 3 Prepare the tissue on the surface of the hard palate superior to the apices of the maxillary premolars and midway between the palatal gingival margin and the median palatal raphe (see Chapter 11 and Table 12.19, Fig. KK).

Step 4. With the handpiece of a computer-controlled local anesthetic delivery device with a 30-gauge short needle in the dominant hand, orient the bevel of the needle toward the hard palate.

Step 5 Determine whether to use the prepuncture technique for surface pain control. *Without prepuncture technique:* Using a new cotton-tipped applicator in the dominant hand, apply firm pressure with the applicator superior to the apices of the maxillary premolars on the surface of the hard palate until tissue is blanched. Maintain pressure with the cotton-tipped applicator throughout the injection for a short time after the agent is deposited. Advise patient that he or she may feel some slight discomfort from the pressure.

Step 6 *For both techniques:* Establish a fulcrum (see Table 12.15, Fig. BB for fulcrum recommendations) and direct the handpiece from the contralateral premolars at a 45° superior to the apices of the maxillary premolars on the hard palate, with the large window facing the clinician.

Step 7 *Without prepuncture technique:* Insert the needle approximately 4 to 7 mm, possibly using the bidirectional rotation needle insertion technique, into the tissue over the hard palate, superior to the apices of the maxillary premolars, as well as being midway between the palatal gingival margin and the median palatal raphe until the maxilla is gently contacted, and maintain pressure with the cotton-tipped applicator throughout the injection and a short time after the agent is deposited (see Table 12.19, Fig. LL1). *With prepuncture technique:* Place the bevel of the needle on the injection site as described above without penetrating the tissue. Apply pressure to the back of the needle and tissue with the cotton-tipped applicator and slowly dispense anesthetic agent. If using a computer-controlled local anesthetic delivery device, depress the foot pedal lightly to start the slow-flow rate. After three audible beeps the system will announce, "cruise control"; continue to administer the anesthetic without penetrating the tissue at the slow-flow rate for about 8 to 10 seconds to produce a topical anesthetic effect (see Table 12.19, Fig. LL2). Insert the needle with the bidirectional rotation needle insertion technique, and after a pause of 5 to 6 seconds with the anesthetic flowing at the slow-flow rate, continue to rotate the needle with a back and forth motion toward the palatal tissue for another 1 to 2 millimeters before pausing. Every 4 to 5 seconds, slowly advance the needle about 1 mm (creating an anesthetic pathway) until you reach the deposit location: the palatal bone.

Step 8 *For both techniques:* Aspirate.

Step 9 *For both techniques:* If negative aspiration is achieved, slowly deposit approximately 1.4 to 1.8 mL of agent at 0.5 mL per minute; tissue in area will blanch even further when the anesthetic is administered. *With prepuncture technique:* Inspect the tissue to make sure the agent is not overblanching it; slow it down or stop if excessive blanching of the palatal tissue occurs (see Table 12.20).

Step 10 *For both techniques:* Carefully withdraw the handpiece and immediately recap the needle using the one-handed scoop method utilizing a needle sheath prop (see Chapter 11).

Step 11 *For both techniques:* Rinse the patient's mouth. Inspect the region and stem any remaining bleeding with pressure using sterile gauze. Wait approximately 3 to 5 minutes until anesthesia takes effect before starting treatment.

TABLE 12.20 Anterior Middle Superior Alveolar Block Complications

Complication	Technique Adjustment
Variable depth and duration of anesthesia	Consider use of ASA, MSA, and PSA blocks as well as GP and NP blocks instead to achieve desired increased clinical effectiveness of depth and duration of anesthesia
Excessive blanching of palatal tissue that may lead to postoperative tissue ischemia and sloughing with delivery device	Slowing or stopping delivery device to let agent dissipate as well as controlling overall amount used

ASA, Anterior superior alveolar; *GP,* greater palatine; *MSA,* middle superior alveolar; *NP,* nasopalatine; *PSA,* posterior superior alveolar.

long axis of the tooth following the contour of the tooth. If the syringe barrel angle is too steep, the needle will be inserted too shallow into the maxillary mucobuccal fold. The needle could possibly be inserted into the firmer tissue of the attached gingiva so the underlying alveolar process of the maxilla will be contacted, causing increased discomfort and possibly trauma to the tissue (see Fig. 12.1) and the target location will be missed, causing a decreased level of clinically effective anesthesia.[1,9] Fig. 12.13 demonstrates *incorrect needle/syringe angulation* for supraperiosteal injections, ASA block and MSA block; Fig. 12.14 demonstrates *correct needle/syringe angulation.*

Common Errors With Posterior Superior Alveolar Block

The most common technique error associated with the PSA block is not obtaining the correct needle and syringe barrel angulation to the injection site or needle insertion point, which must be maintained throughout using three different orientations but only one movement.[1,3] This angulation is upward (or superiorly) at 45° to the maxillary occlusal plane, inward (or medially) at 45° to the midsagittal plane, and backward (or posteriorly) at 45° to the long axis of the maxillary second molar. To achieve these angulations it is important for the syringe barrel to be at the ipsilateral corner of the patient's mouth and resting on the clinician's retraction finger. It is also important for the clinician to retract the tissue vertically rather than horizontally. Note that Fig. 12.15 demonstrates *incorrect syringe angulation* and in contrast, Fig. 12.16 demonstrates *correct syringe angulation.*

Common Errors With Infraorbital Block

The most common technique error associated with the IO block is not aligning the syringe barrel toward the IO foramen in the same ipsilateral linear relationship as the pupil of the eye looking forward. In addition, inserting the needle too shallow into the maxillary mucobuccal fold will cause premature contact with the maxilla and a too inferior deposit of anesthetic agent to the IO foramen, which will result in a less than clinically effective level of anesthesia.[1,3] Note that Fig. 12.17 demonstrates *incorrect syringe/needle angulation* for the IO block and in contrast, Fig. 12.18 demonstrates *correct syringe/needle angulation* for the IO block.

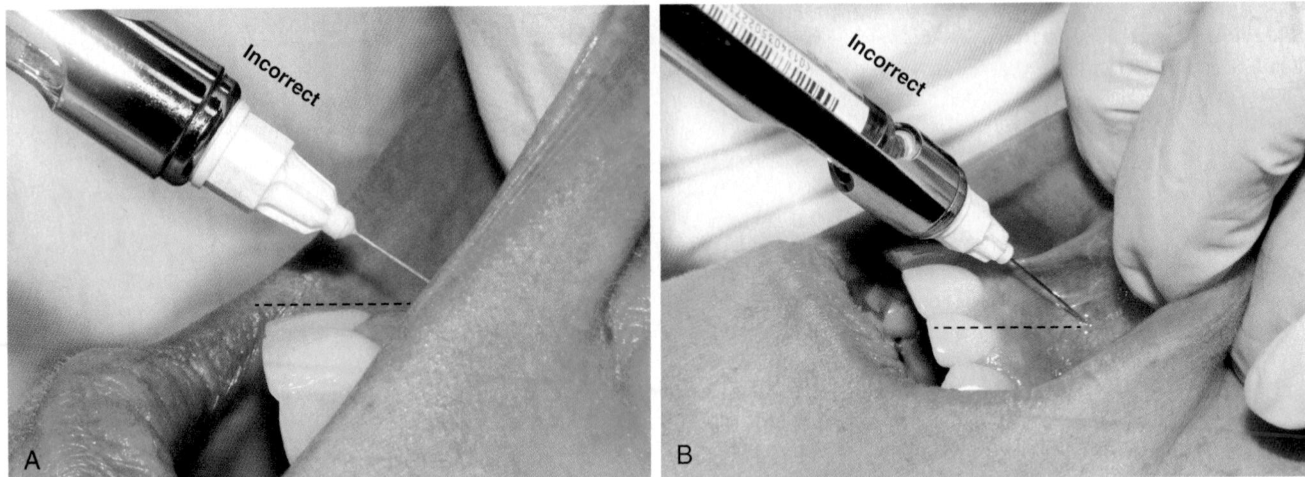

Fig. 12.13 Incorrect angulations of the needle and syringe barrel for maxillary facial injections such as supraperiosteal injections or anterior superior alveolar and middle superior alveolar blocks. (A) **Incorrect angulations:** Syringe barrel angulation is too steep and not parallel with the long axis of the tooth (*dotted line*). (B) **Incorrect angulations:** The injection site or needle insertion point is too shallow and not parallel with the long axis of the tooth (*dotted line*). Bone will be contacted, causing discomfort to the patient, and deposition of agent will be directly over the apex of the tooth and not superior to it, missing each apical foramen.

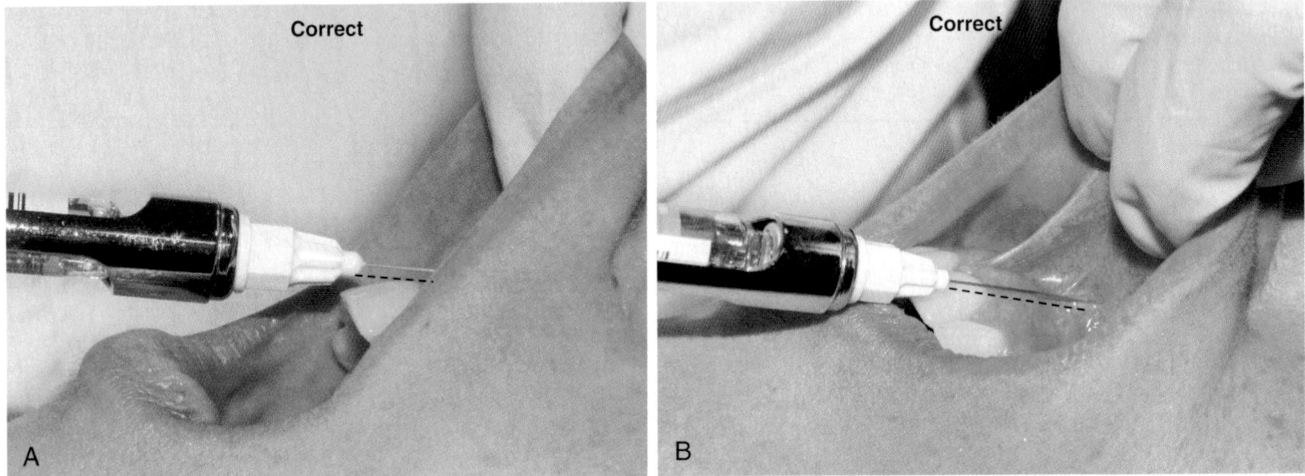

Fig. 12.14 Correct angulations for maxillary facial injections such as supraperiosteal injections or anterior superior alveolar and middle superior alveolar blocks. (A) The syringe barrel angulation is parallel with the long axis of the tooth (*dotted lines*). (B) This allows the needle to be inserted within the correct height of the maxillary mucobuccal fold, allowing the needle to be inserted superior to the apex of the tooth for correct placement of agent so it can enter each apical foramen.

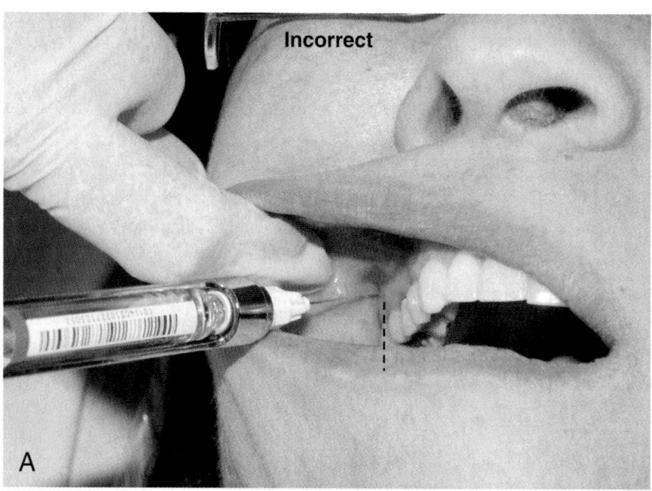

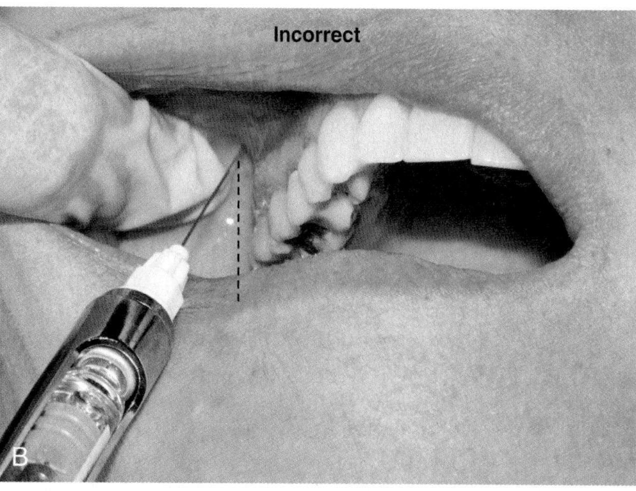

Fig. 12.15 Incorrect angulations of the needle and syringe barrel for posterior superior alveolar block. (A) **Incorrect angulation:** Syringe barrel angulation is greater than 45° backward from the apex of the maxillary second molar (*dotted line*), causing needle tip to be too medial and bone will be contacted. Instead decrease angulation of the syringe barrel angulation to 45°. (B) **Incorrect angulation:** Syringe barrel angulation is not 45° backward from the apices of the maxillary second molar (*dotted line*). Instead the syringe barrel needs to be resting on the clinician's retraction finger and at the ipsilateral corner of the patient's mouth.

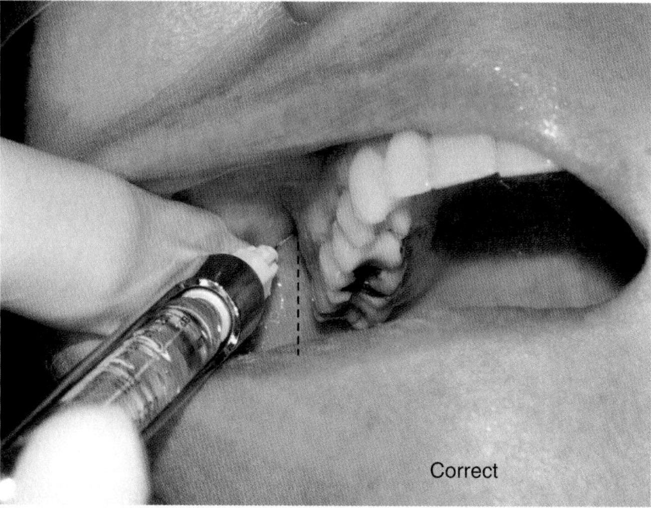

Fig. 12.16 Correct angulation for posterior superior alveolar block since the syringe barrel angulation is 45° upward to the maxillary occlusal plane, 45° inward to the midsagittal plane, and 45° backward to the long axis of the maxillary second molar (*dotted line*). Note stable fulcrum of syringe resting on clinician's retraction finger and at the corner of the patient's mouth.

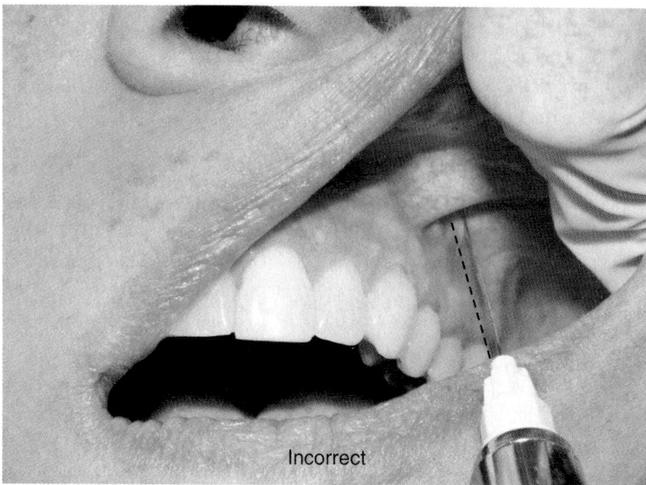

Fig. 12.17 Incorrect angulation for infraorbital block since the syringe barrel is not aligned toward the infraorbital foramen in a linear relationship with the pupil of the eye looking forward; the syringe barrel is also angled toward the maxilla (*dotted line*). Injection site or needle insertion point is too shallow within the maxillary mucobuccal fold. This will cause premature contact of the bone with the needle and an inferior deposition of agent.

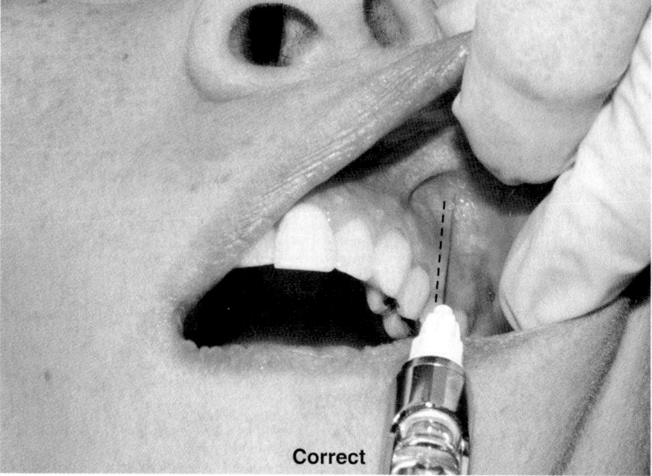

Fig. 12.18 Correct angulation for infraorbital block since the syringe barrel is correctly aligned toward the infraorbital foramen and in a linear relationship with the pupil of the eye looking forward (*dotted line*).

DENTAL HYGIENE CONSIDERATIONS

- Local anesthesia of the maxillae is more clinically effective than that of the mandible because the facial plates of bone over the teeth are less dense than that of the mandible over similar teeth. Since there is less anatomic variation of the maxillae and palatine bones with the associated nerves with respect to local anesthetic landmarks than there is in similar mandibular structures, the maxillary injections are more routine and usually do not need troubleshooting for lack of clinical effectiveness.
- Supraperiosteal injections for maxillary injections are recommended when pulpal anesthesia is needed on a single tooth or when anesthesia of the associated periodontium and gingiva is needed in a localized area.
- The intraseptal injection is an intraosseous supplemental injection recommended when there is a need for additional hemostatic control with the interdental periodontium and gingiva between adjacent teeth.
- The periodontal ligament (PDL) injection is an intraosseous supplemental injection recommended when pulpal anesthesia and associated periodontium and gingiva is indicated on a single tooth.
- To achieve a level of comfort during all maxillary facial nerve blocks, as well as with supraperiosteal injections, there is usually avoidance of contact of the maxilla with the needle except at the final deposition point of the infraorbital (IO) block. Instead, the agent is administered within the height of the maxillary mucobuccal fold of the alveolar mucosa.
- The posterior superior alveolar (PSA) block is recommended for anesthesia of the maxillary molars and associated buccal periodontium and gingiva. In 28% of the cases the mesiobuccal root of the maxillary first molar will not be anesthetized by the PSA but with the MSA.
- The middle superior alveolar (MSA) block is recommended for anesthesia of the maxillary premolars and the mesiobuccal root of the maxillary first molar, and associated buccal periodontium and gingiva. This nerve is present in only 28% of the cases. If the MSA nerve is not present the ASA block will anesthetize the premolars and the PSA block will anesthetize the mesiobuccal root of the first molar.
- The anterior superior alveolar (ASA) block is recommended for anesthesia of the maxillary anterior teeth and associated labial periodontium and gingiva. Bilateral injections of the ASA block or supraperiosteal injections over the contralateral maxillary central incisor may be indicated if the patient is still feeling discomfort during treatment due to crossover-innervation.
- The IO block is recommended for anesthesia of the maxillary anterior teeth and premolars and associated facial periodontium and gingiva.
- If quadrant dental hygiene treatment is planned, it is recommended that the PSA block be administered before any of the other maxillary facial nerve blocks as well as any palatal nerve blocks to allow the necessary time for the larger maxillary molars to become anesthetized. Instrumentation follows the same manner as the administration of the maxillary facial anesthesia block series, first the PSA and MSA blocks and then the ASA block for the maxillary quadrant.
- There is no need to avoid the palatal nerve blocks because of their somewhat greater level of discomfort; the range is still low when administered correctly. In order to maximize patient comfort during a palatal nerve block, pressure anesthesia utilizing a cotton-tipped applicator is recommended. Other clinicians instead use a prepuncture technique with the computer-controlled local anesthesia delivery device.
- The greater palatine (GP) block is recommended for anesthesia of the associated palatal periodontium and gingiva of the maxillary posterior teeth.
- The nasopalatine (NP) block is recommended for anesthesia of the associated palatal periodontium and gingiva for the maxillary anterior teeth bilaterally from maxillary canine to canine.
- Instrumentation follows the same manner as the administration of the palatal injection series of first the GP block and then the NP block for one maxillary quadrant. The clinician may have to additionally administer either a GP or NP block if there is an overlap of nerve fibers in either the canine or premolar region.
- The anterior middle superior alveolar (AMSA) block is recommended for anesthesia of the area innervated by the ASA, MSA, GP, and NP blocks within the maxillary arch. If using the AMSA block, the PSA block is additionally administered first in most cases to complete the coverage maxillary quadrant anesthesia so as to include the maxillary molars. Use of the AMSA block for nonsurgical periodontal therapy may be compromised due to variable depth and duration of anesthesia and lack of hemostatic control.

CASE STUDY 12.1 Considerations With Lesion Formation

A new patient has come into the dental office due to pain with her maxillary right first premolar. Following a complete examination, the supervising dentist determines that the cracked and heavily decayed tooth needs an immediate extraction due to a large periapical lesion formation noted on the radiographs and signs of extreme pulpitis from the pulp tester, even though there are no other intraoral signs at this time.

The supervising dentist asks the dental hygienist to administer the anesthesia since the schedule is running behind and there is not even time to enter the patient history into the computerized patient record. The newly hired dental hygienist hurriedly selects to administer a supraperiosteal injection using the usual volume of agent and without a vasoconstrictor; the treatment plan for anesthesia was formed without further discussing the case with the supervising dentist. When the dentist begins the procedure, the patient says that she is still in pain on the tooth.

Critical Thinking Questions

- Why is the patient still in discomfort?
- How should the dental team have proceeded for a more clinically effective outcome in pain control for the patient?
- What serious complications may still occur for this patient?

CHAPTER REVIEW QUESTIONS

1. Anesthesia of the maxillary teeth is MORE clinically effective than the mandibular teeth BECAUSE the bone of the maxillae overlying the teeth is denser and less porous.
   A. Both the statement and the reason are correct and related.
   B. Both the statement and the reason are correct but NOT related.
   C. The statement is correct, but the reason is NOT correct.
   D. The statement is NOT correct, but the reason is correct.
   E. NEITHER the statement NOR the reason is correct.
2. When performing maxillary nerve anesthesia, which is the ONLY local anesthetic block that requires the clinician to gently contact bone with the needle to confirm clinically effective outcome?
   A. Infraorbital block
   B. Anterior superior alveolar block
   C. Middle superior alveolar block
   D. Posterior superior alveolar block

3. Which block is MOST appropriate to administer so as to allow for clinically effective anesthesia of the associated buccal periodontium and gingiva of the maxillary premolars?
   A. Greater palatine block
   B. Nasopalatine block
   C. Anterior superior alveolar block
   D. Middle superior alveolar block
4. Where is the recommended injection site or needle insertion point for local anesthetic deposition of the agent located when administering a supraperiosteal injection on the surface of the maxilla?
   A. Either facial or lingual surfaces of the cervix of the tooth
   B. Within the height of the maxillary mucobuccal fold
   C. Between the periosteum and alveolar process
   D. Between the gingiva and alveolar process
5. It is ALWAYS important for the clinician to orient the needle as close as possible to the periosteum. This is to confirm the needle glides along the periosteum allowing for more stability.
   A. Both the statement and the reason are correct and related.
   B. Both the statement and the reason are correct but NOT related.
   C. The statement is correct, but the reason is NOT correct.
   D. The statement is NOT correct, but the reason is correct.
   E. NEITHER the statement NOR the reason is correct.
6. Which of the following local anesthetic blocks anesthetizes the mesiobuccal root of tooth #3 (Canadian #1.6) in ONLY approximately 28% of the cases?
   A. Greater palatine block
   B. Nasopalatine block
   C. Anterior superior alveolar block
   D. Middle superior alveolar block
7. Which of the following structures does the infraorbital local anesthetic block USUALLY anesthetize?
   A. Teeth and associated periodontium and gingiva within one maxillary quadrant
   B. Teeth and associated periodontium and gingiva within the maxillary arch
   C. Anterior and middle superior alveolar nerves within one maxillary quadrant
   D. Anterior and middle superior alveolar nerves within the maxillary arch
8. Where is the recommended target area or deposit location for the posterior superior alveolar local anesthetic block?
   A. Posterior superior alveolar nerve entering the infratemporal fossa
   B. Posterior superior alveolar nerve exiting the pterygopalatine fossa
   C. Posterior superior alveolar nerve exiting the parotid salivary gland near the facial nerve
   D. Posterior superior alveolar nerve entering the maxilla through the posterior superior alveolar foramina
9. Which local anesthetic block listed below requires the recommended injection site or needle insertion point to be within the height of the maxillary mucobuccal fold superior to the apices of the maxillary second molar?
   A. Infraorbital block
   B. Anterior superior alveolar block
   C. Middle superior alveolar block
   D. Posterior superior alveolar block
10. If the clinician wanted to anesthetize teeth #9 to #11 (Canadian #2.1 to #2.3) and associated facial and palatal periodontium and gingiva for a limited procedure, it would be BEST to administer which of the following local anesthetic blocks?
   A. Infraorbital block only
   B. Infraorbital and nasopalatine blocks
   C. Infraorbital and greater palatine blocks
   D. Anterior superior alveolar and middle superior alveolar blocks
11. Since the greater palatine block does NOT provide pulpal anesthesia, the use of the middle superior alveolar block and/or posterior superior alveolar block is also indicated when instrumenting on the maxillary premolars.
   A. Both the statement and the reason are correct and related.
   B. Both the statement and the reason are correct but NOT related.
   C. The statement is correct, but the reason is NOT.
   D. The statement is NOT correct, but the reason is correct.
   E. NEITHER the statement NOR the reason is correct.
12. Which of the following local anesthetic blocks requires the needle and syringe barrel angulation to be at 45-degrees within three separate planes during administration?
   A. Infraorbital block
   B. Anterior superior alveolar block
   C. Middle superior alveolar block
   D. Posterior superior alveolar block
13. Where is the recommended injection site or needle insertion point for the nasopalatine block?
   A. Lateral to the incisive papilla
   B. Anterior to the greater palatine foramen
   C. Posterior to the incisive foramen
   D. Near the maxillary labial frenum
14. Where is the recommended injection site or needle insertion point for the middle superior alveolar local anesthetic block?
   A. Height of the mucobuccal fold of the maxillary canine
   B. Apices of the maxillary second premolar
   C. Height of the mucobuccal fold of the maxillary second premolar
   D. Height of the mucobuccal fold of the maxillary first premolar
15. Where is the anesthetic deposit location (or target) for the anterior superior alveolar local anesthetic block?
   A. Superior to the apex of the maxillary canine
   B. Superior to the apex of the maxillary first premolar
   C. Superior to the apex of the maxillary second premolar
   D. Superior to the apex of the maxillary first molar
16. What is the USUAL approximate depth of needle insertion for the anterior superior alveolar local anesthetic block?
   A. 5 millimeters
   B. 10 millimeters
   C. 16 millimeters
   D. 20 millimeters
17. What is the recommended injection site or needle insertion point for the infraorbital block?
   A. Maxillary mucobuccal fold superior to the apex of the maxillary canine
   B. Within the height of the maxillary mucobuccal fold of the maxillary first premolar
   C. Within the height of the maxillary mucobuccal fold of the maxillary second premolar
   D. Maxillary mucobuccal fold at the apices of the maxillary first molar
18. After receiving an infraorbital local anesthetic block, the patient reports slight numbness of the lower eyelid. What should the clinician do next?
   A. Stop treatment and deal with transient facial nerve paralysis

B. Explain to the patient about how it is a common reaction to the block
C. Place a cold compress quickly to prevent hematoma
D. Immediately administer an oral antihistamine

19. Where is the greater palatine foramen usually located?
A. Approximately 10 millimeters medial to the mandibular lingual gingival margin
B. Approximately 10 millimeters medial and directly superior to the palatal gingival margin
C. Lateral to the incisive papilla and palatal to the maxillary central incisors
D. Lateral to the lesser palatine foramen and posterior to the hard plate

20. Pressure anesthesia to control patient discomfort upon injection with the needle can be used during which of the following local anesthetic blocks?
A. Posterior superior alveolar and greater palatine local anesthetic blocks
B. Greater palatine and nasopalatine local anesthetic blocks
C. Nasopalatine and infraorbital local anesthetic blocks
D. Nasopalatine local anesthetic block only

21. Which of the following supplemental injections is RARELY used within the maxillary arch before nonsurgical periodontal therapy?
A. Supraperiosteal injection
B. Intraseptal injection
C. Periodontal ligament injection
D. Both the supraperiosteal and intraseptal injections

22. Which of the following supplemental injections are also intraosseous injections?
A. Supraperiosteal injection
B. Intraseptal injection
C. Periodontal ligament injection
D. Both the intraseptal and periodontal ligament injections

23. What is the injection site or needle insertion point for an intraseptal injection within the maxillary arch?
A. Center of the interdental papilla
B. Superior to the apex of the tooth
C. Depth of the gingival sulcus
D. Within the height of the maxillary mucobuccal fold

24. Which of the following supplemental injections increase hemostasis when used with a less diluted vasoconstrictor such as epinephrine 1:50,000 upon instrumenting within the maxillary arch?
A. Supraperiosteal injection
B. Intraseptal injection
C. Periodontal ligament injection
D. Both the supraperiosteal and intraseptal injections

25. Which of the following supplemental injections within the maxillary arch is palpated before administration to confirm soft tissue entry before the needle is inserted?
A. Supraperiosteal injection
B. Intraseptal injection
C. Periodontal ligament injection
D. Both the supraperiosteal and intraseptal injections

REFERENCES

1. Fehrenbach MJ, Herring SW. *Illustrated anatomy of the head and neck.* ed 6. St Louis: Saunders/Elsevier; 2021.
2. Rodella LF, Buffoli B, Labanca M, Rezzani R. A review of the mandibular and maxillary nerve supplies and their clinical relevance. *Arch Oral Biol.* 2012;57(4):323–334.
3. Malamed S. *Handbook of local anesthesia.* ed 7. St Louis: Mosby/Elsevier; 2018.
4. Kaufman E, Epstein JB, Naveh E, Gorsky M, Gross A, Cohen G. A survey of pain, pressure, and discomfort induced by commonly used oral anesthesia injections. *Anesth Prog.* 2005;54(4):122–127.
5. Fehrenbach MJ, Editor-in-Chief, et al. *Mosby's dental dictionary.* ed 4. St Louis: Mosby/Elsevier; 2020.
6. Bowen DM, Pieren JA. *Darby and Walsh dental hygiene: theory and practice.* ed 5. St Louis: Saunders/Elsevier; 2020.
7. Newman MG, et al. Newman and Carranza's *Clinical periodontology for dental hygienist.* Philadelphia: Saunders; 2021.
8. Nelson S. *Wheeler's dental anatomy, physiology, and occlusion.* ed 9. St Louis: Saunders/Elsevier; 2009.
9. Fehrenbach MJ, Popowics T. *Illustrated dental embryology, histology, and anatomy.* ed 5. St Louis: Saunders/Elsevier; 2020.
10. Fehrenbach MJ. Pain control for dental hygienists: Current concepts in local anesthesia are reviewed. *RDH Magazine,* February 2005.
11. Logan BM, Reynold PA, Hutching RT. *McMinn's color atlas of head and neck anatomy.* ed 4. London: Mosby; 2010.
12. Aboytes DB, Pizanis VG. Reduced depth technique with the posterior superior alveolar block. *J Dent Hyg.* 2018;92:1.
13. Logothetis, DD, Fehrenbach MJ. Local anesthesia options during dental hygiene care, *RDH Magazine,* June 2014.
14. Fehrenbach MJ, contributor. Inflammation and repair. Immunity. In: Ibsen OC, Phelan JA, eds. *Oral pathology for dental hygienists.* St Louis: Saunders/Elsevier; 2018.
15. Fehrenbach MJ, Herring SW. Spread of dental infection. *J Pract Hyg.* September/October 1997:13–19.
16. Fehrenbach MJ, contributor. Extraoral and intraoral patient assessment. In: Bowen DM, Pieren JA, eds. *Darby and Walsh dental hygiene: theory and practice.* Philadelphia: Saunders/Elsevier; 2020.
17. Ahad A, et al. Current status of the anterior middle superior alveolar anesthetic injection for periodontal procedures in the maxilla. *J Dent Anesth Pain Med.* 2019;19(1):1–10.
18. Corbett IP, et al. A comparison of the anterior middle superior alveolar nerve block and infraorbital nerve block for anesthesia of maxillary anterior teeth. *J Am Dent Assoc.* 2010;141(12):1442–1448.
19. Velasco I, Soto R. Anterior and middle superior alveolar nerve block for anesthesia of maxillary teeth using conventional syringe. *Dent Res J.* 2012;9(5):535–540.
20. Ćetković D, et al. The maxillary neurovascular canals as the basis for the local anesthesia efficacy. *J Orthod Endod.* 2018;4:15.

APPENDIX 12.1: SUMMARY OF MAXILLARY INJECTIONS

Supraperiosteal Injection (Also for Mandibular Arch)				
Areas Anesthetized	***Landmarks***	***Administration Sites***	***Technique***	***Adverse Effects***
Teeth Single tooth (or teeth) **Other Structures** Periodontium and gingiva of anesthetized tooth (or teeth) and either facial or lingual soft tissue in area	Selected tooth (or teeth) Mucobuccal fold or lingual tissue of dental arch	**Injection Site** Within height or depth of mucobuccal fold or lingual surface of selected tooth or teeth **Deposit Location** Superior or inferior to apex (or apices) of selected tooth or teeth	Parallel to long axis of tooth (or teeth) superior or inferior to apex (or apices) and then aspirate **Depth of Needle Insertion** Short 27-gauge needle; depth varies based on location of apex (or apices) at approximately 3 to 5 mm **Anesthetic Agent** Approximately 0.6 mL or one-third cartridge; 20 seconds to deposit	Pain from scraping periosteum; pain from injecting too rapidly; inadequate anesthesia from inflammation or infection in area; inadequate anesthesia with dense bone
Intraseptal Injection (Also for Mandibular Arch)				
Areas Anesthetized	***Landmarks***	***Administration Sites***	***Technique***	***Adverse Effects***
None directly from injection; selected teeth are usually already anesthetized by nerve block	Selected adjacent teeth Interdental papilla between selected adjacent teeth	**Injection Site** Center of interdental papilla at approximately 2 mm from tip and equidistant from selected adjacent teeth on dental arch **Deposit Location** Interdental septum or bone of alveolar process	At 45° to long axes of teeth and at 90° to attached gingiva, insert needle in center of interdental papilla and between selected teeth **Depth of Needle Insertion** Short 27-gauge or 30-gauge extra-short needle at approximately 1 to 2 mm into interdental bone after bony contact **Anesthetic Agent** Approximately 0.2 to 0.4 mL or one to two stoppers; 20 seconds to deposit	Anesthetic agent may leak into patient's mouth, especially without adequate levels of interdental septum or bone
Posterior Superior Alveolar (PSA) Block				
Areas Anesthetized	***Landmarks***	***Administration Sites***	***Technique***	***Adverse Effects***
Teeth Maxillary molars in approximately 72% of cases; however, mesiobuccal root of maxillary first molar is not anesthetized in approximately 28% of cases due to presence of MSA nerve **Other Structures** Buccal periodontium and gingiva of anesthetized teeth	Maxillary tuberosity; posterior superior alveolar foramina; maxillary mucobuccal fold; maxillary second molar; zygomatic arch; maxillary occlusal plane	**Injection Site** Within height of maxillary mucobuccal fold of maxillary second molar, posterior to zygomatic arch and with correct angulations to maxillary occlusal plane and long axis of tooth **Deposit Location** PSA foramina on infratemporal surface of maxilla and posterosuperior on maxillary tuberosity	Upward 45° to maxillary occlusal plane, inward 45° to midsagittal plane and backward 45° to long axis of maxillary second molar and then aspirate **Depth of Needle Insertion** Short 25- or 27-gauge needle at three-fourths of needle length **Anesthetic Agent** 0.9 to 1.8 mL or one-half to one cartridge; 60 to 90 seconds to deposit	Needle inserted too far posterior and superior may pierce maxillary artery or pterygoid plexus of veins resulting in hematoma; mandibular anesthesia

(Continued)

Middle Superior Alveolar (MSA) Block				
Areas Anesthetized	***Landmarks***	***Administration Sites***	***Technique***	***Adverse Reactions***
Teeth Maxillary premolars and mesiobuccal root of maxillary first molar **Other Structures** Buccal periodontium and gingiva of anesthetized teeth as well as buccal mucosa and upper lip	Mucobuccal fold; maxillary second premolar	**Injection Site** Within height of maxillary mucobuccal fold of the maxillary second premolar **Deposit Location** Superior to the apex of the maxillary second premolar	Parallel to long axis of maxillary second premolar and superior to apex and then aspirate **Depth of Needle Insertion** Short 27-gauge needle at approximately 5 mm or one-fourth **Anesthetic Agent** Approximately 0.9 to 1.2 mL or one-half to two-thirds of cartridge; 30 to 40 seconds to deposit	Pain from scraping periosteum; pain from injecting too rapidly; inadequate anesthesia from inflammation in area; inadequate anesthesia with dense bone; inadequate anesthesia from injecting inferior to apex; possibly inadequate anesthesia from injecting into area of infection or risking needle tract infection

Anterior Superior Alveolar (ASA) Block				
Areas Anesthetized	***Landmarks***	***Administration Sites***	***Technique***	***Adverse Reactions***
Teeth Maxillary anterior teeth **Other Structures** Labial periodontium and gingiva of anesthetized teeth as well as labial mucosa and upper lip	Mucobuccal fold; canine eminence; maxillary canine	**Injection Site** Within height of maxillary mucobuccal fold of the maxillary canine and just medial to and parallel to the canine eminence **Deposit Location** Superior to apex of maxillary canine	Parallel to long axis of the canine superior to apex and then aspirate **Depth of Needle Insertion** Short 27-gauge needle at approximately 5 to 6 mm or one-fourth of needle **Anesthetic Agent** Approximately 0.9 to 1.2 mL or one-half to two-thirds of cartridge; 30 to 40 seconds to deposit	Pain from scraping periosteum; pain from injecting too rapidly; inadequate anesthesia from inflammation in area; inadequate anesthesia from dense bone over apices; inadequate anesthesia from injecting inferior to apex; possibly inadequate anesthesia from injecting into area of infection or risking needle tract infection; inadequate anesthesia from crossover-innervation from contralateral ASA nerve

Infraorbital (IO) Block				
Areas Anesthetized	***Landmarks***	***Administration Sites***	***Technique***	***Adverse Effects***
Teeth Maxillary anterior teeth and premolars as well as mesiobuccal root of maxillary first molar in approximately 28% of cases **Other Structures** Facial periodontium and gingiva of anesthetized teeth; upper lip to midline; medial part of cheek; side of nose; lower eyelid	*Extraoral:* IO rim; zygomaticomaxillary suture; IO foramen *Intraoral:* maxillary first premolar; maxillary mucobuccal fold	**Injection Site** Within height of maxillary mucobuccal fold superior to apices of maxillary first premolar **Deposit Location** IO foramen at approximately 10 mm inferior to midpoint of IO rim with zygomaticomaxillary suture	Locate infraorbital foramen; maintain pressure with finger over foramen during injection; bevel toward bone; direct needle toward foramen and then aspirate followed by massage of agent into foramen for 2 minutes **Depth of Needle Insertion** Long or short 25- or 27-gauge needle at one-half of long needle or three-fourths of short needle **Anesthetic Agent** Approximately 0.9 to 1.2 mL or one-half to two-thirds of cartridge; minimum of 30 to 40 seconds to deposit	Pain from scraping periosteum; pain from injecting too rapidly; inadequate anesthesia from needle contacting bone inferior to infraorbital foramen; inadequate anesthesia from crossover-innervation from contralateral ASA nerve

Greater Palatine (GP) Block				
Areas Anesthetized	***Landmarks***	***Administration Sites***	***Technique***	***Adverse Reactions***
Teeth None **Other Structures** Posterior hard palate and palatal periodontium and gingiva of ipsilateral maxillary posterior teeth	Maxillary second or third molar; junction of alveolar process of maxilla and posterior hard palate; median palatine raphe (suture); palatal gingival margin; GP foramen	**Injection Site** Palatal tissue 1 to 2 mm slightly anterior to greater palatine foramen **Deposit Location** GP foramen at junction of alveolar process of maxilla and hard palate and superior to apices of maxillary second or third molar as well as midway between median palatine raphe (suture) and palatal gingival margin of determined maxillary molar	Advance syringe from opposite side of mouth at right angle to target area; use pressure anesthesia utilizing cotton-tipped applicator or instead prepuncture technique and then aspirate **Depth of Needle Insertion** Short 27-gauge or extra-short 30-gauge needle at approximately 4 to 6 mm or until contact with palatine bone **Anesthetic Agent** Approximately 0.45 to 0.6 mL or one-fourth to one-third of cartridge until blanching of palatal tissue; minimum of 30 seconds to deposit	Gagging from touching soft palate; patient gags slightly due to soft palate anesthesia; inadequate anesthesia from injecting too far anterior; inadequate anesthesia of maxillary first premolar due to crossover-innervation of NP nerve; excessive blanching of palatal tissue with delivery device that may lead to postoperative tissue ischemia and sloughing with pain
Nasopalatine (NP) Block				
Areas Anesthetized	***Landmarks***	***Administration Sites***	***Technique***	***Adverse Reactions***
Teeth None **Other Structures** Anterior hard palate and palatal periodontium and gingiva of maxillary anterior teeth bilaterally	Maxillary central incisors; anterior hard palate of maxillae; incisive papilla; incisive foramen	**Injection Site** Palatal tissue lateral to incisive papilla and palatal to maxillary central incisors **Deposit Location** At incisive foramen on anterior hard palate of maxillae deep to incisive papilla and palatal to maxillary central incisors	At 45° to 90° to tissue at lateral edge of incisive papilla; watch for blanching of palatal tissue; pressure anesthesia utilizing cotton-tipped applicator or instead prepuncture technique and then then aspirate **Depth of Needle Insertion** Short 27-gauge or extra-short 30-gauge needle at approximately 4 to 5 mm or until bone is lightly contacted **Anesthetic Agent** Approximately 0.45 mL or one-fourth of cartridge until palatal blanching of tissue; minimum of 30 seconds to deposit	Density of tissue and constricted area for anesthetic deposition may cause agent to appear around needle insertion site during anesthetic administration; inadequate anesthesia of maxillary first canine due to crossover-innervations from GP nerve; excessive blanching of palatal tissue with delivery device that may lead to postoperative tissue ischemia and sloughing with pain
Anterior Middle Superior Alveolar (AMSA) Block				
Areas Anesthetized	***Landmarks***	***Administration Sites***	***Technique***	***Adverse Reactions***
Teeth Maxillary anterior teeth and premolars within one maxillary quadrant **Other Structures** Facial periodontium and gingiva of anesthetized teeth to the midline; hard palate and palatal periodontium and gingiva of ipsilateral maxillary posterior teeth and maxillary anterior teeth bilaterally; no regional soft tissue anesthesia of upper lip and face	Maxillary premolars; palatal gingival margin; median palatine raphe (suture)	**Injection Site** Area on hard palate superior to apices of maxillary premolars and midway between palatal gingival margin and median palatal raphe (suture) **Deposit Location** Pores within maxilla of hard palate	Direct handpiece with needle at 45° to apices of maxillary premolars on hard palate until bone of palate is contacted and then aspirate **Depth of Needle Insertion** Short 27-gauge or extra-short 30 gauge needle at approximately 4 to 7 mm until gentle contact with bone of palate **Anesthetic Agent** Approximately 1.4 to1.8 mL until blanching of palatal tissue; 0.5 mL per minute to deposit	Variable depth and duration of anesthesia; excessive blanching of palatal tissue with delivery device leading to possible ischemia and sloughing with pain

13

Mandibular Anesthesia

Margaret Fehrenbach, RDH, MS and Demetra Daskalos Logothetis, RDH, MS

LEARNING OBJECTIVES

1. Discuss the importance of understanding the anatomy of the mandibular nerve and its branches when it comes to the utilization of local anesthesia within the mandibular arch.
2. Discuss the overall clinical effectiveness of mandibular nerve blocks in relationship to anatomy and compare mandibular nerve blocks to similar maxillary nerve blocks.
3. Describe the various types of mandibular nerve blocks.
4. Concerning the inferior alveolar block:
   - Discuss its coverage and common uses.
   - Describe what can occur when bilateral blocks are implemented.
   - Identify the correct tissue inserted by the local anesthetic needle.
   - Demonstrate the correct placement of the needle at the injection site and target area.
   - Demonstrate correct administration of local anesthesia during dental hygiene clinical practice.
   - Discuss the associated troubleshooting paradigm and its implications.
   - Discuss the indications of a clinically effective block and possible complications.
5. Concerning the buccal block:
   - Discuss its coverage and common uses.
   - Demonstrate the correct placement of the needle at the injection site and target area.
   - Demonstrate correct administration of local anesthesia during dental hygiene clinical practice.
   - Discuss the indications of a clinically effective block and possible complications.
6. Concerning the mental block:
   - Discuss its coverage and common uses.
   - Demonstrate the correct placement of the needle at the injection site target area.
   - Demonstrate correct administration of local anesthesia during dental hygiene clinical practice.
   - Discuss the indications of a clinically effective block and possible complications.
7. Concerning the incisive block:
   - Discuss its coverage and common uses.
   - Demonstrate the correct placement of the needle at the injection site and target area.
   - Demonstrate correct administration of local anesthesia during dental hygiene clinical practice.
   - Discuss the indications of a clinically effective block and possible complications.
8. Concerning the Gow-Gates mandibular block:
   - Discuss its coverage and common uses.
   - Demonstrate the correct placement of the needle at the injection site and target area.
   - Demonstrate correct administration of local anesthesia during dental hygiene clinical practice.
   - Discuss the indications of a clinically effective block and possible complications.
   - Discuss the associated troubleshooting paradigm and its implications.
9. Concerning the Vazirani-Akinosi mandibular block:
   - Discuss its coverage and common uses.
   - Demonstrate the correct placement of the needle at the injection site and target area.
   - Demonstrate correct administration of local anesthesia during dental hygiene clinical practice.
   - Discuss the associated troubleshooting paradigm and its implications.
   - Discuss the indications of a clinically effective block and possible complications.
10. List and describe the three supplemental injections that can be administered within the mandibular arch and the maxillary arch.
11. Discuss when mandibular supraperiosteal injections and mandibular intraseptal injections are typically necessary.
12. Concerning periodontal ligament injections that can be used on the mandibular arch and the maxillary arch:
    - Discuss its coverage and common uses.
    - Demonstrate the correct placement of the needle at the injection site and target area within the dental arch.
    - Discuss the indications of a clinically effective injection and possible complications.

INTRODUCTION TO MANDIBULAR ANESTHESIA

The mandibular nerve of the fifth cranial or trigeminal nerve and its branches can be anesthetized in a number of ways by the dental hygienist for patient pain management with hemostatic control depending on the extent of procedure anticipated and the structures needing to be anesthetized (see Table 10.4 in Chapter 10).[1] In addition, the dental hygienist must also understand that administering mandibular anesthesia has its own considerations compared with administering maxillary anesthesia.[2]

First, a supraperiosteal injection of the mandible is not as clinically effective as that of the maxillae because overall the mandible is denser and less porous than the maxillae over similar teeth, especially within the mandibular posterior sextant (see discussion in Chapter 12).[1,3] This increase in density of the mandible compared to the maxillae can be demonstrated with a panoramic radiograph (see Figs. 10.2 and 10.8 in Chapter 10). For this reason, nerve blocks are preferred to supraperiosteal injections in most parts of the mandible, unlike the maxillae.[1,4]

Second, substantial variation exists in the anatomy of local anesthetic landmarks of the mandible as well as the associated nerves, compared with similar structures in the maxillae, complicating mandibular anesthesia for the clinician.[1,2] Thus the need for troubleshooting of cases may occur with a lack of clinical effectiveness of anesthetic administered for the mandible (see Chapter 10).[1,4] This chapter covers some of the most common anatomic variations of the mandible.

MANDIBULAR NERVE BLOCKS

The mandibular nerve blocks anesthetizing various mandibular nerve branches all have an increased level of clinical effectiveness when administered correctly and most involve pulpal anesthesia as well as anesthesia of the various regions of the associated periodontium and gingiva (Fig. 13.1). All the mandibular injections have an associated visual analog scale (VAS) ranging from 0 to 5 utilizing the correct technique by the clinician (see Chapter 1).[5]

Any pulpal anesthesia for these mandibular injections is achieved through anesthesia of each tooth's dental branches as they extend into the pulp by way of the apical foramen from the inferior dental plexus.[1] Both the hard and soft tissue of the associated periodontium and gingiva are anesthetized by way of the interdental and interradicular branches for each tooth (Table 13.1).

The inferior alveolar (IA) block is a nerve block that is recommended for anesthesia of the mandibular teeth and associated lingual periodontium and gingiva to the midline as well as the associated facial periodontium and gingiva of the mandibular anterior teeth and premolars to the midline within one mandibular quadrant. The buccal block is a nerve block that is recommended for anesthesia of the associated buccal periodontium and gingiva of the mandibular molars to complete mandibular quadrant anesthesia.

The mental block is a nerve block that is recommended for anesthesia of the associated facial periodontium and gingiva of the mandibular anterior teeth and premolars to the midline within one mandibular quadrant. More commonly used than the mental block but with a similar technique, the incisive block is recommended for anesthesia of the mandibular anterior teeth and premolars as well as associated facial periodontium and gingiva to the midline within one mandibular quadrant.

The more encompassing Gow-Gates (G-G) mandibular block is a nerve block that anesthetizes the entire mandibular nerve within one mandibular quadrant and thus is highly recommended for quadrant dentistry or with lack of clinical effectiveness of an administered IA block.

Finally, the Vazirani-Akinosi (V-A) mandibular block is a nerve block that has a large area of coverage of the mandibular nerve within one mandibular quadrant similar to the IA block. The V-A block is recommended in a patient with severe trismus or when there is difficulty administering the IA block on certain cases and will be discussed later in the chapter. These two mandibular blocks can also both be used when the patient has a past history of IA block failure owing to anatomic variability or accessory innervation (see Appendix 13.1 for a summary of the mandibular injections).

If quadrant dental hygiene treatment is planned on the mandible after local anesthesia is administered, the clinician must proceed with the anesthesia and then instrumentation first of the mandibular molars (third, second, and then first), then premolars (second and then first), and finally the anterior teeth to allow for complete anesthesia of their nerve core bundles (see Chapter 3 and Figs. 3.10 and 3.11).[6]

If half-mouth treatment is planned, the IA and buccal blocks are administered first, then the maxillary facial injections, and then palatal injections follow in order as discussed in Chapters 11 and 12. Instrumentation, however, proceeds first on the maxillary arch, followed by the mandibular arch, allowing time for the entire mandibular arch to become completely anesthetized because of the larger length and breadth of the mandible (see Fig. 11.5A–B in Chapter 11).

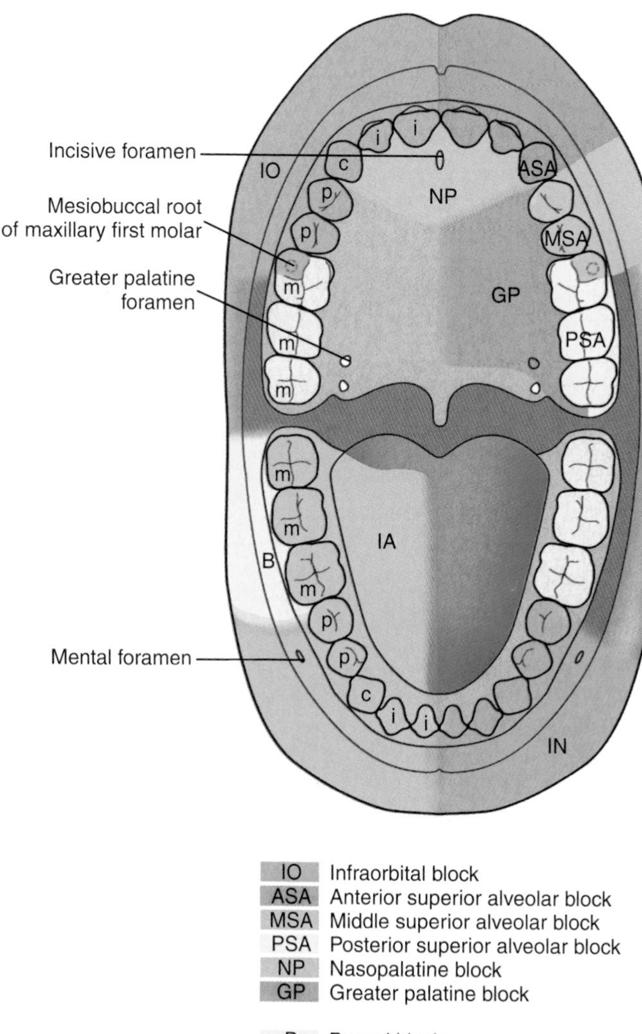

Fig. 13.1 Local anesthetic nerve blocks of the mandibular arch with the related structures anesthetized. Note that the mental blocks as well as the Gow-Gates or Vazirani-Akinosi mandibular blocks are not included; see associated figures for more clarification of these nerve blocks. Note also that the borders of each injection shown are approximate and that substantial overlap exists between nerves that can affect anesthesia. (From Fehrenbach MJ, Herring SW: *Illustrated anatomy of the head and neck,* ed 6, St Louis, 2021, Saunders/Elsevier.)

INFERIOR ALVEOLAR BLOCK

The IA block, also known by clinicians as the *mandibular block,* is the most commonly used injection in dentistry, especially during restorative care but also during nonsurgical periodontal therapy (Table 13.2,

TABLE 13.1 Nerve Blocks for Mandibular Teeth and Associated Structures*

Mandibular Tooth and Structures	IA Block	Buccal Block	Mental Block	Incisive Block
Central Incisor				
Pulpal	X			X
Labial periodontium and gingiva	X		X	X
Lingual periodontium and gingiva	X			
Lateral Incisor				
Pulpal	X			X
Labial periodontium and gingiva	X		X	X
Lingual periodontium and gingiva	X			
Canine				
Pulpal	X			X
Labial periodontium and gingiva	X		X	X
Lingual periodontium and gingiva	X			
First Premolar				
Pulpal	X			X
Buccal periodontium and gingiva	X		X	X
Lingual periodontium and gingiva	X			
Second Premolar				
Pulpal	X			X
Buccal periodontium and gingiva	X		X	X
Lingual periodontium and gingiva	X			
First Molar				
Pulpal with lingual periodontium and gingiva	X			
Buccal periodontium and gingiva		X		
Second Molar				
Pulpal with lingual periodontium and gingiva	X			
Buccal periodontium and gingiva		X		
Third Molar				
Pulpal with lingual periodontium and gingiva	X			
Buccal periodontium and gingiva		X		

IA, Inferior alveolar.
*Anesthesia for anatomic variants is not included as well as the complicated coverage of the Gow-Gates block or Vazirani-Akinosi mandibular block since many branches of the mandibular nerve are anesthetized.
From Fehrenbach MJ, Herring SW: *Illustrated anatomy of the head and neck,* ed 6, St Louis, 2021, Saunders/Elsevier.

Figs. A–F, and Procedure Box 13.1).[4,7] The IA block anesthetizes the mandibular teeth and associated lingual periodontium and gingiva to the midline as well as the associated facial periodontium and gingiva of the mandibular anterior teeth and premolars to the midline within one mandibular quadrant as well as the ipsilateral tongue, floor of the mouth, lower lip, and chin. Thus the IA block anesthetizes the IA nerve and its mental and incisive nerve branches as well as the lingual nerve. However, because not all of the nerve branches of the mandibular nerve are anesthetized with an IA block, it is not considered a true mandibular block; in contrast, the G-G block is considered a true mandibular block because the entire mandibular nerve is anesthetized (see Gow-Gates Mandibular Block, discussed later in this chapter).[1,4]

The IA block's associated VAS specifically ranges from 0 to 5 when correctly administering the block; any discomfort noted is mainly caused by the reaction of the needle near the lingual nerve (discussed later; see also Chapter 1).[4,5] In addition, patients may feel uncomfortable after this injection because the proprioceptor fibers that innervate the tongue, lower lip, and chin are blocked thus numbing these structures.[1] Both the tongue, lower lip, and chin feel swollen or "fat" to the midline because the neurosensory feedback is temporarily absent; any concerned patients given a patient mirror directly following the injection can be assured that this is not the case.

The clinician must remember that the mantle bundles of the IA nerve tend to innervate the posterior mandible so that the mandibular posterior teeth anesthetize earlier, more easily, and for longer (see earlier discussion). In contrast, the core bundles of the IA nerve tend to innervate the anterior mandible. Thus the lower lip, chin, and mandibular anterior teeth anesthetize later and with more difficulty. A lack

TABLE 13.2 Inferior Alveolar Block Review

Indications Fig. A = Distribution of IA block 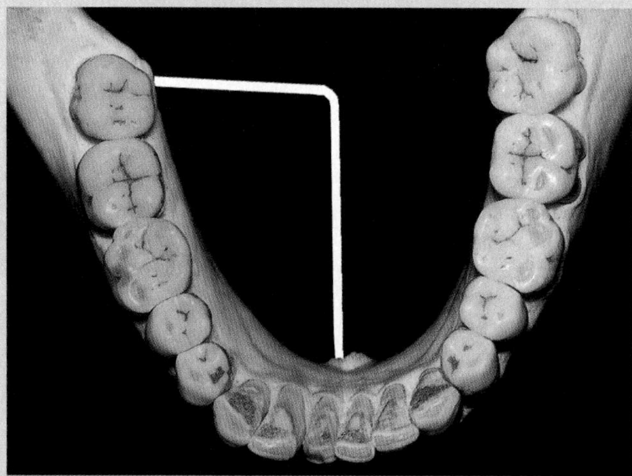 *1,* Intraoral view of distribution of IA block (From Fehrenbach MJ, Herring SW: *Illustrated anatomy of the head and neck,* ed 6, St Louis, 2021, Saunders/Elsevier)	Procedures on mandibular teeth in one mandibular quadrant except for any buccal soft tissue procedures on mandibular molars; will need to administer buccal block to complete mandibular quadrant anesthesia 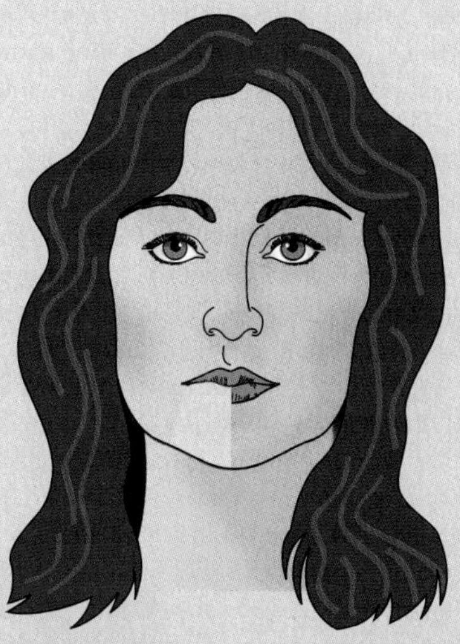 *2,* Facial view of extraoral distribution of IA block as well as G-G and V-A blocks
Nerves anesthetized	IA nerve Mental nerve Incisive nerve Lingual nerve
Teeth anesthetized	Mandibular teeth to midline
Other structures anesthetized	Lingual periodontium and gingiva to midline; facial periodontium and gingiva of mandibular anterior teeth and premolars to midline; lower lip, anterior two-thirds of tongue and floor of the mouth to midline
Administration technique	See Procedure Box 13.1
Needle gauge and length	25-gauge long; smaller diameter gauge would not provide reliable aspiration and short needle would be dangerously inserted to its hub
Target area/Deposit location 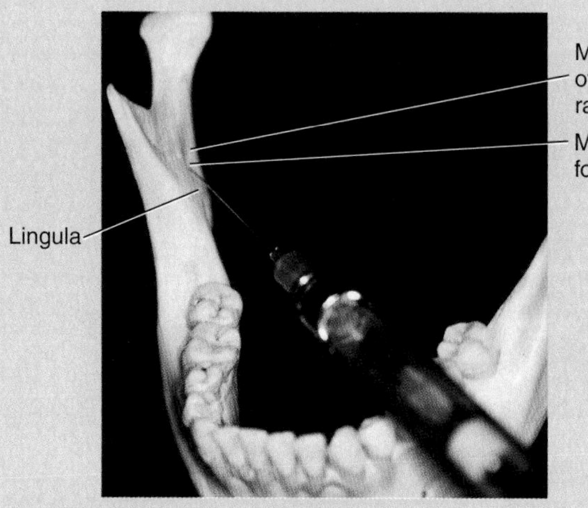 Fig. B = Target area for IA block (From Fehrenbach MJ, Herring SW: *Illustrated anatomy of the head and neck,* ed 6, St Louis, 2021, Saunders/Elsevier)	At mandibular foramen on medial surface of mandibular ramus that is overhung by lingula with IA nerve; lingual nerve by diffusion

(*Continued*)

TABLE 13.2 Inferior Alveolar Block Review (*Cont.*)

Fig. C = Clinician position of right-handed clinician for IA block (same as for buccal block and G-G block)	
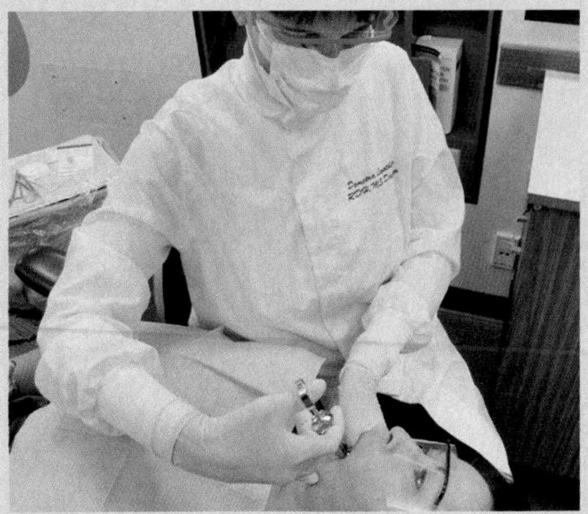 *1,* Right side, right-handed at 8 to 9 o'clock (left-handed at 4 to 3 o'clock)	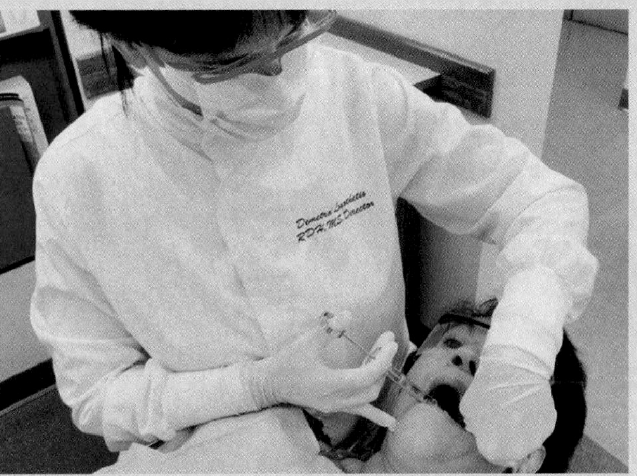 *2,* Left side, right-handed at 10 o'clock (left-handed at 2 o'clock)
Fig. D = Syringe stabilization with fulcrums for IA block	
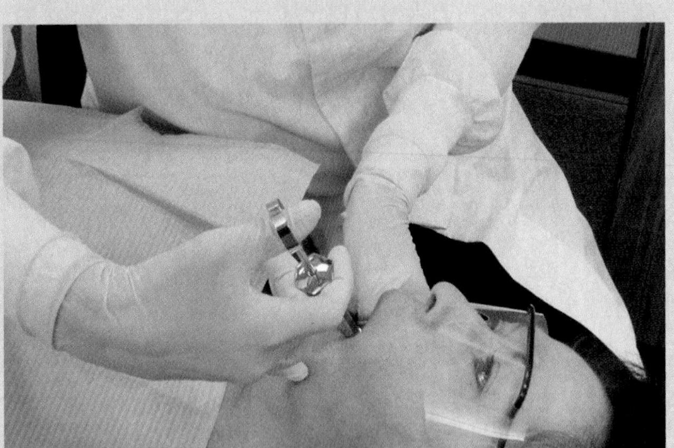 *1,* Pinky finger of dominant hand resting on patient's chin for right side	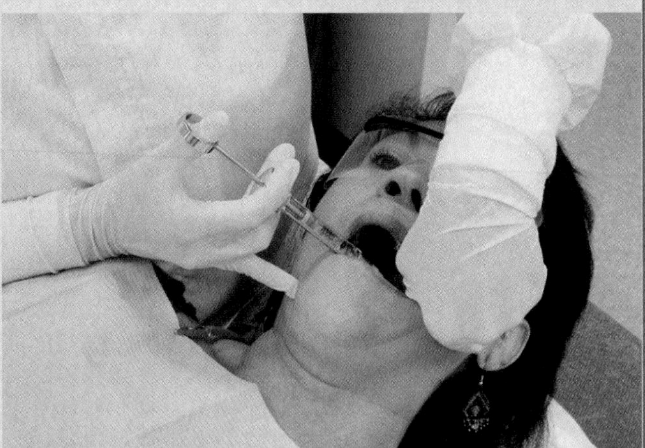 *2,* Pinky finger of dominant hand resting on patient's chin for left side
Landmarks	Medial surface of mandibular ramus Mandibular foramen Lingula Coronoid notch Pterygomandibular fold (raphe) Pterygomandibular space Mandibular occlusal plane
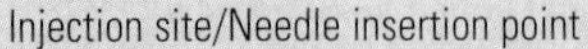 Injection site/Needle insertion point 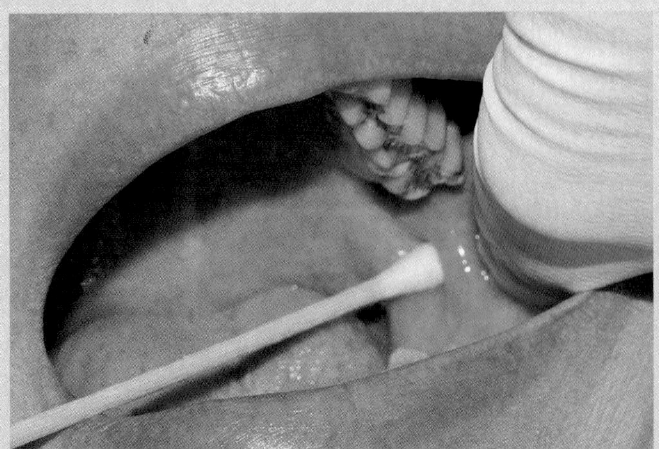 Fig. E = Injection site for IA block	Two-thirds to three-fourths distance from coronoid notch to pterygomandibular fold (raphe) demarcating posterior border of ramus and at center of pterygomandibular space as well as approximately 6 to 10 mm superior to mandibular occlusal plane (for adults)

TABLE 13.2 Inferior Alveolar Block Review (*Cont.*)

Depth of insertion 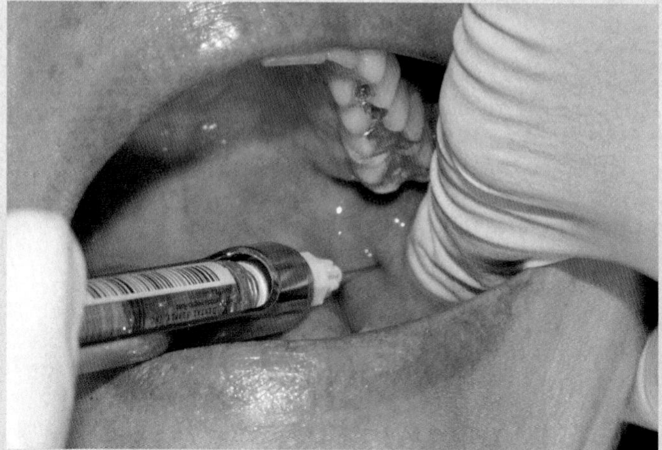 Fig. F = Needle insertion for IA block; note that two-thirds to three-fourths of long needle is needed to reach target location	Approximately 20 to 25 mm or two-thirds to three-fourths of long needle until bone is gently contacted
Amount of anesthetic agent	Approximately 1.8 to 3.6 mL (one to two cartridges); save portion for administration of buccal block (approximately 0.3 mL or one-eighth cartridge) if needed (see Table 13.4)
Length of time to deposit	Approximately 60 to 120 seconds

IA, Inferior alveolar; *G-G,* Gow-Gates; *V-A,* Vazirani-Akinosi.

of labial and mental soft tissue signs and symptoms of anesthesia after an IA block indicates core bundles are not yet adequately anesthetized. Emergence from the block follows the same patterns as induction; however, it does so in the reverse order. These differences must be reflected in the treatment plan by the clinician.

Additional use of the buccal block may be considered when anesthesia of the associated buccal periodontium and gingiva of the mandibular molars is also necessary, which is usually the case with nonsurgical periodontal therapy by the dental hygienist. In some cases, there is overlap of the right and left incisive nerves and the tissue they innervate due to crossover-innervation.[1] Crossover-innervation is the overlap of terminal nerve fibers from the contralateral side of the dental arch (see Chapter 10). The incisive nerve is a branch of the mandibular nerve that innervates the mandibular anterior teeth. If this is the case, a bilateral IA block can be used, but it is not recommended.

Therefore bilateral IA blocks are usually avoided unless absolutely necessary.[1,4] This is because bilateral mandibular injections specifically produce oral anesthesia of the body of the tongue and floor of the mouth. This numbness can cause difficulty with swallowing and speech, especially in patients with full or partial removable mandibular dentures, until the effects of the local anesthetic agent wear off, which may take several hours. Comprehensive dental hygiene treatment planning can usually prevent the need for bilateral IA blocks by treating the mandible in quadrants or even sextants (see Figs. 11.3 and 11.4 in Chapter 11).[6]

More often, the use of a contralateral incisive block or facially or lingually located supraperiosteal injection inferior to the apex (or apices) of the mandibular anterior teeth that fail to achieve initial pulpal anesthesia may be indicated. This would include when the patient feels discomfort during treatment or when a larger scope of anesthesia is necessary, such as the entire mandibular arch (see earlier discussion). However, supraperiosteal injections on the facial surface of the anterior of the mandible are more clinically effective than more posterior injections but less effective than injections over the maxillae in similar locations (see Chapter 12).[3] Again, these differences in clinical effectiveness are caused by differences in the density of the facial cortical plate of the mandible compared to those of the maxillae that vary along the length of the mandible from anterior to posterior.[1]

Target Area and Injection Site for Inferior Alveolar Block

The target area or deposit location for the IA block is the IA nerve exiting the mandibular foramen on the medial surface of the mandibular ramus, overhung anteriorly by the lingula as noted on a panoramic radiograph (Table 13.2, Fig. B; see Fig. 10.8 in Chapter 10). The adjacent anteriorly and medially located lingual nerve will also be anesthetized as the local anesthetic agent diffuses, so there is no need for a separate injection for this nerve.[1,4] However, the agent must be accurately deposited within 1 mm of the target area to achieve overall clinically effective anesthesia, which can be difficult because most of the deeper target anatomy is not visible to the clinician since this is at an approximate depth of 20 to 25 mm. Instead, visible surface landmarks must be relied upon.

The technique discussed is also known as the *Halstead technique,* named after a medical doctor who first gave an intraoral injection of local anesthesia (1886); it is also called the *direct approach* of anesthesia for the IA nerve.[4]

The injection site or needle insertion point for the IA block is at the depth of the pterygomandibular space demarcated by the pterygotemporal depression on the medial border of the mandibular ramus at the correct height and anteroposterior direction determined for the injection (Figs. 13.2 and 13.3; see Table 13.2, Fig. E). Hard tissue landmarks are mainly used to locate the injection site, such as the coronoid notch and the mandibular occlusal plane, to reduce errors caused by patient soft tissue variance.[1]

PROCEDURE BOX 13.1 Inferior Alveolar Block Procedure

Step 1 Assume the correct clinician position for right side, right-handed at 8 to 9 o'clock (left-handed at 4 to 3 o'clock); left side, right-handed at 10 o'clock (left-handed at 2 o'clock; see Table 13.2, Fig. C).

Step 2 Ask the supine patient to open comfortably wide. Use the index finger for intraoral retraction and thumb for extraoral retraction on dominant side and vice versa on nondominant side.

Step 3 Prepare the alveolar mucosa at the location of the pterygotemporal depression overlying pterygomandibular space, lateral to the pterygomandibular fold (see Chapter 11).

Step 4 Using a new cotton-tipped applicator, practice the actual injection pathway, which is usually superior to the mandibular second premolar, with it resting on the contralateral corner of the mouth and parallel and superior to the mandibular occlusal plane. Then palpate the coronoid notch on the anterior border of the mandible from the contralateral side, which is the greatest concavity on the anterior border of the mandibular ramus (see Table 13.2, Fig. E).

Step 5 Palpate the pterygomandibular fold, the tissue that extends from behind the most distal mandibular molar and retromolar pad and horizontally to the posterior border of the mandible.

Step 6 For the height of the injection, imagine a (somewhat) horizontal line that extends posteriorly from the coronoid notch to the pterygomandibular fold as it turns superiorly (upward) toward the palate, demarcating the posterior border of the mandibular ramus (see Figs. 13.4 and 13.5). It is usually approximately 6 to 10 mm superior to the mandibular occlusal plane in most adults; the inside retracting finger or thumb can be kept at this height to help maintain it throughout the injection. For anteroposterior direction, imagine a (somewhat) vertical line approximately two-thirds to three-fourths the distance between the coronoid notch to the pterygomandibular fold as it turns superiorly (upward) toward the palate, demarcating the posterior border of the mandibular ramus. Palpate the pterygopalatine depression overlying the pterygomandibular space at the intersection of these two imaginary lines; note any access problems created by the pterygomandibular fold, buccal fat pad, or tongue (see Table 13.2, Fig. E).

Step 7 Using a 25-gauge long needle with the bevel toward the bone and with the large window of the syringe toward the clinician, direct the syringe from over the contralateral mandibular second premolar, with the syringe barrel resting on the contralateral corner of the mouth, parallel and superior to the mandibular occlusal plane.

Step 8 Establish a fulcrum (see Table 13.2, Fig. D for fulcrum recommendations).

Step 9 Use the needle tip with slight pressure into the space further to ensure its location in the deepest part of the depression created by the pterygomandibular space and at the intersection of these two imaginary lines, using retraction needed if there are access problems, and then proceed to insert the needle within the space (see Table 13.2, Fig. F).

Step 10 Advance the needle into the soft tissue until gentle contact of the bone of the medial surface of the mandibular ramus at the mandibular foramen; do not move the needle except in a forward pathway. This is approximately 20 to 25 mm or two-thirds to three-fourths of the long needle (see Table 13.2, Fig. F). Continue advancement even when the patient experiences a reaction by the lingual nerve ("lingual shock"; see Table 13.3).

Step 11 Aspirate within three planes due to the higher vascularity in the area of anesthetic deposition to ensure that the bevel of the needle is not abutted against the interior of a blood vessel, providing a false aspiration. To accomplish this, first aspirate as usual at the depth of insertion. If aspiration is negative, rotate the syringe barrel gently toward the clinician and reaspirate; if aspiration is negative, rotate the syringe barrel gently back to the original position and aspirate again.

Step 12 If a negative aspiration is achieved after each aspiration, slowly deposit approximately 1.8 to 3.6 mL of agent (one to two cartridges) over approximately 60 to 120 seconds. Aspirate in one plane after each fourth of the cartridge is administered. If administering a buccal block immediately following the inferior alveolar block, a small amount of agent should be saved for the buccal block (administer approximately 1.5 mL if administering one cartridge or one cartridge and most of the second cartridge but save the remaining approximately 0.3 mL or one-eighth of the cartridge). Maintain the height and direction of the syringe barrel throughout the injection.

Step 13 Carefully withdraw the syringe in the same pathway as insertion and immediately administer the buccal block if needed (see Procedure Box 13.2) or carefully recap the needle using the one-handed scoop method utilizing needle sheath prop (see Chapter 11).

Step 14 Place the patient upright or semiupright and wait approximately 3 to 5 minutes until anesthesia takes effect before starting treatment. If there is lack of clinical effective anesthesia or the patient feels uncomfortable during treatment, proceed with the troubleshooting injection paradigm (see Figs. 13.9 and 13.10).

The height of the injection for the IA block is determined by palpating the coronoid notch, the greatest depression on the anterior border of the mandibular ramus, which can be demonstrated using a finger or thumb as well as the cotton-tipped applicator (see Fig. 10.11 in Chapter 10). To determine the injection height, it helps to visualize an imaginary (somewhat) horizontal line that extends posteriorly from the coronoid notch to the pterygomandibular fold as it turns superiorly (upward) toward the soft palate, with the line demarcating the posterior border of the mandibular ramus (Fig. 13.4). Clinicians can palpate extraorally the posterior border of the mandibular ramus but with this intraoral technique that is not usually necessary and allows an immediate and clearer anatomic picture.[8]

This imaginary (somewhat) horizontal line showing the height of IA block injection site is also parallel to and approximately 6 to 10 mm superior to the mandibular occlusal plane in most adults (see Fig. 13.4).[1,4] The clinician's retracting finger or thumb can be kept at this height to help maintain this level throughout the injection because being too far inferior is the most commonly cited reason for missed IA blocks. This will also help keep the needle and syringe barrel parallel to the occlusal plane at all times to ensure correct placement of the needle tip and the agent near the mandibular foramen. Thus it is important not to move the syringe barrel side to side or up and down within the tissue during the dispensing of the agent. The syringe barrel should also not rest on the masticatory surfaces of the mandibular teeth at any time since they can also move and may have an uneven surface.[9]

With a patient having an Angle classification of malocclusion Class III with a prognathic mandible, the clinician should insert the needle at least 10 mm more superior than the usual height of the injection.[10] However, in children and small adults, this imaginary (somewhat) horizontal line for the height of the injection should be more inferiorly located than the usual height and thus closer to the mandibular occlusal plane.[4] In regard to children, this is because the mandible has not reached its full mature size[1] (see Chapter 14). In contrast, in partially edentulous patients with only the mandibular premolars and/or anterior teeth, the mandibular foramen may appear to be more superior because the occlusal plane of the molars is not present as a guide such as when a full dentition is present.[1]

The anteroposterior direction of the IA block injection is determined at the same time as the determination of the correct height of the injection. To determine this anteroposterior direction, it helps to

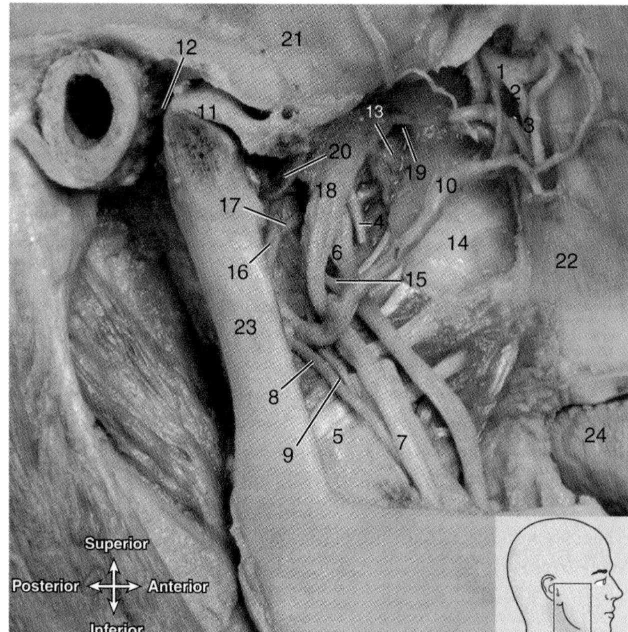

Fig. 13.2 Dissection of the right infratemporal fossa at the injection site or needle insertion point for the inferior alveolar block (*inset:* Note removal of the lateral pterygoid muscle, zygomatic arch, and part of the mandible). Note that the posterior superior alveolar block injection site or needle insertion point is also shown and is discussed in Chapter 12. *1,* Maxillary nerve; *2,* Posterior superior alveolar nerve; *3,* Posterior superior alveolar artery; *4,* (Long) buccal nerve; *5,* Medial pterygoid muscle; *6,* Lingual nerve; *7,* Inferior alveolar nerve; *8,* Inferior alveolar artery; *9,* Mylohyoid nerve; *10,* Maxillary artery; *11,* Joint disc of the temporomandibular joint and mandibular condyle; *12,* Joint capsule; *13,* Medial pterygoid nerve; *14,* Lateral pterygoid plate; *15,* Chorda tympani nerve; *16,* Middle meningeal artery; *17,* Accessory meningeal artery; *18,* Mandibular nerve; *19,* Lateral pterygoid nerve; *20,* Auriculotemporal nerve; *21,* Temporal bone; *22,* Maxilla; *23,* Mandibular ramus; *24,* Tongue. (From Logan BM, Reynold PA, Hutching RT: *McMinn's color atlas of head and neck anatomy,* ed 4, London, 2010, Mosby. In Fehrenbach MJ, Herring SW: *Illustrated anatomy of the head and neck,* ed 6, St Louis, 2021, Saunders/Elsevier.)

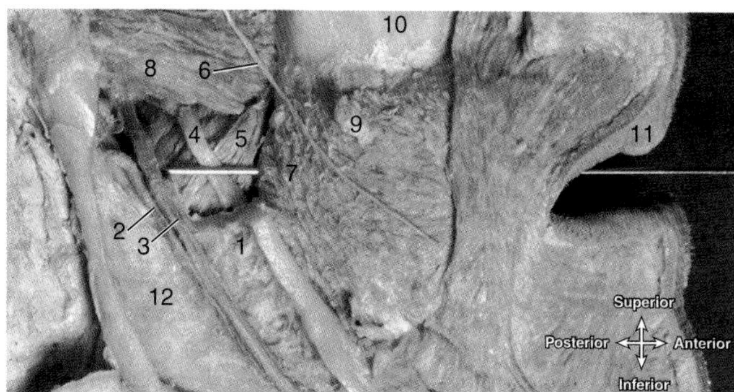

Fig. 13.3 Dissection of the right infratemporal fossa showing the injection site or needle insertion point for the inferior alveolar block. Note how "lingual shock" could occur as the needle passes by the lingual nerve during administration of the block. *1,* Lingula; *2,* Inferior alveolar artery; *3,* Inferior alveolar nerve; *4,* Lingual nerve; *5,* Medial pterygoid muscle; *6,* (Long) buccal nerve; *7,* Buccinator muscle; *8,* Lateral pterygoid muscle; *9,* Parotid duct; *10,* Maxilla; *11,* Upper lip; *12,* Mandibular ramus. (From Logan BM, Reynold PA, Hutching RT: *McMinn's color atlas of head and neck anatomy,* ed 4, London, 2010, Mosby. In Fehrenbach MJ, Herring SW: *Illustrated anatomy of the head and neck,* ed 6, St Louis, 2021, Saunders/Elsevier.)

visualize an imaginary (somewhat) vertical line, approximately two-thirds to three-fourths of the distance between the coronoid notch and the pterygomandibular fold as it turns superiorly (upward) toward the soft palate, demarcating the posterior border of the mandibular ramus (see Fig. 13.4). Clinicians can again palpate extraorally the posterior border of the mandibular ramus but with this intraoral technique that is not usually necessary.[1,8]

This distance determination of two-thirds a distance anteroposteriorly is from the most recent research studies on skulls and not from older sources that only quote three-fourths the distance from the coronoid notch to the posterior border of the mandibular ramus (see Chapter 10).[1] All these recent studies also show that it is always slightly posterior to the middle of the mandibular ramus.

Thus the injection site of the IA block is determined by the intersection of these two imaginary lines, one (somewhat) horizontal and one (somewhat) vertical that meet at the deepest part of the pterygomandibular space, which is also known as the *pterygomandibular triangle* by clinicians. The space is entered into through the pterygotemporal depression, lateral to both the pterygomandibular fold and the sphenomandibular ligament (Figs. 13.5 and 13.6). To accomplish this, the syringe barrel is usually superior to the contralateral mandibular second premolar and at the contralateral corner of mouth.

When administering the injection on the clinician's nondominant side, there is a tendency to place the syringe barrel too far forward or anterior to the injection site, possibly superior to the mandibular canine due to poor visibility of the intraoral landmarks. Using a pathway for the syringe directly from the contralateral corner of mouth to the injection site for both the right and left injection can help avoid this possible blind sight situation.

The 25-gauge needle is inserted into the soft tissue and advanced into the pterygotemporal depression to the depth of the pterygomandibular space with the bevel of the needle toward the bone at approximately 20 to 25 mm or two-thirds to three-fourths of the long needle or until gentle contact with the medial surface of the bone of the mandibular ramus, and then the injection is administered (see Table 13.2, Fig. F).[9,10] The temporalis muscle attaches onto the coronoid process and it is important to avoid this sensitive structure when inserting the needle to avoid post administration muscle soreness.

This may seem extra deep in comparison to injections for other nerve blocks with less depth such as the maxillary injections, but the extra depth is necessary to gain access to the target area (Fig. 13.7; see Fig. 13.5).[4] In addition, the 25-gauge needle is less likely to deflect as would a thinner 30-gauge needle as the needle progresses through the soft tissue to the injection site.[9]

The pterygotemporal depression that demarcates entry into the depth of the pterygomandibular space usually mimics an inverted teardrop in its outer shape: The injection is administered in the center of the superior basin-like part (Fig. 13.8). However, the overall shape and size of the depression can vary and in some cases may not be readily visible to the clinician unless it is palpated with a cotton-tipped applicator prior to the injection.[9,10] Additionally, using the needle tip with slight pressure initially into the pterygotemporal depression before fully entering to the depth of pterygomandibular space may add to the reassurance that the injection site is correctly located.

The needle will naturally withdraw from the periosteum when gentle contact is made with the mandible, so there is no need to withdraw the needle off the medial surface and possibly miss the deeper target area. It is also usually not necessary to deposit small amounts of the local anesthetic agent to anesthetize the adjacent anteriorly and medially located lingual nerve that is contacted at approximately

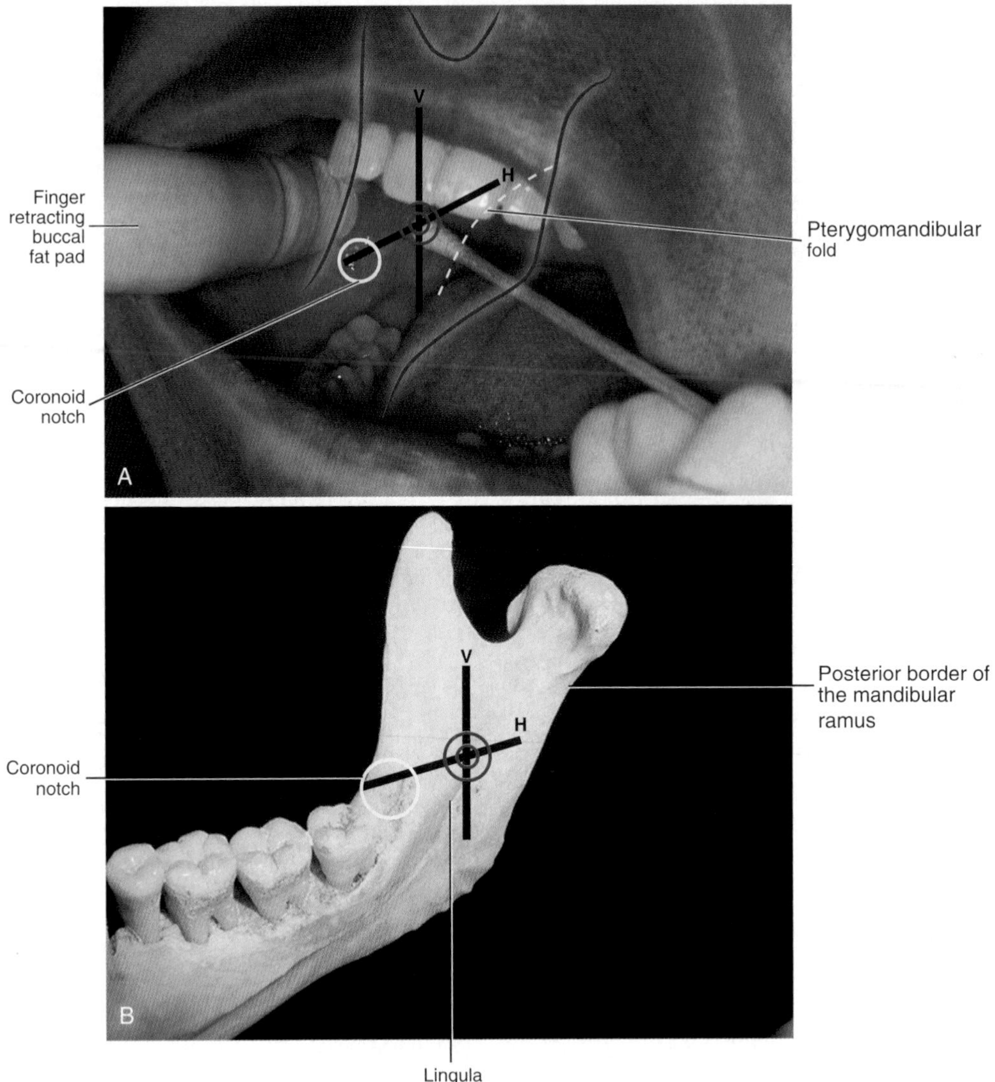

Fig. 13.4 (A) Oral view of the pterygomandibular space with an imaginary (somewhat) horizontal line *(H)* showing the correct injection height, and an imaginary (somewhat) vertical line *(V)* showing the correct anteroposterior direction for the inferior alveolar block. The intersection of these two lines is the injection site or needle insertion point for this block *(bullseye)*, which is at the depth of the pterygomandibular space demarcated by the pterygotemporal depression, lateral to the pterygomandibular fold *(dashed line)* and at the same height as the coronoid notch *(yellow circle)*. (B) Medial surface of the mandible showing the bony landmarks with these imaginary lines. (From Fehrenbach MJ, Herring SW: *Illustrated anatomy of the head and neck*, ed 6, St Louis, 2021, Saunders/Elsevier.)

16 mm after the needle enters the tissue for the IA block because anesthesia of the lingual nerve will occur through diffusion of the local anesthetic agent.[1,4] These small amounts injected early will not reduce any tissue discomfort for the patient. It is also not necessary to save any agent from the target area to deposit for the lingual nerve anesthesia before leaving the soft tissue for the same reason. Administering the agent only after gentle contact with the mandible and at the target area will provide the most anesthetic amount for both nerves.

Often scar tissue is present within the pterygomandibular space when there has been a past history of extensive local anesthesia procedures and/or complicated surgical extraction of the adjacent mandibular third molar. However, this tissue feels firmer, almost "tough," instead of bony hard like the medial surface of the mandible to the clinician as the needle goes through it, but it may still prove difficult to insert the needle on the way to the needed deeper injection site of the mandibular foramen. It is important, therefore, to always use a sharp needle to accomplish all injections and change needles as the situation demands (see Chapter 9).[9]

In addition, the needle may need to be used to gently deflect a pterygomandibular fold even further medially that lies over the pterygotemporal depression if it prevents the needle from entering into the superior basin-like part of the pterygomandibular space from across the mouth. Additionally, an extensive buccal fat pad superior to the site may also need to be strongly retracted by the finger or thumb if it also obscures the pterygotemporal depression. Strong retraction of an active tongue or one that also lies over the pterygotemporal depression can be accomplished by using a mirror (and in some cases, a dental assistant using a mirror); however, never use any fingers to retract any tissue near the pathway of the incoming needle so as to protect from any clinician needle stick injuries. Palpation with a cotton-tipped applicator of the pterygotemporal depression using the correct angulation prior to the injection will allow the clinician to note these needle access problems

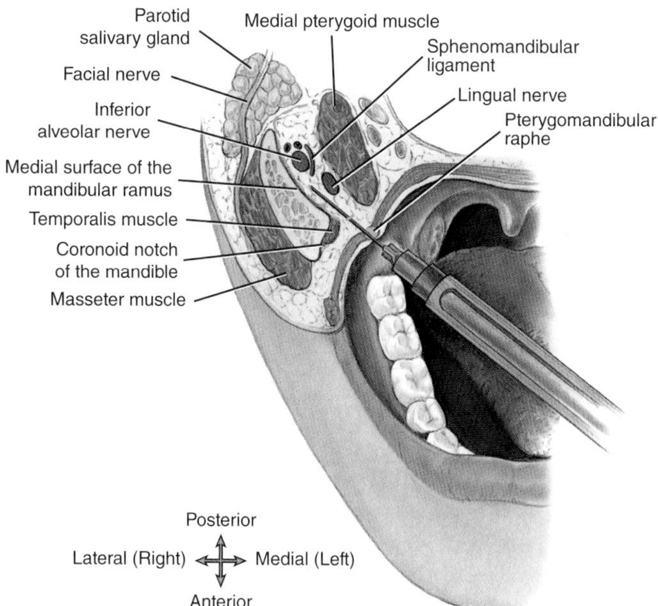

Fig. 13.5 Needle insertion into the depth of the pterygomandibular space *(dashed line)* for an inferior alveolar block until gentle contact with the bone of the medial surface of the mandibular ramus. If the needle is inserted too far posteriorly, it may enter the parotid salivary gland containing the facial nerve, causing the complication of transient facial paralysis due to temporary anesthesia of the facial nerve. Note that the inferior alveolar nerve, artery *(red)*, and vein *(blue)* are wrapped together by a fibrous sheath in a neurovascular bundle, which occupies a small depression on the medial surface of the mandibular ramus. This latter situation explains the higher risk of positive aspiration. (From Fehrenbach MJ, Herring SW: *Illustrated anatomy of the head and neck,* ed 6, St Louis, 2021, Saunders/Elsevier.)

and be able to accommodate them in order to have the needle at the target area (see Fig. 13.8C).[9]

Similar to maxillary supraperiosteal injections and facial nerve blocks as discussed in Chapter 12, there is no need for the clinician to shake the cheek tissue to distract the patient; this so-called "distractor" technique would move the needle and its bevel out of the correct pathway to the target area causing less effective administration, possible trauma, and then pain to the patient. Instead, to reduce patient discomfort, topical anesthesia is used initially and the local anesthetic agent should be deposited slowly.[9]

With the IA block there should be no bending of the needle shank in order to accomplish the necessary needle and syringe barrel angulations as discussed.[4] The needle can break when bent, and there is little control over the needle direction, needle angulation, and needle bevel. And there should not be any change in direction of the needle within the tissue to obtain correct angulation as this may cause deep tissue trauma since the correct angulation should be determined before entering the soft tissue.[9]

Inferior Alveolar Block Troubleshooting Paradigm

Even though the IA block is the most commonly used dental injection, it is not always initially clinically effective; the level for the lack of clinical effectiveness is approximately 15% to 20%.[4] This means that the patient may need to be reinjected to achieve the necessary anesthesia of the tissue. However, the careful clinician will use a troubleshooting injection paradigm in order to achieve clinical effectiveness every time the IA block is used.[1,9,10]

First, the clinician should reassess a panoramic film of the patient if it is available and from this determine again the position of the mandibular foramen (see Fig. 10.8 in Chapter 10). Second, the clinician should reassess the area visually and palpate the landmarks. In addition, consideration should be made to the height of the insertion point, needle and syringe barrel angulation, and depth of insertion. This complex orientation can be practiced using a training needle set up on a syringe (see Chapters 9 and 11) or a topical anesthetic-laced long cotton-tipped applicator to palpate the injection site as if it were the needle and syringe as can be done for all the injections.[9] Lack of consistent clinical effectiveness is in part due to the anatomic variation in the height of the mandibular foramen on the medial side of the mandibular ramus and the great depth of soft tissue insertion required to achieve pulpal anesthesia.[1,4,10]

To further complicate matters, not many patients are symmetrical in their anatomic positioning of landmark structures on both sides so

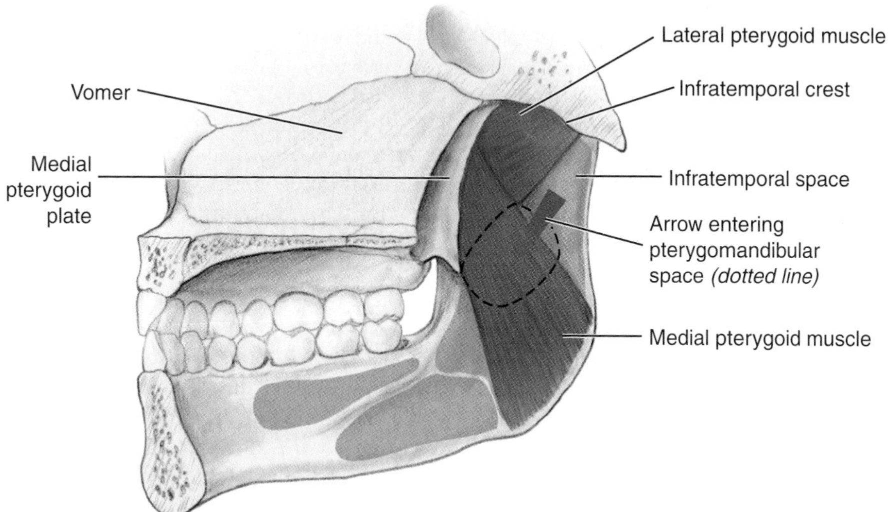

Fig. 13.6 Midsagittal section of the skull with an arrow demonstrating the direction of the anesthetic needle entering the pterygomandibular space *(dotted line)* during the inferior alveolar block. (From Fehrenbach MJ, Herring SW: *Illustrated anatomy of the head and neck,* ed 6, St Louis, 2021, Saunders/Elsevier.)

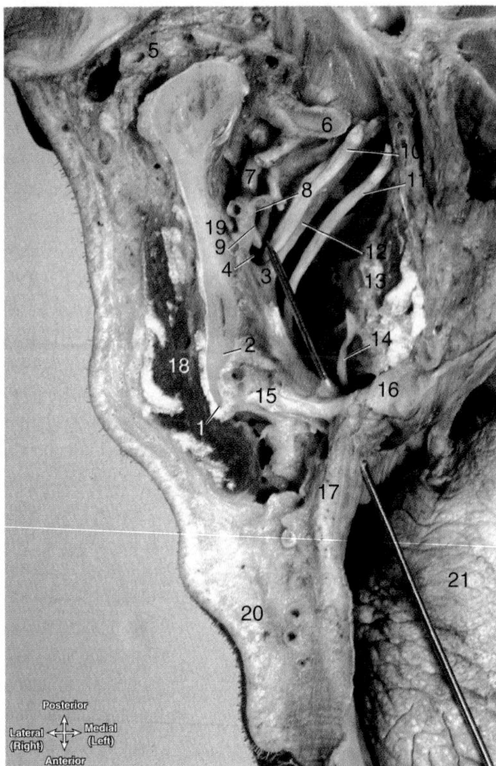

Fig. 13.7 Dissection of the right infratemporal fossa on a transverse section showing the needle at the injection site or needle insertion point for the inferior alveolar block; see also Fig. 13.5. *1,* Coronoid notch superior to external oblique ridge; *2,* Mylohyoid line; *3,* Lingula; *4,* Mandibular foramen; *5,* Parotid salivary gland; *6,* Styloid process; *7,* Maxillary artery; *8,* Inferior alveolar vein; *9,* Inferior alveolar artery; *10,* Inferior alveolar nerve; *11,* Lingual nerve; *12,* Sphenomandibular ligament; *13,* Medial pterygoid muscle; *14,* (Long) buccal nerve; *15,* Temporalis muscle tendon; *16,* Pterygomandibular raphe; *17,* Buccinator muscle; *18,* Masseter muscle; *19,* Medial surface of mandibular ramus; *20,* Buccal fat pad; *21,* Tongue. (From Logan BM, Reynold PA, Hutching RT: *McMinn's color atlas of head and neck anatomy,* ed 4, London, 2010, Mosby. In Fehrenbach MJ, Herring SW: *Illustrated anatomy of the head and neck,* ed 6, St Louis, 2021, Saunders/Elsevier.)

the paradigm for the IA block may be different on each side of the patient's oral cavity. Documenting these anatomic variations as well as any technique adjustments that were implemented in the patient's chart will assist any clinician in subsequent appointments. Other techniques to achieve mandibular anesthesia, such as the G-G or V-A blocks, may also be used when the IA block lacks clinical effectiveness (discussed later). Putting the patient upright or semiupright after the injection also helps the agent diffuse by gravity into the region, similar to that of the mental, incisive, G-G, and V-A blocks.[9] However, recent research suggests that this only increases the anesthetic level within the pulp of the premolars.[11]

If bone is contacted immediately after the needle is inserted into the soft tissue when trying to administer an IA block, it is possible that the insertion point was too inferior and/or too far lateral from the pterygomandibular fold covering the raphe (see Fig. 13.7 and Fig. 13.5). The clinician should remove the needle completely and repalpate to assess the anatomic landmarks. Adjustments should be made accordingly and the needle reinserted.

When this contact occurs at less than 16 mm or half to less than half of the long needle during administration of an IA block the needle tip is located too far anterior on the bone of the medial surface of the mandibular ramus (Fig. 13.9).[1] The needle tip may have either entered the temporalis muscle, which may cause muscle soreness, or come into early contact with the mylohyoid line (or internal oblique ridge) of the mandible.

The correction is made by withdrawing the needle partially or completely and instead bringing the syringe barrel more anterior or closely superior to the mandibular anterior teeth. The correction is by half a tooth at a time, moving anteriorly across the dental arch. This correction moves the needle tip more posteriorly when it is newly directed or reinserted. Injections for the IA block can even be administered in some more complicated cases with the syringe barrel over the contralateral mandibular lateral incisor or canine.

In contrast, if the bone is not contacted on the medial surface of the mandibular ramus when trying to administer an IA block even with the correct depth of insertion by the needle to approximately 20 to 25 mm or two-thirds to three-fourths of the long needle, the needle tip is located too far posterior on the bone of the medial surface of the mandibular ramus (Fig. 13.10).[1] The needle tip may enter the medial pterygoid muscle and be medial to the sphenomandibular ligament instead of lateral to it (see Fig. 13.7 and Fig. 13.5).

The correction is made by withdrawing the needle partially or completely and instead bringing the syringe barrel more posterior or closely superior to the mandibular molars. The correction is by the width of half a tooth at a time, moving posteriorly across the dental arch until bone is contacted at the correct depth. This correction moves the needle tip more anteriorly when it is newly directed or reinserted. The syringe barrel may have to press down even more on the contralateral corner of mouth when directed over the mandibular second molar so there may be some slight temporary discomfort for the patient.

In addition, if the insertion and deposition are too shallow as just discussed and bone is not contacted but the anesthetic is administered in haste, the medially located sphenomandibular ligament can become a barrier (see Figs. 13.5 and 13.7).[1] The ligament can prevent the local anesthetic agent from coming into contact with the deeper mandibular foramen and IA nerve, thus preventing the more profound pulpal anesthesia and allowing only the more superficial lingual nerve to be anesthetized. In addition, the needle within the medial pterygoid muscle may cause trismus.[1]

At all times, it is important not to deposit the local anesthetic agent in haste if bone is not contacted on an insertion of the needle for an IA block.[9] The needle tip may be too posterior and thus resting within the parotid salivary gland near the seventh cranial or facial nerve, resulting in serious complications (see Figs. 13.5 and 13.7; discussed further in the next section).[1,4]

If there is still lack of clinical effectiveness of anesthesia mainly on the mandibular first molar, even after proceeding with the troubleshooting injection paradigm, there may be accessory innervation present for this tooth. Current thinking supports the mylohyoid nerve as the nerve that may be involved in this accessory mandibular innervation (see Chapter 10).[1,4,12,13]

To directly correct this situation of accessory innervation after administration of the IA block, local anesthesia of the mylohyoid nerve using a mandibular supraperiosteal injection is indicated.[1,4] This reinjection technique directs the needle into the lingual tissue inferior to the apex of the mesial root of the mandibular first molar, near the mylohyoid line on the medial surface of the body of the mandible (Fig. 13.11). Alternatively, a periodontal ligament injection could be administered directly into the periodontium of the tooth.

The clinician may also want to attempt a true mandibular block for a patient with a past history of IA block failure or add an additional block when failure has occurred that has an increased level of overall

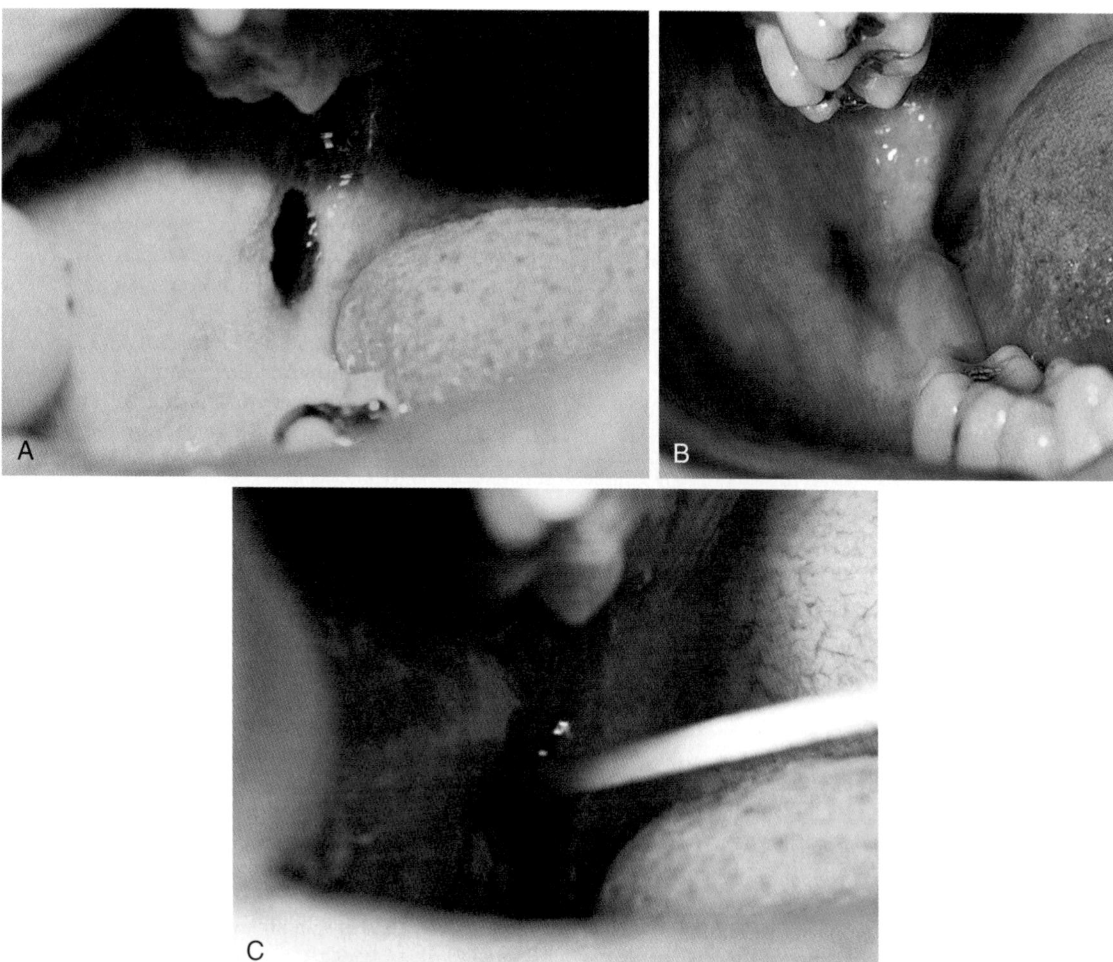

Fig. 13.8 Pterygotemporal depression that overlies the depth of the pterygomandibular space usually mimics an inverted teardrop; the injection site for the inferior alveolar block is in its superior basin-like part. (A) Depression has been temporarily dyed to show its location and shape. (B) Hematoma within the space showing a bluish-tinged depression, a possible risk of local anesthesia, again shows its most common location and shape. (C) Slight pressure with the opposite end of the cotton-tipped applicator into the pterygotemporal depression to enter the depth of the pterygomandibular space that can also be used before administration by the tip of the needle to help determine the correct needle insertion point. (Courtesy Margaret J. Fehrenbach, RDH, MS.)

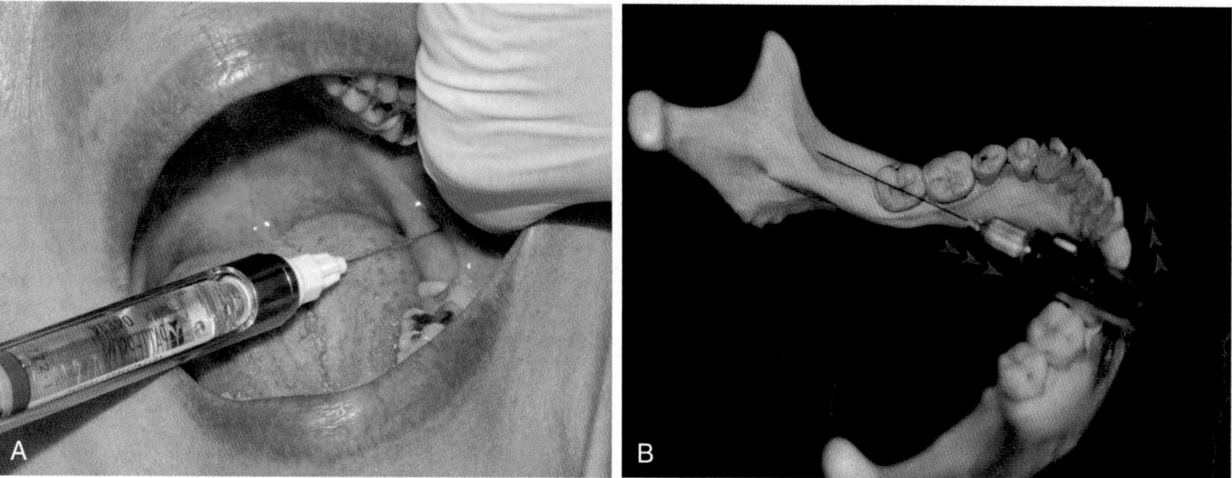

Fig. 13.9 Troubleshooting inferior alveolar block. If bone is contacted immediately after the needle is inserted when trying to administer an inferior alveolar block, the needle tip is located too far anterior on the mandibular ramus. (A) Intraoral view of the long needle contacting bone early at approximately one-half of the long needle. (B) The correction is made after partially or completely withdrawing the needle and moving the syringe barrel more closely superior to the mandibular anterior teeth when it is redirected or reinserted *(arrows);* with the correction the needle tip is more posterior. (B, Courtesy Margaret J. Fehrenbach, RDH, MS.)

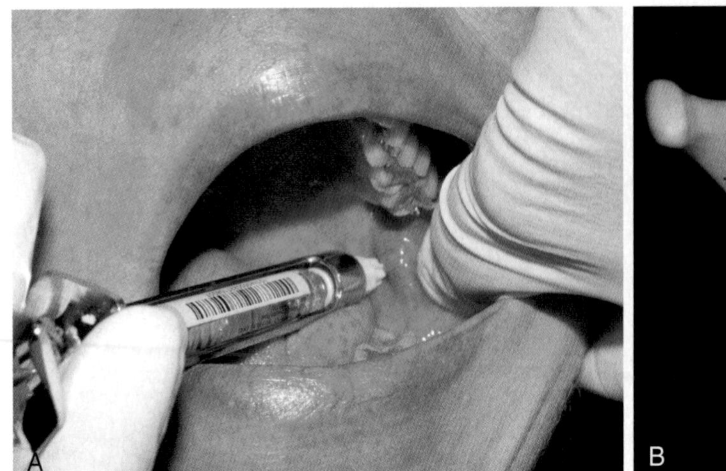

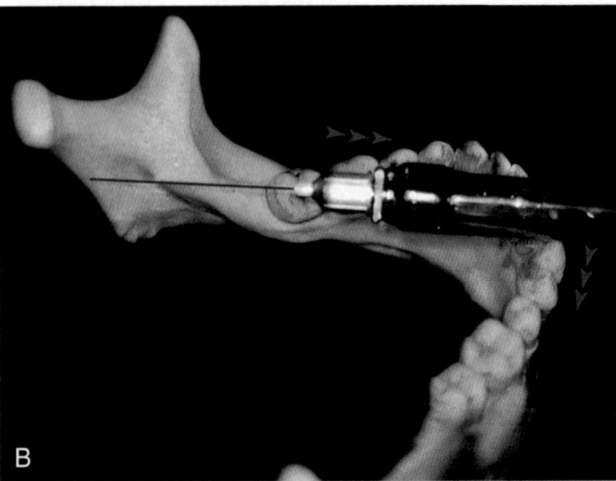

Fig. 13.10 Troubleshooting inferior alveolar block. If bone is not contacted when trying to administer an inferior alveolar block, the needle tip is located too far posterior on the mandibular ramus. (A) Intraoral view of the long needle not contacting bone and needle incorrectly inserted to its hub. (B) The correction is made after partially or completely withdrawing the needle and moving the syringe barrel more closely superior to the mandibular molars when it is redirected or reinserted *(arrows)*; with this correction the needle tip is more anterior. (B, Courtesy Margaret J. Fehrenbach, RDH, MS.)

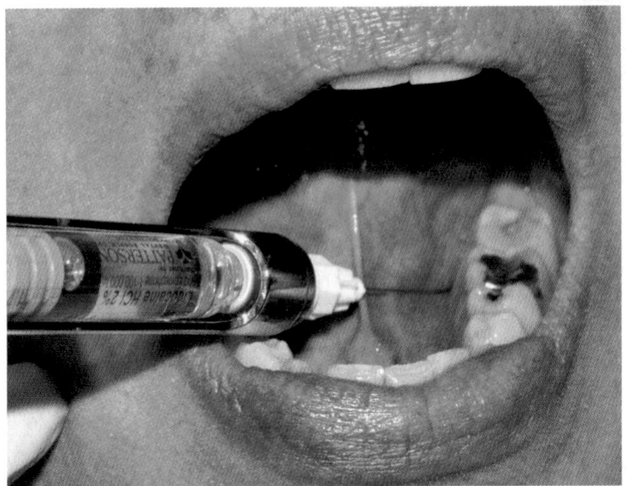

Fig. 13.11 Supraperiosteal injection into the lingual tissue on the medial surface of the mandible to obtain pulpal anesthesia of the mandibular first molar following a less than clinically effective inferior alveolar block, possibly anesthetizing the accessory innervation of the tooth by the mylohyoid nerve.

clinical effectiveness than the IA block and provide additional anesthesia for the mylohyoid nerve by administering either the G-G or V-A blocks (discussed later in this chapter).

Another less common reason for incomplete anesthesia following an IA block is a bifid IA nerve, which can be detected by noting a second mandibular canal upon radiographic assessment such as with cone-beam computed tomography (CBCT). In many such rare cases, a second mandibular foramen, more inferiorly located, exists; however, studies show that it occurs in less than approximately 1% of the population (see Chapter 10).[1,4] To work effectively with this anatomic anomaly, the local anesthetic agent is deposited more inferior to the usual anatomic landmarks for the target area of the IA block or the G-G block is administered instead.

Indications of Clinically Effective Inferior Alveolar Block and Possible Complications

Indications of a clinically effective IA block include harmless numbness and tingling of the lower lip because the mental nerve, a branch of the IA nerve, is anesthetized. This is only an indication that the IA nerve has been initially anesthetized, but it is not a reliable indicator of the depth of anesthesia, especially concerning pulpal anesthesia.[1,4]

Another indication of anesthesia is harmless numbness and tingling of the body of the tongue and floor of the mouth, which indicates that the lingual nerve, a branch of the mandibular nerve, is anesthetized.[1,4] Important to note is that this anesthesia of the tongue may occur without concurrent anesthesia of the IA nerve due to the barrier presented by the shallower sphenomandibular ligament (see previous discussion of this ligament). Possibly the needle was not advanced deeply enough into the tissue to anesthetize the deeper IA nerve. It is also important to remember that the most reliable indicator of a clinically effective IA block is the absence of discomfort during dental procedures.

In addition, "lingual shock" as the needle passes by the lingual nerve may occur during administration of the IA block (Table 13.3; see Fig. 13.2).[1,13] The patient may make an involuntary movement, varying from a slight opening of the eyes to jumping up in the chair. This reaction is only momentary and anesthesia will quickly occur. Gently informing the patient that this reaction may occur before the injection can help alleviate any alarm the patient may experience.[9] Moreover, effective preanesthetic communication can help the patient understand that reactions like these are common occurrences of the anesthesia within the mandible.

Since this reaction from contacting the lingual nerve occurs frequently when administering the IA block, the clinician must be prepared to maintain control of the injection even as the patient responds to this involuntary reaction. Stable fulcrums and slowly continuing on the intended path to the target location will provide the necessary control. Trying to pull the needle out or adjusting the needle within the tissue will not avoid the sensitive lingual nerve.[9] In addition, trying to deposit any amounts of agent as the needle advances through the

TABLE 13.3 Complications with Inferior Alveolar Block

Complication	Technique Adjustment
"Lingual shock" when moving needle through tissue and past lingual nerve	Reaction is only momentary and unavoidable
Inadequate anesthesia possibly caused by depositing agent inferior to mandibular foramen	Reinject at more superior injection site
Incomplete anesthesia of mandibular central or lateral incisors due to crossover-innervation from contralateral incisive nerve	Additionally administer supraperiosteal injection on contralateral mandibular central incisor (see Figs. 13.18 and 13.19 and Chapter 12) or additionally administer contralateral incisive block (see Table 13.8)
Incomplete anesthesia of mandibular first molar possibly caused by accessory innervation by mylohyoid nerve that is not usually anesthetized by IA block	Additionally administer supraperiosteal injection into lingual tissue with 27-gauge short needle inferior to apices of mandibular first molar at approximately 3 to 5 mm or one-fourth of needle, aspirate and deposit approximately 0.3 mL or one-fourth of cartridge over approximately 20 seconds (see Fig. 13.11 and Procedure Box 12.1 in Chapter 12)
Transient facial paralysis when facial nerve is mistakenly anesthetized due to incorrect administration of anesthetic agent into parotid salivary gland containing facial nerve because mandible was not contacted	To prevent always gently contact mandible before depositing anesthetic agent and if not able to initiate troubleshooting injection paradigm (see Fig. 13.10)
Hematoma	Apply pressure with sterile gauze to area if needed; reassure patient after treatment is completed

tissue to the mandibular foramen will not prevent the reaction and may end up reducing the amount of agent available for anesthesia at the target area and thus reduce overall clinical effectiveness.[1] Small drops of local anesthetic agent inadvertently will be given off as the needle moves through the tissue.

One serious shorter-term complication with an IA block is transient facial paralysis if the facial nerve is mistakenly anesthetized (see Table 13.3).[1,4,13,14] This can occur because of incorrect administration of anesthetic into the parotid salivary gland containing the seventh cranial or facial nerve when the bone of the medial surface of the mandibular ramus was not contacted as was discussed earlier (see Figs. 13.5 and 13.7). This causes unilateral loss of motor function to the muscles of facial expression.[1] The patient will experience the inability to close the eyelid and drooping of the ipsilateral corner of the mouth on the affected side. However, the loss of motor function is temporary and fades within a few hours once the action of the agent resolves (see Chapter 16). Contacting the medial surface of the mandibular ramus during the inferior alveolar block injection or being careful about depth with Vazirani-Akinosi mandibular block will usually prevent this complication.

This injection also has a higher risk of positive aspiration in approximately 10% to 15% of cases due to the nearness of the IA blood vessels to the target nerves (see Table 13.3 and Fig. 13.2).[1,4] The inferior alveolar nerve, artery, and vein are wrapped together by a fibrous sheath in a neurovascular bundle, which occupies a small depression on the medial surface of the mandibular ramus. This is the highest positive aspiration rate of all block injections of either dental arch.

Another related complication such as a hematoma may occur due to these blood vessels being pierced by the needle even when the block is administered correctly.[1,3,14] If hematoma occurs in the area of the pterygomandibular space, let the patient see the bruising from the hematoma when the dental treatment is finished, discussing that it is a basic risk of anesthesia and is temporary (see Fig. 13.8B and Chapter 16).[1,4] Muscle soreness or limited movement of the mandible such as with trismus is rarely seen with this block when administered correctly. However, related self-inflicted trauma, such as lower lip biting and resulting swelling can also occur due to anesthesia of the lower lip, and the patient should not eat until the anesthesia wears off; this is especially true for children or those with physical or developmental disabilities (see Figs. 14.2 and 16.7 in Chapters 14 and 16).[1,4] Additionally, a warning concerning this trauma needs to be gently communicated to the parent or guardian (see earlier discussion).

Trauma can occur during an administration of the IA block, possibly to the lingual nerve, causing paresthesia of the nerve (see Table 13.3).[4,15] Paresthesia is an abnormal sensation from an area such as burning or prickling, like a "pins-and-needles" feeling that can range in level as well as in time span (see Chapter 16). Some studies demonstrate that this paresthesia may be due to lack of adequate padding by fascia around the lingual nerve or possibly neurotoxicity from the local anesthetic agent; especially in patients that receive multiple injections to the area.[16] Other studies do not reach any set conclusions but state that nerve damage can occur during nerve blocks.

Paresthesia can also occur with the spread of dental infection from a contaminated needle, but in most cases it occurs due to a complicated oral surgical extraction of impacted mandibular third molars or mandibular posterior implant placement.[1] In these cases, the avoidance of further local anesthesia in the area is recommended to allow for resolution of any nerve damage.[4,16] Finally, if the needle is contaminated, there may be a needle tract infection in the pterygomandibular space, which can spread to the cervical spaces.[1,14,17]

BUCCAL BLOCK

The buccal block or *long buccal block* anesthetizes the (long) buccal nerve and thus the associated buccal periodontium and gingiva of the mandibular molars within one mandibular quadrant (Table 13.4, Figs. G–K, and Procedure Box 13.2). Many times this block is not necessary if the buccal tissue is not impacted by the dental procedures provided such as restoration of occlusal caries without use of a rubber dam.[4] However, for nonsurgical periodontal therapy of the mandibular molars by a dental hygienist, especially with furcation involvement and root concavities when visibility due to hemostatic control is necessary, this block is often necessary and should be administered immediately following the IA block to complete mandibular quadrant anesthesia.[3,6,12] Therefore, the two nearby injection sites can be prepared simultaneously with topical anesthetic but always making sure to cover each separate site.[9]

This is a very clinically effective dental block because the (long) buccal nerve is readily located on the surface of the tissue and not within bone.[1,4] However, because there is contact with the mandible, the buccal block's associated VAS specific range is 2 to 4 if the clinician uses the correct technique, which is a somewhat higher-end range than the IA block, but the injection itself does not take as long to administer since the agent volume needed is considerably less (see Chapter 1).[5]

Target Area and Injection Site for Buccal Block

The target area or deposit location for the buccal block is the (long) buccal nerve on the anterior border of the mandibular ramus in the area of the retromolar pad overlying the retromolar triangle (see Table 13.4, Fig. G). This catches the buccal nerve as it passes anteriorly to the anterior border of the mandibular ramus, crossing the external oblique ridge before it enters the buccal region. Thus the injection site is the buccal mucosa that is distal and buccal to the most distal mandibular molar (see Table 13.4, Fig. J). The syringe barrel is parallel and directly superior to the mandibular occlusal plane on the side of injection.

The needle is advanced until it gently contacts the mandible and then the injection is administered (see Table 13.4, Fig. K). However, "scrunching" or pushing the softer tissue of the buccal fat pad down over the usually bony injection site after initially retracting the outer cheek may make the needle entry more comfortable to the patient. And careful placement of retraction finger or thumb away from the injection pathway will ensure clinician safety when administering the injection.

Because the buccal tissue is so tightly adhered to the bone and the injection is quite shallow, the tissue may balloon with the agent, which due to injecting too rapidly.[4] Also the agent may leak out of the injection site, but rinsing the patient's mouth immediately after safely capping the needle will help reduce the bitter taste of the anesthetic agent.

Indications of Clinically Effective Buccal Block and Possible Complications

Usually there are no overt indications of a clinically effective buccal block because of the location and small size of the anesthetized region. There is usually only absence of discomfort with dental procedures. Self-inflicted trauma can occur as a cheek bite so the patient should not eat until the anesthesia wears off (Table 13.5).[4,8] The complication of a hematoma rarely occurs because positive aspiration is approximately 0.7%.[4]

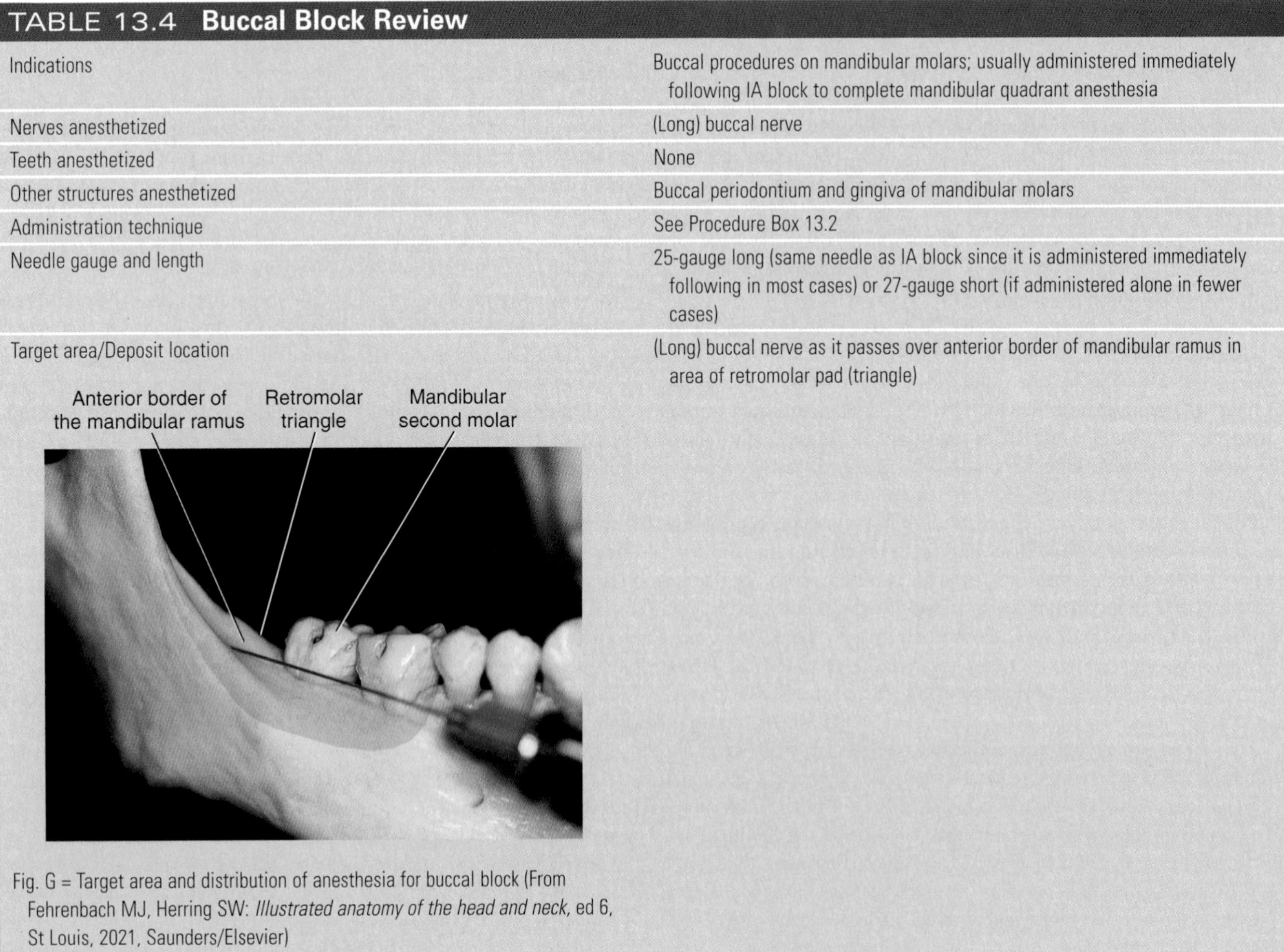

TABLE 13.4 Buccal Block Review

Indications	Buccal procedures on mandibular molars; usually administered immediately following IA block to complete mandibular quadrant anesthesia
Nerves anesthetized	(Long) buccal nerve
Teeth anesthetized	None
Other structures anesthetized	Buccal periodontium and gingiva of mandibular molars
Administration technique	See Procedure Box 13.2
Needle gauge and length	25-gauge long (same needle as IA block since it is administered immediately following in most cases) or 27-gauge short (if administered alone in fewer cases)
Target area/Deposit location	(Long) buccal nerve as it passes over anterior border of mandibular ramus in area of retromolar pad (triangle)

Fig. G = Target area and distribution of anesthesia for buccal block (From Fehrenbach MJ, Herring SW: *Illustrated anatomy of the head and neck*, ed 6, St Louis, 2021, Saunders/Elsevier)

TABLE 13.4 **Buccal Block Review (*Cont.*)**

Fig. H = Clinician position of right-handed clinician for buccal block (same as IA block and G-G block)

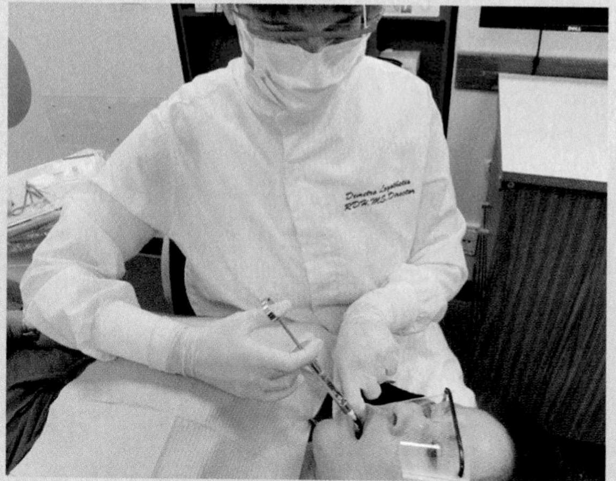

1, Right side, right-handed at 8 to 9 (left-handed at 10 o'clock)

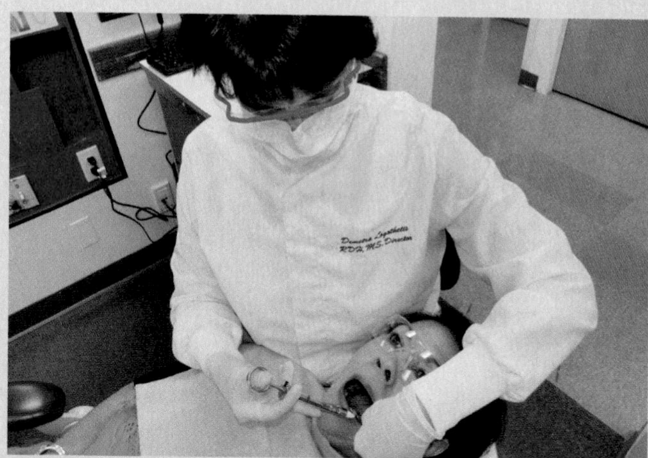

2, Left side, right-handed at 4 to 3 (left-handed at 2 o'clock).

Fig. I = Syringe stabilization with fulcrums for buccal block

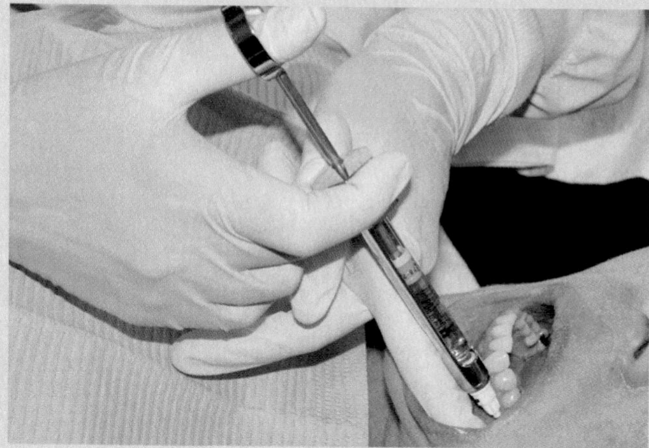

1, Retracting with index finger of nondominant hand and resting syringe barrel on top of finger

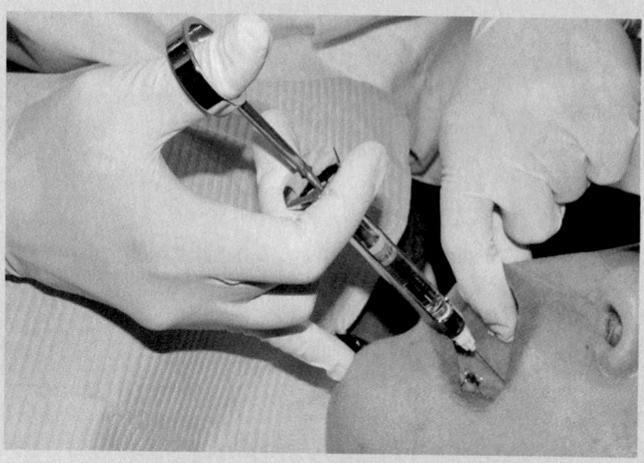

2, Resting pinky finger of dominant hand on patient's chin right side

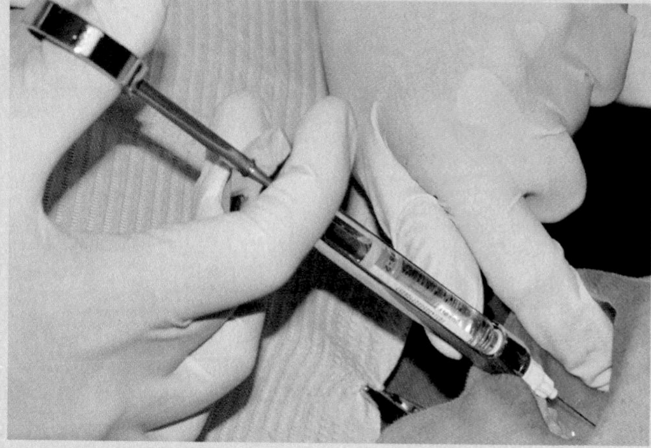

3, Resting syringe barrel on thumb of nondominant hand

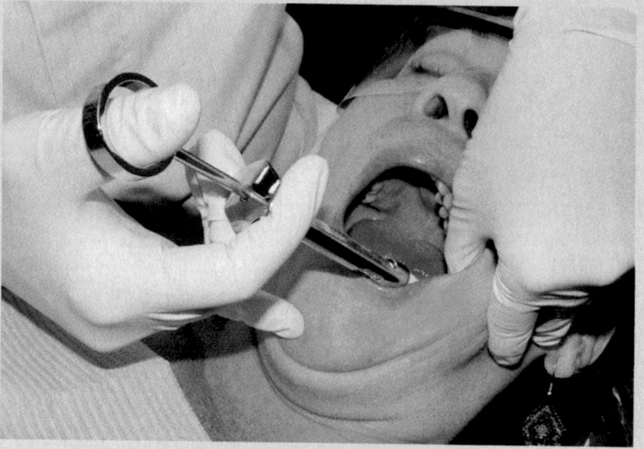

4, Resting pinky finger of dominant hand on patient's chin left side

Landmarks	Most distal mandibular molar Anterior border of mandibular ramus Retromolar pad (triangle)

(*Continued*)

TABLE 13.4 Buccal Block Review (*Cont.*)

Injection site/Needle insertion point 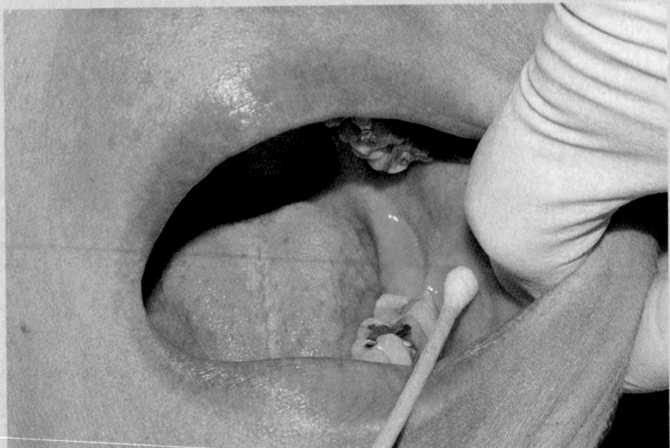 Fig. J = Injection site for buccal block	Buccal mucosa distal and buccal to most distal mandibular molar
Depth of insertion 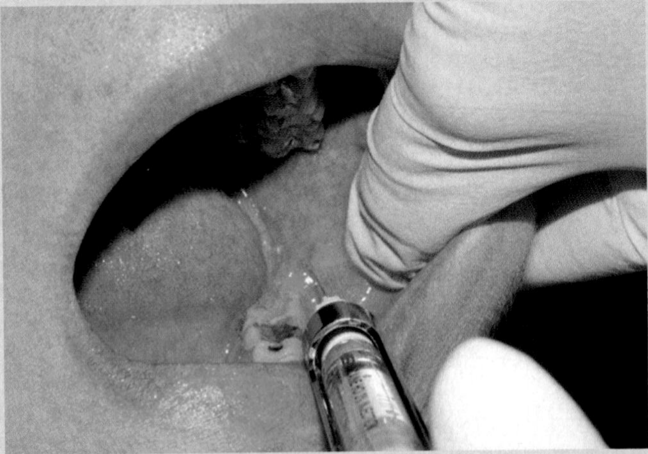 Fig. K = Needle insertion for buccal block	Approximately 2 to 4 mm until bone is gently contacted
Amount of anesthetic agent	Approximately 0.3 mL or one-eighth cartridge
Length of time to deposit	Approximately 10 seconds

IA, Inferior alveolar; *G-G*, Gow-Gates.

PROCEDURE BOX 13.2 Buccal Block Procedure

Step 1 Administer the buccal block immediately following the administration of the inferior alveolar (IA) block if both are needed and keep the same clinician position as the IA block: For right side, right-handed at 8 to 9 o'clock (left-handed at 4 to 3 o'clock); left side, right-handed at 10 o'clock (left-handed at 2 o'clock; see Table 13.4, Fig. H).

Step 2 Ask the supine patient to keep the mouth open or again open the mouth but not as wide as for the previous IA block. Retract the buccal soft tissue laterally, pinching it between both the index finger and thumb (as when administering the IA block; one inner and one outer), pulling the tissue taut.

Step 3 Prepare the buccal mucosa distal and buccal to the most distal mandibular molar (see Chapter 11).

Step 4 Using 25-gauge long (same needle set up as the IA block if administered together) or using a 27-gauge short needle (if administered alone), orient the bevel toward the bone and large window toward the clinician.

Step 5 With the taut buccal soft tissue, push the buccal fat pad into the injection site so that the bony injection will be somewhat padded, being careful to keep the retracting index finger or thumb out of the pathway of the needle (see Table 13.4, Fig. J).

Step 6 Establish a fulcrum (see Table 13.4, Fig. I for fulcrum recommendations).

Step 7 Direct the syringe barrel parallel and directly superior to the mandibular occlusal plane.

Step 8 Insert the needle into alveolar mucosa distal and buccal to the most distal mandibular molar in the quadrant until gently contacting bone at a depth of approximately 2 to 4 mm (see Table 13.4, Fig. K).

Step 9 Aspirate.

Step 10 If negative aspiration is achieved, slowly deposit approximately 0.3 mL of agent (one-eighth) over approximately 10 seconds; if the tissue balloons this is due to injecting too rapidly. The clinician should stop the deposition, remove the needle or slow down the deposition, and massage the area if needed.

Step 11 Carefully withdraw the syringe and immediately recap the needle using the one-handed scoop method utilizing a needle sheath prop (see Chapter 11).

Step 12 Rinse the patient's mouth and wait until anesthesia takes effect before starting treatment: approximately 3 to 5 minutes if administered with the IA block or approximately 1 minute if administered alone.

TABLE 13.5 Complications With Buccal Block

Complication	Technique Adjustment
Leakage of agent at injection site due to bevel of needle only partially in tissue with bitter taste of anesthetic agent	Correct by deeper depth of insertion upon reinsertion; rinse patient's mouth afterward
Ballooning of tissue caused by rapid deposit of agent	Correct by slowing down injection procedure

MENTAL BLOCK

The mental block anesthetizes the mental nerve and thus the associated facial periodontium and gingiva of the mandibular anterior teeth and premolars to the midline as well as the tissue of the ipsilateral lower lip and chin (Table 13.6, Figs. L–P, and Procedure Box 13.3). If pulpal anesthesia is necessary for the mandibular anterior teeth or premolars, administration of an incisive block or IA block (discussed earlier) as well as the use of a G-G block or V-A block (discussed later) may be considered instead. The additional use of a facially or lingually located supraperiosteal injection in the tissue inferior to the apices of these teeth on the medial border of the mandible may be indicated since the mental block also does not provide any anesthesia of the associated lingual periodontium and gingiva of the involved teeth.

In contrast, the incisive block is more commonly used for nonsurgical periodontal therapy by the dental hygienist.[6] However, the mental block may be used for maintenance or recare appointments involving the mandibular anterior teeth when neither pulpal anesthesia nor anesthesia of the associated lingual periodontium and gingiva is necessary, such as when dealing with facially located Stillman clefts that do not involve any dentinal hypersensitivity.[1,3]

Target Area and Injection Site for Mental Block

The target area or deposit location for the mental block is the mental nerve entering the mental foramen (see Table 13.6, Fig. L). This block catches the mental nerve before it merges with the incisive nerve within the mandibular canal to form the IA nerve. The mental foramen is usually located on the lateral surface of the mandible inferior to the apices of the mandibular premolars as recently noted with dental CBCT studies[18] (Fig. 13.12). The mental foramen in adults faces posterosuperiorly.

The mental foramen can be located on a radiograph before administering the mental block to allow for a better determination of its position during palpation (Fig. 13.13).[1,2,8,12] However, studies show that the mental foramen can be as far posterior as the apices of the mandibular first molar or as far anterior as the apex of the mandibular canine, so palpation should begin as far posterior as the mandibular first molar and proceed to the mandibular canine.[1,19,20]

To locate the mental foramen for the mental block, palpate first at the depth of the mandibular mucobuccal fold inferior to the apices of the mandibular first molar and move inferiorly to the apex of the

TABLE 13.6 Mental Block Review

Indications	Procedures on mandibular anterior teeth and premolars without any need for pulpal anesthesia and when anesthesia of lingual periodontium and gingiva is not needed
Nerves anesthetized	Mental nerve
Teeth anesthetized	None
Other structures anesthetized	Facial periodontium and gingiva of mandibular anterior teeth and premolars to midline; lower lip and skin of chin to midline
Administration technique	See Procedure Box 13.3
Needle gauge and length	27-gauge short
Target area/Deposit location	At mental foramen and inferior to apices of mandibular premolars or location determined by radiographs and/or palpation

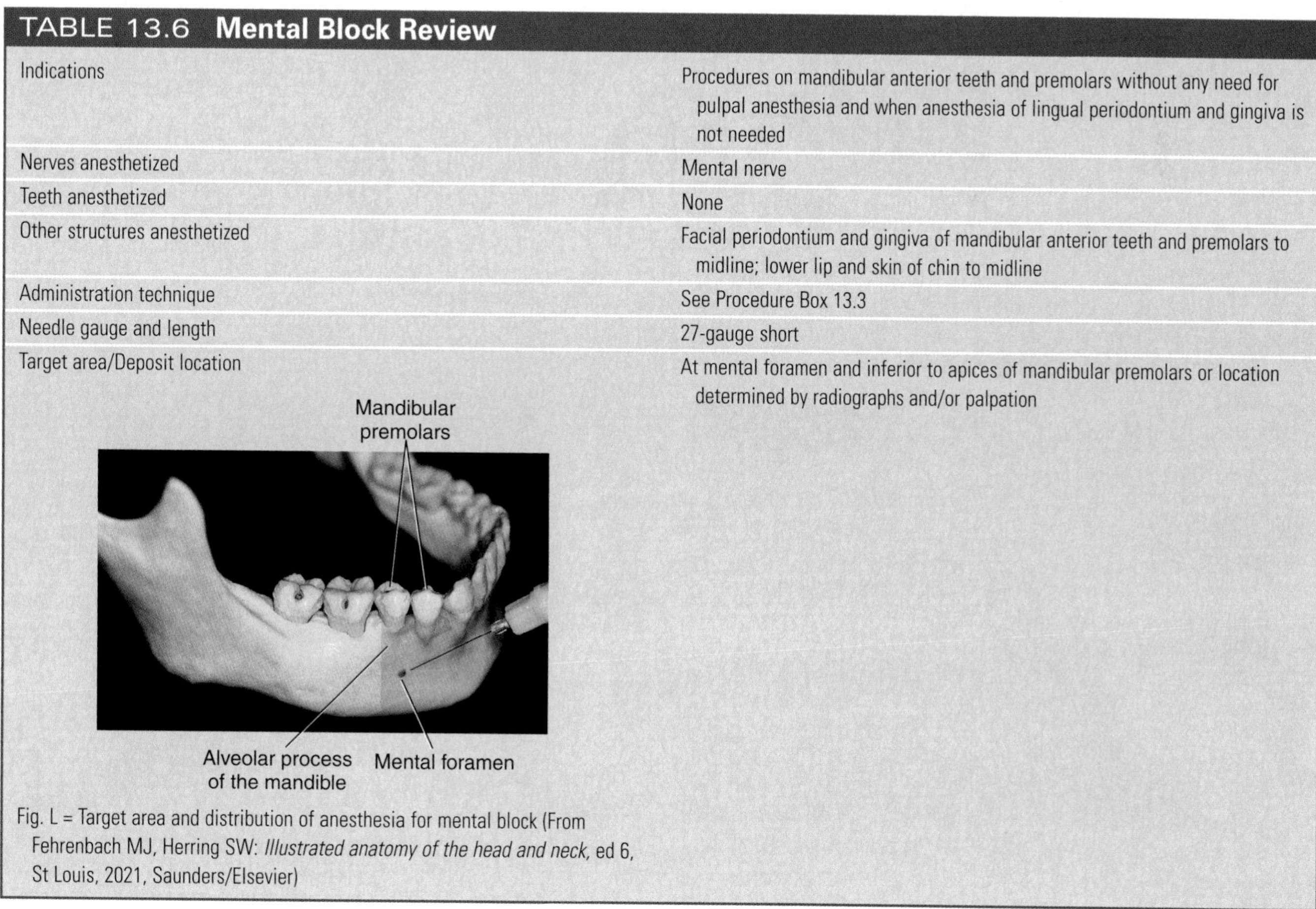

Fig. L = Target area and distribution of anesthesia for mental block (From Fehrenbach MJ, Herring SW: *Illustrated anatomy of the head and neck*, ed 6, St Louis, 2021, Saunders/Elsevier)

(Continued)

TABLE 13.6 Mental Block Review (*Cont.*)

Fig. M = Clinician position for either mental block or incisive block with two approaches, horizontal or vertical

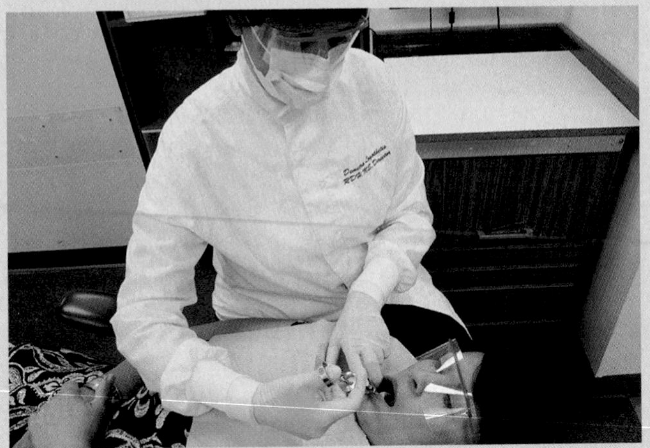

1, Horizontal approach: right side, right-handed at 8 to 9 o'clock (left-handed at 4 to 3 o'clock)

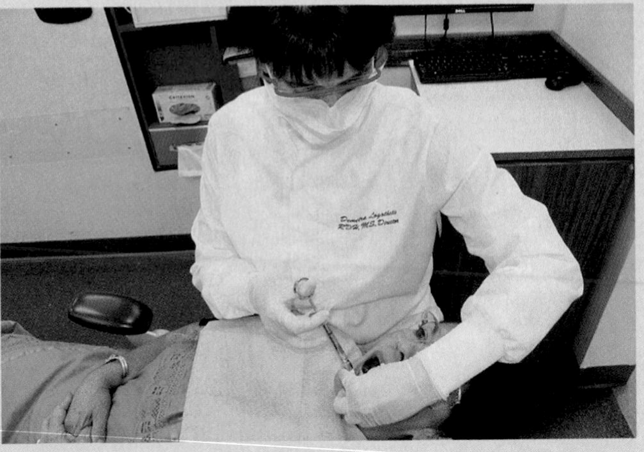

2, Horizontal approach: left side, right-handed at 8 to 9 o'clock (left-handed at 4 to 3 o'clock)

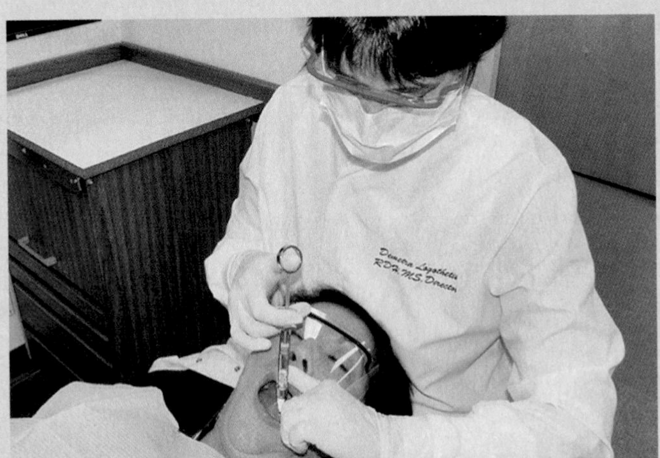

3, Vertical approach: right side or left side and right-handed or left-handed at 12 to 1 o'clock

Fig. N = Syringe stabilization with fulcrums for either mental block or incisive block with two approaches, horizontal or vertical

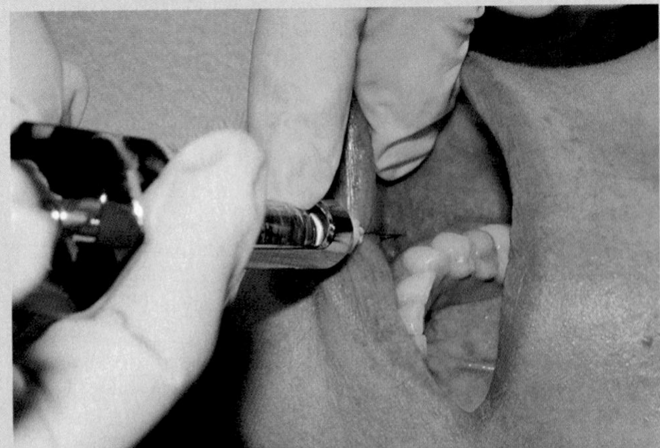

1, Horizontal approach: right side, syringe barrel resting on index finger of nondominant hand

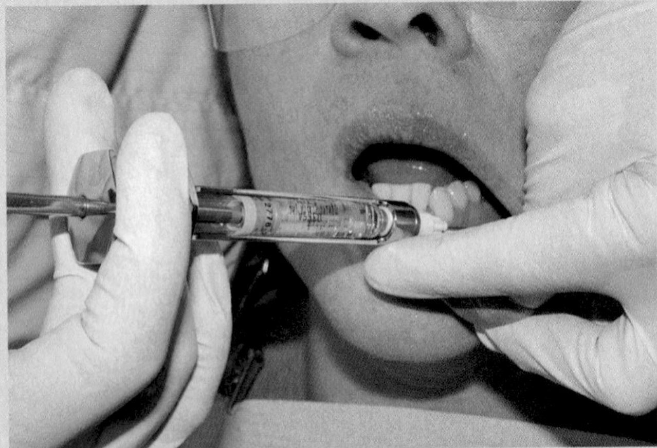

2, Horizontal approach: left side, syringe barrel resting on index finger of nondominant hand

TABLE 13.6 Mental Block Review (*Cont.*)

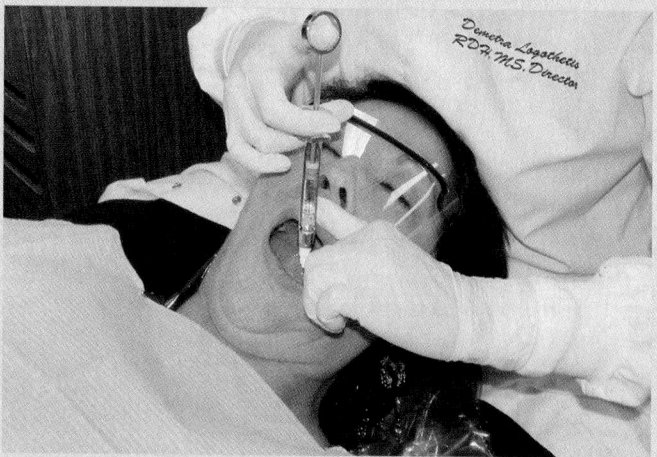

3, Vertical approach: both right and left side, syringe barrel resting on thumb of nondominant finger

Landmarks	Mandibular premolars Mental foramen Mandibular mucobuccal fold
Fig. O = Injection site or needle insertion point for either mental block or incisive block with two approaches, horizontal or vertical	Anterior to mental foramen at depth of mandibular mucobuccal fold inferior to apices of mandibular premolars or location determined by radiographs and/or palpation
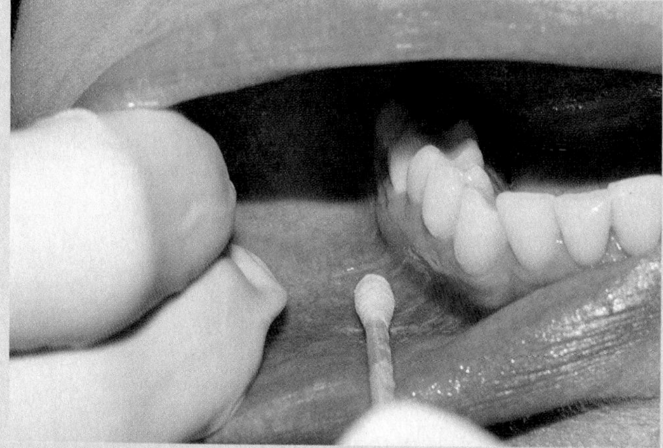 *1,* Injection site for either mental block or incisive block, horizontal approach	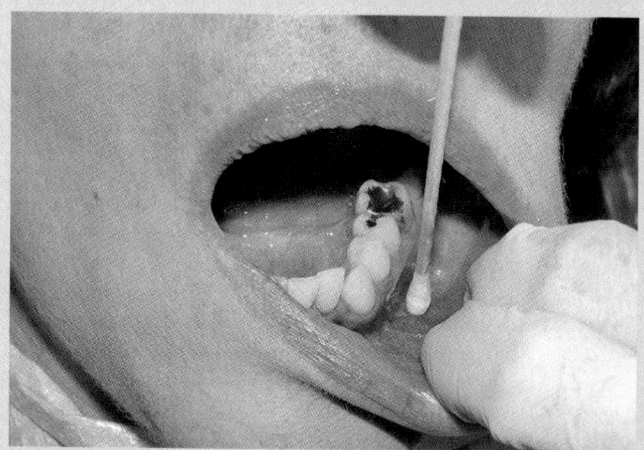 *2,* Injection site for either mental block or incisive block, vertical approach
Fig. P = Depth of insertion for either mental block or incisive block with two approaches, horizontal or vertical	Approximately 5 to 6 mm or one-fourth of short needle
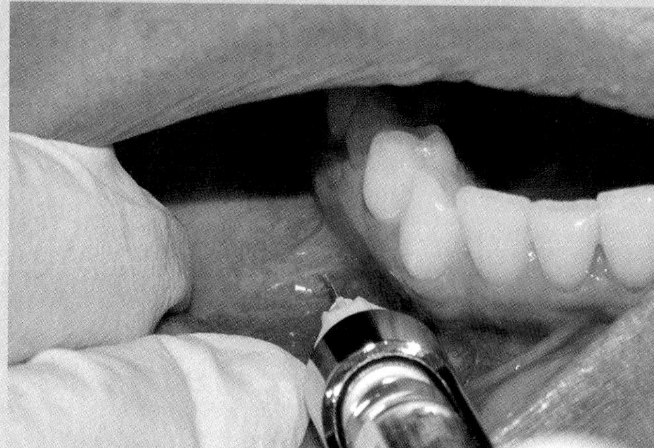 *1,* Needle insertion for either mental block or incisive block, horizontal approach	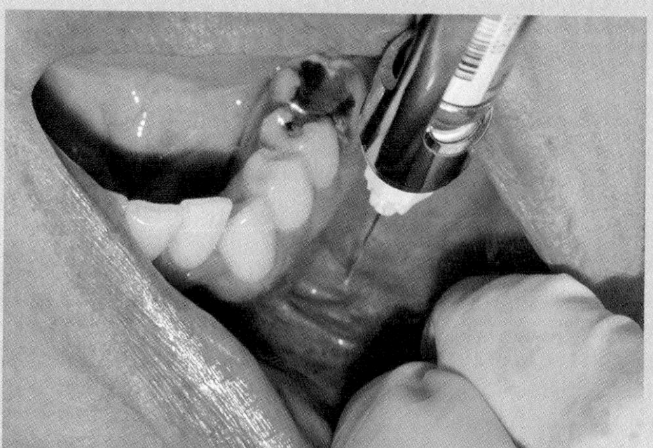 *2,* Needle insertion for either mental block or incisive block, vertical approach
Amount of anesthetic agent	Approximately 0.6 mL or one-third of cartridge
Length of time to deposit	Approximately 20 seconds

PROCEDURE BOX 13.3 Mental Block Procedure

Step 1 Determine syringe approach and assume the correct clinician positioning (see Table 13.6, Fig. M). For horizontal approach: For right side, right-handed at 8 to 9 o'clock (left-handed at 4 to 3 o'clock); for left side, right-handed at 8 to 9 o'clock (left-handed at 4 to 3 o'clock). For vertical approach: For right side or left side for right-handed or left-handed at 12 to 1 o'clock.

Step 2 Ask the supine patient to open and retract the lower lip outward, pulling the tissue taut; sterile gauze may be used to help retract slippery tissue.

Step 3 Locate the mental foramen by placing cotton-tipped applicator tip first at depth of the mandibular mucobuccal fold inferior to the apices of the mandibular first molar and moving to inferior to the apex of the mandibular canine or at a site indicated by a radiograph until a depression is felt on the surface of the mandible, surrounded by smoother bone (see Fig. 13.13 and Table 13.6, Fig. O). Too much pressure on the site before the injection may be uncomfortable for the patient.

Step 4 Prepare the alveolar mucosa anterior to the mental foramen at the depth of the mandibular mucobuccal fold (see Chapter 11).

Step 5 Using a 27-gauge short needle, orient the bevel toward the bone and large window toward the clinician.

Step 6 For horizontal approach: Establish a fulcrum, and then direct the syringe from the anterior of the mouth to the posterior in a horizontal manner, with the syringe barrel resting on the lower lip and index finger or thumb of the retraction hand (see Table 13.6, Fig. N1–2). Insert the needle at the depth of the mandibular mucobuccal fold, directing the needle anterior to the mental foramen at approximately 5 to 6 mm or one-fourth of a short needle (see Table 13.6, Fig. P1).

For vertical approach: Establish a fulcrum using the thumb of the retraction hand (see Table 13.6, Fig. N3), and then direct the syringe vertically with the patient's cheek toward the needle insertion site anterior to the mental foramen at approximately 5 to 6 mm or one-fourth of a short needle (see Table 13.6, Fig. P2).

Step 7 Aspirate within two planes.

Step 8 If negative aspiration is achieved, slowly deposit approximately 0.6 mL or one-third of cartridge over approximately 20 seconds; if the tissue balloons, the clinician is injecting too rapidly and should stop the deposition, remove the needle, and massage the area.

Step 9 Carefully withdraw the syringe and immediately recap the needle using the one-handed scoop method utilizing a needle sheath prop (see Chapter 11).

Step 10 Place the patient upright or semiupright, rinse the mouth, and wait approximately 2 to 3 minutes until anesthesia takes effect before starting treatment.

mandibular canine or at a site indicated by a radiograph until a depression is felt on the lateral surface of the mandible surrounded by smoother bone (see Fig. 13.1 and Table 13.6, Fig. O). The patient will comment that pressure in this area produces slight soreness because the mental nerve is compressed against the mandible near the foramen; however, care must be taken not to apply too much pressure directly to the site before administration of the agent.

Currently there are two pathways or methods of anesthetizing this nerve to consider.[4] The syringe barrel can be directed either from the anterior of the mouth to the posterior in a horizontal position with the syringe barrel resting on the lower lip, or vertically aligned with the patient's cheek with needle being inserted parallel with the long axis of the tooth. Both techniques provide the necessary anesthesia. However, the horizontal pathway is now considered the preferred method because it keeps the syringe out of the patient's line of sight and thus offers a psychological advantage over the vertical approach.[19,20] In addition, it offers a direct view of the large window during aspiration and less risk of puncturing through the lower lip when advancing the needle or causing unseen trauma to the deeper periosteum.[9]

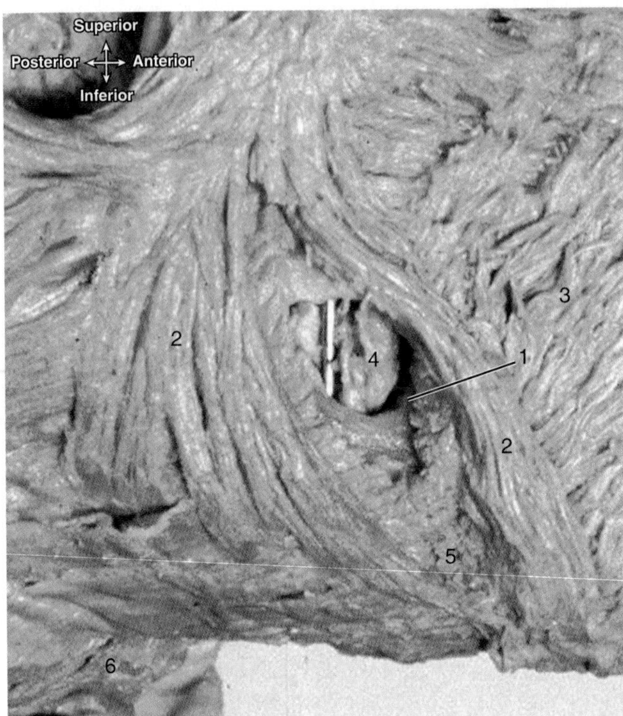

Fig. 13.12 Dissection showing a probe deep at the injection site or needle insertion point for either the mental block or incisive block. *1,* Mental foramen; *2,* Depressor anguli oris muscle; *3,* Depressor labii inferioris muscle; *4,* Mental nerve and vessels; *5,* Lower chin; *6,* Neck. (From Logan BM, Reynold PA, Hutching RT: *McMinn's color atlas of head and neck anatomy,* ed 4, London, 2010, Mosby. In Fehrenbach MJ, Herring SW: *Illustrated anatomy of the head and neck,* ed 6, St Louis, 2021, Saunders/Elsevier.)

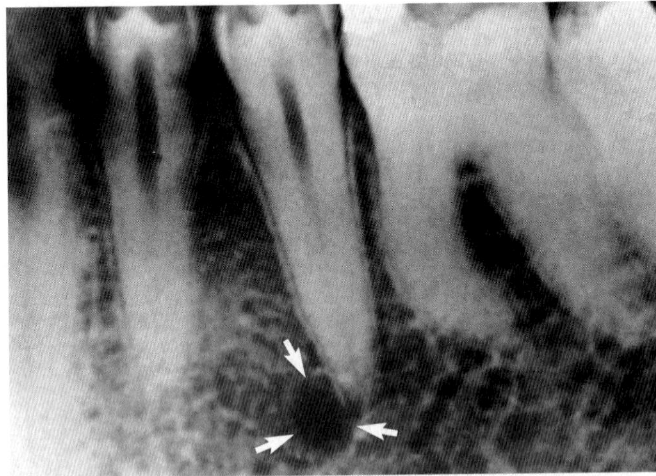

Fig. 13.13 Radiographs can be used to assist in locating the mental foramen (*arrows*) before administering both the mental block and incisive block. Note that the mental foramen is usually located on the lateral surface of the mandible inferior to the apices of the mandibular premolars (From Bowen DM, Pieren, JA: *Darby and Walsh Dental hygiene theory and practice,* ed 5, St Louis, 2020, Saunders/Elsevier.)

TABLE 13.7 Complication With Mental Block

Problem	Technique Adjustment
Hematoma	Apply pressure with gauze to area

The injection site or needle insertion point for a mental block is anterior to the mental foramen on the lateral surface of the mandible at the depth of the mandibular mucobuccal fold (see Fig. 12.1 in Chapter 12 and Table 13.6, Fig. O).[3,8] The needle is advanced without contacting the bone of the mandible and then the injection is administered (see Table 13.6, Fig. P). The tissue may balloon with the agent, which is due to injecting too rapidly, so the clinician will need to slow down the administration.

There is no need to enter the mental foramen to achieve anesthesia; in fact, the needle cannot enter the mandibular canal using the recommended positions of the needle.[4] Using the horizontal angulation approach, the clinician sits more along the side of the patient, where visibility is better and the patient does not see the needle.[19,20] The vertical angulation approach recommends that the clinician sit behind the patient. This approach may alarm the patient if the syringe with the needle in place is seen; however, asking patients to close their eyes may alleviate this problem.[9] Studies show that putting the patient upright or semiupright after the injection helps with the diffusion of the agent by gravity into the region.[9] However, recent research suggests that this only increases the anesthetic level within the pulp of the premolars.[11]

Indications of Clinically Effective Mental Block and Possible Complications

The indications of a clinically effective mental block are harmless numbness and tingling of the lower lip and absence of discomfort during dental procedures. The risk of positive aspiration is approximately 5.7%, which is the second highest rate of all the block injections due to the nearness of the mental blood vessels (Table 13.7).[1,4] However, the complication of a hematoma rarely occurs.

INCISIVE BLOCK

The incisive block anesthetizes the incisive nerve and thus mandibular anterior teeth and premolars as well as associated facial periodontium and gingiva to the midline with the ipsilateral lower lip and chin (Table 13.8, Fig. Q, and Procedure Box 13.4; see Table 13.6, Figs. M–P). However, if anesthesia of the associated lingual periodontium and gingiva of these teeth is also necessary, the additional use of the supraperiosteal injection in the lingual tissue on the medial surface of the mandible inferior to the apices of these teeth may also be considered (see Fig. 13.11 and discussion in Chapter 12) or an IA block would be administered instead.

The incisive block has increased clinical effectiveness because the incisive nerve is readily accessible.[4] The incisive block is also used when there is crossover-innervation of the contralateral incisive nerve and there is still discomfort on the mandibular anterior teeth following administration of an IA block as discussed earlier (see Chapter 10).[19,20] This block is also used bilaterally when providing nonsurgical periodontal therapy on a maintenance case with sensitive mandibular anterior teeth from previous care or if the patient does not have any mandibular posterior teeth present. Finally, the injection is also helpful on the more difficult nonsurgical periodontal therapy cases that are treated by the dental hygienist in sextants (see Fig. 11.3).

Target Area and Injection Site for Incisive Block

The target area or deposit location for the incisive block is the incisive nerve within the mental foramen. This block catches the incisive nerve as it merges with the mental nerve and before it continues on in the mandibular canal to form the IA nerve (see Table 13.8, Fig. Q).

The mental foramen is usually located on the lateral surface of the mandible inferior to the apices of the mandibular premolars (see Fig. 13.12). The mental foramen in adults faces posterosuperiorly.[1] The mental foramen can be located on a radiograph before administering the block to allow for a better determination of its position during palpation (see Fig. 13.13). However, studies show that the mental foramen can be as far posterior as the apices of the mandibular first molar or as far anterior as the apex of the mandibular canine, so palpation should begin as far posterior as the mandibular first molar and proceed to the mandibular canine.[1,19,20]

To locate the mental foramen for the incisive block, palpate first at the depth of the mandibular mucobuccal fold inferior to the apices of the mandibular first molar and move inferiorly to the apex of the mandibular canine or at a site indicated by a radiograph until a depression is felt on the lateral surface of the mandible surrounded by smoother bone (see Figs. 12.1 and 13.13 and Table 13.6, Fig. O). The patient will comment that pressure in this area produces slight soreness because the mental nerve is compressed against the mandible near the foramen; however, care must be taken not to apply too much pressure directly to the site before administration of the agent.

The syringe barrel for the incisive block can be directed either from the anterior of the mouth to the posterior in a horizontal position with the syringe barrel resting on the lower lip, or vertically aligned with the patient's cheek in the same manner as the mental block. As with the mental block discussed earlier, the horizontal approach is the preferred method based on many important considerations that were already listed earlier.[19,20]

The injection site or needle insertion point for an incisive block is anterior to the mental foramen at the depth of the mandibular mucobuccal fold (see Fig. 12.1 in Chapter 12 and Table 13.6, Fig. O). The needle is advanced without contacting the bone of the mandible and then the injection is administered (see Table 13.6, Fig. P). The tissue may balloon with the agent, which is due to injecting too rapidly so the clinician will need to slow down the administration and then later massage the area if needed.

It is not necessary to have the needle enter the mental foramen to achieve anesthesia; in fact, the needle cannot enter the mandibular canal using the recommended positions of the needle.[1,4] However, more local anesthetic agent is deposited within the tissue for the incisive block than for the mental block, and gentle pressure to the site is applied intraorally after the injection.[4] This pressure forces more local anesthetic agent into the mental foramen, thus anesthetizing first the shallow mental nerve and then the deeper incisive nerve.

Anesthesia of the tissue innervated by the mental nerve will precede that of the deeper incisive nerve's tissue; thus the soft tissue anesthesia precedes pulpal anesthesia so the careful clinician needs to wait for the latter when instrumenting sensitive root surfaces.[1] Also putting the patient upright or semiupright after the injection and then gently applying recommended pressure to the mental foramen has been shown in studies to help with further diffusion of the agent by gravity into the region.[9] However, recent research suggests that this only increases the anesthetic level within the pulp of the premolars.[11]

Indications of Clinically Effective Incisive Block and Possible Complications

The indications of a clinically effective incisive block are the same as those for a mental block with harmless tingling and numbness of the

TABLE 13.8 Incisive Block Review

Indications	Facial procedures on mandibular anterior teeth and premolars, when anesthesia provided for IA block is not needed (no scheduled mandibular molars instrumentation) or with cross-innervation following IA block; in some cases will need lingual anesthesia to complete anesthesia
Nerves anesthetized	Mental nerve Incisive nerve
Teeth anesthetized	Mandibular anterior teeth and premolars to midline
Other structure anesthetized	Facial periodontium and gingiva of anesthetized mandibular teeth to midline; lower lip and skin of chin to midline
Administration technique	See Procedure Box 13.4
Needle gauge and length	27-gauge short
Clinician position	Horizontal approach: right side, right-handed at 8 to 9 o'clock (left-handed at 4 to 3 o'clock); left side, right-handed at 8 to 9 o'clock (left-handed at 4 to 3 o'clock) Vertical approach: right side or left side for right-handed or left-handed at 12 to 1 o'clock (same as mental block; see Table 13.6, Fig. M)
Target area/Deposit location Fig. Q = Target area and distribution of anesthesia for incisive block (From Fehrenbach MJ, Herring SW: *Illustrated anatomy of the head and neck*, ed 6, St Louis, 2021, Saunders/Elsevier) 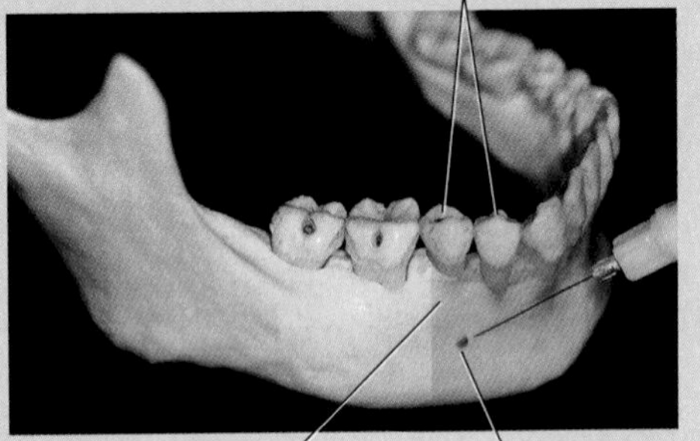	At mental foramen inferior to apices of mandibular premolars or location determined by radiographs and/or palpation
Syringe stabilization with fulcrums	Horizontal approach: right side, syringe barrel resting on index finger of retraction hand Horizontal approach: left side, syringe barrel resting on index finger of retraction hand Vertical approach: both right and left side, syringe barrel resting on thumb of retraction finger (same as mental block, see Table 13.6, Fig. N)
Landmarks	Mandibular premolars Mental foramen Mandibular mucobuccal fold
Injection site/Needle insertion point	Anterior to mental foramen at depth of mandibular mucobuccal fold inferior to apices of mandibular premolars or location determined by radiographs and/or palpation (same as mental block; see Table 13.6, Fig. O)
Depth of insertion	Approximately 5 to 6 mm or one-fourth of a short needle (same as mental block; see Table 13.6, Fig. P)
Amount of anesthetic agent	Approximately 0.6 to 0.9 mL or one-third to one-half of cartridge
Length of time to deposit	Approximately 20 seconds

IA, Inferior alveolar.

PROCEDURE BOX 13.4 Incisive Block Procedure

Step 1 Determine syringe approach and assume the correct clinician positioning (see Table 13.6, Fig. M). For horizontal approach: For right side, right-handed at 8 to 9 o'clock (left-handed at 4 to 3 o'clock); for left side, right-handed at 8 to 9 o'clock (left-handed at 4 to 3 o'clock). For vertical approach: For right side or left side for right-handed or left-handed at 12 to 1 o'clock.

Step 2 Ask the supine patient to open and retract the lower lip outward, pulling the tissue taut; sterile gauze may be used to help retract slippery tissue.

Step 3 Locate the mental foramen by placing cotton-tipped applicator tip first at the depth of the mandibular mucobuccal fold inferior to the apices of the mandibular first molar and moving to the apex of the mandibular canine or at a site indicated by a radiograph until a depression is felt on the lateral surface of the mandible, surrounded by smoother bone (see Fig. 13.13 and Table 13.6, Fig. O). Too much pressure on the site before the injection may be uncomfortable for the patient.

Step 4 Prepare the alveolar mucosa anterior to the mental foramen at the depth of the mandibular mucobuccal fold (see Chapter 11).

Step 5 Using a 27-gauge short needle orient the bevel toward the bone and large window toward the clinician.

Step 6 For horizontal approach: Establish a fulcrum, and then direct syringe from the anterior of the mouth to the posterior in a horizontal manner, with the syringe barrel resting on the lower lip and index finger or thumb of the retraction hand (see Table 13.6, Fig. N1–2). Insert the needle at the depth of the mandibular mucobuccal fold, directing the needle anterior to the mental foramen on the lateral surface of the mandible, approximately 5 to 6 mm or one-fourth of a short needle (see Table 13.6, Fig. P1).

For vertical approach: Establish a fulcrum using the thumb (see Table 13.6, Fig. N3) of the retraction hand, and then direct the syringe vertically with the patient's cheek toward the needle insertion site anterior to the mental foramen on the lateral surface of the mandible, approximately 5 to 6 mm or one-fourth of a short needle (see Table 13.6, Fig. P2).

Step 7 Aspirate within two planes.

Step 8 If negative aspiration is achieved, slowly deposit approximately 0.6 to 0.9 mL or one-third to one-half of the cartridge over approximately 20 seconds; if the tissue balloons, the clinician is injecting too rapidly and should stop the deposition and remove the needle.

Step 9 Carefully withdraw the syringe and immediately recap the needle using the one-handed scoop method utilizing a needle sheath prop (see Chapter 11).

Step 10 Place the patient upright or semiupright and apply firm pressure intraorally to the injection site for a minimum of 2 minutes to assist the agent into the mental foramen and then rinse the patient's mouth.

Step 11 (Optional) If anesthesia of the associated lingual periodontium and gingiva is necessary in the area of the incisive block, an additional supraperiosteal injection can be administered by inserting a 27-gauge short needle inferior to the apex (or apices) of the selected tooth or teeth on the medial surface of the mandible and slowly depositing approximately 0.6 or one-third of a cartridge over approximately 20 seconds (see Fig. 13.11 and Procedure Box 12.1 in Chapter 12).

Step 12 Wait approximately 2 to 3 minutes until anesthesia takes effect before starting treatment.

TABLE 13.9 Complications With Incisive Block

Complication	Technique Adjustment
Inadequate anesthesia due to inadequate volume of anesthetic into mental foramen or inadequate duration of pressure over mental foramen following injection	Correct by reinjecting in same location but with additional anesthetic agent and applying firm pressure to deposition site for minimum of 2 minutes
Hematoma	Apply pressure with gauze to area if needed

lower lip, except that there is pulpal anesthesia and anesthesia of the associated facial periodontium and gingiva of the involved teeth, and there is an absence of discomfort during more invasive dental procedures. As with a mental block, it has the same higher risk of positive aspiration due to the nearness of the incisive blood vessels, approximately 5.7%, which is the second highest rate of all the block injections (Table 13.9).[1,4] However as with a mental block, a hematoma rarely occurs.

GOW-GATES MANDIBULAR BLOCK

The G-G block is considered a true mandibular block because it anesthetizes the entire V_3 or mandibular nerve in most patients.[1,4] Thus, the nerves anesthetized with a G-G block are the IA, lingual, mental, incisive, mylohyoid, and auriculotemporal nerves as well as the (long) buccal nerve approximately 75% of the time (Table 13.10, Figs. R–U, and Procedure Box 13.5; see Table 13.2, Fig. A–2). The G-G block will anesthetize the mandibular teeth to the midline and associated lingual periodontium and gingiva as well as the associated facial periodontium and gingiva of the mandibular anterior teeth and premolars to the midline and probably the buccal periodontium and gingiva of the mandibular molars within one mandibular quadrant with the same extraoral tissue as the IA block.

Therefore the G-G block is usually indicated for use in quadrant dentistry and in cases when the IA block has shown failure to achieve overall clinical effectivenes.[21,22] Thus it can prove optimum for use before nonsurgical periodontal therapy since it usually has wide soft tissue coverage with just one injection. Pain levels using the VAS are similar to the other mandibular quadrant blocks, the IA and V-A blocks.[23] One of the major advantages of the block is that its clinical effectiveness is at an increased level than that of an IA block, even taking into account a slightly more complicated procedure since it uses mainly extraoral landmarks.

And with additional experience with the G-G block the clinician can achieve this increased level of clinical effectiveness.[21,22] Studies show that this clinical effectiveness once achieved may be related to the block also providing anesthesia to the mylohyoid nerve that has been shown to be involved in many case of accessory innervation with the IA block (see earlier discussion).[1,4] Thus it can be used when the patient has a past history of IA block failure owing to anatomic variability or accessory innervation.

Target Area and Injection Site for Gow-Gates Mandibular Block

The target area or deposit location for the G-G block is the anteromedial border of the neck of the mandibular condyle, just inferior to the insertion of the lateral pterygoid muscle and lateral to the medial pterygoid muscle as well as medial to the mandibular ramus (see Table 13.10, Fig. S).

TABLE 13.10 Gow-Gates Mandibular Block Review

Indications 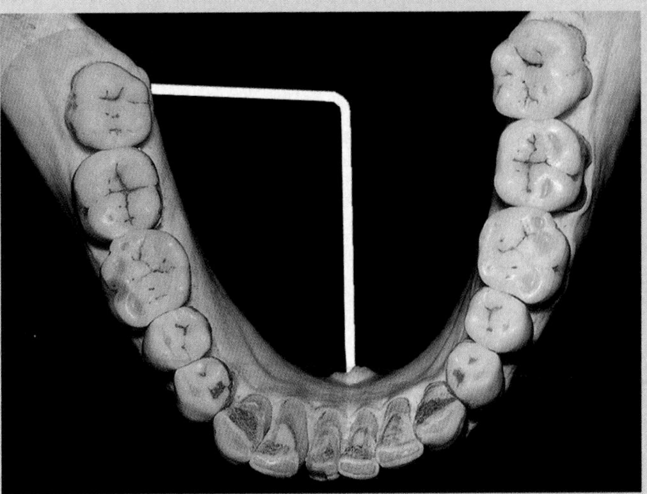 Fig. R = Distribution of anesthesia for G-G block, which probably includes that of buccal periodontium and gingiva of mandibular molars (shown) (this is same distribution as V-A block but also with auriculotemporal nerve anesthesia) (From Fehrenbach MJ, Herring SW: *Illustrated anatomy of the head and neck,* ed 6, St Louis, 2021, Saunders/Elsevier)	When IA block is less than clinically effective or extensive quadrant coverage is needed for procedures since anesthetizes entire mandibular nerve resulting in wide coverage; may need to administer buccal block to complete mandibular quadrant anesthesia
Nerves anesthetized	IA nerve Lingual nerve (Long) buccal nerve (most cases) Mental nerve Incisive nerve Mylohyoid nerve Auriculotemporal nerve
Teeth anesthetized	Mandibular teeth to midline
Other structures anesthetized	Lingual periodontium and gingiva of anesthetized mandibular teeth as well as facial periodontium and gingiva of anesthetized mandibular anterior teeth and premolars to midline and probably buccal periodontium and gingiva of anesthetized mandibular molars; lower lip, anterior two-thirds of tongue and floor of the mouth to midline; skin over zygomatic bone and posterior part of buccal and temporal regions; additional innervation by way of mylohyoid nerve to muscles and also can serve as afferent nerve for mandibular first molar; see also Fig. A2
Administration technique	See Procedure Box 13.5
Needle gauge and length	25-gauge long
Clinician position	Right side, right-handed at 8 to 9 (left-handed at 10 o'clock); left side, right-handed at 4 to 3 (left-handed at 2 o'clock) (same as IA block; see Table 13.2, Fig. C)
Target area/Deposit location Neck of mandibular condyle Mandibular foramen Fig. S = Target area for G-G block (From Fehrenbach MJ, Herring SW: *Illustrated anatomy of the head and neck,* ed 6, St Louis, 2021, Saunders/Elsevier)	Anteromedial border of neck of mandibular condyle

TABLE 13.10 Gow-Gates Mandibular Block Review (*Cont.*)

Syringe stabilization with fulcrums	Resting pinky of dominant hand on patient's chin (same as IA block; see Table 13.2, Fig. D)
Landmarks	*Extraoral:* Intertragic notch (lower border of tragus) Corner of mouth *Intraoral:* Mesiolingual cusp of maxillary second molar Buccal mucosa just distal to maxillary second molar
Injection site/Needle insertion point 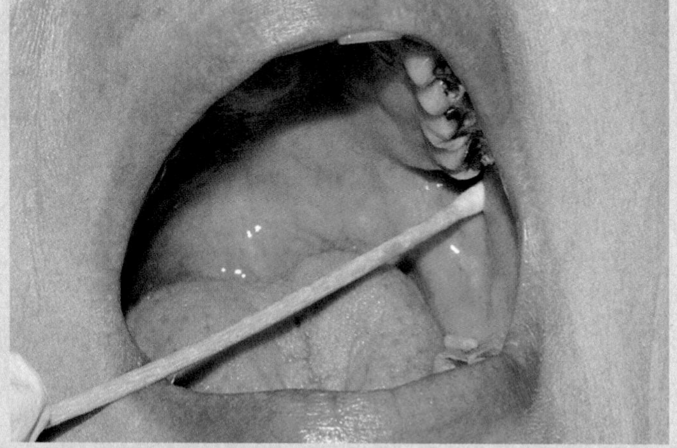 Fig. T = Injection site for G-G block	Buccal mucosa on medial surface of mandibular ramus just distal to height of mesiolingual cusp of maxillary second molar
Depth of insertion 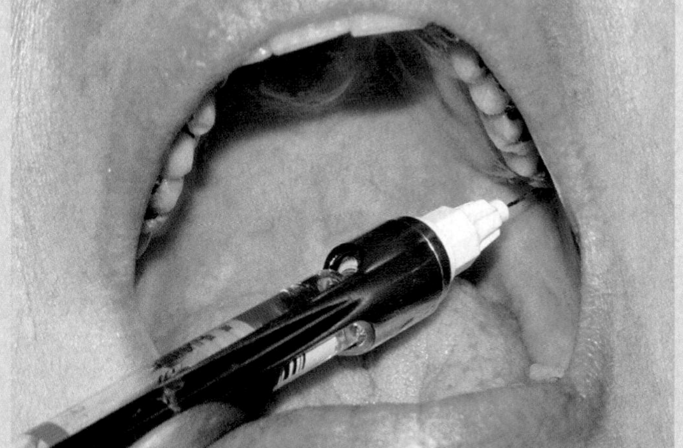 Fig. U = Needle insertion for G-G block	Approximately 25 mm or three-fourths of long needle until bone is gently contacted
Amount of anesthetic agent	Approximately 1.8 mL or full cartridge
Length of time to deposit	Approximately 60 to 90 seconds

IA, Inferior alveolar; *G-G,* Gow-Gates; *V-A,* Vazirani-Akinosi.

The extraoral landmarks of the ipsilateral intertragic notch and corner of the mouth are first located (Fig. 13.14). The tragus is the smaller flap of tissue of the auricle of the ear anterior to the external acoustic meatus, with the antitragus being the other flap of tissue opposite the tragus. Between the tragus and antitragus is a deep notch, the intertragic notch. The pathway of the needle parallels an imaginary extraoral line connecting the ipsilateral intertragic notch of the ear and corner of the mouth.

Thus the injection site is located intraorally on the buccal mucosa of the medial surface of the mandibular ramus, just distal to the height of the mesiolingual cusp of the maxillary second molar (see Table 13.10, Fig. T). Initially the needle is used to determine the height for the injection by placing the needle just inferior to the mesiolingual cusp of the maxillary second molar (Fig. 13.15). The injection height of the G-G block is more lateral when compared to that of the IA block since it is on the lateral margin of pterygotemporal depression and just medial to

PROCEDURE BOX 13.5 Gow-Gates Mandibular Block Procedure

Step 1 Assume the correct clinician positioning at right side, right-handed at 8 to 9 o'clock (left-handed at 10 o'clock); left side, right-handed at 4 to 3 o'clock (left-handed at 2 o'clock, same as inferior alveolar [IA] block; see Table 13.2, Fig. C).

Step 2 Locate the extraoral landmarks: intertragic notch at the lower border of the tragus and corner of mouth. Ask the supine patient to open wide. Locate the intraoral landmarks: mesiolingual cusp of maxillary second molar and buccal mucosa just distal to the maxillary second molar; when a maxillary third molar is present, the site of injection is just distal to that tooth (see Fig. 13.14 and Table 13.10, Fig. S).

Step 3 Prepare the buccal mucosa at the injection site on the medial surface of the mandibular ramus, just distal to the height of the mesiolingual cusp of the maxillary second molar (see Chapter 11).

Step 4 Using a 25-gauge long needle orient the bevel of the needle toward the bone and large window toward the clinician and then direct the syringe with the barrel superior to the contralateral mandibular canine-to-premolar region, such that the angulation of the syringe parallels an imaginary line connecting the ipsilateral corner of mouth and the lower border of the tragus at the intertragic notch. Initially place the needle just inferior to the mesiolingual cusp of the maxillary second molar to determine the height for the injection (see Fig. 13.14 and Table 13.10, Fig. T).

Step 5 The needle is next located distal to the maxillary second molar, maintaining the established height (see Fig. 13.15). The height of insertion is also superior to the mandibular occlusal plane at approximately 10 to 25 mm, depending on the patient's size.

Step 6 Establish a fulcrum by resting the pinky finger of the dominant hand on the patient's chin, same as IA block (see Table 13.2, Fig. D).

Step 7 The needle is inserted parallel to the determined imaginary line until gentle contact is made with the neck of the condyle at approximately 25 mm or three-fourths the length of the long needle (see Table 13.10, Fig. U).

Step 8 Aspirate within two planes.

Step 9 If negative aspiration is achieved slowly deposit approximately 1.8 mL or one cartridge over approximately 60 to 90 seconds.

Step 10 Carefully withdraw the syringe and immediately recap the needle using the one-handed scoop method utilizing a needle sheath prop (see Chapter 11).

Step 11 The patient should continue to keep open for approximately 1 to 2 minutes until indications of IA nerve anesthesia are present.

Step 12 Rinse the mouth and wait approximately 5 minutes or more until anesthesia takes effect before starting treatment. If there is lack of clinical effective anesthesia or the patient feels uncomfortable during treatment, proceed with the troubleshooting injection paradigm.

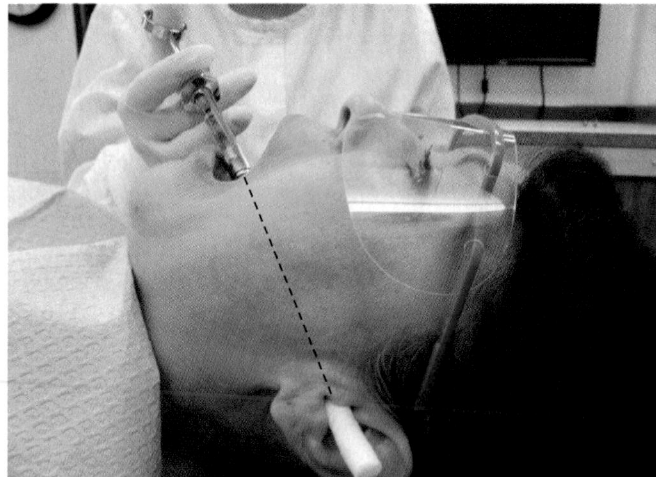

Fig. 13.14 Imaginary extraoral line (*dashed line*) for determining the pathway of the needle for the Gow-Gates mandibular block. The extraoral line connects the ipsilateral intertragic notch (cotton roll placed in the notch for demonstration purposes) of the ear and the contralateral corner of the mouth.

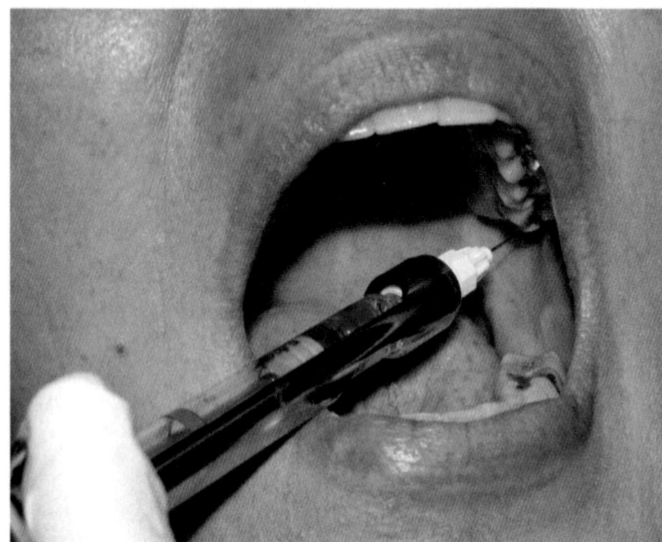

Fig. 13.15 Using the needle to assess the height of the injection for the Gow-Gates mandibular block by initially placing the needle just inferior to the mesiolingual cusp of the maxillary second molar.

the attachment of the temporalis muscle. Again it is important to avoid the sensitive structure of the temporalis muscle with the needle to prevent post administration muscle soreness. The injection height is also more superior to the mandibular occlusal plane than that of an IA block, approximately 10 to 25 mm, depending on the patient's size.[1,21]

When a maxillary third molar is present, the injection site will be just distal to that tooth. Some clinicians find that holding the non-dominant hand in the shape of a "C" with the finger or thumb inside the mouth retracting the cheek and relatively close to the site of the entry point of the needle but with the middle finger outside the mouth placed firmly over the intertragic notch does help aim the pathway of the needle.

The 25-gauge long needle is inserted into the buccal mucosa distal to the maxillary second molar at the established height. The 25-gauge needle is less likely to deflect as would a thinner 30-gauge needle as the needle progresses through the soft tissue to the injection site (see later discussion).[9] The needle is then advanced while maintaining the needle pathway and injection height until gentle contact is made with the anterolateral part of the neck of the mandibular condyle at approximately 25 mm or three-fourths of the long needle and the injection is administered (see Table 13.10, Fig. U). This injection is similar in depth to the IA block so it may be a more superiorly located injection but it is not a deeper one. The syringe barrel is maintained superior to the contralateral mandibular canine-to-premolar region and aligned parallel to the determined needle pathway; however, the syringe is also at the contralateral corner of the mouth, which again is similar to the IA block.

The needle naturally withdraws from the periosteum when contact is made with the neck, so there is no need to withdraw further as recommended by some clinicians and miss the target area. If there is no bony contact, the injection should not be administered. By contacting the bone of the neck of the mandibular condyle, the needle avoids causing traumatic injury to the area blood vessels, temporomandibular joint capsule, and otic ganglion.[21] Interestingly, this target area of the G-G block is a relatively avascular region as well as lacking in muscular tissue compared to that encountered with the IA block.

It is also recommended that the patient open the mouth as comfortably wide as possible during the entire injection.[21,22] The condyle assumes a more frontal position with the mouth open and the injection site is closer to the mandibular nerve trunk, which is preferred for this injection.[1,13] In contrast, with a more closed mouth, the condyle will move out of the injection site and the soft tissue will become thicker thus preventing overall effective anesthesia.

Later after administering the injection, leaving the mouth open for approximately 1 to 2 minutes until IA nerve anesthesia occurs is important until the complete diffusion of the agent occurs since the open mouth allows the IA nerve to be closer to the injection site at the neck of the mandibular condyle.[1,21,22] Using a bite block to keep the mouth open after the injection may be helpful as well as sitting the patient upright or semiupright; this change in position will also help the agent diffuse by gravity into the region.[22] However, recent research suggests that this only increases the anesthetic level within the pulp of the premolars.[11]

Gow-Gates Mandibular Block Troubleshooting Paradigm

Similar to the IA block (and also the V-A block), a troubleshooting paradigm may be used to achieve clinical effectiveness with the G-G block. This injection is most often missed if attempted too inferiorly due to the more common past experience of the clinician with administration of the IA block at its more inferior target area. Centering the focus on the maxillary arch instead of the mandibular arch aids the clinician in undertaking this block.

In addition, the unique angulation of the G-G block needs to be palpated with the cotton-tipped applicator even before the injection is administered. This angle of injection varies according to the degree to which the tragus diverges from the ear.[1,21] As a rule, the flatter the tragus lies in relation to the facial surface, the more anterior or more closely superior to the contralateral mandibular canine the syringe barrel position should be. In contrast, the closer the tragus is to 90 degrees to the facial surface, the more posterior or more closely superior to the contralateral mandibular second premolar the syringe barrel position should be.

If bone is not contacted on the neck of the mandibular condyle even with the correct depth of insertion by the needle to approximately 25 mm or three-fourths of the long needle, a greater depth of the needle may be required for larger patients or those with a markedly flaring mandibular ramus.[1,21]

If this is not the case with the patient, the lack of bony contact can be due to deflection of the needle in a mesial direction. The correction is made by withdrawing the needle completely and instead bringing the syringe barrel more posterior or more closely superior to the contralateral mandibular second molar.[1] This correction moves the needle tip more anterior when it is reinserted or more closely superior to mandibular canine, which should ensure contact with the bone of the neck. The correction is by the width of half a tooth at a time, moving posteriorly across the dental arch until bone is contacted at the correct depth. In contrast with the IA block, multiple tries with this block do not produce related muscle soreness in the patient since the needle passes through little or no muscle tissue.

Indications of Clinically Effective Gow-Gates Mandibular Block and Possible Complications

Indications of a clinically effective G-G block are anesthesia of the mandibular teeth and numbness of the associated facial and lingual periodontium and gingiva. Inadvertently, the anterior two-thirds of the tongue, floor of mouth, body of the mandible, and inferior mandibular ramus as well as the facial skin over the zygomatic bone and the posterior buccal and temporal regions will undergo numbness.[1]

If the associated buccal periodontium and gingiva of the mandibular molars do not have an adequate level of anesthesia, the buccal block can be additionally administered following the G-G block to complete the mandibular quadrant anesthesia similar to that needed with the IA block.[1,4] As the buccal nerve is approximately 23 mm from the injection site at the condyle, there is a significant reduction in the concentration of the anesthetic agent consequently affecting the buccal block.[1]

The two main disadvantages of the G-G block are the numbness of the lower lip as well as the temporal and buccal regions as discussed and the longer time necessary for the anesthetic to take effect, approximately 5 to 10 minutes.[1,21,22] The increased time of onset is due to the larger size of the nerve trunk being anesthetized and the distance of the trunk from the site of deposition, which is approximately 5 to 10 mm.[1] Thus this block may be contraindicated in a patient who may not be willing to undergo increased soft tissue anesthesia or wait time. This block is also contraindicated in patients with limited ability to open the mouth or trismus.[1] However, trismus is rarely an additional complication (see Chapter 16); for those patients with trismus, a V-A block would instead be indicated.

Another disadvantage, other than the large area anesthetized and its clinical effectiveness, is that the injection also lasts longer than the IA block because the area of the injection is less vascular and a larger volume of anesthetic may be used.[1,21] Thus this block may be contraindicated for certain patients who do not like the feeling of numbness to last too long or may undergo related self-inflicted trauma such as that with the IA block with children or those with physical or developmental disabilities. Additionally, a warning concerning this trauma needs to be gently communicated to the parent or guardian (see earlier discussion).[19,20] This longer duration is useful for more advanced cases of periodontal disease with its increased levels of dentinal hypersensitivity and postinstrumentation bleeding.

The risk of positive aspiration is lower for the G-G block since the IA blood vessels are further away from the target site than they are with the IA block as discussed earlier. Thus with less than approximately 2% positive aspiration, hematoma is also rare (Table 13.11).[19] However, if there is a positive aspiration and blood enters the cartridge before the injection, the needle is too far inferior to the target area; the internal maxillary artery or its larger tributaries have been traumatized.[22]

In addition, because of the lower vascularization in the area, the agent is less likely to undergo rapid absorption into adjacent blood vessels prolonging the presence of the anesthesia in the area, which means that an agent without vasoconstrictor may be used to greater and longer lasting effect with the G-G block. In fact, some clinicians of this technique recommend that no vasoconstrictor be used at all, which may be useful in patients that have a contraindication to the use of vasoconstrictors due to their medical history (see Chapter 7).

TABLE 13.11 Complications With Gow-Gates Mandibular Block

Complication	Technique Adjustment
Buccal periodontium and gingiva of mandibular molars does not have adequate level of anesthesia	Buccal block can be additionally administered following block (see Table 13.4)
Hematoma	Apply pressure with gauze to area if needed; reassure patient

VAZIRANI-AKINOSI MANDIBULAR BLOCK

The nerves anesthetized with the V-A block include the IA, lingual, mental, incisive, and mylohyoid nerves within the pterygomandibular space as well as the (long) buccal nerve approximately 75% of the time (Table 13.12, Figs. V–Y, Procedure Box 13.6; see Table 13.2 Fig. A2 and Table 13.10 Fig. R). Thus it is not considered a true mandibular block because it does not anesthetize the entire mandibular nerve and its branches as does the G-G block.[1,4,21] Instead the V-A block is more similar to the IA block in anesthetic coverage. Therefore the V-A block will anesthetize the mandibular teeth to the midline and associated lingual periodontium and gingiva as well as the associated facial periodontium and gingiva of the mandibular anterior teeth and premolars to the midline but also possibly the buccal periodontium and gingiva of the mandibular molars within one mandibular quadrant with the same extraoral tissue as the IA block.

In contrast to these other mandibular quadrant blocks, the V-A block is a closed-mouth mandibular block. Thus this block has a major advantage over these other mandibular blocks since it allows clinically adequate anesthesia of a patient that has severe trismus, which is a limited mandibular opening as a result of infection, trauma, or postinjection complication (see Chapter 16).[1,4,21]

The V-A block is also useful when soft tissue structures such as the tongue or buccal fat pad persistently obstruct the view of the necessary and usually visible intraoral landmarks for the IA block (see earlier discussion).[1] In addition, this block can be used for the fearful patient that does not want to open for anesthesia or may not be able to hold their mouth open for the length of either the IA block or G-G block.[1] Pain levels using the VAS are similar to the other mandibular quadrant blocks, the IA and G-G blocks.[23] In fact, one clinical trial found that the V-A block was "subjectively most acceptable to the patient."[23-25]

Finally, this mandibular block can be used if the patient has a past history of IA block failure owing to anatomic variability or accessory innervation.[1,4,21] There is increased clinical effectiveness with the V-A block than the IA block with many cases and this is theorized to occur since the mylohyoid nerve is anesthetized, which is a nerve that has been associated with accessory innervation of the mandibular first molar.[1,4,21,24] However, the V-A block is contraindicated in patients with an acute infection or inflammation within either the pterygomandibular space or maxillary tuberosity region.[1,18,21]

Additional administration of the buccal block to anesthetize the associated buccal periodontium and gingiva of the mandibular molars may also be indicated to complete the mandibular quadrant anesthesia similar to that needed by the IA block.[1,4] Now that the patient is relaxed by the loss of trismus or reduction of fear, the buccal block usually administered following the major block will now be easier to administer to the patient since it is an intraoral block that is not hampered by soft tissue structures (see earlier discussion).

Target Area and Injection Site for Vazirani-Akinosi Mandibular Block

The target area or deposit location for the V-A mandibular block is the medial surface of mandibular ramus within the pterygomandibular space approximately halfway between the mandibular foramen and the neck of the mandibular condyle as well as being adjacent to the maxillary tuberosity (see Table 13.12, Fig. V).

The patient is asked to gently occlude the posterior teeth, with the muscles of mastication remaining as relaxed as possible. If the muscles are clenched, the pterygomandibular space will be obliterated, which will prevent the agent from contacting the nerves within it.[1,21] However, the intraoral landmarks must be visible during the injection so retraction of the cheek and its buccal fat laterally is needed and using a retractor instrument is highly recommended. The intraoral landmarks

TABLE 13.12 Vazirani-Akinosi Mandibular Block Review

Indications	Procedures on patient with trismus or when IA block is less than clinically effective or extensive quadrant coverage is needed for procedures since anesthetizes most of mandibular nerve, including mylohyoid nerve; may need to administer buccal block to complete mandibular quadrant anesthesia (see Table 13.10, Fig. R for distribution)
Nerves anesthetized	IA nerve Lingual nerve (Long) buccal nerve (most cases) Mental nerve Incisive nerve Mylohyoid nerve
Teeth anesthetized	Mandibular teeth to the midline
Other structures anesthetized	Lingual periodontium and gingiva of anesthetized mandibular teeth as well as facial periodontium and gingiva of anesthetized mandibular anterior teeth and premolars to midline and probably buccal periodontium and gingiva of the anesthetized mandibular molars; lower lip, anterior two-thirds of tongue, and floor of the mouth to midline; additional innervation by way of mylohyoid nerve to muscles that can also serve as afferent nerve for mandibular first molar; see also Table 13.2, Fig. A2
Administration technique	See Procedure Box 13.6
Needle gauge and length	25-gauge long
Clinician position	For both right and left sides at 8 o'clock for right-handed clinician or 4 o'clock for left-handed clinician

TABLE 13.12 **Vazirani-Akinosi Mandibular Block Review Review (*Cont.*)**

Target area/Deposit location
Fig. V = Target area or deposit location for V-A block

Center of pterygomandibular space and at approximately equidistant between mandibular foramen and neck of mandibular condyle as well as being adjacent to maxillary tuberosity

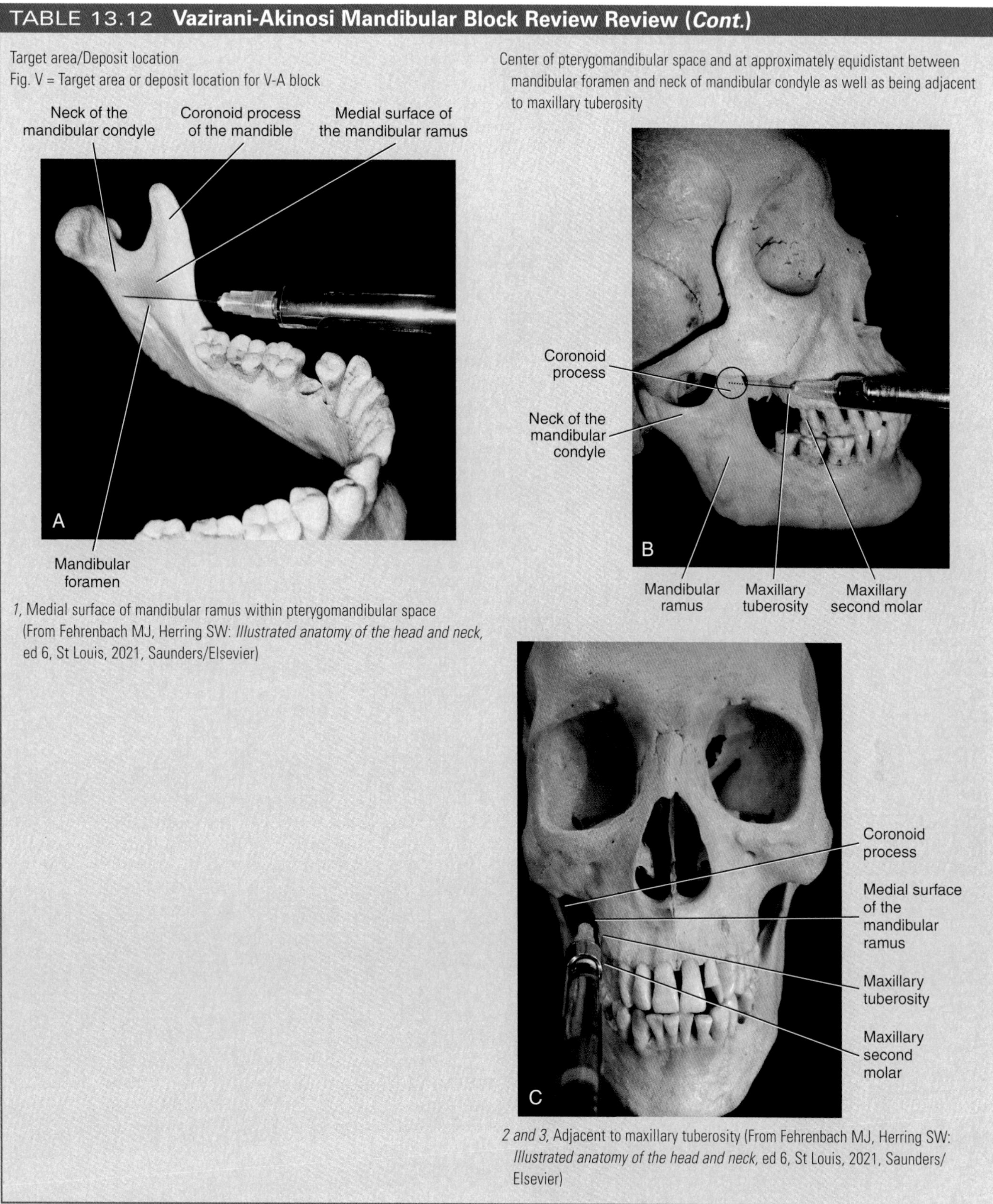

1, Medial surface of mandibular ramus within pterygomandibular space (From Fehrenbach MJ, Herring SW: *Illustrated anatomy of the head and neck*, ed 6, St Louis, 2021, Saunders/Elsevier)

2 and 3, Adjacent to maxillary tuberosity (From Fehrenbach MJ, Herring SW: *Illustrated anatomy of the head and neck*, ed 6, St Louis, 2021, Saunders/Elsevier)

for the V-A block are the medial surface of the mandibular ramus, maxillary tuberosity, and mucogingival junction of the maxillary third or second molar.

The injection site or needle insertion point is the buccal mucosa between the medial surface of the mandibular ramus and the maxillary tuberosity, with the syringe parallel to the maxillary occlusal plane (see Table 13.12, Fig. X). Thus this injection is administered at a site more inferiorly located than the G-G block but more superiorly located than the IA block. The injection height of the V-A block is determined by placing the needle at the same height as the mucogingival junction of the maxillary third or second molar directly across the way from the tooth (Fig. 13.16).

TABLE 13.12 **Vazirani-Akinosi Mandibular Block Review Review (*Cont.*)**	
Syringe stabilization with fulcrum 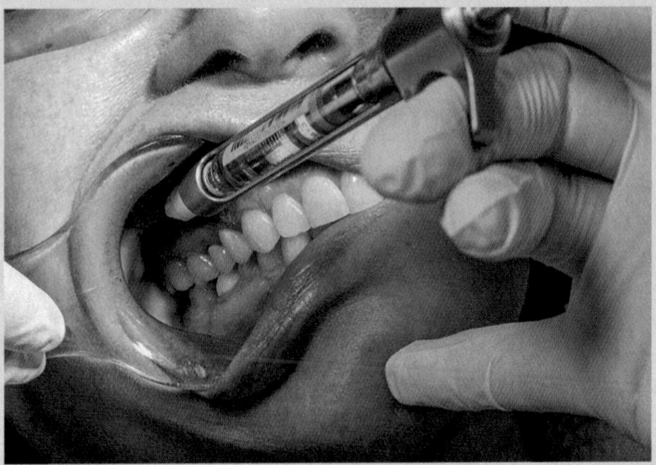 Fig. W = Resting pinky of dominant hand on patient's chin	
Landmarks	Coronoid process Maxillary occlusal plane Medial surface of mandibular ramus Pterygomandibular space Maxillary tuberosity Mucogingival junction of maxillary third or second molar
Injection site/Needle insertion point 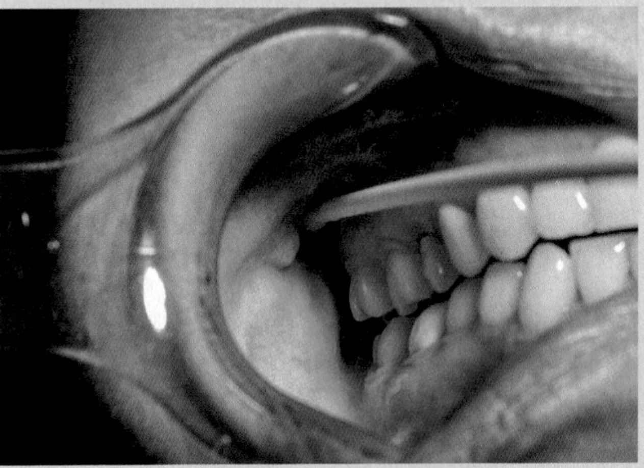 Fig. X = Injection site for V-A block	Medially past coronoid process and then into buccal mucosa on medial surface of mandibular ramus at same height as mucogingival junction of maxillary third or second molar directly across the way and with bevel oriented away from bone of mandibular ramus so it faces toward midline
Depth of insertion 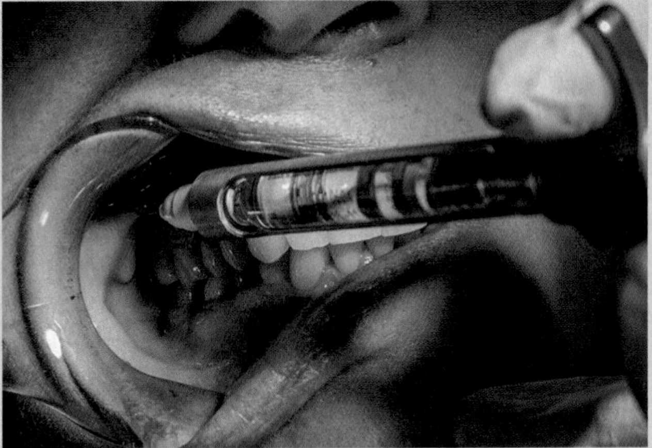 Fig. Y = Needle insertion for V-A block	Approximately 25 mm or two-thirds to three-fourths of long needle without contacting bone with hub of syringe ending up opposite mesial aspect of maxillary second molar
Amount of anesthetic agent	Approximately 1.8 mL or full cartridge
Length of time to deposit	Approximately 60 to 90 seconds

IA, Inferior alveolar; *G-G*, Gow-Gates; *V-A*, Vazirani-Akinosi.

PROCEDURE BOX 13.6 Vazirani-Akinosi Mandibular Block Procedure

Step 1 Assume the correct clinician positioning for both right and left sides at 8 o'clock for right-handed or 4 o'clock for left-handed.
Step 2 Ask the supine patient to gently occlude the posterior teeth, with the muscles of mastication remaining as relaxed as possible. After retracting the cheek with a retractor instrument as much as possible, locate the intraoral landmarks: medial surface of the mandibular ramus, maxillary tuberosity, and mucogingival junction of the maxillary third or second molar (see Table 13.12, Fig. V).
Step 3 Prepare the buccal mucosa at the injection site or needle insertion point on the medial surface of mandibular ramus within the pterygomandibular space adjacent to the maxillary tuberosity (see Chapter 11).
Step 4 Using a 25-gauge long needle orient the bevel of the needle away from the bone of the mandibular ramus so that it faces toward the midline with the large window toward the clinician.
Step 5 Direct the syringe barrel parallel to the maxillary occlusal plane and medially past the coronoid process. Then the needle is located at the same height as the mucogingival junction of the maxillary third or second molar directly across the way to determine the height of the injection (see Fig. 13.16).
Step 6 Establish a fulcrum by resting the pinky finger of the dominant hand on the patient's chin (see Table 13.12, Fig. W).
Step 7 The needle is then inserted into the buccal mucosa at the established height. The needle is then advanced posteriorly and slightly laterally without contacting the bone of the medial surface of the mandibular ramus, with the hub of the syringe ending up opposite the mesial aspect of the maxillary second molar (see Table 13.12, Fig. Y). The depth is approximately half the mesiodistal length of the mandibular ramus as measured from the maxillary tuberosity at approximately 25 mm or two-thirds to three-fourths of a long needle for the average adult with the distance measured from the maxillary tuberosity; in smaller or larger patients, this depth of insertion should be adjusted.
Step 8 Aspirate within two planes.
Step 9 If negative aspiration is achieved, slowly deposit approximately 1.8 mL or one cartridge over 60 to 90 seconds.
Step 10 Carefully withdraw the syringe and immediately recap the needle using the one-handed scoop method utilizing a needle sheath prop (see Chapter 11).
Step 11 Place the patient upright or semiupright, rinse the mouth, and wait approximately 3 to 5 minutes until anesthesia takes effect before starting treatment. If there is lack of clinical effective anesthesia or the patient feels uncomfortable during treatment, proceed with the troubleshooting injection paradigm.

The needle with the bevel oriented away from the bone of the mandibular ramus and facing toward the midline is directed medially past the coronoid process and then inserted into the buccal mucosa at the established height. The temporalis muscle attaches here on the coronoid process and the needle must again not penetrate this sensitive structure to avoid post administration muscle soreness. Thus in a lateromedial plane the point of insertion is medial to the coronoid process and lateral to the maxillary tuberosity.

The needle is then advanced posteriorly and slightly laterally without contacting the bone of the medial surface of the mandibular ramus unlike the IA block, with the hub of the syringe ending up opposite the mesial aspect of the maxillary second molar (see Table 13.12, Fig. Y). The needle will naturally deflect toward the mandibular ramus so that the needle will remain nearby to the IA nerve for an increased level of clinical effectiveness.[21]

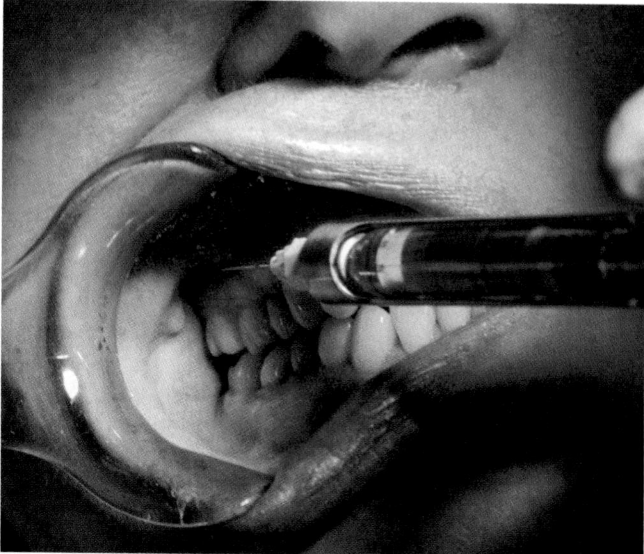

Fig. 13.16 Determining the injection height of the Vazirani-Akinosi mandibular block by placing the needle at the same height as the mucogingival junction of the maxillary third or second molar directly across the way.

Due to the closed-mouth situation, it may be difficult to fully visualize the path of the needle, so depth of the needle is always a concern and must be carefully controlled; the depth is approximately half the mesiodistal length of the mandibular ramus as measured from the maxillary tuberosity (see discussion next). The depth of insertion is approximately 25 mm or two-thirds to three-fourths of a long needle for the average-sized adult with the distance again measured from the maxillary tuberosity; in smaller or larger patients, this depth of insertion should be adjusted to more or less.[21] Thus the depth of insertion will vary with the anteroposterior size of the patient's mandibular ramus.

As with the IA block, there should be no bending of the needle shank toward the lateral with the V-A block to accomplish the necessary needle and syringe barrel angulations as discussed.[4] The needle can break when bent and there is little control over the needle direction, needle angulation, and needle bevel. And there should not be any change in direction of the needle within the tissue to obtain correct angulation as this may cause deep tissue trauma since the correct angulations should be determined before entering the soft tissue.

With the needle tip within the center of the pterygomandibular space, the injection is administered (Fig. 13.17; see Chapter 10). The goal of the block is to fill the pterygomandibular space with the agent so as to get complete contact of the agent with the IA and lingual nerves within the space.[1,21] In addition, putting the patient upright or semiupright after the injection also helps the agent diffuse by gravity into the region.[9] However, recent research suggests that this only increases the anesthetic level within the pulp of the premolars.[11]

Vazirani-Akinosi Mandibular Block Troubleshooting Paradigm

Similar to the IA and G-G blocks, a troubleshooting paradigm may be used to achieve clinical effectiveness with the V-A block. Although no bone should be contacted with this block as discussed, if the mandibular ramus obstructs needle placement, it often occurs early. It is usually due to contact with the outer coronoid process since the insertion point is located too far laterally; it may be corrected by reinserting the needle at a more medial position.[1,21]

However, if the needle is located too medially, it will end resting medial to the sphenomandibular ligament and only the superficial

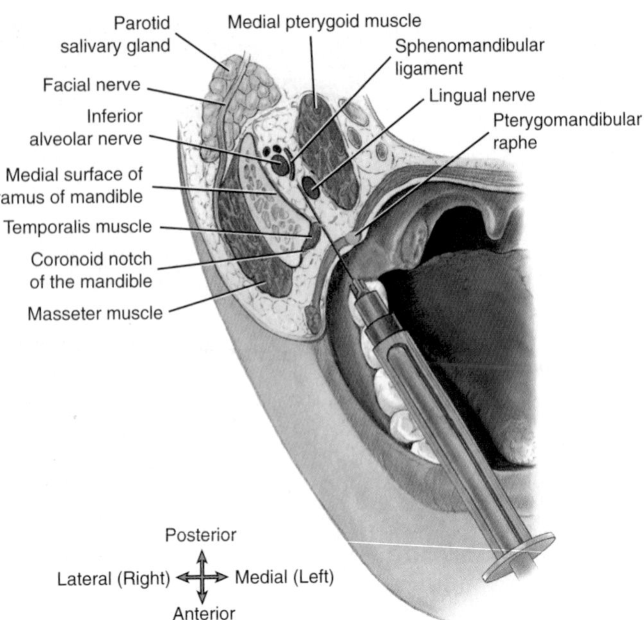

Fig. 13.17 Needle insertion into the midsection of the pterygomandibular space *(dashed line)* during a Vazirani-Akinosi mandibular block without contacting the bone of the medial surface of the mandibular ramus unlike the inferior alveolar block (see Fig. 13.5). The depth of the needle is approximately half the mesiodistal length of the mandibular ramus as measured from the maxillary tuberosity. However, if the needle is inserted too far posteriorly, it may enter the parotid salivary gland containing the terminal branches of the facial nerve causing the complication of transient facial paralysis. (From Fehrenbach MJ, Herring SW: *Illustrated anatomy of the head and neck,* ed 6, St Louis, 2021, Saunders/Elsevier.)

lingual nerve will become anesthetized and not the deeper IA nerve similar to the IA block (see Fig. 13.17).[1,21] This latter case mainly occurs when injecting on the nondominant side of the mouth due to even less visibility of the intraoral landmarks. Again the clinician needs to establish the correct and most clinically effective pathway of the needle and syringe barrel to achieve placement within the pterygomandibular space. Thus administering the agent too early and with the needle too shallow will cause this same situation with its lack of depth to the anesthesia.

Out of a concern for the risk of complications, the clinician may also inject the agent at too inferior a position, again similar to the IA block. To correct this situation, the insertion of the needle can be at or slightly superior to the level of the mucogingival junction of the maxillary second or third molar across the way.[1,20]

If there is still discomfort during dental procedures, the V-A block can be readministered if there is still trismus present. If trismus has subsided for the patient but discomfort is still present, then an IA block or G-G block can be administered instead.[4,20]

Indications of Clinically Effective Vazirani-Akinosi Mandibular Block and Possible Complications

Indications of a clinically effective V-A block allow for anesthesia and numbness that is very similar to that of the IA block. And since motor nerve paralysis develops as quickly as or quicker than sensory anesthesia, the patient with trismus begins to notice increased ability to open the jaws shortly after the administration of anesthetic.[1,21]

If there is still discomfort during dental procedures, the V-A block can be readministered if there is still trismus present. If trismus has subsided for the patient but discomfort is still present, then either the IA block or G-G block can be administered instead.[4,20]

TABLE 13.13 Complications With Vazirani-Akinosi Mandibular Block

Complication	Technique Adjustment
Transient facial paralysis when facial nerve is mistakenly anesthetized due to incorrect administration of anesthetic agent into parotid salivary gland containing facial nerve because needle was inserted with too much depth	To prevent, avoid contact with bone of medial surface of mandibular ramus and control depth of needle within pterygomandibular space so that it is not more than approximately 25 mm or two-thirds to three-fourths of long needle for average adult with distance measured from maxillary tuberosity; in smaller or larger patients this depth of insertion should be adjusted
Hematoma	Apply pressure with gauze to area if needed; reassure patient

Additional administration of the buccal block to anesthetize the associated buccal periodontium and gingiva of the mandibular molars may also be indicated to complete the mandibular quadrant anesthesia similar to that needed by the IA block.[1,4] Now that the patient is relaxed by the loss of trismus or even fear, the buccal block will now be easier to administer to the patient since it is a quick intraoral block that is not hampered by soft tissue structures (see earlier discussion).

There is a decreased risk of positive aspiration as well as hematoma formation compared to the IA block since the IA artery and vein are further away from the injection site with the V-A block than they are with the IA block. It is also less traumatic overall than the G-G block with the mouth needing to stay open for a long time (see earlier discussions).[1,20,24]

However, depth of the needle must be considered to avoid administration of anesthetic into the parotid salivary gland with the facial nerve (Table 13.13; see Fig. 13.17).[1,4,21] This may cause the complication of transient facial paralysis. See earlier discussion related to similar complications of an IA block and see Chapter 15.

MANDIBULAR SUPPLEMENTAL INJECTIONS

There are three supplemental injections that can be administered within the mandibular arch as well as the maxillary arch (see Chapter 12). The mandibular supplemental injections all have a moderate to high level of clinical effectiveness when administered correctly.[4] The supplemental injections have an associated VAS ranging from 0 to 6 when using the correct technique by the clinician (see Chapter 1).[5] The higher-end range is due to two of these injections entering into the cancellous bone of the alveolar process and not always being administered following a nerve block. However, the administration of all of these injections is of short duration.

The supraperiosteal injection is recommended when pulpal anesthesia is needed on a single tooth or when anesthesia of the associated periodontium and gingiva is needed in a localized area. The next two injections are intraosseous injections since the agent is deposited into the alveolar process that supports the teeth. The intraseptal injection is recommended when there is a need for additional hemostatic control with the interdental periodontium and gingiva between adjacent teeth. The periodontal ligament (PDL) injection is recommended when pulpal anesthesia as well as associated periodontium and gingiva is indicated on a single tooth.

If there is any pulpal anesthesia for these supplemental injections present, such as that for the supraperiosteal or PDL injections, it is achieved through anesthesia of each tooth's dental branches as they extend into the pulp by way of each apical foramen from the dental plexus.[1] Both the hard and soft tissue of the associated periodontium and gingiva are anesthetized by way of the interdental and interradicular branches for each tooth.

MANDIBULAR SUPRAPERIOSTEAL INJECTION

The supraperiosteal injection (or local infiltration) was discussed in detail in Chapter 12. However, one of the most common uses for this injection on the mandible is when there is incomplete anesthesia of the mandibular central or lateral incisors following an IA, mental, or incisive block.[1,10] This usually is due to crossover-innervation or overlap of terminal fibers of the inferior dental plexus from the contralateral incisive nerve (Fig. 13.18). This is similar to the crossover-innervation of the anterior superior alveolar nerve that can involve the maxillary arch. Because the alveolar process is slightly less dense and more porous surrounding the mandibular anterior teeth, a supraperiosteal injection may be more clinically effective than the same injection on the mandibular posterior teeth (see earlier discussion).

To correct this situation, the facially located supraperiosteal injection for the contralateral mandibular central incisor is administered. The injection site is at the depth of the mandibular mucobuccal fold inferior to the apex of the mandibular central incisor in the contralateral quadrant. This will anesthetize the terminal nerve fibers of the inferior dental plexus crossing over from the other side. This can be accomplished using either a horizontal or vertical approach similar to that used for both the mental or incisive nerve blocks but with the horizontal approach being preferred since it has easier access to the mandible (Fig. 13.19). Administering an incisive block will also accomplish the same effect but to a wider degree of anesthetic coverage (see earlier discussion).

The supraperiosteal injection can also be used when the mandibular first molar is additionally innervated by the mylohyoid nerve so that there is incomplete anesthesia following administration of an IA block as discussed earlier (see Fig. 13.11).[1,4,10] This injection can be performed anywhere along the medial surface of the mandible as needed, especially for limited procedures. Because the root lengths of teeth vary, the depth of needle insertion will vary. For the mandibular arch, the clinician should review the average root lengths of the mandibular teeth to help make this adjustment of needle depth more accurate (Table 13.14).[3,12]

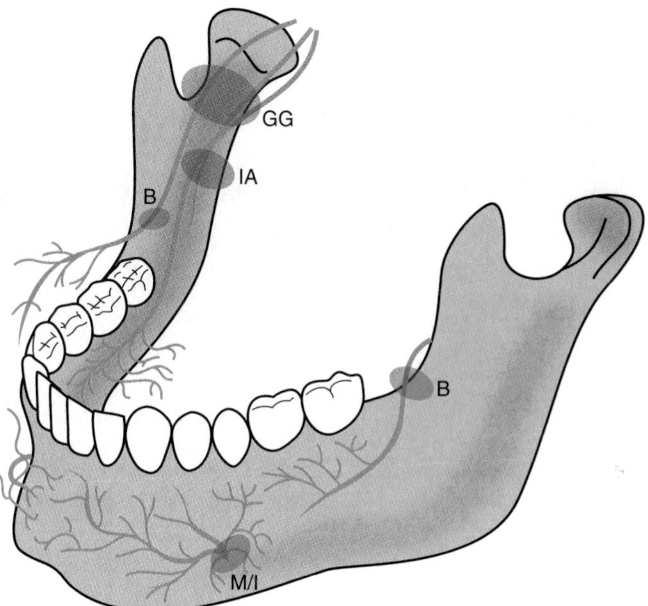

Fig. 13.18 The anesthetic deposition sites for mandibular anesthesia demonstrated by circles (*B*, Buccal; *G-G*, Gow-Gates; *IA*, inferior alveolar; *M/I*, mental/incisive). Note crossover of incisive nerve may occur at the midline requiring a supraperiosteal injection on the contralateral side.

Mandibular Intraseptal Injection

A supplemental injection, the intraseptal injection is used when there is a stronger need for hemostatic control of the interdental papilla of the attached gingiva between adjacent teeth. Thus a less diluted but smaller amount of vasoconstrictor, such as 1:50,000 epinephrine, can be used in this localized area (see Chapter 4).[4] The injection can be used in either dental arch (see Chapter 12).

Typically, the mandibular posterior sextant is the focus for this injection within the mandibular arch (Fig. 13.20), but it is also useful for the mandibular anterior sextant if there has been advanced periodontal disease. However, cases of extreme reduced height of the interdental bone level may prove inadequate and the agent will leak out of the opposite side of the dental arch and into the patient's mouth. The intraseptal injection is usually administered following the nerve block for the region to allow for less discomfort. Additionally, it already has the usual dilution of vasoconstrictor (such as 1:100,000 epinephrine) present to stem any bleeding from the intraosseous injection. For more detailed discussion of the intraseptal injection and its use on the maxillary arch as well as advantage and disadvantages, see Chapter 12.

Mandibular Periodontal Ligament Injection

A supplemental injection, the PDL injection, is used when pulpal anesthesia and associated periodontium and gingiva is indicated on a single tooth mainly within the mandibular arch; the injection can also be used on the maxillary arch but is rarely administered. Because of the increased density and less porosity of the facial cortical plate of the mandible, supraperiosteal injections are usually less clinically effective within the mandibular arch, which is predominantly noted in the posterior region.[1,3] Instead the PDL injection provides a short duration of pulpal anesthesia and anesthesia of the associated facial or lingual periodontium and gingiva and without causing collateral numbness of the tongue or lower lip (Table 13.15, Figs. Z–AA, and Procedure Box 13.7).

In most cases, the PDL injection is not commonly used during nonsurgical periodontal therapy because it is contraindicated in areas of inflammation or infection at the injection site such as occurs commonly with periodontal disease.[1,4] Instead the nerve blocks or possibly supraperiosteal or intraseptal injections are used since the advantages of these methods outweigh any advantages of the PDL injection in most cases.

Target Area and Injection Site for Periodontal Ligament Injection

The target area or deposit location is the nearby terminal nerve endings at the apex (or apices) of the tooth so the agent can also flow into the bone marrow spaces of the alveolar bone proper of the alveolar process surrounding the teeth (see Table 13.15, Fig. Z). It is important to note that the studies show that the agent should not be forced apically through the PDL fibers because of the increased hydrostatic pressure being exerted in a confined space; this amount of pressure could possibly cause an avulsion of the tooth.[4]

The injection site or needle insertion point is directly into the depth of the gingival sulcus, with the needle and syringe parallel to the long axis of the tooth to be treated (see Table 13.15, Fig. Z). The

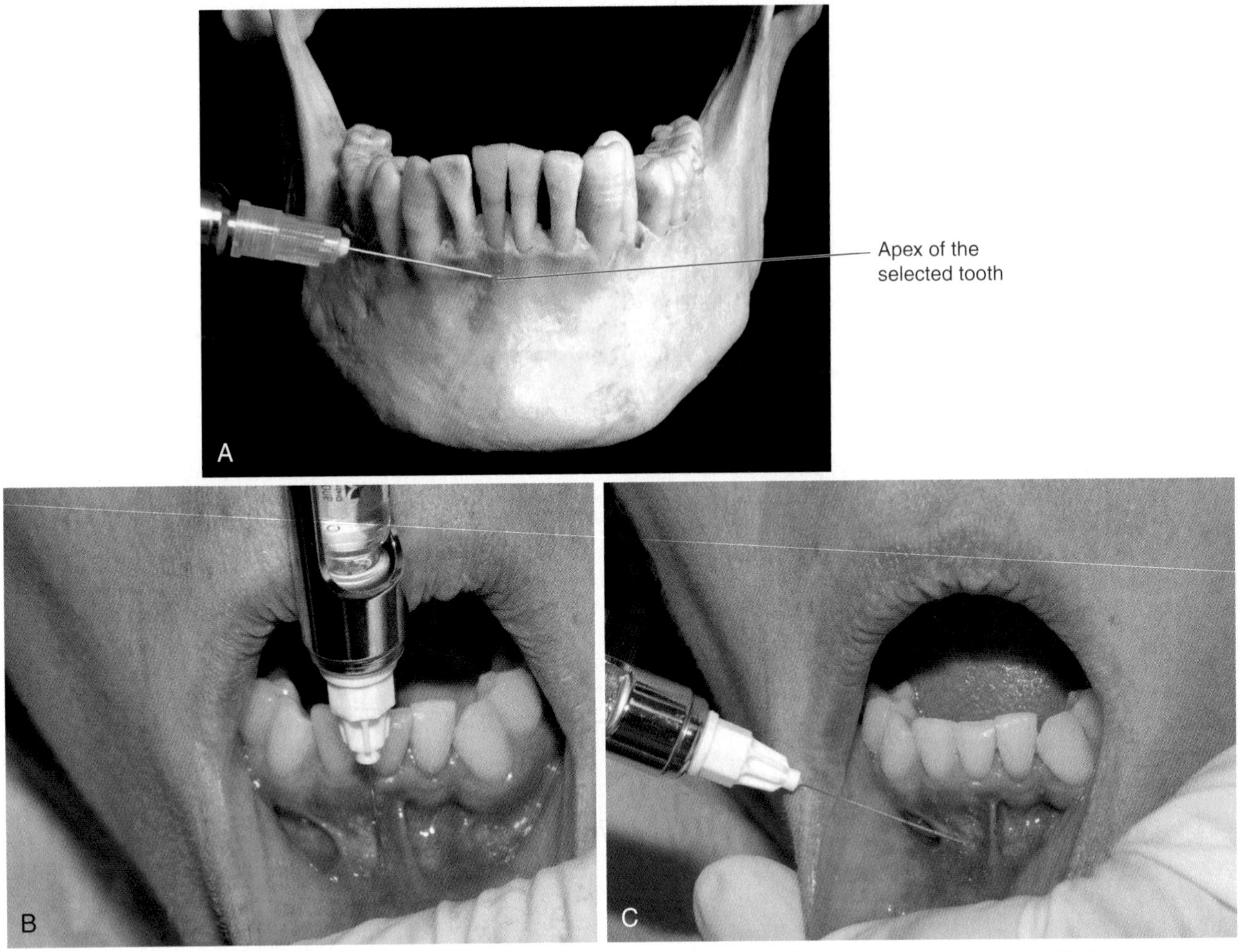

Fig. 13.19 Mandibular supraperiosteal injection. (A) Target area and distribution of anesthesia for mandibular supraperiosteal injection. (B) Vertical approach. (C) Horizontal approach. (A, Courtesy Margaret J. Fehrenbach, RDH, MS.)

TABLE 13.14 Mandibular Teeth Average Root Length(s)

Tooth	Average Root Length(s) (mm)
Central incisor	12.5
Lateral incisor	14.0
Canine	16.0
First premolar	14.0
Second premolar	14.5
First molar	14.0
Second molar	13.0
Third molar	11.0

All data from Nelson S: *Wheeler's dental anatomy, physiology, and occlusion,* ed 9, St Louis, 2009, Saunders/Elsevier. In Fehrenbach MJ, Popowics T: *Illustrated dental embryology, histology, and anatomy,* ed 5, St Louis, 2020, Saunders/Elsevier.

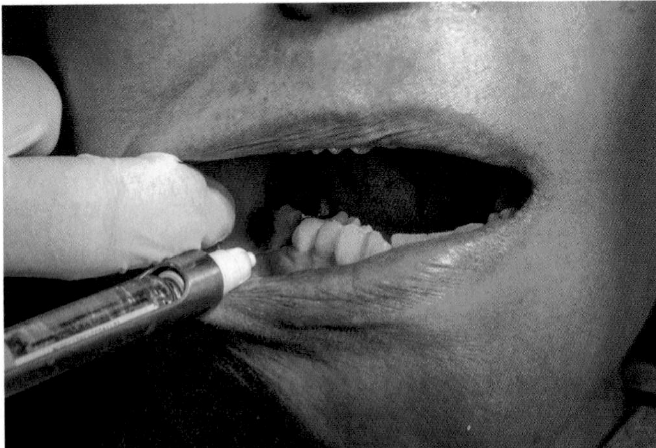

Fig. 13.20 Injection site or needle insertion point for a buccal intraseptal injection between mandibular first and second molar.

landmarks are the root(s) of the selected tooth. There is no need to use topical anesthesia on the attached gingival surface since the injection into hard bony tissue.[4] Stabilize the syringe along the long axis of the root to be anesthetized, and with the bevel of needle on the root surface, advance the needle apically until resistance is met.

Applying pressure, push the needle slightly deeper at approximately 1 to 2 mm into the cancellous bone of the alveolar bone proper of the alveolar process, and then the injection is administered (see Table 13.15, Fig. AA). Use of a computer-controlled local anesthesia delivery device with an extra-short or short needle (see Chapter 9) may be warranted with this injection since it slowly delivers the anesthetic agent, but standard or specialized syringes may also be used, typically with extra-short or short needles.[4]

Indications of Clinically Effective Periodontal Ligament and Possible Complications

If the injection is going to be clinically effective, there will be significant resistance to the deposition of the agent, at least with the standard syringe.[4] Blanching of the attached gingival surface will immediately be noted as the agent enters the tissue. Intravascular injection is extremely unlikely to occur so aspiration is not necessary. Since the PDL injection has a shorter duration than a nerve block, it may be repeated if necessary to permit completion of the dental procedure.[4]

If the agent is not retained in the tissue upon administration, it may be due to the bone loss within the gingival sulcus changing its architecture. To correct, remove the needle and reenter at a different site until the correct amount is deposited and retained in the tissue. Without the extensive soft tissue anesthesia, noted with other injections, especially most nerve blocks, patients may be concerned that they are not adequately anesthetized. The clinician will need to assure patients that indeed the localized region is anesthetized. The advantages and disadvantages of the PDL injection are listed in Table 13.16.

TABLE 13.15 Periodontal Ligament Injection Review

Indications	Procedures requiring pulpal anesthesia of selected tooth with anesthesia of associated periodontium and gingiva
Nerves anesthetized	Terminal nerve endings at apex (or apices) of selected tooth and into bone marrow spaces of alveolar bone proper
Teeth anesthetized	Selected tooth
Other structures anesthetized	Associated periodontium and gingiva
Administration technique	See Procedure Box 13.7
Needle gauge and length	27-gauge extra-short or short for standard or specialized syringe; also 30-gauge extra-short or short with computer-controlled local anesthetic delivery device
Target area/Deposit location	Alveolar bone proper of alveolar process of selected tooth or teeth

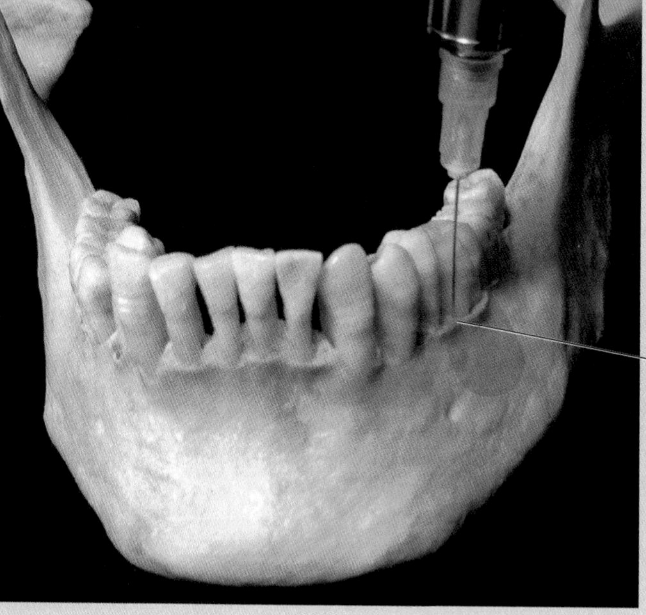

Fig. Z = Example: Distribution of anesthesia for PDL injection (Courtesy Margaret J. Fehrenbach, RDH)

Clinician position	Varies with different teeth; clinician should be positioned for greatest visibility
Syringe stabilization with fulcrums	Against patient's teeth, lips, or face
Landmarks	Selected tooth Root(s) of selected tooth

(*Continued*)

TABLE 13.15 Periodontal Ligament Injection Review (*Cont.*)

Injection site/Needle insertion point 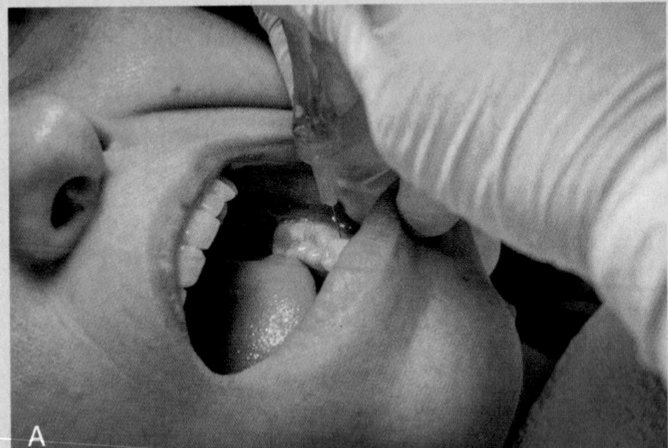 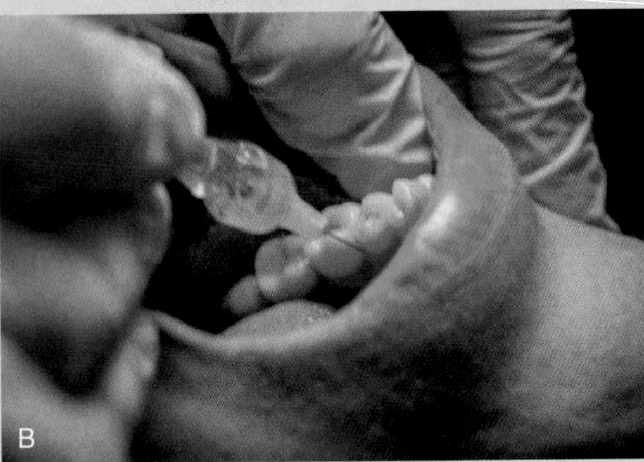 Fig. AA = Example: PDL injections within mandibular arch. (A) Buccal. (B) Lingual	Long axis of tooth either mesial or distal with single-rooted tooth; mesial or distal to each root for multirooted tooth
Depth of insertion	Approximately 1 to 2 mm into alveolar bone proper after bony contact (see Table 13.15, Fig. AA)
Amount of anesthetic agent	Approximately 0.2 mL or one stopper with standard or computer-controlled local anesthesia delivery device; one squeeze for specialized syringe
Length of time to deposit	Approximately 20 seconds

PDL, Periodontal ligament.

PROCEDURE BOX 13.7 Periodontal Ligament Injection Procedure

Step 1 Ask the supine patient to open and then retract the patient's lip, pulling the tissue taut using the thumb and index finger of the nondominant hand (one inside and one outside); sterile gauze may be used to help retract slippery tissue.

Step 2 Assemble the standard or specialized syringe with a 27-gauge short or extra-short needle or use computer-controlled delivery device with an extra-short or short needle after careful consideration of the situation. Using the syringe in the dominant hand orient the bevel of the needle toward the alveolar process.

Step 3 Clinician and patient positions as well as fulcrums vary from tooth to tooth.

Step 4 Stabilize the syringe and angle the needle along the long axis of the tooth on the mesial surface or distal surface at 30 degrees.

Step 5 Direct the syringe until the depth of the gingival sulcus is reached and resistance is felt (see Table 13.15, Fig. AA). Applying pressure, push the needle slightly deeper at approximately 1 to 2 mm into the alveolar bone proper of the alveolar process.

Step 6 Deposit approximately 0.2 mL of agent or one stopper with standard or computer-controlled local anesthesia delivery device; one squeeze for specialized syringe. There will be significant resistance to the deposition of the agent, at least with the standard syringe. Blanching of the attached gingival surface will immediately be noted as the agent enters the tissue.

Step 7 Carefully withdraw the syringe and immediately recap the needle using the one-handed scoop method utilizing a needle sheath prop (see Chapter 11).

Step 8 Rinse the patient's mouth. Inspect the region and stem any remaining bleeding with pressure using sterile gauze. Onset of action is immediate, and treatment may commence. Note that multirooted teeth require a periodontal ligament injection for each root present. The periodontal ligament injection may be repeated if necessary to permit completion of the dental procedure without patient discomfort.

TABLE 13.16 Advantages and Disadvantages of Periodontal Ligament Injection

Advantages	Disadvantages
• Single dose and minimal volume of anesthetic and hemostatic agent with intravascular injection extremely unlikely to occur, which are considerations with medically compromised patients since there is decreased risk of toxicity with approximately 0.2 mL • Minimizes bleeding in localized area of treatment • Alternative or supplemental method when other options are ineffective or can be considered • Immediate (<30 seconds) onset of action • Postoperative complications such as paresthesia are unlikely since lingual nerve is not anesthetized in most cases • Absence of lip or tongue numbness, which is particularly beneficial to children and those with physical or developmental disabilities to decrease risk of self-inflicted trauma	• Contraindicated in areas with localized infection or severe inflammation such as with advanced periodontal disease, severe caries, or endodontic lesions* • Short duration of pulpal anesthesia when patient may need it to be longer due to dentinal hypersensitivity; however injection can be repeated • Multiple injections may be needed • Excessive pressure needed for injection may cause tissue damage or tooth avulsion and posttreatment soreness or may cause breakage of cartridge in standard syringe • Needle placement may be difficult without experience and with certain crowded dentitions or if patient has lost adjacent alveolar bone proper • Anesthetic agent may leak into patient's mouth especially without adequate levels of alveolar bone proper of alveolar process

*Most common reason cited for not using periodontal ligament injection during nonsurgical periodontal therapy unless outweighed by the advantages such as medical history of the patient.

DENTAL HYGIENE CONSIDERATIONS

- Substantial variation exists in the anatomy of local anesthetic landmarks of the mandible and its nerves complicating mandibular anesthesia.
- The inferior alveolar (IA) block is recommended for anesthetizing mandibular teeth and associated lingual periodontium and gingiva to the midline as well as the associated facial periodontium and gingiva of the mandibular anterior teeth and premolars to the midline within one mandibular quadrant.
- If there is a lack of clinical effective anesthesia following the first attempt of a seemingly correct IA block, the dental hygienist should reattempt the injection at a slightly superior level than the first injection because being too far inferior is the most commonly cited reason for missed IA blocks.
- If bone is contacted immediately after the needle is inserted into the soft tissue when trying to administer an IA block, it is possible that the insertion point was too inferior and/or too far lateral from the pterygomandibular fold covering the raphe. The correction is made by removing the needle completely and repalpating to assess the anatomic landmarks, and adjustments made accordingly.
- If bone is contacted at less than 16 mm or half to less than half of the long needle during administration of the IA block, the needle tip is located too far anterior on the bone of the medial surface of the mandibular ramus. The correction is made after withdrawing the needle partially or completely from the tissue and bringing the syringe barrel more closely superior to the mandibular anterior teeth when it is redirected or reinserted; with this correction, the needle tip is more posterior.
- If bone is not contacted when trying to administer an IA block even with the usual depth of insertion by the needle, the needle tip is located too far posterior on the mandibular ramus. The correction is made withdrawing the needle partially or completely from the tissue and bringing the syringe barrel more closely superior to the mandibular molars when it is redirected or reinserted; with this correction the needle tip is more anterior. If bone is not contacted during the IA block, the anesthetic may be inadvertently deposited in the parotid salivary gland causing transient facial paralysis with the facial nerve.
- Lack of clinically effective anesthesia during the IA block of the mandibular first molar may be due to the accessory innervation by the mylohyoid nerve; anesthesia of the mylohyoid nerve using a supraperiosteal injection on the lingual border of the mandible may be indicated.
- Incomplete anesthesia following an IA block may be because of a bifid IA nerve, which can be detected by noting a second more inferiorly located mandibular canal on an intraoral radiograph. Agent needs to be deposited more inferior to the usual anatomic landmarks for the IA block to correct this.
- The reaction of the "lingual shock" may occur as the needle passes by the lingual nerve during the IA block; communication to the patient that this may occur may alleviate the patient's fear if it happens during injection.
- The IA block has the highest positive aspiration rate of all the block injections; aspirating within three planes and reaspiration after every one-fourth of a cartridge deposited is recommended. A hematoma may also occur due to the nearness of the blood vessels to the target nerves.
- Paresthesia may occur following an IA block, usually from trauma to the lingual nerve and with the spread of dental infection from a contaminated needle, but in most cases it occurs due to complicated oral surgery.
- The buccal block is recommended for anesthesia of the associated buccal periodontium and gingiva of the mandibular molars within one mandibular quadrant. This block should be administered immediately following the IA block to complete mandibular quadrant anesthesia.
- For mandibular quadrant dental hygiene treatment, the clinician must proceed with instrumentation first of the mandibular molars (third, second, and then first), then premolars (second and then first), and finally the anterior teeth to allow for complete anesthesia of the core bundles of the anterior sextant of the dental arch.
- If half-mouth treatment is planned, the IA and buccal blocks are administered first, then the maxillary facial injections, followed by the palatal injections; instrumentation should proceed first on the maxillary arch, to be followed by the mandibular arch.
- The mental block is recommended for anesthesia of the associated facial periodontium and gingiva of the mandibular anterior teeth and premolars to the midline.
- The incisive block is recommended for anesthesia of the mandibular anterior teeth and premolars and associated facial periodontium and gingiva to the midline. The incisive block is also used when there is crossover-innervation of the contralateral incisive nerve and there is still discomfort on the mandibular anterior teeth following administering an IA block.
- The Gow-Gates (G-G) mandibular block is recommended for extensive procedures during quadrant dentistry or with lack of clinical effectiveness of the IA block since it anesthetizes the entire mandibular nerve within one mandibular quadrant.
- The Vazirani-Akinosi (V-A) mandibular block is recommended when a similar region of anesthesia is needed as the IA block but with a closed-mouth situation or when there is difficulty administering the IA block. Possible complications for

the V-A block include the anesthetic inadvertently deposited in the parotid salivary gland causing transient facial paralysis with the facial nerve.

- The supraperiosteal injection is recommended when pulpal anesthesia is needed on a single tooth or when anesthesia of the associated periodontium is needed in a localized area. Supraperiosteal injections of the mandible are not as clinically effective as that of the maxillae because overall the mandible is denser or less porous than the maxillae. Supraperiosteal injections are more clinically effective on mandibular anterior teeth and can be administered to the contralateral quadrant if crossover-innervation is present in the midline.
- The intraseptal injection is an intraosseous supplemental injection recommended when there is a need for additional hemostatic control of the interdental papilla of the attached gingiva between adjacent teeth.
- The periodontal ligament (PDL) injection is an intraosseous supplemental injection recommended when pulpal anesthesia as well as associated periodontium and gingiva is indicated on a single tooth. The PDL injection is more commonly used on the mandibular teeth for single tooth anesthesia but is not usually used prior to nonsurgical periodontal therapy.

CASE STUDY 13.1 Considerations Following Inferior Alveolar Block

A patient of record has come into the dental office for scheduled nonsurgical periodontal therapy of the mandibular right quadrant. The dental hygienist prepares to administer both an inferior alveolar block and buccal block. However, when administering the inferior alveolar block, the dental hygienist has a difficult time contacting bone of the mandible regardless of properly readjusting the syringe barrel more posteriorly upon reentry so the needle will be at the correct injection site. The patient has had extensive past dental work in the area and there is resultant firmer tissue at the injection site.

Following the third attempt of readjustment, the dental hygienist feels frustration and is concerned about the schedule getting behind, but is still unsure if the bone of the medial surface of the mandible has been contacted. Hoping for the best, a full cartridge of anesthetic agent is deposited, and minutes later the ipsilateral corner of the patient's mouth begins to droop.

Critical Thinking Questions

- What is the reason why the ipsilateral corner of the patient's mouth begins to droop?
- How could the dental hygienist have prevented this occurrence?
- What should now be done to care for the patient?

CHAPTER REVIEW QUESTIONS

1. What is the approximate needle insertion depth into soft tissue in MOST cases for the inferior alveolar local anesthetic block?
   A. 5 to 10 millimeters
   B. 11 to 15 millimeters
   C. 16 to 19 millimeters
   D. 20 to 25 millimeters
2. The mandibular nerve or third division is a branch of which cranial nerve?
   A. X
   B. V
   C. VII
   D. IV
3. The posterior mandibular sextant is denser and less porous than the mandibular anterior sextant, which allows for MORE clinically effective molar anesthesia.
   A. Both the statement and the reason are correct and related.
   B. Both the statement and the reason are correct but NOT related.
   C. The statement is correct, but the reason is NOT correct.
   D. The statement is NOT correct, but the reason is correct.
   E. NEITHER the statement NOR the reason is correct.
4. Which injection is USUALLY administered along with the inferior alveolar block to provide complete anesthesia of a mandibular quadrant on a patient before nonsurgical periodontal therapy WITHOUT any overlapping coverage?
   A. Buccal block
   B. Mental block
   C. Gow-Gates mandibular block
   D. Vazirani-Akinosi mandibular block
5. Which of the following local anesthesia blocks will NOT provide pulpal anesthesia to tooth #23 (Canadian #3.2) before restorative dental procedures?
   A. Inferior alveolar block
   B. Incisive block
   C. Gow-Gates mandibular block
   D. Buccal block
6. After administering a mental local anesthetic block, the patient reports slight numbness of the chin. What should the clinician do next for the patient?
   A. Stop treatment and explain facial nerve paralysis to the patient
   B. Explain to the patient that this is the usual reaction and continue with treatment
   C. Place a cold compress to prevent hematoma from occurring
   D. Immediately administer an oral antihistamine to reduce inflammation
7. After a few minutes following the administration of a mental local anesthetic block, a patient reports that some of her contralateral mandibular anterior teeth feel numb. What caused the patient's contralateral mandibular anterior teeth to become anesthetized?
   A. Diffusion of the anesthetic agent to the incisive nerve
   B. Trauma to the nerves within the inferior dental plexus
   C. Overlapping of lingual nerve fibers in the inferior dental plexus
   D. Rapid constriction of the mental artery in the area
8. What injection uses the mesiolingual cusp of the maxillary second molar as a landmark during administration?
   A. Gow-Gates mandibular block
   B. Inferior alveolar block
   C. Mental block
   D. Buccal block
   E. Vazirani-Akinosi mandibular block
9. When administering the inferior alveolar block, the syringe barrel in MOST cases should be in what relation to the mandibular occlusal plane?
   A. Perpendicular plane
   B. Parallel plane
   C. At 45 degrees
   D. At 90 degrees

10. When administering the inferior alveolar block, the syringe barrel in MOST cases should usually be superior to which mandibular tooth?
   A. Premolar on the injection side
   B. Premolar on the contralateral side
   C. First molar on the contralateral side
   D. First molar on the injection side
11. If anesthesia of the lingual periodontium and gingiva is required for #25–27 (Canadian #4.1–4.3), an incisive block is clinically effective BECAUSE it anesthetizes both the associated facial and lingual periodontium and gingiva of the mandibular anterior teeth.
   A. Both the statement and the reason are correct and related.
   B. Both the statement and the reason are correct but NOT related.
   C. The statement is correct, but the reason is NOT correct.
   D. The statement is NOT correct, but the reason is correct.
   E. NEITHER the statement NOR the reason is correct.
12. Which of the following local anesthetic blocks has the HIGHEST risk of hematoma for the patient after administration?
   A. Posterior superior alveolar block
   B. Inferior alveolar block
   C. Gow-Gates mandibular block
   D. Mental or incisive blocks
13. While administering the inferior alveolar block, the clinician contacts bone at a depth of approximately 10 millimeters on an average-sized adult patient. What should the clinician do next?
   A. Aspirate correctly and then deposit anesthetic agent at the site
   B. Slightly withdraw the needle and redirect the syringe barrel more anteriorly
   C. Slightly withdraw the needle and redirect the syringe barrel more posteriorly
   D. Slightly withdraw the needle and redirect the syringe barrel more perpendicularly to the mandibular occlusal plane
14. While administering the inferior alveolar block, the clinician does NOT contact bone. What should the clinician do?
   A. Aspirate correctly and then deposit anesthetic agent at the site
   B. Slightly withdraw the needle and redirect the syringe barrel more anteriorly
   C. Slightly withdraw the needle and redirect the syringe barrel more posteriorly
   D. Slightly withdraw the needle and redirect the syringe barrel more perpendicular to the mandibular occlusal plane
15. The target area for the incisive block is the same as the mental block, but when administering the mental block, the clinician MUST place pressure to the injection site following the injection for clinically effective local anesthesia.
   A. Both statements are correct.
   B. Both statements are NOT correct.
   C. The first statement is correct; the second statement is NOT correct.
   D. The first statement is NOT correct; the second statement is correct.
16. There is NO need to palpate for the mental foramen prior to administering the mental local anesthetic block because the mental foramen is USUALLY in the same location on all patients.
   A. Both the statement and the reason are correct and related.
   B. Both the statement and the reason are correct but NOT related.
   C. The statement is correct, but the reason is NOT correct.
   D. The statement is NOT correct, but the reason is correct.
   E. Neither the statement NOR the reason is correct.
17. Which of the following local anesthetic blocks anesthetizes the mylohyoid, mental, and the auriculotemporal nerves?
   A. Gow-Gates mandibular block
   B. Inferior alveolar block
   C. Mental block
   D. Buccal block
   E. Vazirani-Akinosi mandibular block
18. Which mandibular local anesthetic blocks require the clinician to gently contact bone with the anesthetic needle?
   A. Inferior alveolar block and infraorbital block
   B. Inferior alveolar block and Gow-Gates mandibular block
   C. Buccal block and mental block
   D. Gow-Gates mandibular block and mental block
19. Which of the following situations is NOT related to incomplete anesthesia on the usual areas of the mandible on an adult patient after administering an inferior alveolar local anesthetic block?
   A. Bifid inferior alveolar nerve
   B. Accessory innervation by the mylohyoid nerve
   C. Crossover-innervation from the incisive nerve
   D. Angle classification of malocclusion Class III case
   E. Patient experiencing "lingual shock" during the injection
20. Which of the following local anesthetic blocks uses BOTH the mandibular occlusal plane and pterygomandibular raphe as landmarks for administration?
   A. Gow-Gates mandibular block
   B. Inferior alveolar block
   C. Mental block
   D. Incisive block
21. Which of the following supplemental injections is MAINLY used within the mandibular arch?
   A. Supraperiosteal injection
   B. Intraseptal injection
   C. Periodontal ligament injection
   D. Both the supraperiosteal and intraseptal injections
22. Which of the following supplemental injections are NOT intraosseous injections?
   A. Supraperiosteal injection
   B. Intraseptal injection
   C. Periodontal ligament injection
   D. Both the intraseptal and periodontal ligament injections
23. What is the injection site or needle insertion point for a periodontal ligament injection within the mandibular arch?
   A. Center of the interdental papilla
   B. Inferior to the apex (or apices) of the tooth
   C. Depth of the gingival sulcus
   D. Depth of the maxillary mucobuccal fold
24. Which of the following supplemental injections increase hemostasis when used with a LESS diluted vasoconstrictor upon instrumenting within the mandibular arch?
   A. Supraperiosteal injection
   B. Intraseptal injection
   C. Periodontal ligament injection
   D. Both the supraperiosteal and intraseptal injections
25. Which of the following supplemental injections within the mandibular arch is palpated to ensure soft tissue entry before the needle is inserted?
   A. Supraperiosteal injection
   B. Intraseptal injection
   C. Periodontal ligament injection
   D. Both the supraperiosteal and intraseptal injections

REFERENCES

1. Fehrenbach MJ, Herring SW. *Illustrated anatomy of the head and neck.* ed 6. St Louis: Saunders/Elsevier; 2021.
2. Rodella LF, et al. A review of the mandibular and maxillary nerve supplies and their clinical relevance. *Arch Oral Biol.* 2012;57(4):323–334.
3. Fehrenbach MJ, Popowics T. *Illustrated dental embryology, histology, and anatomy.* ed 5. St Louis: Saunders/Elsevier; 2020.
4. Malamed S. *Handbook of local anesthesia.* ed 7. St Louis: Mosby/Elsevier; 2018.
5. Kaufman E, Epstein JB, Naveh E, Gorsky M, Gross A, Cohen G. A survey of pain, pressure, and discomfort induced by commonly used oral anesthesia injections. *Anesth Prog.* 2005;54(4):122–127.
6. Bowen DM, Pieren JA. *Darby and Walsh dental hygiene: theory and practice.* ed 5. St Louis: Saunders/Elsevier; 2020.
7. Perry DA, Beemsterboer PL, Taggart EJ. *Clinical periodontology for dental hygienists.* ed 4. Philadelphia: Saunders/Elsevier; 2014.
8. Fehrenbach MJ. Extraoral and intraoral patient assessment. In: Bowen DM, Pieren JA, eds. *Darby and Walsh dental hygiene theory and practice.* Philadelphia: Saunders/Elsevier; 2020.
9. Fehrenbach MJ. Pain control for dental hygienists: current concepts in local anesthesia are reviewed, *RDH Magazine,* February 2005.
10. Lee CR, Yang HJ. Alternative techniques for failure of conventional inferior alveolar nerve block. *Dent Anesth Pain Med.* 2019;19(3):125–134.
11. Crowley C, et al. Anesthetic efficacy of supine and upright positions for the inferior alveolar nerve block: a prospective, randomized study. *J Endod.* 2018;44(2):202–205.
12. Nelson S. *Wheeler's dental anatomy, physiology, and occlusion.* ed 9. St Louis: Saunders/Elsevier; 2009.
13. Logan BM, Reynold PA, Hutching RT. *McMinn's color atlas of head and neck anatomy.* ed 3. London: Mosby; 2004.
14. Fehrenbach MJ. Inflammation and repair. Immunity. In: Ibsen OC, Phelan JA, eds. *Oral pathology for dental hygienists.* St Louis: Saunders/Elsevier; 2018.
15. Khoury JN, et al. Applied anatomy of the pterygomandibular space: improving the success of inferior alveolar nerve blocks. *Aust Dent J.* 2011;56(2):112–121.
16. Iwanaga J, et al. Anatomical study of the lingual nerve and inferior alveolar nerve in the pterygomandibular space: complications of the inferior alveolar nerve block. *Cureus.* 2018;10(8):e3109.
17. Fehrenbach MJ, Herring SW. Spread of dental infection. *J Dent Hyg.* September/October 1997;13–19.
18. Goyushov S, et al. Assessment of morphological and anatomical characteristics of mental foramen using cone beam computed tomography. *Surg Radiol Anat.* 2018;40(10):1133–1139.
19. Fehrenbach MJ. The incisive block: underutilized but ultimately useful. *California Dent Hyg J.* 2011;27(2):13–16.
20. Logothetis DD, Fehrenbach MJ. Local anesthesia options during dental hygiene care. *RDH Magazine.* June 2014.
21. Haas DA. Alternative mandibular nerve block techniques: a review of the Gow-Gates and Akinosi-Vazirani closed-mouth mandibular nerve block techniques. *J Am Dent Assoc.* 2011;142(Suppl 3):8S–12S.
22. Fehrenbach MJ. Gow-Gates mandibular nerve block: an alternative in local anesthetic use. *Access (ADHA).* 2002;34–37.
23. Johnson TM, et al. Teaching alternatives to the standard inferior alveolar nerve block in dental education: outcomes in clinical practice. *J Dent Ed.* 2007;71(9):1145–1152.
24. Kiran R, et al. Comparison of efficacy of Halstead, Vazirani Akinosi and Gow Gates techniques for mandibular anesthesia. *J Maxillofac Oral Surg.* 2018;17(4):570–575.
25. Fehrenbach MJ, Logothetis DD. The underused block: Vazirani-Akinosi mandibular block. *RDH Magazine.* February 2016.

APPENDIX 13.1: SUMMARY OF MANDIBULAR INJECTIONS

Inferior Alveolar Block

Areas Anesthetized	*Landmarks*	*Administration Sites*	*Technique*	*Adverse Effects*
Teeth Mandibular teeth to midline **Other Structures** Lingual periodontium and gingiva to midline; facial periodontium and gingiva of mandibular anterior teeth and premolars to midline; lower lip; anterior two-thirds of tongue; floor of the mouth to midline	Medial surface of mandibular ramus Mandibular foramen Lingula Coronoid notch Pterygomandibular fold (raphe) Pterygotemporal depression Pterygomandibular space Mandibular occlusal plane	**Injection Site** Two-thirds to three-fourths distance from coronoid notch to pterygomandibular fold (raphe), demarcating posterior border of ramus and at center of pterygotemporal depression to enter pterygomandibular space as well as approximately 6 to10 mm superior to mandibular occlusal plane **Deposit Location** At mandibular foramen on medial surface of mandibular ramus that is overhung by lingula with IA nerve; lingual nerve by diffusion	Insert needle into pterygotemporal depression to enter depth of pterygomandibular space and at intersection of two imaginary lines moving through soft tissue until bone is gently contacted and aspirate **Depth of Insertion** Long 25-gauge needle at approximately 20 to 25 mm or two-thirds to three-fourths of needle until bone is gently contacted **Anesthetic Agent** Approximately 1.8 to 3.6 mL or one to two cartridges; 60 to 120 seconds to deposit	Transient facial paralysis from deposition in parotid salivary gland; hematoma; lingual shock when moving needle through tissue; inadequate anesthesia possibly caused by depositing agent inferior to mandibular foramen; incomplete anesthesia of first molar due to mylohyoid nerve; incomplete anesthesia from crossover-innervation of incisive nerve

Buccal Block

Areas Anesthetized	*Landmarks*	*Administration Sites*	*Technique*	*Adverse Effects*
Teeth None **Other Structures** Buccal periodontium and gingiva of mandibular molars	Most distal mandibular molar Anterior border of mandibular ramus Retromolar pad (triangle)	**Injection Site** Buccal mucosa distal and buccal to most distal mandibular molar **Deposit Location** (Long) buccal nerve as it passes over anterior border of mandibular ramus in area of retromolar pad	Direct syringe barrel parallel to occlusal plane but directly superior to mandibular molars and then aspirate **Depth of Insertion** Long 25-gauge if after IA or short 27-gauge if no IA at approximately 2 to 4 mm of needle until bone is gently contacted **Anesthetic Agent** Approximately 0.3 mL one-eighth of cartridge; 10 seconds to deposit	Leakage of agent at injection site with bitter taste of anesthetic agent; ballooning of tissue caused by rapid deposit of agent

(*Continued*)

Mental Block

Areas Anesthetized	*Landmarks*	*Administration Sites*	*Technique*	*Adverse Reactions*
Teeth None **Other Structures** Facial periodontium and gingiva of mandibular anterior teeth and premolars to midline; lower lip and skin of chin to midline	Mandibular premolars Mental foramen Mandibular mucobuccal fold	**Injection Site** Anterior to mental foramen at depth of mandibular mucobuccal fold inferior to apices of mandibular premolars or location determined by radiographs and/or palpation **Deposit Location** At mental foramen and inferior to apices of mandibular premolars or location determined by radiographs and/or palpation	**Horizontal Approach:** insert needle at depth of mucobuccal fold, directing needle anterior to mental foramen; **Vertical Approach:** direct syringe vertically with patient's cheek anterior to mental foramen and aspirate **Depth of Insertion** Short 27-gauge needle at approximately 5 to 6 mm or one-fourth of needle **Anesthetic Agent** Approximately 0.6 mL or one-third of cartridge; 20 seconds to deposit	Hematoma

Incisive Block

Areas Anesthetized	*Landmarks*	*Administration Sites*	*Technique*	*Adverse Reactions*
Teeth Mandibular anterior teeth and premolars to midline **Other Structures** Facial periodontium and gingiva of anesthetized mandibular teeth to midline; lower lip and skin of chin to midline	Mandibular premolars Mental foramen Mandibular mucobuccal fold	**Injection Site** Anterior to mental foramen at depth of mandibular mucobuccal fold inferior to apices of mandibular premolars or location determined by radiographs and/or palpation **Deposit Location** At mental foramen inferior to apices of mandibular premolars or location determined by radiographs and/or palpation	**Horizontal Approach:** insert needle at depth of mucobuccal fold, directing needle anterior to mental foramen; **Vertical Approach:** direct syringe vertically with patient's cheek anterior to mental foramen and then aspirate; deposit agent and massage agent into foramen for 2 minutes **Depth of Insertion** Short 27-gauge needle at approximately 5 to 6 mm or one-fourth of needle **Anesthetic Agent** Approximately 0.6 to 0.9 mL or one-third to one-half of cartridge; 20 seconds to deposit	Hematoma; inadequate anesthesia due to inadequate volume of anesthetic into mental foramen or inadequate duration of pressure and massage over mental foramen after injection

Gow-Gates Mandibular Block				
Areas Anesthetized	***Landmarks***	***Administration Sites***	***Technique***	***Adverse Effects***
Teeth Mandibular teeth to midline **Other Structures** Lingual periodontium and gingiva of anesthetized mandibular teeth as well as facial periodontium and gingiva of anesthetized mandibular anterior teeth and premolars to midline and in most cases buccal periodontium and gingiva of anesthetized mandibular molars; lower lip; anterior two-thirds of tongue; floor of the mouth to midline; skin over zygomatic bone and posterior part of buccal and temporal regions; additional innervation by way of mylohyoid nerve to muscles and also can serve as afferent nerve for mandibular first molar	**Extraoral** Intertragic notch (lower border of tragus) Corner of mouth **Intraoral** Mesiolingual cusp of maxillary second molar Buccal mucosa just distal to maxillary second molar	**Injection Site** Buccal mucosa on medial surface of mandibular ramus, just distal to height of mesiolingual cusp of maxillary second molar **Deposit Location** Anteromedial border of neck of mandibular condyle	Insert needle parallel to determined imaginary line until gentle bony contact is made with neck of condyle **Depth of Insertion** Long 25-gauge needle at approximately 25 mm or three-fourths of needle until bone is gently contacted **Anesthetic Agent** Approximately 1.8 mL or one cartridge; 60 to 90 seconds to deposit	Buccal periodontium and gingiva of mandibular molars does not have adequate level of anesthesia; hematoma

Vazirani-Akinosi Mandibular Block				
Areas Anesthetized	***Landmarks***	***Administration Sites***	***Technique***	***Adverse Effects***
Teeth Mandibular teeth to midline **Other Structures** Lingual periodontium and gingiva of anesthetized mandibular teeth as well as facial periodontium and gingiva of anesthetized mandibular anterior teeth and premolars to midline and possibly buccal periodontium and gingiva of anesthetized mandibular molars; lower lip; anterior two-thirds of tongue; floor of the mouth to midline; additional innervation by way of mylohyoid nerve to muscles that can also serve as afferent nerve for mandibular first molar	Coronoid process Maxillary occlusal plane Medial surface of mandibular ramus Pterygomandibular space Maxillary tuberosity Mucogingival junction of maxillary third or second molar	**Injection Site** Medially past coronoid process and then into buccal mucosa on medial surface of mandibular ramus at same height as mucogingival junction of maxillary third or second molar directly across the way and with bevel oriented away from bone of mandibular ramus so it faces toward midline **Deposit Location** Center of pterygomandibular space and at approximately halfway between mandibular foramen and neck of mandibular condyle as well as being adjacent to maxillary tuberosity	Direct syringe barrel parallel to maxillary occlusal plane and medially past coronoid process. Place needle at same height as mucogingival junction of maxillary third or second molar to determine height of injection. Insert needle into buccal mucosa **Depth of Insertion** Long 25-gauge needle at approximately 25 mm or two-thirds to three-fourths of needle without contacting bone, with hub of syringe ending up opposite mesial aspect of maxillary second molar and then aspirate **Anesthetic Agent** Approximately 1.8 mL or one cartridge; 60 to 90 seconds to deposit	Transient facial paralysis when facial nerve is mistakenly anesthetized; hematoma

(Continued)

Periodontal Ligament Injection (for mandibular supraperiosteal and intraseptal injections, see Appendix 12.1)				
Areas Anesthetized	***Landmarks***	***Administration Sites***	***Technique***	***Adverse Reactions***
Teeth Selected tooth **Other Structures** Associated periodontium and gingiva	Selected tooth Root(s) of selected tooth	**Injection Site** Long axis of tooth either mesial or distal with single-rooted tooth; mesial or distal to each root for multirooted tooth **Deposit Location** Alveolar bone proper of alveolar process	Direct syringe until depth of gingival sulcus is reached and resistance is felt. Applying pressure, push needle slightly deeper at approximately 1 to 2 mm into alveolar bone proper **Depth of Insertion** Extra-short or short 27-gauge needle at approximately 1 to 2 mm into alveolar bone proper after bony contact **Anesthetic Agent** 0.2 mL, one stopper of anesthetic; 20 seconds to deposit	Postoperative soreness; may cause tissue damage

IA, Inferior alveolar.

SPECIAL APPENDIX: SUMMARY OF MAXILLARY AND MANDIBULAR INJECTION TECHNIQUES WITH DISTRIBUTION OF ANESTHESIA

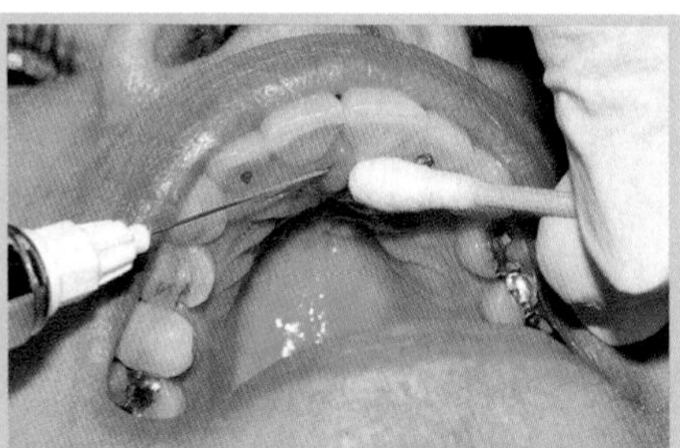

NP: 4 to 5 mm of short needle
0.45 mL (1/4 cartridge) of agent

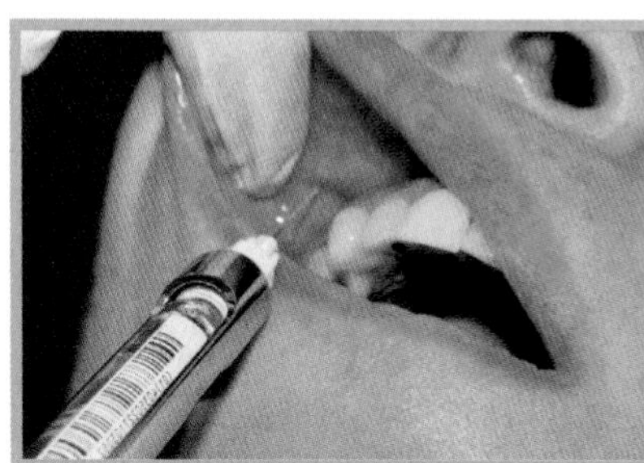

IO: 3/4 of short needle or
1/2 of long needle
0.9 to 1.2 mL (1/2 to 2/3 cartridge) of agent

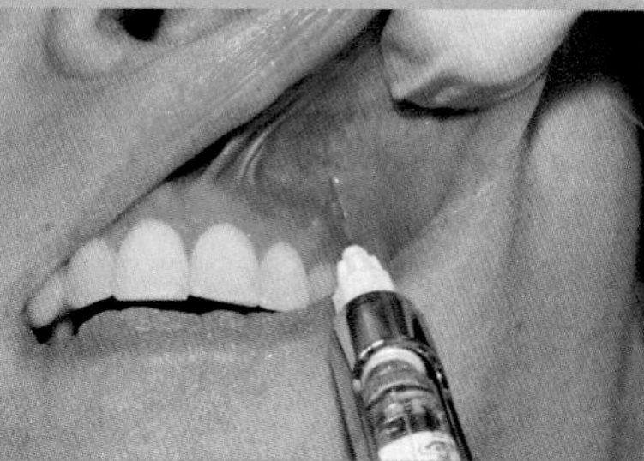

ASA: 5 to 6 mm of short needle
0.9 to 1.2 mL (1/2 to 2/3 cartridge) of agent

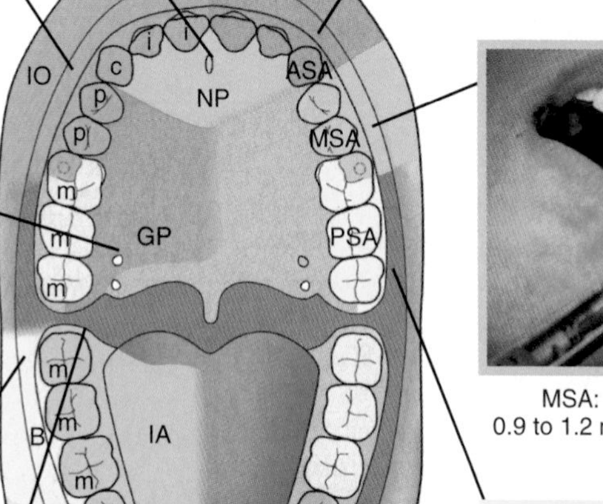

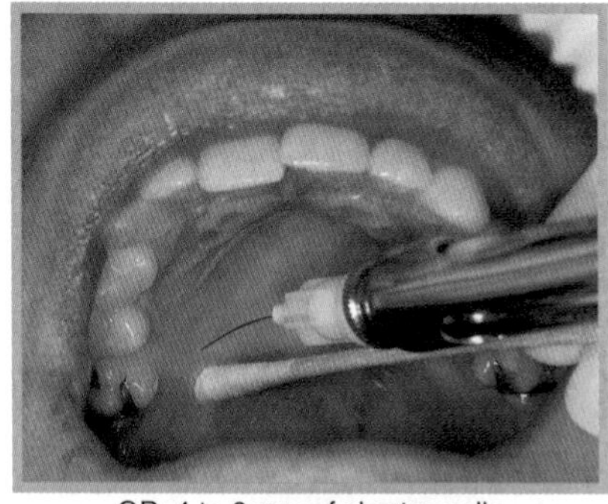

GP: 4 to 6 mm of short needle
0.45 to 0.6 mL (1/4 to 1/3 cartridge) of agent

MSA: 5 mm or 1/4 of short needle
0.9 to 1.2 mL (1/2 to 2/3 cartridge) of agent

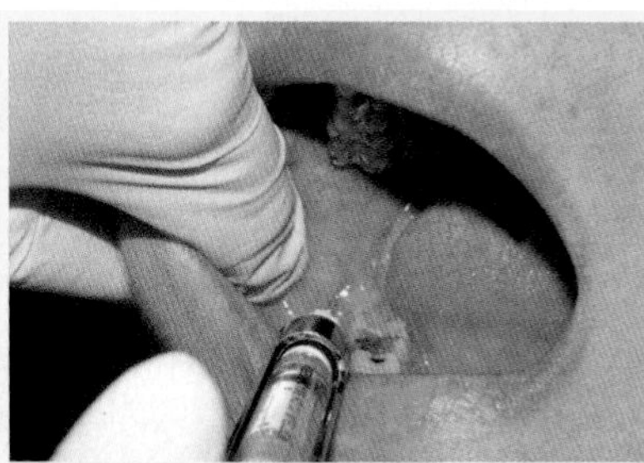

B: 2 to 4 mm of short needle
0.3 mL (1/8 of cartridge) of agent

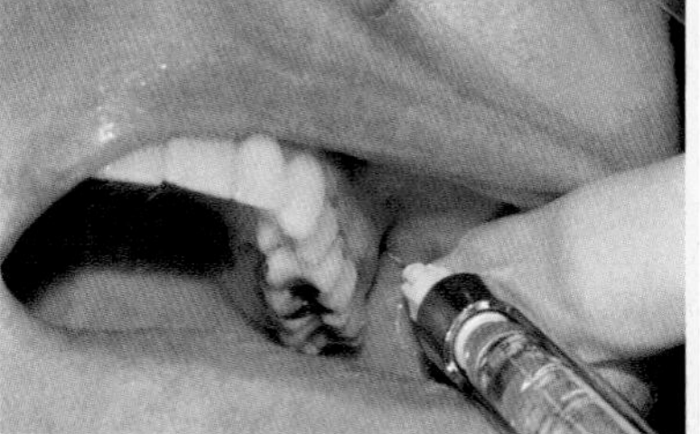

PSA: 3/4 of short needle
0.9 mL to 1.8 mL (1/2 to 1 cartridge) of agent

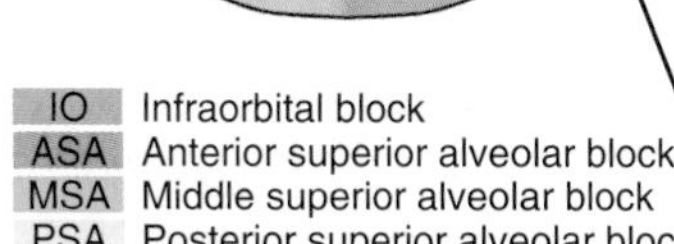

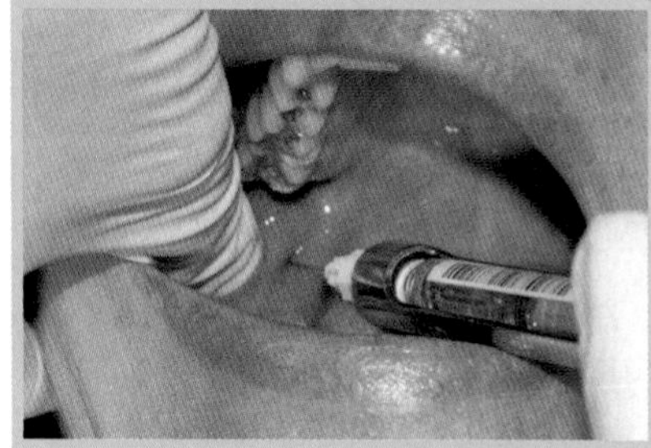

IA: 2/3 to 3/4 of long needle
1.8 to 3.6 mL (one to two cartridges) of agent

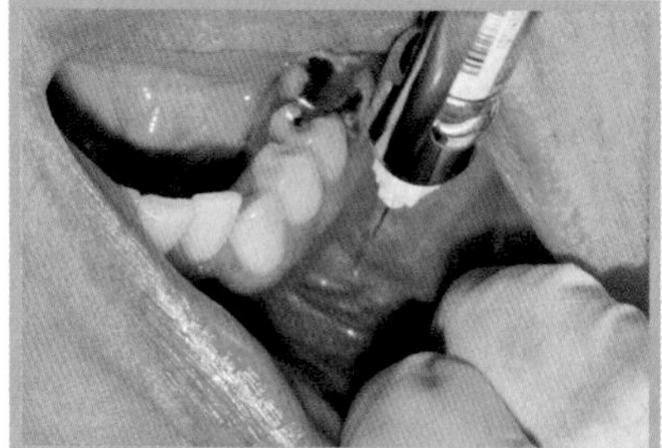

M/I: 5 to 6 mm of short needle
0.6 mL (1/3 cartridge) of agent for M and 0.6 to 0.9 mL (1/3 to 1/2 cartridge) of agent for I

Developed by Donna S. Low CRDH, MS, Pasco-Hernando State College. Center image from Fehrenbach MJ, Herring SW: *Illustrated anatomy of the head and neck,* ed 6, St Louis, 2021, Saunders/Elsevier.

14

Local Anesthesia for the Child and Adolescent

Demetra Daskalos Logothetis, RDH, MS

LEARNING OBJECTIVES

1. Discuss why systemic toxicity is more common in children than in adults.
2. Describe how to prevent systemic toxicity in children and effectively calculate maximum recommended doses (MRDs) in children, including obese children.
3. Describe each anesthetic agent and the benefits and risks of each for the pediatric population.
4. Describe the prevention and management of postoperative soft tissue injuries in children.
5. Describe the local anesthesia delivery techniques for children, including patient preparation and administration protocol.

INTRODUCTION

Successful treatment of all patients is dependent on relieving their pain, discomfort, and anxiety for all dental procedures. This is facilitated by profound anesthesia; pain control is an important part of the treatment and management of children. This is one of the most important challenges a clinician will face when treating children. If the child experiences pain during dental treatment, it may affect their future as dental patients. Unpleasant dental experiences during childhood have resulted in many cases of adult dental phobias. Unfortunately, the local anesthetic injection has been documented as producing the greatest negative response in children, and the dental hygienist should be sensitive to children's anxieties and help them cope with dental injections. The need for local anesthesia to be administered by the dental hygienist to a pediatric patient is rare, because these patients typically do not require nonsurgical periodontal therapy. However, in some instances, the dentist performing restorative work on children may ask the dental hygienist to administer the local anesthetic. Moreover, if the patient has back-to-back appointments, first with the dental hygienist and second with the dentist for restorative work, it may be more time efficient for the dental hygienist to administer the local anesthesia for the restorative work before moving the patient into the dentist's chair. The dental hygienist should review the care plan, taking into consideration the necessity of lowering the child's maximum recommended dose (MRD). The care plan should minimize the extent of treatment completed in one appointment.

This chapter will guide the dental hygienist through topics related to the effective administration of local anesthesia for the child and adolescent patient.

LOCAL ANESTHETIC SYSTEMIC TOXICITY IN CHILDREN

Local anesthetic agents are used routinely in dentistry, and practitioners use them with so much confidence that adverse reactions are rare.[1] However, one of the most common adverse reactions is systemic toxicity, typically a result of administering the anesthetic agent over the patient's MRD, or from inadvertent intravascular injections. A typical local anesthetic overdose manifests itself as a generalized tonic-clonic seizure regardless of which anesthetic is being administered. A single cartridge rapidly injected intravenously would likely induce severe seizure activity. Proper technique for all injections as discussed in Chapter 11 can prevent this from occurring (see Chapter 17).

Overdose reactions occur more frequently in children than adults and are an even greater risk in this population when concomitant central nervous system (CNS) depressants, such as opioid/sedative medications, are also administered.[2-4] This increased risk of systemic toxicity in children results from physiologic differences between children and adults. Children have disproportionately large heads (75% the size of their adult counterparts) compared with their total body size because the head develops quickly during early childhood (Fig. 14.1). When seated in a dental chair the child looks deceptively large, especially with a bib or blanket over their body.[5] This appearance may prompt the practitioner to administer more anesthetic based upon appearances rather than actual body weight, when indeed this child has only 20% the body weight of the adult counterpart, and only 25% of the blood volume, increasing the risk of local anesthetic systemic toxicity (LAST). In addition, children have larger tongues, tonsils, and adenoids than adults, increasing the risk of losing airway patency.[5]

Most adverse drug reactions occur within 5 to 10 minutes of injection. LAST initially manifests as excitation followed by depression of the CNS and, to a lesser extent, of the cardiovascular system (CVS). These early subjective symptoms of the CNS include dizziness, anxiety, and confusion. Objective signs include muscle twitching, tremors, talkativeness, and slowed speech followed by overt seizure activity. Unconsciousness and respiratory arrest may occur.

The initial CVS response to LAST is an increase in heart rate and blood pressure. As blood plasma levels of the anesthetic increase, vasodilatation occurs, followed by depression of the myocardium with subsequent fall in blood pressure. Bradycardia and cardiac arrest may follow. See Chapter 17 for in-depth information on signs, symptoms, and treatment of LAST.

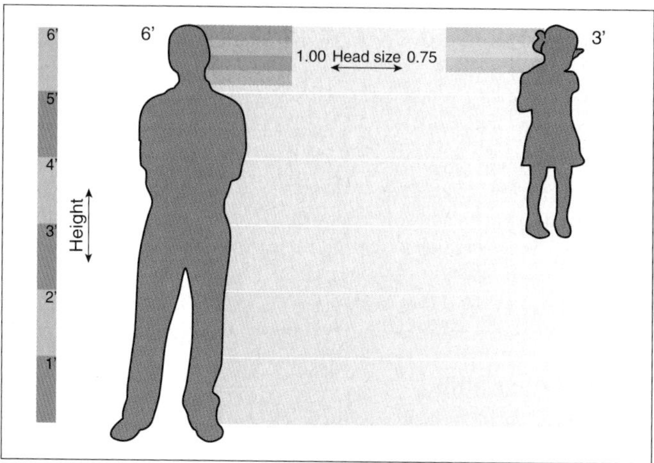

Fig. 14.1 Diagram illustrating the comparison of height to head size between a 3.5-year-old child and an adult.

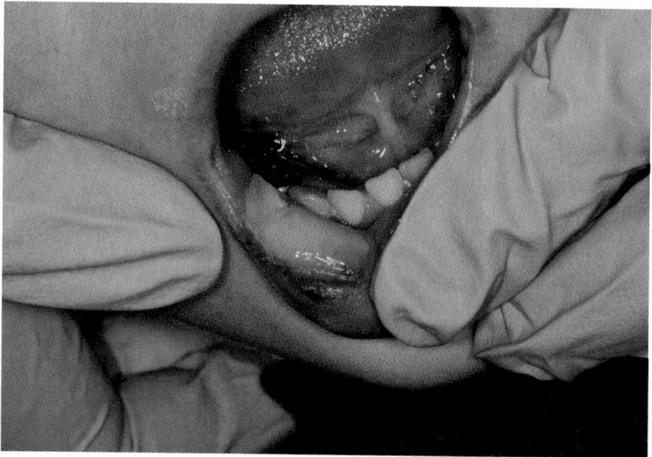

Fig. 14.2 Masticatory trauma of the lip after an inferior alveolar block. (From Casamassimo PS, Fields HW, McTigue DJ, Nowak AJ: *Pediatric dentistry infancy through adolescence*, ed 6, St Louis, 2019, Elsevier.)

Preventing Local Anesthetic Systemic Toxicity: Calculating Maximum Recommended Dose

To prevent the overestimation of body weight in a child, a standard scale should be used to provide the clinician with the child's accurate body weight. Adhering to MRDs for children set by the American Academy of Pediatric Dentistry (AAPD; see Chapter 8) and only anesthetizing the quadrants currently being treated will decrease the possibility of LAST. Administration of large volumes of anesthetic is not necessary in younger patients because of the anatomic differences between adults and children (see Local Anesthesia Delivery Techniques). Smaller volumes will produce the profound anesthesia needed for treatment of pediatric patients of lighter weight. Moreover, when considering MRDs for children, it is also important to consider that children's organ function may be immature, decreasing the effectiveness of the organs to biotransform the administered anesthetic, thus increasing the risk of overdose. This is particularly important when calculating the child's MRD based on weight for an overweight (or obese) child. For example, a 156-lb child could receive 400 mg of lidocaine, or 8.3 cartridges when using the AAPD maximum doses. This amount of anesthetic may not be biotransformed effectively due to immature organs and may alter the distribution and elimination of the drug, which may increase the risk of complications. Therefore the lowest effective dose should be administered in this situation, significantly lowering the MRD based on body weight. Determining the MRD based on the standard tables and utilizing Clark's rule (see Chapter 8) will not apply in this situation. It has been suggested that in situations of obese children an ideal body weight (IBW) index should be used rather than actual body weight.[6,7] IBW tables can be easily found online as a reference.

Clinicians should never exceed MRDs for weight or age. Studies have shown that exceeding the MRD in children, either by administering the local anesthetic agent alone or combined with a narcotic, may result in permanent brain damage or death.[2,8] Clinicians should be knowledgeable of maximum doses based on weight and age. See Chapter 8 for pediatric MRD and drug calculation guidelines. In addition, it is suggested that the dose of local anesthetic be adjusted downward when the child is sedated with opioids.[9] Another important consideration is the use of a topical anesthetic applied before the local anesthetic injection. It should be factored into the total administered dose as it can infiltrate into the vascular system. After injection, the patient should be observed for any possible toxic response, as early recognition and intervention are the keys to a successful outcome.

LOCAL ANESTHETIC AGENT SELECTION FOR CHILDREN

Local anesthetic selection is equally important when treating children. Frequently, 3% mepivacaine plain is used when anesthetizing children in dental offices with the misconception that using a local anesthetic without a vasoconstrictor will provide a shorter duration of soft tissue anesthesia than a local anesthetic with a vasoconstrictor, such as 2% lidocaine 1:100,000 epinephrine, and therefore reducing the risk of postoperative lip, cheek, and tongue biting[9-12] (Fig. 14.2). This is a considerable concern as this injury is the most common local anesthetic complication in children and adolescents; 3% mepivacaine offers shorter pulpal anesthesia compared with 2% lidocaine with epinephrine, but soft tissue anesthesia is almost identical between the two anesthetics (see Chapter 5). Therefore using 3% mepivacaine plain over 2% lidocaine with epinephrine does not provide any benefit to the prevention of postoperative lip/mouth trauma. In addition, the use of 3% mepivacaine plain does make it easier to reach or exceed MRDs. Because 3% mepivacaine has a higher concentration of anesthetic (54 mg/cartridge) than a 2% formulation (36 mg/cartridge), this means that 3% mepivacaine contains 50% more local anesthetic drug than a cartridge of 2% lidocaine;[3] thus it would take less volume (or fewer cartridges) of a more concentrated drug (3% mepivacaine) to reach its respective MRD. Moreover, 3% mepivacaine without a vasoconstrictor has higher documented toxicity reports that may result from the lack of a vasoconstrictor.[11,12] A vasoconstrictor (such as epinephrine) reduces the systemic absorption of a local anesthetic, and several pharmacokinetic studies have demonstrated that the average peak blood levels after maxillary supraperiosteal injections were three times higher with 3% mepivacaine plain compared with 2% lidocaine with epinephrine.[12] Lidocaine 1:100,000 epinephrine remains the preferred drug of choice for approximately 77% of dentists for pediatric patients. However, since the introduction of articaine hydrochloride in the United States in June 2000, 17% of dentists report that articaine is their preferred choice.[13] Because articaine has an elimination half-life of 27 minutes, it is the least likely of all the amide local anesthetics to induce a toxic overdose resulting from administering too much anesthetic. Studies have shown that articaine 4% 1:100,000 epinephrine is a safe and effective local anesthetic for use in pediatric dentistry.[14,15] For pediatric patients under the age of 4, the safety and efficacy of articaine have not been established.[14,15]

Long-acting local anesthetic agents, such as bupivacaine, are not recommended for children because of their prolonged soft tissue anesthesia of approximately 240 to 540 minutes. The prolonged anesthetic effect will increase the risk of soft tissue injury, and there are no procedures in pediatric dentistry that warrant 1.5 hours of pulpal anesthesia and over 4 hours of soft tissue anesthesia.

Postoperative Soft Tissue Injury

Self-inflicted soft tissue injury, such as lip, cheek, or tongue biting, is a significant concern for children who receive regional local anesthesia in the dental office, and these injuries are considered to be a common local complication. These injuries can range from mild to severe, and the most common area of injury is the lower lip (Fig. 14.2). It has been reported that these injuries occur 3% to 16% of the time. From 4 to 7 years of age, the rate was 16%, from 8 to 11 years the rate was 13%, and from 12 years or above, 7%.[16,17]

Preventive Measures of Soft Tissue Injury

There are several preventive measures that can be followed to decrease the occurrences of soft tissue injury:

- Select a local anesthetic agent with a duration of action that is appropriate for the length of the dental treatment.
- Advise the parent or caretaker about the possibility of injury caused by biting or chewing the lip, tongue, or cheek.
- Advise the parent or caretaker to delay having the child eat or drink hot beverages until the effects of the anesthesia have worn off.
- It is suggested to reinforce the verbal warning by placing cotton rolls in the mucobuccal fold, and place warning stickers on the patient's head.
- Administer phentolamine mesylate (OraVerse) at the end of the procedure. Phentolamine mesylate is a pharmaceutical agent indicated for the reversal of soft tissue anesthesia when a local anesthetic with a vasoconstrictor was administered. The FDA has approved its use for children 3 years of age and above, weighing 15 kilograms or 33 pounds or above.
- It is an alpha-adrenergic antagonist that will increase the speed of anesthetic reversal by producing vasodilation and increasing blood flow through the area when injected into the same site as the original injection. See Chapter 16 for more in-depth information on phentolamine mesylate.

Management of Self-Inflicted Soft Tissue Trauma

The injured tissue may appear red or red with white, and typically edema is present.

- The day of the injury: Instruct the parent to apply an ice pack to the area to reduce swelling.
- The following day: Instruct the parent to place a warm pack to the lesion to encourage circulation to promote healing.
- Lubricant (petroleum jelly) may be applied to prevent drying, cracking, and pain.
- Antibiotics are usually not necessary, only in rare cases when infection occurs.

LOCAL ANESTHESIA DELIVERY TECHNIQUES

Local anesthetic techniques for children do not differ significantly from those used in adults, and the basic injection techniques discussed in Chapter 11 apply to children as well. The main differences between children and adults are anatomic. The maxillary and mandibular bone in children is less dense compared with adults, allowing more rapid and complete diffusion of anesthetic agent through the bone. In addition, less needle depth is needed to reach the target locations for most injection techniques because children are smaller. Moreover, providing effective patient management techniques will ensure that the clinician can provide a pain-free successful injection.

BOX 14.1 Sample Dialogue

Today I am going to be putting your tooth to sleep, after a little pinch is felt near the tooth. So that you do not feel this pinch very much, I am going to first place the goofy, bubble gum (or other selected topical anesthetic) tooth jelly that you selected next to your tooth. I will then wipe it away and it will make that area feel sleepy. I am going to show you everything I do so you can see how easy it is. Afterward you will feel just a little pinch for a couple of seconds before your tooth falls asleep. Once your tooth falls asleep, you will not be able to feel anything, and your lip and tongue will feel fat and funny for a little while. Do you have any questions about what we will be doing today?

Patient Preparation

All preadministration protocols discussed in Chapters 7 and 11 should be used when administering local anesthetics to children. The armamentarium needed is identical to the adult administration; however, with small children, a short needle may be used for all injections because less tissue will need to be penetrated (see Chapter 9).

In children, behavior management is essential to achieving successful administration of local anesthesia. A relaxed, calm patient will ease the anesthetic delivery process. The clinician's ability to effectively communicate with the child at a level appropriate to the child's development is vital to creating an atmosphere of trust between the child and the clinician. Word choices are critical and trigger words, such as shot, needle, hurt, pain, bee sting, and so on, should be avoided. However, the dental hygienist should not deny that the procedure might hurt a little because this denial may cause the child to lose trust in the clinician. Box 14.1 offers a sample dialogue to use before the administration of the local anesthetic injection. Using the strategy of show-tell-do communication by demonstrating to the child what you will be doing and explaining the process in a tone that is reassuring yet assertive is often effective. Give the child a few simple, clear, nonthreatening expectations so he or she understands his or her role in the procedure. Praise good behavior and reward if possible. Praise in front of parents works well. Never belittle a child or compare negative behavior with another child's good behavior.

Administration Protocol

Position the Patient in the Dental Chair

The child should be positioned in supine positioning to reduce the incidence of syncope that can result from anxiety.

Apply Topical Anesthetic

Topical anesthetic should be used for effective prevention of discomfort during needle insertion. Topical anesthetics are available in all flavors, and allowing children to smell and choose their favorite flavor will help them become familiar with the agent and help put them at ease.

Stabilization and Communication

During the administration of local anesthetic, it is important for the clinician to control and limit the patient's movement. The head and body of the child should be stabilized while the clinician is communicating to the patient to focus attention away from the minor discomfort that may be felt during the injection process. Using a dental assistant is recommended. To stabilize the patient's head, hands, and body, the clinician may administer local anesthesia at a 9 o'clock position while the dental assistant is stabilizing the patient's head by gently holding it in place and stabilizing the patient's hands by placing his or hers gently on top (Fig. 14.3A), or at an 11 o'clock position to stabilize the patient's head while the dental assistant is stabilizing the patient's hands by placing his or hers on top (Fig. 14.3B). This position works

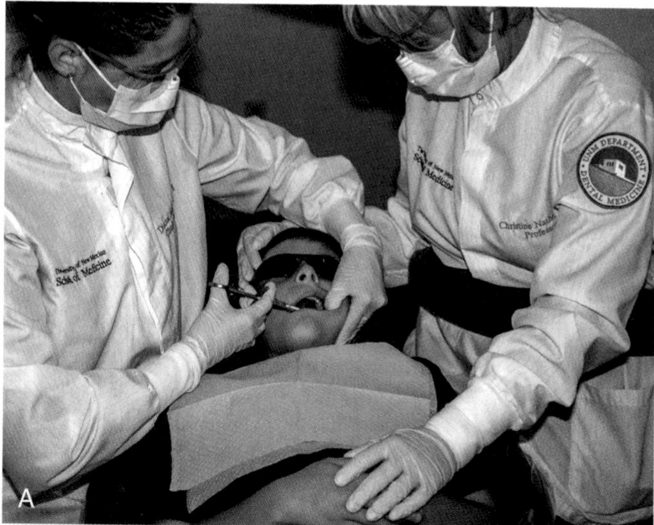

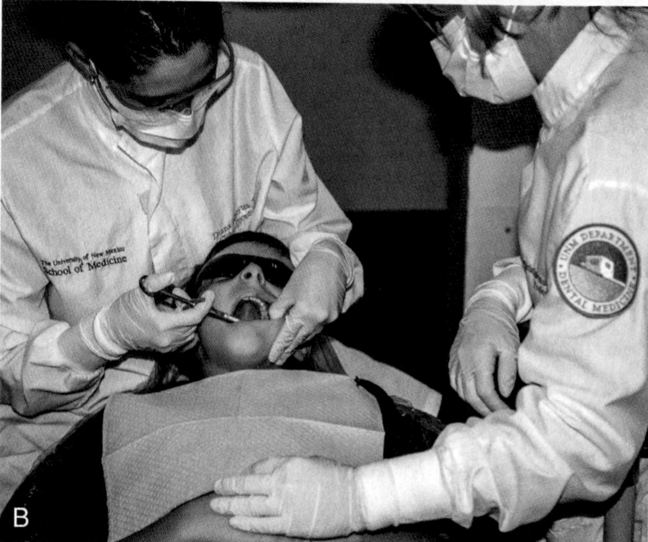

Fig. 14.3 (A) The dental hygienist is positioned at 9 o'clock during the administration of the local anesthetic on the contralateral side to the dental hygienist's dominate hand, while the dental assistant is stabilizing the patient's head by gently holding it in place and stabilizing the patient's hands by placing hers gently on top. (B) The dental hygienist is positioned at 11 o'clock to stabilize the patient's head, while the dental assistant is stabilizing the patient's hands by placing hers gently on top.

well for injecting anterior regions. When administering local anesthesia to a cooperative child, the dental hygienist may work without a dental assistant and should be positioned at a 10 o'clock or 11 o'clock position. The head is stabilized by the clinician supporting the head against his or her body with the nondominant hand and arm while controlling the jaw by resting the fingers against the mandible for added support and retraction of the lips and cheek (Fig. 14.4).

Continued reassuring communication throughout the anesthesia administration is critical to the successful injection. The clinician can discuss the process using children's terminology, or by praising, storytelling, or even singing. Use your imagination to create a fun, nonintimidating environment.

Maxillary Anesthesia

Maxillary supraperiosteal injections, as described in Chapter 12, can be used for all primary and permanent molars and are administered in the mucobuccal fold identical to the procedures outlined for permanent

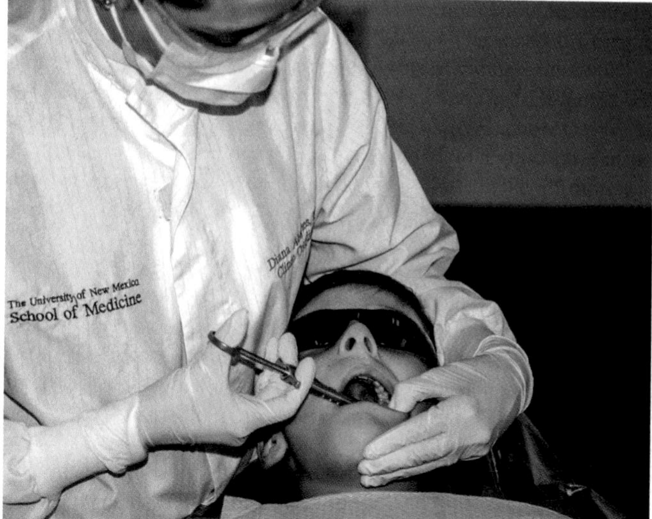

Fig. 14.4 The dental hygienist is positioned at a 10 o'clock to 11 o'clock position to administer local anesthetic to a cooperative child without a dental assistant to stabilize the patient's head by gently wrapping her arm around the patient's head. In addition, the clinician gently supports the mandible with her fingers.

dentition. Anatomic differences of primary dentition compared with permanent dentition are shorter roots allowing for a shallower insertion of the needle, approximately 2 mm at the most. An extra-short needle (12 mm) is typically adequate to reach the target location in many children (Fig. 14.5). The posterior alveolar (PSA) block is generally not recommended or needed because of the effectiveness of supraperiosteal injections in children. However, in some children, the thick zygomatic process may overlie the buccal roots of the second primary and first permanent molars in primary and early mixed dentition. Clinical effectiveness of the supraperiosteal injection may not be achieved in these instances, warranting a PSA block. Should a PSA block be indicated, the depth of insertion should be greatly reduced (approximately ¼ the depth of a short needle) for children and adolescent patients to prevent hematomas (Fig. 14.6).

The administration of palatal injections is painful for adults and children. Using the prepuncture technique described in Chapter 11 will help reduce the painful sensations. In addition, the use of the computer-controlled local anesthetic delivery (C-CLAD) system will also increase comfort for pediatric patients due to the ability of the device to deliver a slow, steady anesthetic flow. For the nasopalatine (NP) block, the target location (Fig. 14.7) and technique are identical to that described for adults in Chapter 12. For the greater palatine (GP) block, the target location is the GP foramen (Fig. 14.8). To locate, the clinician should bisect an imaginary line drawn from the gingival border of the most posterior molar that has erupted to the midline. The needle is inserted from the contralateral side toward the last molar (Fig. 14.9). If only primary dentition is present, the insertion point is approximately 10 mm posterior to the distal surface of the second primary molar. The key to a successful, comfortable injection is administering the agent slowly.

Mandibular Anesthesia

Supraperiosteal injection techniques are more clinically effective in mandibular primary molars compared with mandibular permanent molars because of the decrease in density of the mandibular bone in younger children. This allows many simple restorative procedures and some extractions to be accomplished using mandibular supraperiosteal injections (see Chapters 12 and 13). It has been reported that

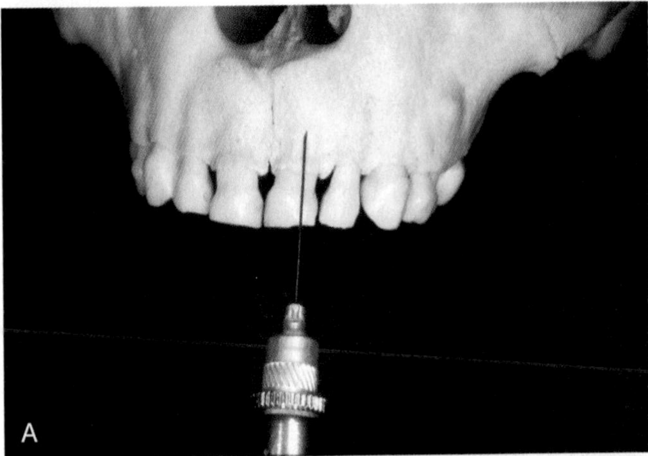

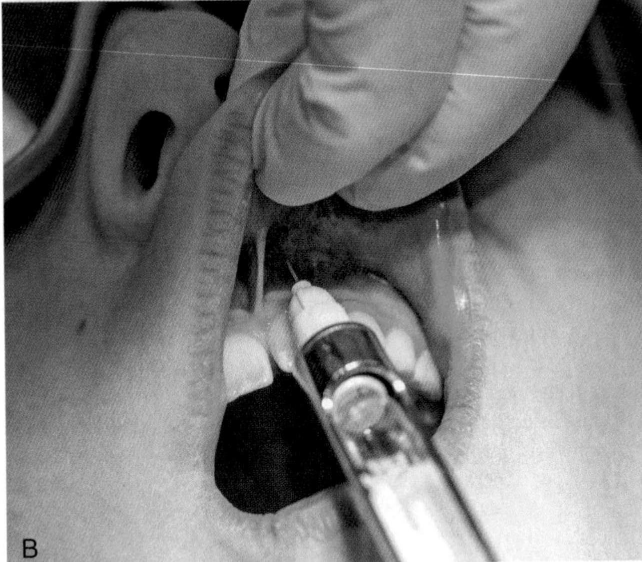

Fig. 14.5 (A) A child's maxilla illustrating a short needle at the target location for a supraperiosteal injection of the maxillary central incisor. (B) Supraperiosteal injection of the maxillary central incisor on a child using an extra-short needle. Only 2 mm of needle depth is needed to reach the target location. (A, From Dean JA: *McDonald and Avery's dentistry for the child and adolescent,* ed 10, St Louis, 2016, Elsevier.)

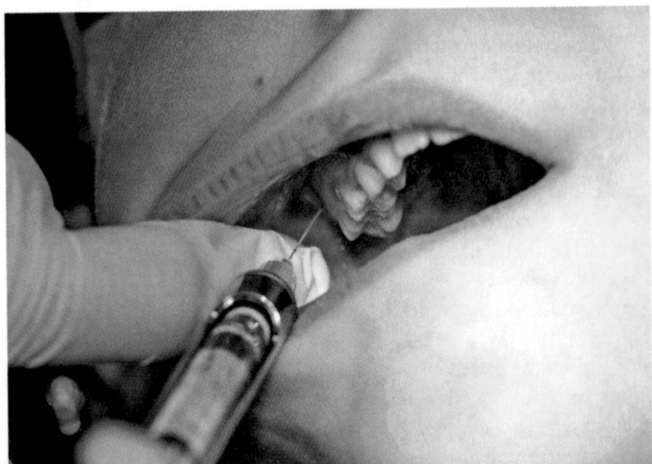

Fig. 14.6 Posterior superior alveolar block on a child using a short needle, decreasing the depth of the needle for the child to approximately ¼ the depth of the short needle.

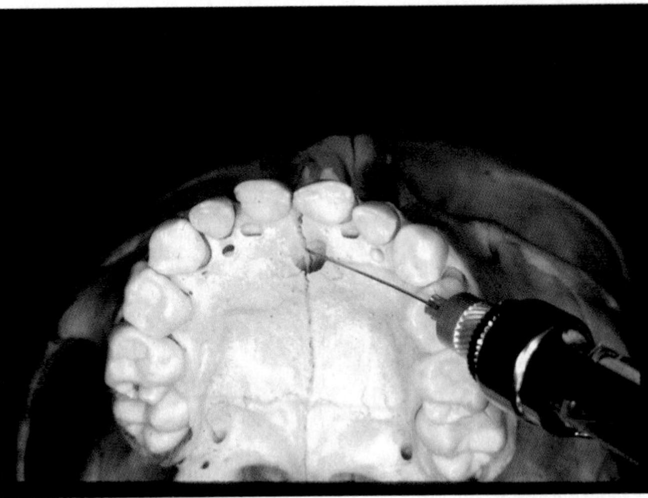

Fig. 14.7 Target location for the nasopalatine block on a child's palate. The target location is the incisive foramen. (From Dean JA: *McDonald and Avery's dentistry for the child and adolescent,* ed 10, St Louis, 2016, Elsevier.)

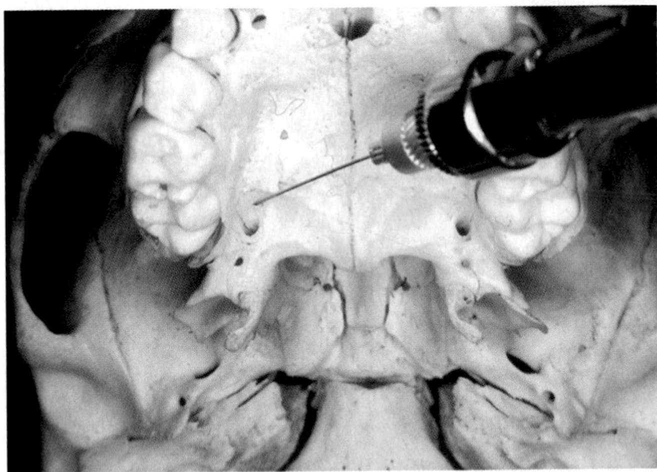

Fig. 14.8 Target location for the greater palatine block on a child's palate. The target location is the greater palatine foramen. (From Dean JA: *McDonald and Avery's dentistry for the child and adolescent,* ed 10, St Louis, 2016, Elsevier.)

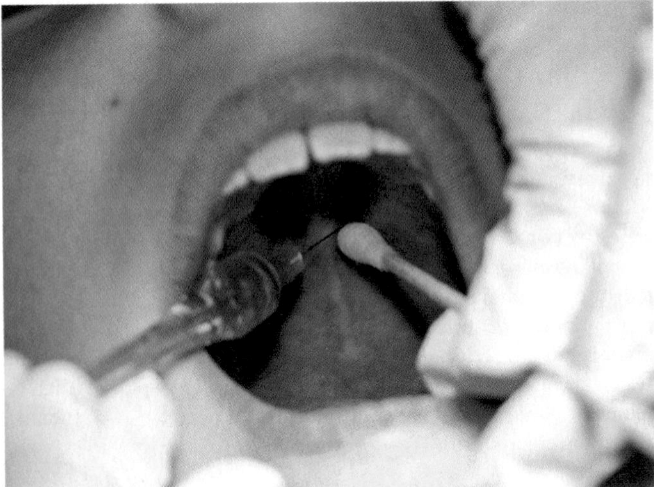

Fig. 14.9 Greater palatine block on a child. The computer-controlled local anesthetic delivery device and prepuncture technique with a cotton-tipped applicator is being used to increase patient comfort. The needle is inserted from the contralateral side toward the greater palatine foramen.

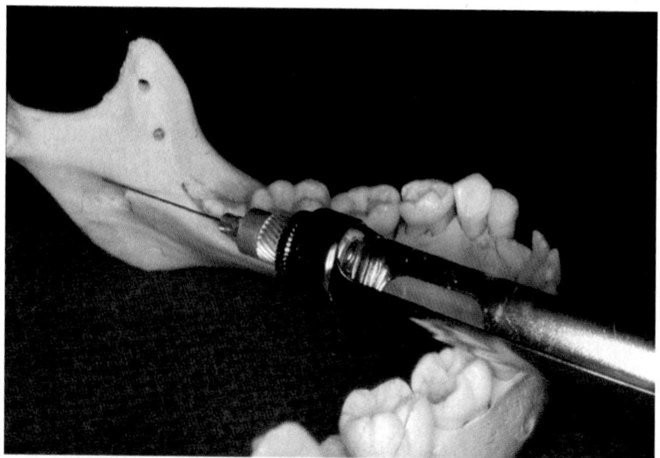

Fig. 14.10 A child's mandible illustrating the mandibular foramen at the same level as the occlusal plane and the anesthetic needle at its target location. (From Dean JA: *McDonald and Avery's dentistry for the child and adolescent,* ed 10, St Louis, 2016, Elsevier.)

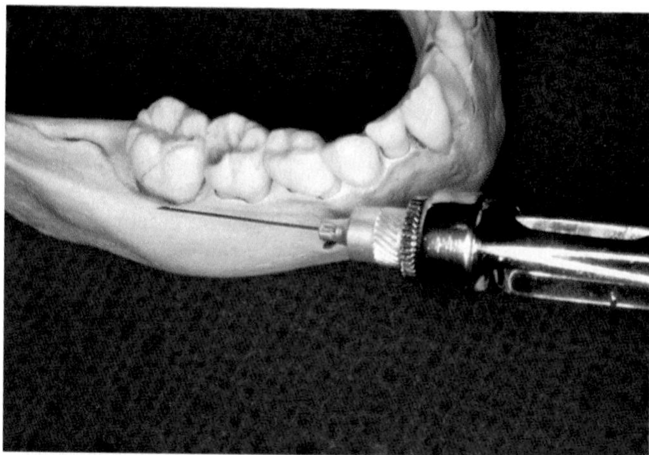

Fig. 14.12 A child's mandible illustrating the target location of the long buccal block. (From Dean JA: *McDonald and Avery's dentistry for the child and adolescent,* ed 10, St Louis, 2016, Elsevier.)

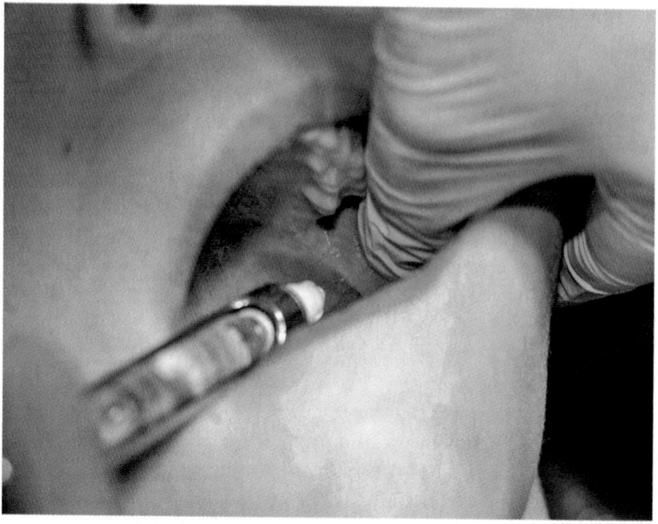

Fig. 14.11 Inferior alveolar block on a child. The technique is similar to that on an adult with the barrel of the syringe at the contralateral corner of the mouth, but instead of using a long needle, a short needle at approximately the depth of 15 mm is enough to reach the target location.

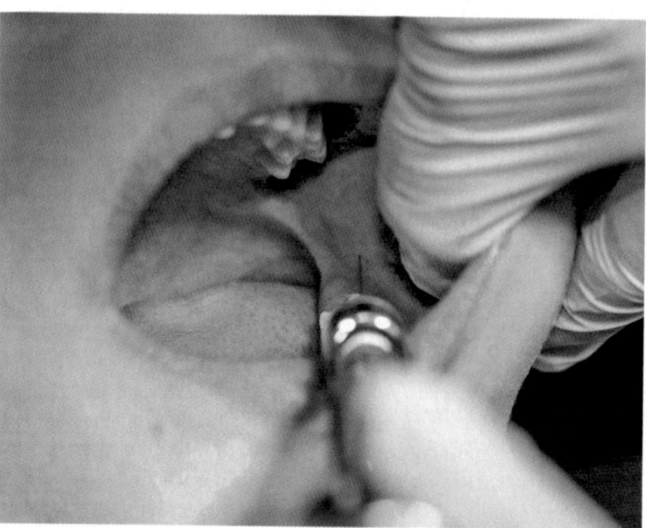

Fig. 14.13 Long buccal block. The technique is similar to that on an adult by inserting the needle in the mucobuccal fold at the point distal and buccal to the last most posterior tooth in the quadrant.

children between the ages of 6 and 9 received effective pain control from buccal supraperiosteal injections equivalent to that of an inferior alveolar (IA) block.[18,19] However as children increase in age, this success rate diminishes. The technique used for mandibular supraperiosteal injections is the same as described for the maxilla (see Chapter 12).

When more extensive procedures are needed on children, the IA block should be administered. The IA block has a greater success rate in children than in adults because the mandibular foramen is situated at or lower than the occlusal plane of primary teeth, compared with an average of 10 mm above the occlusal plane in adults[13,20] (Fig. 14.10). Because the mandibular foramen is more inferior in children compared with adults, injections that are administered "too low" are more likely to be successful.[20] The technique for the IA block is similar to that of the adult patient, as described in Chapter 13 with a few minor differences. The barrel of the syringe should be directed between the two primary mandibular molars on the contralateral side of the arch, and parallel to the occlusal plane for children, instead of over the two premolars on the contralateral side as in adults. The average depth of needle insertion is approximately 15 mm but may vary depending on the size of the mandible and its changing proportions depending on the age of the patient. Because the soft tissue is less thick overlying the IA nerve, a 25- or 27-gauge short needle may be used in younger children (Fig. 14.11).[20] The needle should be changed to a long needle as the patient increases in size and the short needle can no longer reach the target location.[13] Bone should be contacted before deposition of anesthetic. The buccal nerve may also need to be anesthetized for the removal of mandibular permanent molars or when a rubber dam needs to be placed. The technique is similar to the adult patient by placing the needle tip distal and buccal to the last molar in the quadrant (Figs. 14.12 and 14.13; see Chapter 13).

DENTAL HYGIENE CONSIDERATIONS

- Careful consideration should be made to maximum recommended doses (MRDs) of local anesthetic in children who are taking opioid/sedative medications.
- Systemic toxicity is more common in children.
- To prevent the overestimation of body weight in a child, a standard scale should be used to provide the clinician with the child's accurate body weight.
- An ideal body weight (IBW) index should be used when calculating MRDs in obese children. These can be easily found online.
- It is recommended that the American Academy of Pediatric Dentistry (AAPD) MRDs be used rather than the manufacturer doses in children.
- There is very little difference between 3% mepivacaine plain and 2% lidocaine 1:100,000 in soft tissue duration. Therefore using 3% mepivacaine plain over 2% lidocaine with epinephrine does not provide any benefit to the prevention of postoperative lip/mouth trauma.
- 3% mepivacaine without a vasoconstrictor has higher documented toxicity reports because of its higher concentration compared with 2% lidocaine and because of the lack of a vasoconstrictor.
- Articaine has an elimination half-life of 27 minutes, and it is the least likely of all the amide local anesthetics to induce a toxic overdose.
- For pediatric patients under the age of 4, the safety and efficacy of articaine have not been established.
- Long-acting local anesthetic agents, such as bupivacaine, are not recommended for children because of their prolonged soft tissue anesthesia.
- Phentolamine mesylate is an effective reversal agent for soft tissue anesthesia when a local anesthetic containing a vasoconstrictor is used, and is approved by the FDA for children 3 years of age and above, weighing 33 pounds or above.
- Inferior alveolar blocks are more successful in children compared with adults because the mandibular foramen is more inferior.
- In children, supraperiosteal injections are more effective in both the maxillary and mandibular arch because of the less dense bone on the mandible.

CASE STUDY 14.1 The Apprehensive Child

A 6-year-old, 100-lb patient is in the office today for a cleaning followed by a restoration on tooth #30. During the cleaning the patient was wriggly and a little apprehensive. The dentist asked the dental hygienist to administer the anesthetic for tooth #30 before the patient is moved to the dentist's chair for the restoration.

Critical Thinking Questions

- What should the dental hygienist do about the apprehensiveness of the patient before the administration of the local anesthetic?
- What local anesthetic agent would be appropriate for this child and why?
- What is the maximum recommended dose based on the selected solution?
- Which injection(s) should be administered for the treatment?

CHAPTER REVIEW QUESTIONS

1. One of the most common adverse reaction to the administration of a local anesthetic is systemic toxicity. It is usually a result of the administration of the local anesthetic above the patient's maximum recommended dose.
   A. Both the statement and the reason are CORRECT and related.
   B. Both the statement and the reason are correct but NOT related.
   C. The statement is correct, but the reason is NOT correct.
   D. The statement is NOT correct, but the reason is CORRECT.
   E. NEITHER the statement nor the reason is CORRECT.
2. Overdose reactions occur more frequently in children than adults. Early signs and symptoms of central nervous system overdose are increased heart rate and blood pressure.
   A. Both statements are correct.
   B. Both statements are NOT correct.
   C. The first statement is correct; the second statement is NOT correct.
   D. The first statement is NOT correct; the second statement is correct.
3. When calculating maximum recommended doses (MRDs) for children, these doses should be calculated by using:
   A. Manufacturer's MRDs
   B. American Academy of Pediatric Dentistry MRDs
   C. Estimated doses
   D. Estimated patient weight
4. When calculating the maximum recommended doses (MRDs) for obese children, all of the following should be used EXCEPT one. Which one is the EXCEPTION?
   A. Manufacturer's MRDs
   B. American Academy of Pediatric Dentistry MRDs
   C. Clark's rule
   D. IBW index
5. Which of the following is an anatomic difference between children and adults?
   A. The cortical plates are denser in children compared with adults
   B. The roots of primary dentition are shorter
   C. The roots of primary dentition are longer
   D. The inferior alveolar foramen is more superior in children compared with adults
6. Which of the following is a successful management tool when soft tissue injury occurs from biting the lip?
   A. Apply an ice pack on the day of the injury.
   B. Apply an ice pack the next day.
   C. Apply a warm pack on the day of the injury.
   D. Ask the dentist to administer antibiotics.
7. Which of the following is an effective way to use a dental assistant during the administration of local anesthetics to a child?
   A. To help stabilize the patient during the injection by gently placing their hands on top of the child's hand

B. By holding the needle cap for the clinician to easily recap the needle after the procedure
C. Describing the procedure by showing the patient the syringe and needle
D. By making the patient laugh during the injection

8. Why are inferior alveolar blocks more successful in children compared with adults?
A. Because of the density of bone in children
B. Because you can use a short needle when injecting children
C. Because of the location of the mandibular foramen in adults
D. Because of the location of the mandibular foramen in children

9. When administering the inferior alveolar local anesthetic block in children, the syringe barrel in most cases should be in what relation to the mandibular occlusal plane?
A. Perpendicular
B. Parallel
C. At a 45-degree angle
D. At a 90-degree angle

10. When administering the inferior alveolar local anesthetic block in children, the syringe barrel in most cases should usually be superior to which mandibular tooth?
A. Premolar on the injection side
B. Premolar on the contralateral side
C. First molar on the contralateral side
D. First molar on the injection side

11. 2% Lidocaine 1:100,000 is preferred over 3% mepivacaine for children. This is because of the vasoconstrictor decreasing the risk of local anesthetic systemic toxicity.
A. Both the statement and the reason are CORRECT and related.
B. Both the statement and the reason are correct but NOT related.
C. The statement is correct, but the reason is NOT correct.
D. The statement is NOT correct, but the reason is CORRECT.
E. NEITHER the statement nor the reason is CORRECT.

12. Which of the following local anesthetic blocks has the highest risk of hematoma for the child after administration?
A. Posterior superior alveolar block
B. Inferior alveolar block
C. Gow-Gates mandibular block
D. Mental or incisive blocks

13. What is the typical depth of needle insertion in children for a supraperiosteal injection?
A. No more than 5 mm
B. No more than 4 mm
C. No more than 3 mm
D. No more than 2 mm

14. The inferior alveolar foramen in children is:
A. More anterior than in adults
B. More lateral than in adults
C. More inferior than in adults
D. More superior than in adults

15. Bupivacaine is indicated for children because it provides long-acting pain control.
A. Both the statement and the reason are CORRECT and related.
B. Both the statement and the reason are correct but NOT related.
C. The statement is correct, but the reason is NOT correct.
D. The statement is NOT correct, but the reason is CORRECT.
E. NEITHER the statement nor the reason is CORRECT.

16. Phentolamine mesylate should be administered immediately after the dental procedure because this helps to prevent self-mutilation of the lip by children who are at risk.
A. Both the statement and the reason are CORRECT and related.
B. Both the statement and the reason are correct but NOT related.
C. The statement is correct, but the reason is NOT correct.
D. The statement is NOT correct, but the reason is CORRECT.
E. NEITHER the statement nor the reason is CORRECT.

17. All of the following are management tools when administering a local anesthetic to a child EXCEPT one. Which one is the EXCEPTION?
A. Application of topical anesthetic
B. Supine positioning
C. Restraining the child tightly
D. Communication using easily understandable terminology

18. All of the following are reasons to administer a long buccal block to a child EXCEPT one. Which one is the EXCEPTION?
A. Application of a rubber dam
B. An extraction
C. A class I restoration
D. A class II restoration

19. Computer-controlled local anesthetic delivery devices should not be used on children because the device delivers a rapid anesthetic flow.
A. Both the statement and the reason are CORRECT and related.
B. Both the statement and the reason are correct but NOT related.
C. The statement is correct, but the reason is NOT correct.
D. The statement is NOT correct, but the reason is CORRECT.
E. NEITHER the statement nor the reason is CORRECT.

20. It is not necessary to contact bone when administering an inferior alveolar block to children because there is no risk of injecting into the parotid gland on a child.
A. Both the statement and the reason are CORRECT and related.
B. Both the statement and the reason are correct but NOT related.
C. The statement is correct, but the reason is NOT correct.
D. The statement is NOT correct, but the reason is CORRECT.
E. NEITHER the statement nor the reason is CORRECT.

REFERENCES

1. Jeske AH, Blanton PL. Misconceptions involving dental local anesthesia. Part 2: Pharmacology. *Tex Dent J.* 2002;119(4):310–314.
2. Hersh EV, Helpin ML, Evans QB. Local anesthetic mortality: report of case. *ASDC J Dent Child.* 1991;58(6):489–491.
3. Moore PA. Preventing local anesthesia toxicity. *J Am Dent Assoc.* 1992;123(9):60–64.
4. Goodson JM, Moore PA. Life-threatening reactions after pedodontic sedation: an assessment of narcotic, local anesthetic, and antiemetic drug interaction. *J Am Dent Assoc.* 1983;107(2):239–245.
5. Saraghi M, Moore PA, Hersh EV. Local anesthetic calculation: avoiding trouble with pediatric patients. *Gen Dent.* 2015;63(1):48–52.
6. Bouillon T, Shafer SL. Does size matter? *Anesthesiology.* 1998;89(3):557–560.
7. Leykin Y, Pellis T, Lucca M, Lomangino G, Marzano B, Gullo A. The pharmacodynamic effects of rocuronium when dosed according to real body weight or ideal body weight in morbidly obese patients. *Anesth Analg.* 2004;99(4):1056–1089.
8. Tarsitano JJ. Children, drugs, and local anesthesia. *J Am Dent Assoc.* 1965;70:1153–1158.

9. Moore PA. Adverse drug reactions in dental practice: interactions associated with local anesthetics, sedatives, and anxiolytics. *J Am Dent Assoc.* 1999;130(4):541–544.
10. Saraghi M, Moore PA, Hersh EV. Local anesthetic calculations: avoiding trouble with pediatric populations. *Gen Dent.* 2015;63(1):48–52.
11. Moore PA, Hersh EV. Local anesthesia: pharmacology and toxicity. *Dent Clin North Am.* 2010;54(4):587–599.
12. Goebel WM, Allen G, Randall F. The effect of commercial vasoconstrictor preparations on the circulating venous serum level of mepivacaine and lidocaine. *J Oral Med.* 1980;35(4):91–96.
13. Malamed S. *Handbook of local anesthesia.* ed 7. St Louis: Elsevier; 2020.
14. Leith R, Lynch K, O'Connell AC. Articaine use in children: a review. *Eur Arch Paediatr Dent.* 2012;13:293–296.
15. Malamed SF, Gagnon S, Leblanc D. A comparison between articaine HCl and lidocaine HCl in pediatric dental patients. *Pediatric Dentistry.* 2000;22(4):307–311.
16. Boynes SG, Riley AE, Milbee S, Bastin MR, Price ME, Ladson A. Evaluating complications of local anesthesia administration and reversal with phentolamine mesylate in a portable pediatric dental clinic. *Gen Dent.* 2013;61(5):70–76.
17. College C, Feigal R, Wandera A, Strange M. Bilateral versus unilateral mandibular block anesthesia in a pediatric population. *Pediatr Dent.* 2000;22(6):453–457.
18. Sharaf AA. Evaluation of mandibular infiltration versus block anesthesia in pediatric dentistry. *ASDC J Dent Child.* 1997;64(4):276–281.
19. Oulis CJ, Vadiakis GP, Vasilopoulou A. The effectiveness of mandibular infiltration compared to mandibular block anesthesia in treating primary molars in children. *Pediatr Dent.* 1996;18(4):301–305.
20. Olsen NH. Anesthesia for the child patient. *J Am Dent Assoc.* 1956;53(5):548–555.

15

Nitrous Oxide/Oxygen Administration

Diana Burnham Aboytes, RDH, MS

LEARNING OBJECTIVES

1. Describe the role of nitrous oxide/oxygen (N_2O/O_2) as an adjunct to local anesthesia injections.
2. Discuss indications and contraindications of N_2O/O_2.
3. Discuss advantages and disadvantages of N_2O/O_2.
4. Recite the steps associated with administration of N_2O/O_2.
5. Differentiate between signs and symptoms of ideal sedation versus heavy and oversedation.
6. Describe components of documentation in a patient's record.

INTRODUCTION

Nitrous oxide remains the most commonly used inhalation agent in dentistry.[1] Used in combination with oxygen, nitrous oxide serves as both an anxiolytic and analgesic agent, making it a great option to assist in the management of pain, fear, and anxiety associated with dental treatment. Part of the fear and anxiety associated with dentistry comes from receiving the local anesthesia injections (see Chapter 1). Although nitrous oxide/oxygen does not substitute the need for local anesthesia, its delivery as an adjunct may be a great option by increasing a patient's pain threshold and overall tolerance of the local anesthesia injections. Patients may require N_2O only during the local anesthesia administration, however some may opt for administration during the entire non-surgical periodontal therapy procedure.

The purpose of this chapter is to serve as a reference regarding nitrous oxide/oxygen administration and its use alongside other pain management modalities such as local anesthetics. It is not intended to serve as a substitute for comprehensive educational and clinical training.

HISTORY

Nitrous oxide gas is one of many gases first discovered by Joseph Priestly, an English chemist, early in the 1770s. Thereafter, another chemist, Sir Humphrey Davy, began experimenting with pure nitrous oxide. He was quick to discover that it produced a feeling of euphoria and pleasure. He coined the term "laughing gas," as those who inhaled the gas found that they could not help but laugh under its influence. The euphoric effect made pure nitrous oxide a staple for recreational use at social gatherings and community exhibitions for the next several decades.

It was not until 1844 when a dentist named Dr. Horace Wells attended one of these exhibitions and during the presentation noticed one of the participants suffer a large injury to his leg that went unnoticed. It was then that Dr. Wells suspected that nitrous oxide might have analgesic properties. The next day, Dr. Wells tested his suspicion by having one of his own teeth extracted while under the influence of nitrous oxide. Dr. Wells is considered a pioneer of nitrous oxide use in dentistry and continued its use as a standard part of his dental procedures up until his death in 1848. It was not until 1864, after years of reviewed medical documents, interviews, and attestations that the American Dental Association officially proclaimed Dr. Wells the discoverer or "father of anesthesia."[2,3]

Since then, administration of nitrous oxide has been modified and updated. No longer is pure nitrous oxide used. The administration includes a combination of simultaneous use of nitrous oxide and oxygen of various concentrations.[4] Improvements in equipment for delivery and monitoring have contributed to its long-documented safety record and over 175 years of successful use.[5–7]

> **Important Point to Remember**
>
> As a safety feature, current dental nitrous oxide systems do not allow the delivery of a 100% pure concentration of nitrous oxide and always delivers approximately 30% oxygen to the patient.

CHARACTERISTICS OF NITROUS OXIDE

Nitrous oxide (molecular formula N_2O) is one of several types of inhaled anesthetic gases used in dentistry (Fig. 15.1).[8] Nitrous oxide is a colorless, odorless, nonflammable gas that occurs naturally or can be manufactured.[8] It is commonly known as *laughing gas* and is used during a variety of medical and dental procedures. It is nonallergenic and does not irritate the lungs, making it suitable for a variety of people ranging from young children to the geriatric population. It is the least potent of inhaled gases, but it still has the ability to produce depression of the central nervous system resulting in state of conscious sedation.

Sedation Continuum

Sedation is a continuum and ranges from minimal sedation to general anesthesia (Fig. 15.2). A continuum is a sequence of elements that vary only by a slight difference without clearly defined points, yet the beginning and end are opposite extremes. Sedation can be achieved using oral, intravenous, and inhalation agents. The American Society of Anesthesiologists (ASA), in a document written in the 1980s and recently updated in 2019, describes the levels of sedation based on the typical response of the patient (Table 15.1).[9] This is meant to serve as a guide for providers to assess and monitor a patient's depth of sedation. The depth or level of sedation needed varies by individual patient

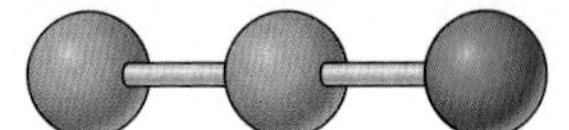

Fig. 15.1 Nitrous oxide (N_2O) molecule.

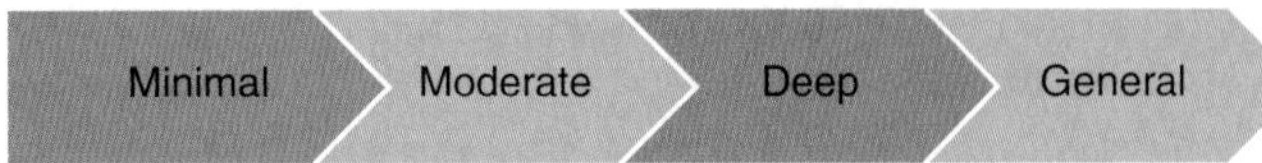

Fig. 15.2 Sedation continuum.

and the procedure being performed. The level of sedation a dental hygienist needs for procedures in their scope is different than the level needed by a dentist or a dental anesthesiologist operating in an ambulatory surgical center.

Minimal sedation, defined as less than 50% N_2O, is the first stage in the continuum. During this stage, the anxiolytic properties are evident as the patient's anxiety is reduced and the patient is able to relax. Patients can still respond normally to verbal commands. Cardiovascular function, ventilation, and the airway are unaffected. The gag reflex may slightly be reduced, but the protective cough reflex remains fully intact. Most dental hygiene procedures, including local anesthesia administration can be completed using minimal sedation.

A moderate level of sedation produces greater depressed consciousness and is referred to as conscious sedation.[9,10] Patients are still able to respond with purpose to both verbal and tactile stimulation. Spontaneous ventilation remains adequate and no intervention of the airway is required.

The deep sedation/analgesia and general anesthesia levels of sedation are beyond the scope of administration for a dental hygienist. Patients become less responsive, spontaneous ventilation is inadequate, and an intervention to maintain airway may be required.[9] Emphasis should be placed on the recognition of signs and symptoms associated with this level of sedation to prevent a patient from reaching this depth.

ROLE IN PAIN MANAGEMENT

Indications Versus Contraindications

Nitrous oxide/oxygen (N_2O/O_2) is indicated for patients who experience mild to moderate anxiety associated with dental appointments. The anxiolytic properties help relieve the stresses that come with the sights, sounds, and smells of an appointment. This can increase tolerance for the length of the appointment and patient compliance during the procedure. It can be used to help diminish a hypersensitive gag reflex, helping facilitate taking impressions or radiographs.[11]

Overall, there are no absolute or true contraindications to N_2O/O_2, especially with at least 20% to 30% O_2 being delivered.[6–7,12] Each patient, however, should be evaluated to ensure that benefits of administration use outweigh any risks. Examples of relative contraindications include patients with chronic obstructive pulmonary disease (COPD), pregnancy in the first trimester, cystic fibrosis, a recent ear surgery, and an eye surgery in which a gas bubble was used.[6,7] The use of N_2O/O_2 is contraindicated for patients who present with any upper respiratory problems, such as rhinitis, or those with changes in nasal anatomy, such as deviated septum in which they cannot breathe through their nose. Also consideration should be taken with patients who are claustrophobic and not comfortable with the nasal hood on their face.

TABLE 15.2 Advantages Versus Disadvantages for the Administration of Nitrous Oxide

Advantages	Disadvantages
Ease of administration	Low-potency drug
Works quickly, allowing for immediate treatment	Does not work on everyone
Able to titrate and control depth of sedation	Will not manage severe anxiety or dental phobia
Quick recovery	
Able to drive to/from appointments	

Advantages Versus Disadvantages

There are many advantages associated with the use of N_2O/O_2 (Table 15.2). Administration of N_2O/O_2 has a quick onset of action, allowing for immediate treatment. The depth of sedation can be controlled through titration, and as fast as it starts working, it can also be quickly reversed. This allows for rapid patient recovery, allowing the patient to drive themselves to and from the dental appointment. The ease of administration makes it acceptable for use with all patient populations including pediatric and geriatric patients.

The main disadvantage is that N_2O is a low-potency drug. There is a small percentage (~5%) of people that are considered hyporesponders, and N_2O will not work on these individuals.[6,7] Additionally, it may not be strong enough to work on patients with severe anxiety or dental phobia. These patients may require additional sedative agents to be used in combination with N_2O/O_2.

TABLE 15.1 Continuum of Depth of Sedation

	Minimal Sedation Anxiolysis	Moderate Sedation/Analgesia ("Conscious Sedation")	Deep Sedation/ Analgesia	General Anesthesia
Responsiveness	Normal response to verbal stimulation	Purposeful* response to verbal or tactile stimulation	Purposeful* response after repeated or painful stimulation	Unarousable even with painful stimulus
Airway	Unaffected	No intervention required	Intervention may be required	Intervention often required
Spontaneous ventilation	Unaffected	Adequate	May be inadequate	Frequently inadequate
Cardiovascular function	Unaffected	Usually maintained	Usually maintained	May be impaired

*Reflex withdrawal from a painful stimulus is NOT considered a purposeful response.

From American Society of Anesthesiologists: *Continuum of depth of sedation.* www.asahq.org/standards-and-guidelines/continuum-of-depth-of-sedation-definition-of-general-anesthesia-and-levels-of-sedationanalgesia. Last amended October 2019.

DELIVERY SYSTEMS

Centralized System Versus Portable System

There are different types of delivery systems available to meet the needs of each practice. Centralized systems are built directly into the foundation of the dental office. N_2O and O_2 cylinders are set up in a separate room and gases are plumbed through the building and into the individual clinical operatories (Fig. 15.3). Portable delivery systems contain all the necessary components housed together and can be moved from room to room for administration (Fig. 15.4). Regardless of the type of system, they all contain some basic components for operation. Always refer to the manufacturer instructions for specifics of each type of unit.

Equipment

The cylinders hold the gases until they are ready for use. In the United States, the N_2O cylinder is blue, whereas the O_2 cylinder is green.

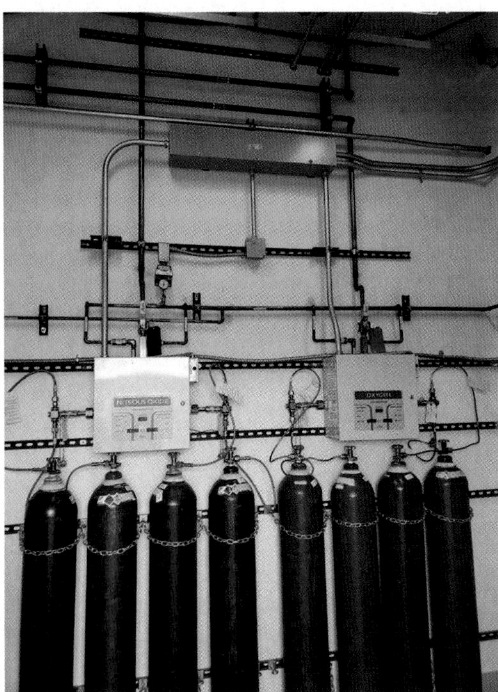

Fig. 15.3 Nitrous oxide (blue) and oxygen (green) cylinders of a centralized system.

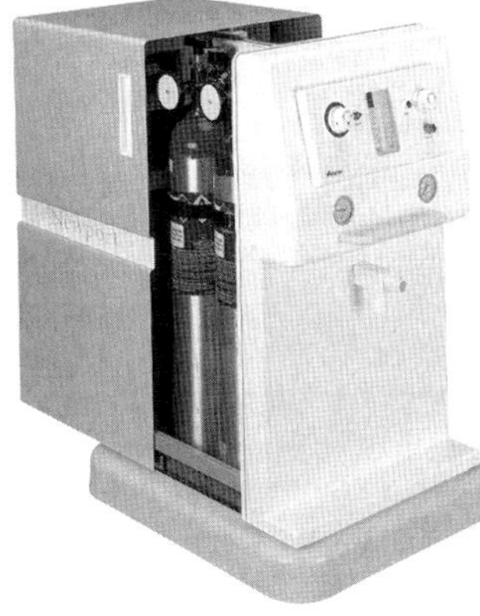

Fig. 15.4 Portable delivery system: All components are self-contained. (From Clark M, Brunick A: *Handbook of nitrous oxide and oxygen sedation,* ed 4, St Louis, 2015, Elsevier.)

Cylinders come in a variety of sizes depending on the unit and range from sizes A to HH. When N_2O is manufactured and placed into cylinders, it is stored as a compressed liquid. As it is released from the cylinder, it changes back to a gas (Fig. 15.5).

On portable delivery systems, the yokes are responsible for holding the cylinders in place. The control knob or knobs on some units are used to start and adjust the flow of gases. The flowmeter identifies the flow rate, in liters per minute, of the individual gas being administered. Each system contains a reservoir bag that contains a reserve of gases that can be used if a patient takes a larger breath and requires more volume during respiration (Fig. 15.6). With every breath the bag inflates and deflates. It is important to notice if the bag is underinflated or overinflated. Additionally, the system has an O_2 flush button that, when pressed, can quickly allow O_2 through the unit and reservoir bag, getting O_2 to the patient.

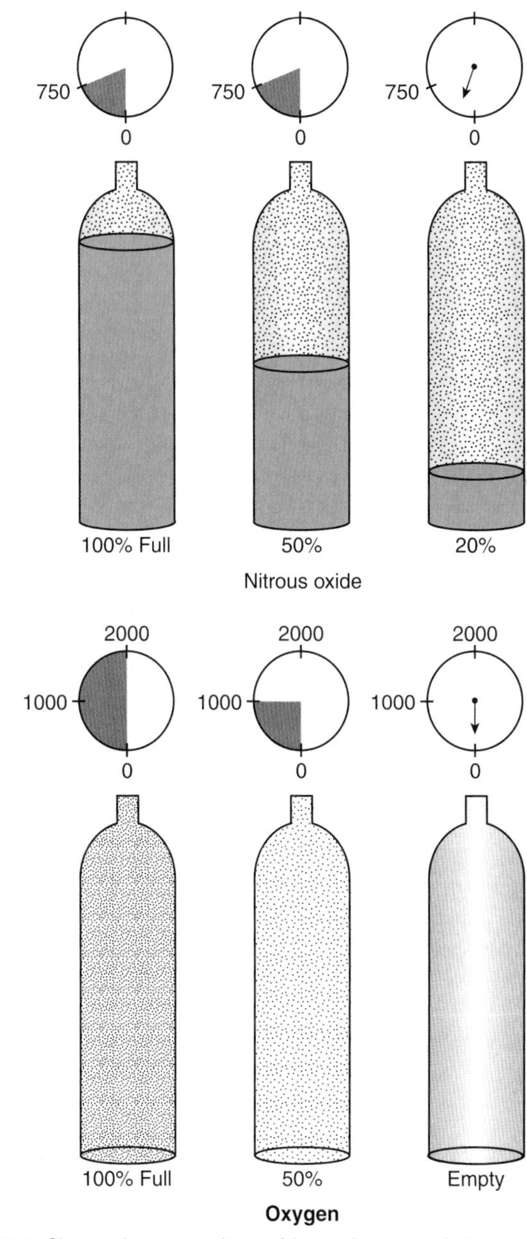

Fig. 15.5 Shows the comparison of how nitrous oxide is stored as a liquid and gas, whereas oxygen is stored solely as gas. (From Clark M, Brunick A: *Handbook of nitrous oxide and oxygen sedation,* ed 4, St Louis, 2015, Elsevier.)

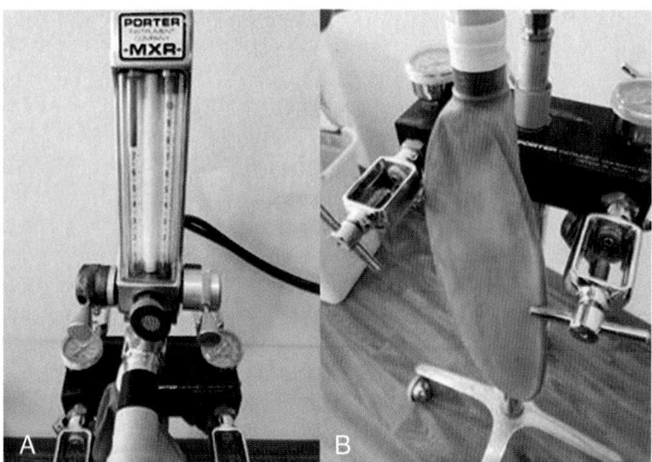

Fig. 15.6 Components of delivery system. (A) Shows the flowmeter, control knobs, pressure gauges, and yokes. (B) Shows the reservoir bag between the yokes.

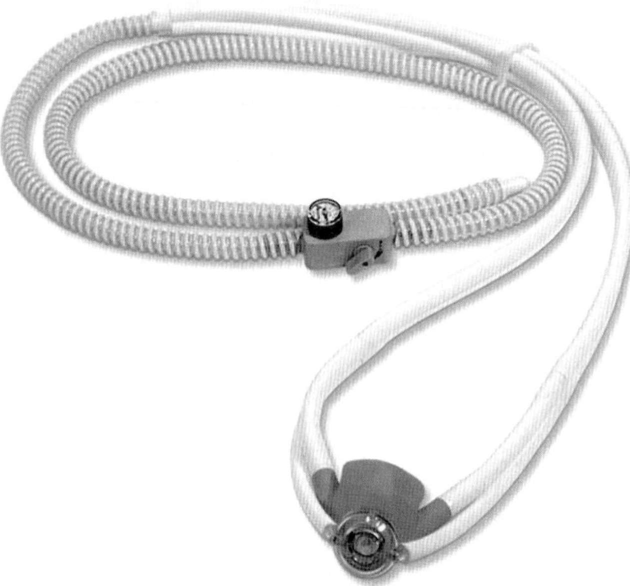

Fig. 15.7 Nasal hood shown attached to the scavenging system. (From Clark M, Brunick A: *Handbook of nitrous oxide and oxygen sedation*, ed 4, St Louis, 2015, Elsevier.)

The nasal hood attaches to the tubing and is the piece of equipment that fits over the patient's nose and is essential for delivering the gases. Nasal hoods come in a variety of sizes, and a proper fit increases the effectiveness of the gases delivered to the patient and decreases the chances of leaks into the surrounding environment. Attached to the nasal unit is an important part of the equipment called the scavenger system (Fig. 15.7). This system removes excess N_2O gas from the immediate area, protecting the clinician. The scavenging unit consists of the control valve and hoses that connect directly to the high-volume evacuation (HVE) system. It is standard that dental units for N_2O/O_2 delivery come equipped with a scavenger system.

Safety Features

Nitrous oxide units available for use in dentistry come with a variety of safety features. First, multiple components of the nitrous delivery unit are color-coded, including the gas cylinders, tubing, pressure gauges, and wall outlets. Green represents O_2 and blue represents N_2O. The

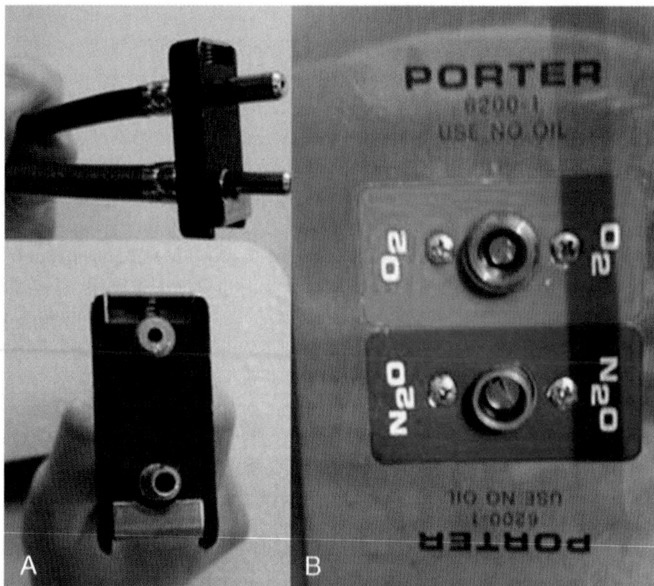

Fig. 15.8 Shows the diameter index safety system that prevents the tubing from being incorrectly connected to the wrong gas. (A) Shows the different diameters of the connectors. (B) The wall outlet is designed to receive the specific diameter of the connector.

diameter index system includes connectors that are intentionally different diameters to ensure that the tubing is connected properly from the delivery unit to the intended wall outlet (Fig. 15.8). Both types of delivery systems typically have an audible alarm to indicate when gases are running low and/or auto-shut off features in the event that O_2 runs out.

ADMINISTRATION

Assemble all armamentarium in preparation for administration (see Procedure 15.1). Confirm that the N_2O delivery system is turned on and/or cylinder tanks are opened. Attach the tubing of the scavenger system to the high volume evacuation (HVE) system. Because nasal hoods come in a variety of sizes, proper size may not be able to be selected until the patient is seated. Ensuring an accurate fit increases patient comfort and success of administration and reduces the chance of leaks.

Complete a medical history including reconciliation of current medications. Obtain vital signs, including blood pressure, pulse, and respiration rate. Additionally, according to the ASA *Practice Guidelines for Non-Anesthesiologists*, a pulse oximeter is required to measure the O_2 saturation of the blood for any patient receiving greater than 50% N_2O, as this is considered more than minimal sedation (Fig. 15.9).[13] A pulse oximeter is an instrument that measures the O_2 saturation of the circulating blood. A typical O_2 saturation level is greater than 95%.[14]

Important Point to Remember

The use of a pulse oximeter is considered a best practice when using N_2O/O_2 and is required at concentrations greater than 50% to assess and continue monitoring a patient during treatment.

Start the flow of O_2 (100%) prior to placing the nasal hood on the patient. This step helps alleviate the patient's worry about not being able to breathe properly once the hood is placed. Place the nasal hood on the patient, allowing the patient to adjust over the nose for a comfortable fit. Check and listen for any leaks around the edge of the hood (Fig. 15.10). Assess the patient's tidal volume in order to determine the

PROCEDURE 15.1 Steps for the Administration of Nitrous Oxide/Oxygen

Step 1 Gather armamentarium and prepare unit for use, including scavenging tubing into high-volume evacuation (HVE) system.

Step 2 Review health history including medication reconciliation. Obtain patient consent.

Step 3 Obtain baseline vital signs, including of oxygen saturation level using a pulse oximeter.

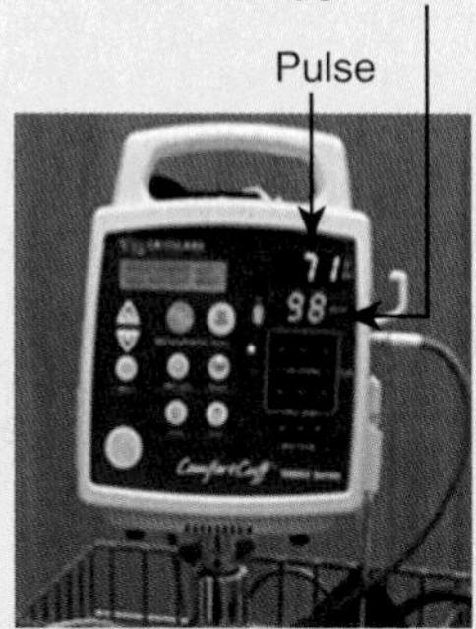

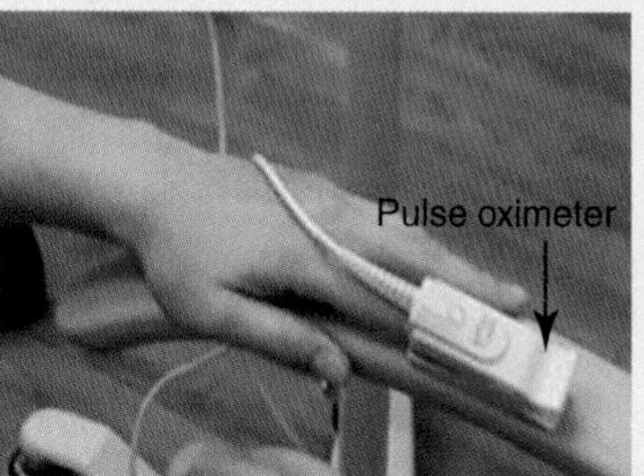

Step 4 Turn on flow of oxygen.

Step 5 Place nasal hood on patient's nose. Allow patient to adjust and hold in place.

Step 6 Assess minute volume and determine flow rate (6–8 L/minute for adults).

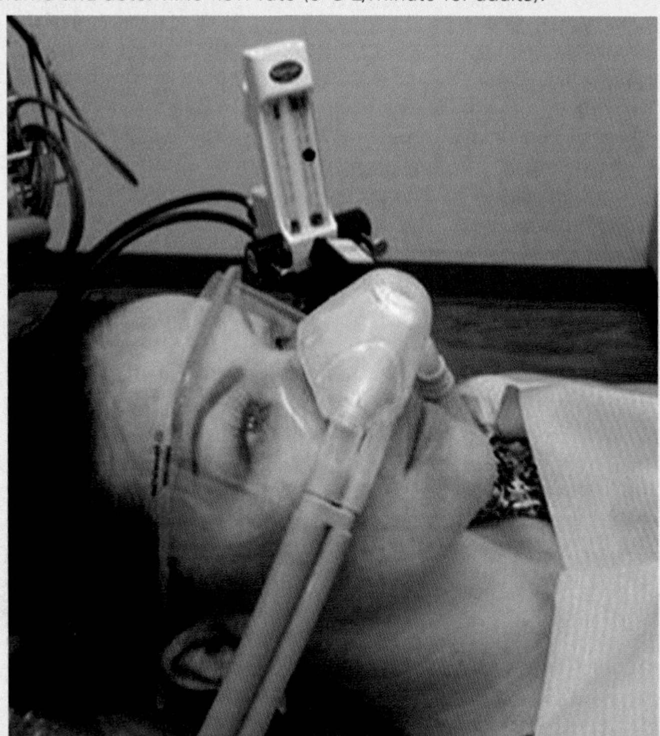

Step 7 Begin titration of nitrous oxide, starting with approximately 20% concentration. (Make a note of time.)

Step 8 Wait 1–2 minutes, and then assess patient signs and symptoms for ideal conscious sedation (see Fig. 15.13).

Step 9 If required, titrate again using increments of 5%–10% over time until ideal level of sedation is reached.

NEVER LEAVE THE PATIENT UNATTENDED DURING ADMINISTRATION.

Step 10 Begin treatment.

Step 11 Upon completion of treatment, turn off the flow of nitrous oxide, leaving only 100% oxygen flowing to the patient.

Step 12 Administer 100% oxygen to the patient for 3–5 minutes or longer if the patient is still feeling effects of N_2O. (Take note of the time.) Ensure postoperative vital signs are comparable to preoperative values.

Step 13 Document procedure and details of administration in the patient's chart (see Box 15.2).

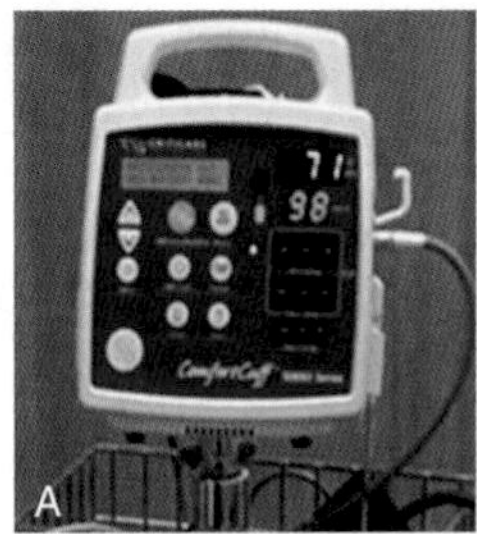
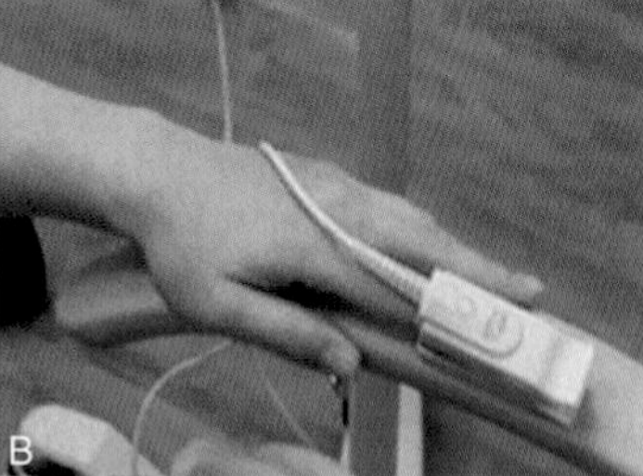

Fig. 15.9 (A) Shows the oxygen saturation of 98%, pulse 71. (B) The pulse oximeter placed on index finger. Leave in place to monitor during the procedure.

total flow rate. Tidal volume is the quantity of air that is inhaled and exhaled during normal respiration. Minute volume is based on the patient's respiration rate per minute. To meet the demands of an average volume, adults will require a flow rate of approximately 6 L to 8 L per minute, and children will range between 4 L and 6 L per minute.

Techniques: Constant Liter Flow Versus Constant Oxygen Flow

Once flow rate has been determined, the administration of N_2O can begin (Fig. 15.11). There are two techniques that can be utilized: the constant liter flow and the constant O_2 technique. With the constant liter flow technique, the total liters of gases being delivered (N_2O and O_2) remains constant. For example, if the total flow rate determined is 7 L/minute, then as the liters of N_2O increase by 1 L/minute, the liters of O_2 will decrease by 1 L/minute. This inverse relationship ensures that the total flow rate remains constant (Fig. 15.12). The constant O_2 technique is used when trying to keep the liters of O_2 constant. N_2O is added until desired effect is reached, but O_2 is *not* decreased. This increases the total flow rate or total liters being administered. For example, if the flow rate determined is 7 L/minute and titration begins with 1 L/minute of N_2O, the total flow rate is now 8 L/minute because, with this technique, the liter of O_2 is not decreased.

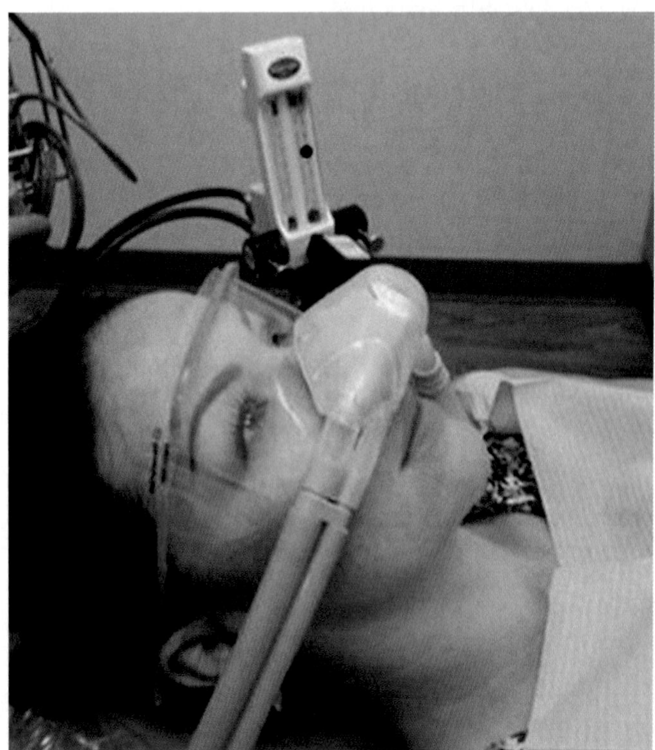

Fig. 15.10 Shows only 100% oxygen flowing. The nasal hood is placed on the patient and assessed to confirm a good fit with no leaks.

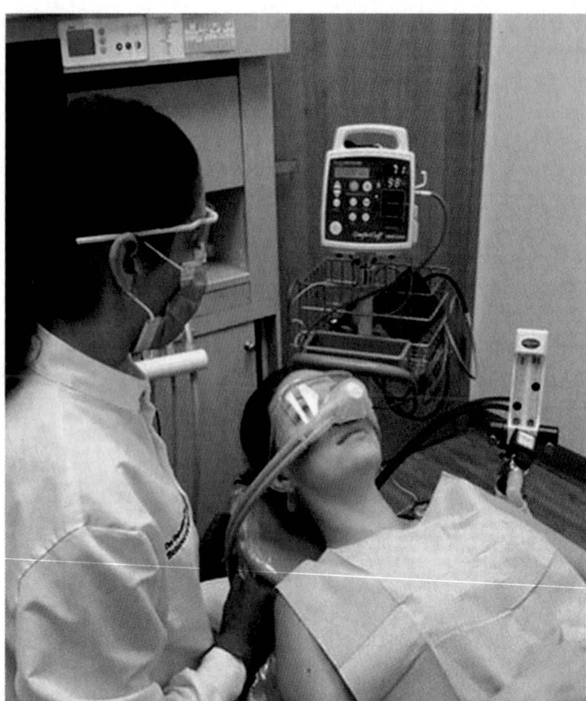

Fig. 15.11 Begin the flow of nitrous oxide (N_2O) using a titration method. Wait 1 to 2 minutes and assess the patient's signs and symptoms. Continue titration of N_2O until the desired level is reached.

Regardless of the technique used, it is the best practice to use a titration technique to administer the N_2O. Titration is the incremental dosing of a drug until the desired effect is reached. This dose should be individualized to the patient, as the effective dose for one patient may not be the same for another and reactions to the agent may vary. The mantra "start low and go slow" applies here, and adhering to the titration principle decreases risk of adverse events. Start with a 20% concentration of N_2O (leaving 80% O_2) and wait approximately 1 to 2 minutes.[6] Continue to titrate and increase dosage in increments of 5% to 10% over time until the ideal level of conscious sedation is reached (Fig. 15.13).

Important Point to Remember

It is important to understand the liters being delivered are not necessarily the percent concentration. For example, 2 L N_2O/minute does not automatically equate to 20% gas concentration.

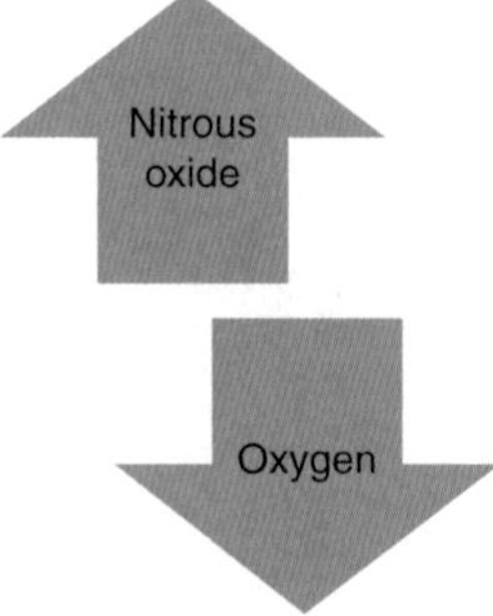

Fig. 15.12 Shows the inverse relationship of the constant liter flow technique. As liter per minute of nitrous oxide (N_2O) increase, equal liter per minute of oxygen (O_2) is decreased, keeping total liter flow rate the same.

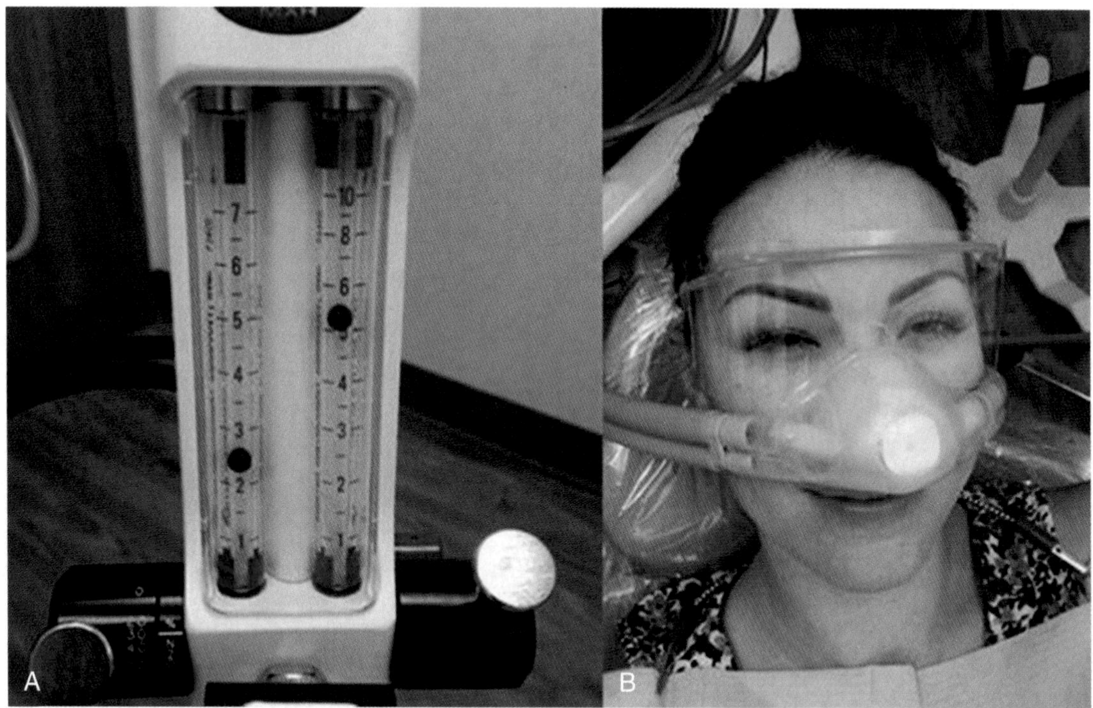

Fig. 15.13 (A) Shows 2.5 L/minute nitrous oxide (N_2O; 31%) and 5.5 L/minute O_2 (oxygen; 69%) being delivered. (B) Patient showing ideal signs, including relaxed, heavy eyes and a smile.

Upon completion of the procedure, terminate the flow of N_2O, leaving on only O_2. Continue to administer a 100% concentration of O_2 until the patient is no longer experiencing signs or symptoms. Typically 3 to 5 minutes is sufficient; however some patients may require more time. This is a valuable step to ensure that a patient is fully recovered from the effects of N_2O. If using N_2O/O_2 just during the local anesthesia injections, placing the patient back on 100% O_2 while waiting for the local anesthesia to take effect may work out perfectly. Take postoperative vital signs and ensure comparable values to those taken preoperatively. This is an objective assessment measure of recovery. Be sure to take note of how much time the patient was back on pure O_2 in order to properly document in the patient's chart.

Calculations

To determine the percentage concentration of the gas, take the liters of gas and divide by the total volume of gases being delivered. Multiply by 100, and this will be the percentage of the concentration of gas delivered.

For example, if a patient is receiving 3 L/min of N_2O and 5 L/min of O_2 = 8 L/min total:

To calculate the % of nitrous oxide delivered: $\frac{3\text{L/min}\,N_2O}{8\text{L/min (both gases)}}$

$3/8 = 0.375 \rightarrow \times 100 = 37.5\%\ N_2O$

To calculate the % of oxygen delivered: $\frac{5\text{L/min}\,O_2}{8\text{L/min (both gases)}}$

$5/8 = 0.625 \rightarrow \times 100 = 62.5\%\ O_2$

EFFECTS OF NITROUS OXIDE

Physiology and Pharmacology

N_2O/O_2 is administered via the nose by inhalation. The gases make their way into the respiratory system by traveling down the trachea and through the left and right bronchi where eventually they reach the air sacs of the alveolus (Fig. 15.14).

As the concentration of N_2O increases in the lungs, the partial pressure increases in alveolus. Partial pressure is the force exerted by a gas. The higher pressure in the alveolus causes diffusion of the N_2O out of the alveolus and into the blood circulation (Fig. 15.15). Nitrous oxide does not bind to hemoglobin and is rapidly transported through circulation.[15]

Upon completion of the procedure, when the patient is returned to a 100% concentration of O_2, the concentration of N_2O becomes greater in the blood than in the lungs. This causes diffusion of the nitrous oxide in the opposite direction going from the blood back into the alveoli of the lungs where a large amount of N_2O can be exhaled.

Signs and Symptoms

It is important that a provider recognize the signs and symptoms of the desired level of sedation (Table 15.3). Minimal sedation may produce lightheadedness, tingling, or numbness of the oral soft tissues, hands, and feet. One major component of minimal sedation is that the protective reflexes remain intact.

It is also extremely important to recognize the signs and symptoms of a heavy level of sedation and/or oversedation (Table 15.4). As patients move into heavy levels of sedation, it may be increasingly difficult for them to keep their mouth or eyes open, and they are less responsive to commands and stimuli. Patients may begin to experience uncontrollable emotions and laugh, cry, or become agitated or irritated. An oversedated patient may feel nauseated or even vomit, tremble, or move uncontrollably, and could potentially lose consciousness.

Important Point to Remember

Though it is referred to as laughing gas, if a patient is laughing uncontrollably, it is a sign of oversedation.

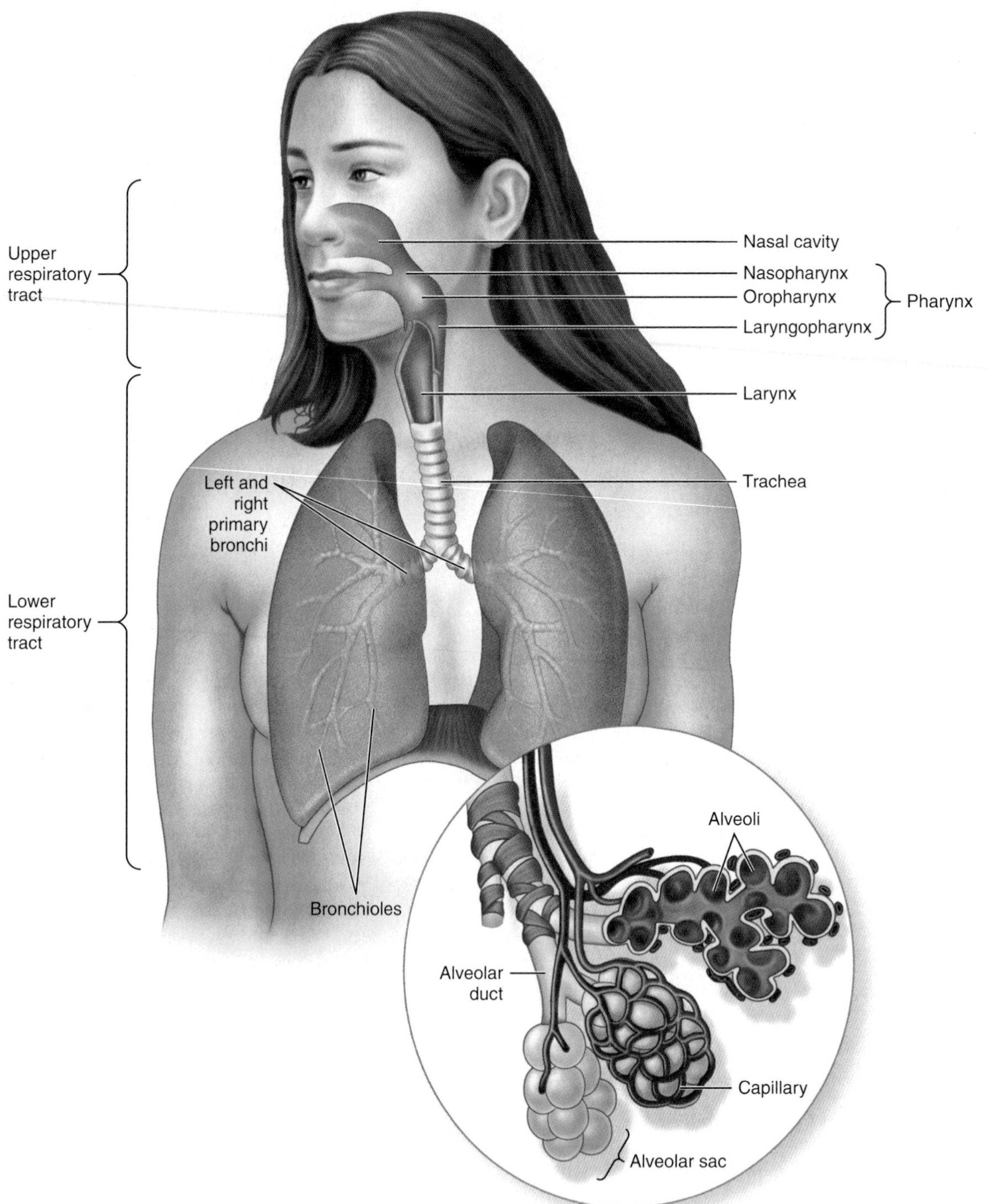

Fig. 15.14 Reviews respiratory anatomy. Nitrous oxide is inhaled via the nose, down through trachea into the bronchi and into alveolar air sacs. (From Malamed S: *Sedation,* ed 5, St Louis, 2018, Elsevier.)

PROFESSIONAL CONSIDERATION

Documentation

Upon completion of the administration of N_2O/O_2, proper documentation is essential. The Current Dental Terminology (CDT) code D9230, "analgesia, inhalation of nitrous oxide," is used to add a charge or send out an insurance claim. Insurance may or may not cover and reimburse for this code, thus patients should be prepared to pay out of pocket for this additional service.

Information regarding the specifics of the appointment should be included in the patient's chart. Health history and vital signs, including O_2 saturation when more than 50% N_2O delivered, must be documented. In the progress note, record the minute volume, the amount of N_2O delivered, and the duration. The amount can be documented using liters per minute or by the percentage concentration of the gases. Also, document the time that the patient was returned back to 100% O_2. Additional information worth noting is the patient's response during the process. Creating a template can save time and prove useful in

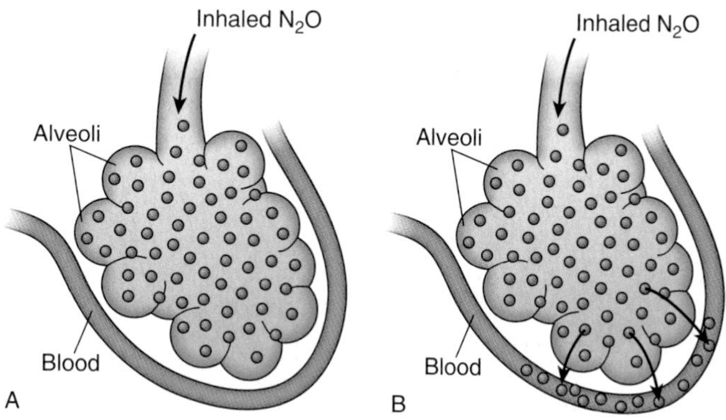

Fig. 15.15 (A) Shows the concentration of nitrous oxide (N_2O) gas increases in alveolus as N_2O is inhaled. (B) Diffusion of N_2O occurs from the air sac and into blood circulation.

TABLE 15.3 Signs and Symptoms of Ideal Sedation

Signs of Ideal Sedation	Symptoms of Ideal Sedation
Able to respond to commands	Lightheadedness or heavy feeling
Slower eye movement	Tingling/numbness of perioral area
Relaxed posture and facial features	Tingling of fingers and toes
	A warm feeling

TABLE 15.4 Signs and Symptoms of Heavy and Oversedation

Heavy Sedation	Oversedation
Sweating	Nausea
Uncontrollable emotions	Vomiting
• Laughter	Loss of consciousness
• Crying	
• Agitation/irritation	
Sleepiness	

TABLE 15.5 Example of Treatment Note After the Administration of Nitrous Oxide/Oxygen

Date	Treatment	Signature
3/17/21	**HH:** Reviewed and updated. Medications: Reviewed—none being taken. Vitals: 132/89 pulse: 90 resp: 18 O_2Sat: 98% **Tx rendered:** NSPT/SRP of UR and LR quadrants. N_2O/O_2 administered to ease moderate anxiety during local anesthesia injections. Flow rate determined: 7 L/minute. Administered: N_2O 3 L/minute (43%) and O_2 4 L/minute (57%) for 13 minutes (or 11:00–11:13). O_2 saturation monitored and maintained at 97% during treatment. Administered 5% lidocaine topical, 2% lidocaine (72 mg), 1:100,000 epinephrine (0.036 mg) for the Rt. PSA, IO, NP, GP, IA, B blocks using 25-gauge long needle and 27-gauge short needle. Upon completion of local anesthesia injections administered 100% O_2 for 5 minutes (or 11:13–11:18). Patient responded well to N_2O/O_2, tolerated local anesthesia injections well.	D Aboytes

order to capture all the necessary information in a clear, organized manner. See Table 15.5 for an example of patient documentation.

Scope Of Practice: N_2O/O_2 Rules and Regulations

In many states, the administration of N_2O/O_2 falls within the scope of practice of the dental hygienist. Educational and clinical requirements vary in each state. However, a dental hygienist allowed to administer N_2O/O_2 in one state may not be able to do so in another state. Additionally levels of dental supervision need to be taken into consideration. It is important to always follow the rules and regulations set per the Dental Practice Act in the state where you are practicing.

DENTAL HYGIENE CONSIDERATIONS

- Nitrous oxide is always used in combination with oxygen.
- Nitrous oxide serves as both an anxiolytic and analgesic agent, making it a great option to assist in the management of pain, fear, and anxiety associated with dental treatment.
- The level of sedation a dental hygienist needs for procedures in their scope is different than the level needed by a dentist or a dental anesthesiologist operating in an ambulatory surgical center.
- Minimal sedation, defined as less than 50% N_2O, is the first stage in the continuum, and many dental hygiene procedures can be completed in this level.
- Upon completion of treatment, administer a 100% concentration of oxygen to the patient until the patient is no longer experiencing signs or symptoms and postoperative vital sign values are within an acceptable range of preoperative values.

CASE STUDY 15.1 Complications From the Administration of Nitrous Oxide

Your patient today informs you that she is fine with the deep cleaning but is scared of "the shots." You discuss the use of nitrous oxide/oxygen (N_2O/O_2) with the patient, and she is willing to try it. You begin administering 45% N_2O, and 2 minutes upon delivery of N_2O/O_2, the patient reports feeling lightheaded and her lips are tingling. Then, 15 minutes into the procedure, the patient is no longer responding to your voice and appears to have fallen asleep. With a stern shake, you are able to wake her, and she tells you that she is beginning to feel nauseated.

Critical Thinking Questions:

- What is the first course of action?
- At what point is a deeper level of sedation noted?
- What could have been done to prevent this event?

CHAPTER REVIEW QUESTIONS

1. Who did the American Dental Association consider the discoverer of anesthesia?
   A. Horace Wells
   B. Humphrey Davy
   C. G.V. Black
   D. Joseph Priestly
2. Which of the following is the molecular formula for nitrous oxide?
   A. N_2
   B. N_2O_2
   C. N_2O
   D. N_2O/O_2
3. All of the following are considered signs or symptoms of an ideal level of sedation EXCEPT one. Which one is the EXCEPTION?
   A. Tingling fingers
   B. Relaxed muscle tone
   C. Uncontrolled laughter
   D. Numbness of lips
4. Which of the following terms describes the incremental dosing of a drug until the desired effect is reached?
   A. Hypoxia
   B. Titration
   C. Oximeter
   D. Continuum
5. Which of the following parts of the delivery system is responsible for reducing the amount of nitrous oxide in the operatory and exposure to the clinician?
   A. Reservoir bag
   B. Flowmeter
   C. Nasal hood
   D. Scavenging system
6. If the total flow rate delivered is 6 L/minute, and the patient is being delivered 2 L/minute of nitrous oxide (N_2O), what is the concentration of N_2O being delivered?
   A. 28.5%
   B. 66.6%
   C. 50.1%
   D. 33.3%
7. The use of which of the following is considered a best practice to measure the oxygen saturation in the blood when concentrations are greater than 50%?
   A. Scavenging system
   B. Pulse oximeter
   C. Flowmeter
   D. Yokes
8. What is the typical color of the nitrous oxide gas cylinder?
   A. Blue
   B. Green
   C. Yellow
   D. Black
9. Which of the following is considered a relative contraindication to the administration of N_2O?
   A. First trimester of pregnancy
   B. Moderate level of anxiety
   C. A hypersensitive gag reflex
   D. Inability to tolerate a long appointment
10. Which of the following concentrations of N_2O is considered more than minimal sedation?
    A. 20%
    B. 25%
    C. 45%
    D. 55%
11. Which of the following statements is true regarding completion of the procedure and termination of the flow of N_2O?
    A. A patient should be placed on 100% oxygen for a minimum of 3 to 5 minutes.
    B. The 100% oxygen is not a necessary step.
    C. It is better to go straight to ambient room air.
    D. Let the patient decide whether he or she would like if oxygen is desired at the end.
12. Which of the following characteristics is true of N_2O?
    A. Allergenic
    B. Flammable
    C. Highly potent
    D. Colorless
13. During which level of sedation can a patient begin to feel the anxiolytic effects of N_2O?
    A. Moderate
    B. Minimal
    C. Deep
    D. General
14. The administration of N_2O/O_2 is considered what type of sedation?
    A. Oral sedation
    B. Intravenous sedation
    C. Inhalation sedation
    D. Unconscious sedation
15. Most dental hygiene procedures can be completed under which level of sedation?
    A. Minimal
    B. Moderate

C. Deep
D. General

16. Which of the following should be documented in the patient's health record after the administration of N_2O/O_2?
A. Pre- and postoperative vital signs
B. Duration of time nitrous oxide is administered
C. Reaction of the patient
D. All of the above

17. Nitrous oxide is considered a high-potency drug. It especially works great on patients with severe dental anxiety and dental phobia.
A. The first statement is true, and the second statement is false.
B. The first statement is false, and the second statement is true.
C. Both statements are true.
D. Both statements are false.

18. Which of the following is the code that can be used to charge a patient or submit a claim for nitrous oxide administration?
A. D9230
B. D9430
C. D1110
D. D4381

19. Which of the following terms describes the amount of air passing into and out of lungs during normal respiration?
A. Titration
B. Tidal volume
C. Hypoxia
D. Analgesia

20. Which of the following is considered normal blood oxygen saturation as measured by pulse oximeter?
A. 97%
B. 85%
C. 75%
D. 70%

REFERENCES

1. Satuito M, Tom J. Potent inhalational anesthetics for dentistry. *Anesth Prog.* 2016;63(1):42–49. doi:10.2344/0003-3006-63.1.42.
2. Jacobsohn PH. What others said about Wells. *J Am Dent Assoc.* 1994;125(12):1583–1584.
3. Menczer LF, Mittleman M, Wildsmith JA. Horace Wells. *J Am Dent Assoc.* 1985;110:773.
4. Andrews E. The oxygen mixture, a new anæsthetic combination. *Am J Dent Sci.* 1869;2(9):440–446.
5. Brunick A, Clark M. Nitrous oxide and oxygen sedation: an update. *Dent Assist.* 2010;79(4):22–23, 26, 28–30; quiz 32, 34. PMID 20853735.
6. Clark M, Brunick A. *Handbook of nitrous oxide and oxygen sedation.* ed 4. St. Louis: Elsevier; 2015.
7. Malamed S. *Sedation: A guide to patient management.* ed 6. St. Louis: Elsevier; 2018.
8. National Center for Biotechnology Information. PubChem Database. Nitrous oxide, CID =948. https://pubchem.ncbi.nlm.nih.gov.compound/nitrous-oxide.
9. American Society of Anesthesiologists. Continuum of depth of sedation: definition of general anesthesia and levels of sedation/analgesia. Last amended October 2019. www.asahq.org/standards-and-guidelines/continuum-of-depth-of-sedation-definition-of-general-anesthesia-and-levels-of-sedationanalgesia.
10. Kapur A, Kapur V. Conscious sedation in dentistry. *Ann Maxillofac Surg.* 2018;8(2):320–323.
11. Chidiac JJ, Chamseddine L, Bellos G. Gagging prevention using nitrous oxide or table salt: a comparative pilot study. *Int J Prosthet.* 2001;14:364.
12. Bowen DM, Pieren JA. *Darby and Walsh dental hygiene: theory and practice.* ed 5. St. Louis: Elsevier; 2020.
13. American Society of Anesthesiologists Task Force on Sedation and Analgesia by Non-Anesthesiologists. Practice guidelines for sedation and analgesia by non-anesthesiologists. *Anesthesiology.* 2002;96:1004–1017.
14. Hafen BB, Sharma S. *Oxygen saturation.* [Updated June 2, 2019.] Treasure Island, FL: StatPearls Publishing; 2020. https://www.ncbi.nlm.nih.gov/books/NBK525974/.
15. Becker D, Rosenburg M. Nitrous oxide and the inhalation anesthetic. *Anesth Prog.* 2008;55(4):124–130.

PART 5

Complications, Risk Management, and Exposure Prevention

CHAPTER 16 Local Complications, 347

CHAPTER 17 Systemic Complications and Emergency Management, 362

CHAPTER 18 Risk Management and Exposure Prevention, 377

16

Local Complications

Demetra Daskalos Logothetis, RDH, MS

LEARNING OBJECTIVES

1. Define local anesthetic complications and describe the three primary categories for local anesthetic complications.
2. Discuss the possible complications (as well as management and prevention) of local anesthetic administration, such as needle breakage, pain during injection, burning during injection, hematoma, transient facial paralysis, paresthesia, trismus, infection, edema, soft tissue trauma, postanesthetic intraoral lesions, and sloughing of tissue.

INTRODUCTION

Local anesthetics allow dentistry to be practiced without patient discomfort. Serious complications associated with the use of these drugs are rare. However, regardless of appropriate preanesthetic patient assessment, effective patient communication, and use of proper technique according to all the recommended guidelines and procedures prior to the administration of the local anesthetic agent, localized and systemic responses to anesthetic injections may still occur. **Localized complications** occur in the region of the injection and can be attributed to the anesthetic needle, administration technique, and/or anesthetic drug administered (Table 16.1). **Systemic complications** (see Chapter 17) are attributed to the drug administered. According to Bennett, there are three primary categories for local anesthetic complications.[1]

1. **Primary complication** such as burning during the injection, is experienced by the patient at the time of the injection. For example, the patient experiences the burning sensation at the time of drug administration.
2. **Secondary complication** is apparent after the injection is completed. It is caused by the injection of the local anesthetic drug, but it is experienced shortly after the injection or later. Secondary complications can be either mild or severe.
   - **Mild complications** resolve without requiring treatment. For example, burning during injection is temporary and resolves shortly after the deposition of the agent.
   - **Severe complications** require a plan of treatment to resolve the complication. For example, anaphylaxis requires immediate treatment and drug intervention.
3. Transient or permanent
   - **Transient complications** may appear severe at the time of their observance but will eventually resolve without any residual effect. For example, a hematoma may cause severe swelling and bruising, but will resolve over time without leaving any residual effects.
   - **Permanent complications** leave a residual effect. For example, nerve damage associated with the inferior alveolar (IA) block may last a few weeks, months, or indefinitely.

LOCAL COMPLICATIONS

See Table 16.2 for a summary of local complications, prevention, and management.

Needle Breakage

Reported incidences of accidental breakage of disposable stainless steel needles are uncommon and are usually reported when thinner 30-gauge needles are used (see Chapter 9).[2,3] The most common cause of needle breakage is from sudden unexpected movement of the patient during the injection or poor technique by applying excessive lateral pressure on the needle. A needle that is deeply embedded into tissue increases the risk, and, when it is broken, the needle fragment is more difficult to retrieve. If the end of the needle fragment remains outside the mucosa, it is readily retrievable with a hemostat, and no emergency exists. However, if the needle fragment is embedded in the tissue, it is extremely difficult to remove and will most likely require specialized radiographic and surgical procedures to locate and remove, usually by an oral maxillofacial surgeon (Fig. 16.1). Needle fragments that remain encased in scar tissue may be better left untouched because a difficult surgical procedure is required for removal.

Prevention of Needle Breakage

Patient communication. Effective communication by the dental hygienist to the patient before administration of the local anesthetic drug may help alleviate the patient's fear of the unknown and could significantly reduce the possibility of sudden unexpected movements by the patient. The dental hygienist should thoroughly explain the procedure before the injection is administered and continue the communication throughout the procedure, helping the patient anticipate the dental hygienist's actions.

Long, large-gauge needle. Long 25-gauge needles should be used when penetrating significant soft tissue because they are less likely to break than thinner, smaller-gauge needles. Documented incidences of needle breakage have been reported mainly when using 30-gauge, and occasionally 27-gauge, needles.[1,2]

Do not bend needle. Bending the needle weakens its integrity, increasing the possibility of breakage. All intraoral injections can be

TABLE 16.1 Local Complications

Complications Associated With the Anesthetic Needle or Administration Technique	Complications Associated With the Anesthetic Agent
Broken needle	Burning during injection
Pain during injection	Edema
Burning during injection	Infection
Hematoma	Soft tissue injuries
Transcient facial paralysis	Tissue sloughing
Paresthesia	
Trismus	
Infection	
Edema	
Postanesthetic intraoral lesions	

performed successfully without bending the needle. Bending the needle also prevents the proper recapping of the needle (see Chapters 9 and 11), increasing the likelihood of postexposure. The Occupational Health and Safety Administration (OSHA) bloodborne pathogens standard [29 CFR 1910.1030(d)(2)(vii)(A)] states that contaminated needles and other contaminated sharps shall not be bent, recapped, or removed unless the employer can demonstrate that no alternative is feasible or that such action is required by a specific medical or dental procedure. Standard [1910.1030(d)(2)(vii)(B)] states that such bending, recapping, or needle removal must be accomplished through the use of a mechanical device or a one-handed technique.

Advance needle slowly. Slow advancement of the needle results in gentle contact of the bone, decreasing the possibility of needle breakage. In addition, sudden forceful bone contact may startle the patient, causing sudden unexpected movement.

TABLE 16.2 Local Complications Associated With the Administration of Local Anesthetics

Complication	Causes	Prevention	Management
Needle breakage	Sudden, unexpected movement Poor technique	Patient communication Long large-gauge needle Do not bend needle Advance needle slowly Never force needle No sudden direction changes, only change needle directions when needle is almost completely withdrawn from tissue Never insert to hub	Remain calm Keep hands in patient's mouth to prevent closure Remove needle fragment if visible Refer to oral and maxillofacial surgeon if unable to retrieve the complete needle length Document incident
Pain during injection	Careless technique Dull needle Barbed needle Traumatizing bone Rapid deposit	Use proper technique Sharp needles Topical anesthetic Sterile anesthetics Inject slowly Room temperature agent	Effective communication Reassure patient that pain is only temporary
Burning during injection	Normal response to acidic local anesthetic agent deposited into normal physiologic pH of the tissue Contamination of local anesthetics Heated anesthetic Expired agent Rapid deposit	Never store in disinfecting solution Store at room temperature Check expiration date Do not use cartridge warmers Inject slowly Consider buffering the local anesthetic	Reassure patient that burning will last only a few seconds
Hematoma	Inadvertent puncturing of a blood vessel Overinsertion of needle during PSA block Improper technique Multiple needle insertions	Short 25-gauge needle for PSA Know dental anatomy Modify injection technique for patient size Minimize the number of needle insertions Maintain proper technique	Swelling; apply direct pressure Apply ice to the region; warm packs the next day Discuss possibility of soreness and limited movement to patient Instruct patient that swelling and discoloration will disappear after 7–14 days Dismiss patient when bleeding has stopped
Transient facial paralysis	Inadvertent deposition of local anesthetic in parotid salivary gland during IA block or V-A block Parotid salivary gland is located on the posterior border of the mandibular ramus and seventh cranial or facial nerve travels through gland Temporary loss of function of muscles of facial expression due to anesthesia of innervating facial nerve	Use proper technique for IA or V-A blocks Contact bone on the medial surface of the mandibular ramus before depositing agent for the IA block Redirect barrel of syringe more posteriorly if bone is not contacted for the IA block Control depth of needle at not more than 25 mm for the V-A block; less for smaller adults Avoid flexible 30-gauge needles	Reassure patient that paralysis is temporary and will last only a few hours Ask patient to remove contact lenses if applicable Close eyelid manually Arrange for patient transportation home Document

TABLE 16.2 **Local Complications Associated With the Administration of Local Anesthetics (*Cont.*)**

Complication	Causes	Prevention	Management
Paresthesia	Irritation to nerve after injection of contaminated agent (less nerve fascia) Edema places pressure on nerve Trauma, electrical shock, or even hemorrhage around nerve sheath Higher concentrations of local anesthetic agent may increase risk for paresthesia Controversy on role of articaine	Store dental cartridges properly Avoid placing cartridges in disinfectant solution Use proper technique: Do not move needle around in deep tissue and change needle directions when needle is almost completely withdrawn from tissue Consider the risks verses the benefits of using 4% anesthetic agents Consider use of alternative nerve blocks (G-G or VA) to IA block if needed	Reassure patient Arrange examination with dentist Consultation with oral and maxillofacial surgeon Record incident Inform insurance carrier of incident
Trismus	Trauma to muscles in infratemporal space Multiple needle insertions Using contaminated needles Depositing contaminated agent Depositing large amounts of agent in restricted areas Hemorrhage Low-grade infection	Store anesthetic properly Use sharp, sterile, needles Use appropriate injection technique Use minimal amount of agent Deposit agent slowly	Arrange for exam from dentist if needed Heat therapy Jaw exercises Severe pain or increased level of inflammation, treat as an infection If pain and loss of function persist despite the recommended therapy refer the patient to an oral and maxillofacial surgeon for consultation Record incident
Infection	Contamination of the anesthetic needle before injection Improper handling of local anesthetic Administration of contaminated agent Improper tissue preparation Administering local anesthetics through areas of dental infection (needle tract)	Use sterile needles Sheathe needle before and immediately after injection Be aware of the location of the uncovered needle at all times to prevent contaminating the needle Use appropriate infection control protocols Store anesthetic properly Wipe off diaphragm Topical antiseptic Do not administer local anesthetics through areas of dental infection	Treat initially as trismus; if patient does not respond in 3 days, systemic antibiotic therapy may be prescribed by patient's dentist or physician
Edema	Trauma during injection Administration of contaminated agent Hemorrhage Infection Allergic response; may produce airway obstruction	Appropriate infection control Appropriate technique Adequate preanesthetic assessment	Usually resolves within several days without any required treatment Edema caused by infection may require systemic antibiotic therapy prescribed by patient's dentist or physician
Soft tissue injuries	Lips, tongue, cheeks traumatized by patient while numb Typically seen in children and in special needs patients	Select anesthetic with appropriate duration for treatment Warn patient not to eat, drink hot fluids, or test anesthesia by biting Instruct parent or guardian of danger Place cotton rolls between teeth and soft tissue Warning stickers can be used to remind patient and guardian of dangers associated with being numb Consider administering phentolamine mesylate to reverse anesthetic	Analgesics for pain Recommend warm saline rinses to decrease swelling and discomfort Natural oils can be used to coat the lips to minimize discomfort Systemic antibiotic therapy may be prescribed by patient's dentist or physician
Tissue sloughing	Prolonged use of topical anesthetics Sterile abscess may develop after prolonged ischemia, usually on palate caused by vasoconstrictor	Use topical agent for only 1–2 minutes and in a small area Avoid high concentrations of vasoconstrictors	Usually requires no treatment unless prolonged with sterile abscess formation that will need incision and drainage
Postanesthetic intraoral lesions	Trauma to area of injection	Use appropriate administration techniques	Topical anesthetic agents or pastes for discomfort

G-G, Gow-Gates; *IA*, inferior alveolar; *PSA*, posterior superior alveolar; *V-A*, Vazirani-Akinosi.

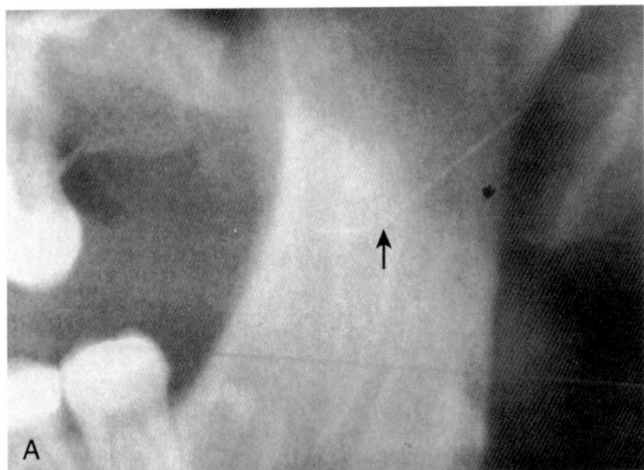

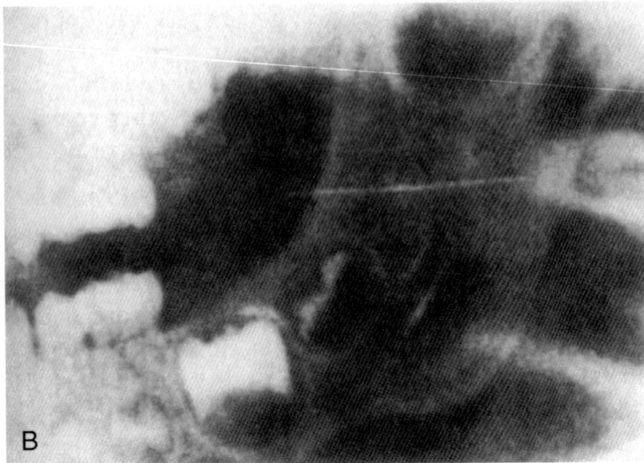

Fig. 16.1 (A) Radiograph of a broken dental needle (note bend in needle). (From Malamed S: *Handbook of local anesthesia,* ed 7, St Louis, 2020, Elsevier.). (B) Radiograph of a broken dental needle in the pterygomandibular space. (From Marks RB, Carlton DM, McDonald S: Management of a broken needle in the pterygomandibular space report of a case, *J Am Dent Assoc* 109:263–264, 1984.)

Never force needle. The needle should never be forced against significant resistance such as bone.

No sudden direction changes. Direction changes of the needle may be indicated during certain injections such as the IA block. Changes in needle direction should never be initiated when the needle is inserted deeply in soft tissue. The needle should be withdrawn almost completely and then redirected (see Chapter 13). Use caution when injecting younger, immature children or extremely anxious adult patients as they are more likely to move unexpectedly during the injection.

Never insert needle to hub. The most vulnerable part of the needle is at the hub, and it is the location where most needle breakages are likely to occur. Inserting the needle to the hub increases the risk for breakage in this area and makes it virtually impossible to retrieve the needle. To increase the chances of retrieving a needle fragment, a portion of the needle's shaft in front of the hub should always be visible during the injection.

Management of Needle Breakage

Needle fragment visible. If needle breakage occurs and the needle fragment is visible, the following are recommendations for the dental hygienist to follow:

1. Remain calm. If the patient senses panic, he or she will close the mouth, causing the needle fragment to embed into the tissue.
2. Keep one's hands in the patient's mouth to prevent closure and ask the patient to continue to open widely.
3. If the needle fragment is visible, attempt to remove it with the hemostat or cotton pliers.

Needle fragment not visible. If the needle fragment is not visible and cannot be retrieved, the following are recommendations for the dental hygienist to follow:

1. Remain calm and inform the patient of the incident in a manner that will alleviate his or her fear and apprehension.
2. The dental hygienist, in consultation with the dentist, should immediately refer the patient to an oral maxillofacial surgeon for consultation and possible further treatment.
3. Document the incident and sequence of events in the patient's permanent record. It is important to include the patient's reaction to the situation.
4. Keep the remaining needle fragment for structural evaluation.
5. Surgical procedures are indicated if the needle fragment is not deeply embedded in tissue and easily located by radiographic or clinical examination.
6. If the needle is deeply embedded in tissue, the oral maxillofacial surgeon may recommend that the needle remain in the tissue without further attempt for removal. Needles that are embedded and not removed are reported to develop fibrous connective tissue or scars around them that restrict the migration of the needle fragment, but in rare instances they may migrate. Broken needle fragments that are left within the patient's soft tissue are more likely to progress to litigation.[3]

Pain During Injection

As discussed in Chapter 1, patients' reactions to pain may vary according to their pain reaction thresholds.[4] Therefore, it is impossible for the dental hygienist to ensure that every injection will be pain-free. However, it is the dental hygienist's responsibility to make every effort to take the necessary precautions to prevent pain during injection. Pain during administration of local anesthetics may be caused by several reasons: careless technique, a dull needle, a barbed needle caused during manufacturing, traumatizing bone, and rapid deposition of the anesthetic agent. The following recommendations will help reduce pain during injection.

Proper Technique

The dental hygienist should adhere to the proper techniques discussed in Chapters 11, 12, and 13. Carefully following the recommended guidelines will decrease patient discomfort and strengthen the patient's confidence in the practitioner. This allows future dental appointments requiring anesthesia to be less stressful on the patient and the practitioner.

Sharp Needles

Dull needles cause pain on insertion, a situation usually caused by repeated injections using the same needle. For most dental hygiene procedures requiring anesthesia, several injections are administered to achieve the necessary anesthesia. Therefore it is essential that the needle be changed after three to four needle insertions.

Topical Anesthetic

Applying topical anesthetic for 1 to 2 minutes before the injection will block the free nerve endings supplying the mucosal surfaces. This procedure will significantly reduce the pain caused by needle insertion.

Anesthetics Placed in Disinfecting Solution

Anesthetics that have been placed in disinfecting solution or have been frozen will cause burning and pain during the injection. Anesthetic cartridges should never be placed in disinfecting solution. The dental hygienist should carefully evaluate every cartridge before the syringe is set up to ensure that no large bubbles are present and that the rubber stopper is intact and does not show any signs of contamination. If the cartridge contains large bubbles or the rubber stopper is extruded, the cartridge should not be used and should be discarded (see Chapter 9).

Inject Slowly

Injecting the anesthetic slowly during the injection is one of the most valuable methods to reduce pain. It prevents the tissue from tearing and improves patient comfort. Because the anesthetic agent is more acidic than the patient's tissue, the patient will also feel stinging when the anesthetic is administered. To decrease or avoid this sensation, the anesthetic agent should be deposited slowly at a rate of 1 mL of agent per minute.

Room Temperature Agents

Anesthetic cartridges should be stored in a dark place at room temperature in their original containers. Cartridge warmers should not be used.

Burning During Injection

The patient may experience a commonly occurring burning sensation during the deposition of the anesthetic agent, usually caused by the local anesthetic agent and the vasoconstrictor being more acidic than the patient's tissue. The burning sensation only lasts a few seconds until anesthesia manifests and does not last after the anesthetic wears off.

However, more severe burning sensations may be caused by other factors not related to the usual short-term response of the anesthetic being deposited into the tissue. These factors include contaminated agent, heated cartridges, expired agent, and too rapid deposition of the agent into tissue. Responses to these factors may result in postanesthetic trismus, edema, and possibly paresthesia.

Prevention of Burning During Injection

To prevent normal burning during injection due to the pH of the vasoconstrictor, as well as abnormal burning sensation during the injection, the dental hygienist should adhere to the following guidelines:

- Never store cartridges in disinfecting solution; always store in a dark place at room temperature.
- Check expiration date; discard outdated agents.
- Do not use cartridge warmers.
- Inject slowly at a rate of 1 mL of agent per minute, taking approximately 2 minutes for an entire cartridge.
- Consider buffering the local anesthetic agent to decrease the normal burning sensation during the administration of the local anesthetic (see Chapters 3 and 9).

Hematoma

A hematoma develops when a blood vessel, particularly an artery, is punctured or lacerated by the needle. This is observed as asymmetric swelling and discoloration of the tissue resulting from the effusion of blood into extravascular spaces (Fig. 16.2).

Although hematomas may appear serious, the lesions are usually just a cosmetic nuisance. Trismus and mild pain may also occur. Hematomas can occur without a positive aspiration, by nicking a blood vessel with the needle during the pathway to the target location, or while removing the needle after the anesthetic has been deposited. And in most cases positive aspirations do not produce hematomas and only result in unnoticeable slight leakage of blood in the tissue.[3-5]

Hematomas particularly result after administration of a posterior superior alveolar (PSA) block caused by overinsertion of the needle that traumatized the pterygoid plexus of veins or even the nearby maxillary artery (Fig. 16.2A–B). Additionally, a hematoma resulting from a PSA block is usually the largest because of the infratemporal fossa being able to accommodate large volumes of blood that clinically appears as extraoral bruising. However, the IA nerve block also commonly cause hematomas (Fig. 16.2C). Hematomas occur less often after an infraorbital (IO) block because pressure is applied to the foramen immediately after the injection.[3] Hematomas are least likely to develop after palatal blocks. Hematomas resulting from an IA block appear most commonly as intraoral bruising but may also demonstrate as extraoral bruising (Fig. 16.2C).

Prevention of Hematoma

Although hematomas can occur even when proper technique is used, to decrease the risk, the dental hygienist should follow these guidelines:

1. Know dental anatomy as to where major blood vessels are located near the target areas for nerve blocks.
2. Screen patient for any medically compromised conditions involving the vascular system, such as anticlotting medications and anemia.
3. Minimize the number of needle insertions by using nerve blocks instead of supraperiosteal injections and carefully planning dental hygiene treatment (see Chapter 11).
4. Follow all recommended injection techniques for all local anesthetic injections, such as performing aspiration(s) with the syringe for most injections.
5. Always use a short needle and possibly modify the needle insertion depth using a more conservative technique for the PSA block for children, small adults, and patients with smaller facial characteristics as discussed in Chapters 12 and 14.

Management of Hematoma

1. At the first sign of swelling, apply pressure directly to the area for a minimum of 2 minutes. This involves the medial aspect of the mandibular ramus for the IA block and the mental foramen for the mental or incisive block. And because it is difficult to locate the blood vessels for the PSA block, pressure should be applied intraorally as far posterior as possible without getting near the soft palate and producing a gag reflex.
2. Apply ice to the region of the developing hematoma to reduce the swelling. Ice will constrict the blood vessels, decreasing the effusion of blood into the extravascular spaces, and also provide some analgesic effects for the patient.
3. Communicate to the patient that soreness and limited movement of their jaw may occur. Instruct the patient to use warm moist towels applied to the region the next day for 20 minutes every hour to assist in the resorption of blood. This will also provide comfort to the patient should soreness occur.
4. Be sure to inform the patient that there are generally no serious complications associated with hematomas, and that swelling and discoloration should disappear after 7 to 14 days. Dental hygiene treatment should resume after the swelling and discoloration have disappeared.
5. Do not dismiss the patient until bleeding has stopped. Document the incident in the patient's record, including instructions presented to the patient and the patient's response.
6. Follow up as indicated.

Transient Facial Paralysis

Transient facial paralysis can be caused by the inadvertent deposition of local anesthetic agent during the IA block, as well as the Vazirani-Akinosi (V-A) block, into the deeper parotid salivary gland located at

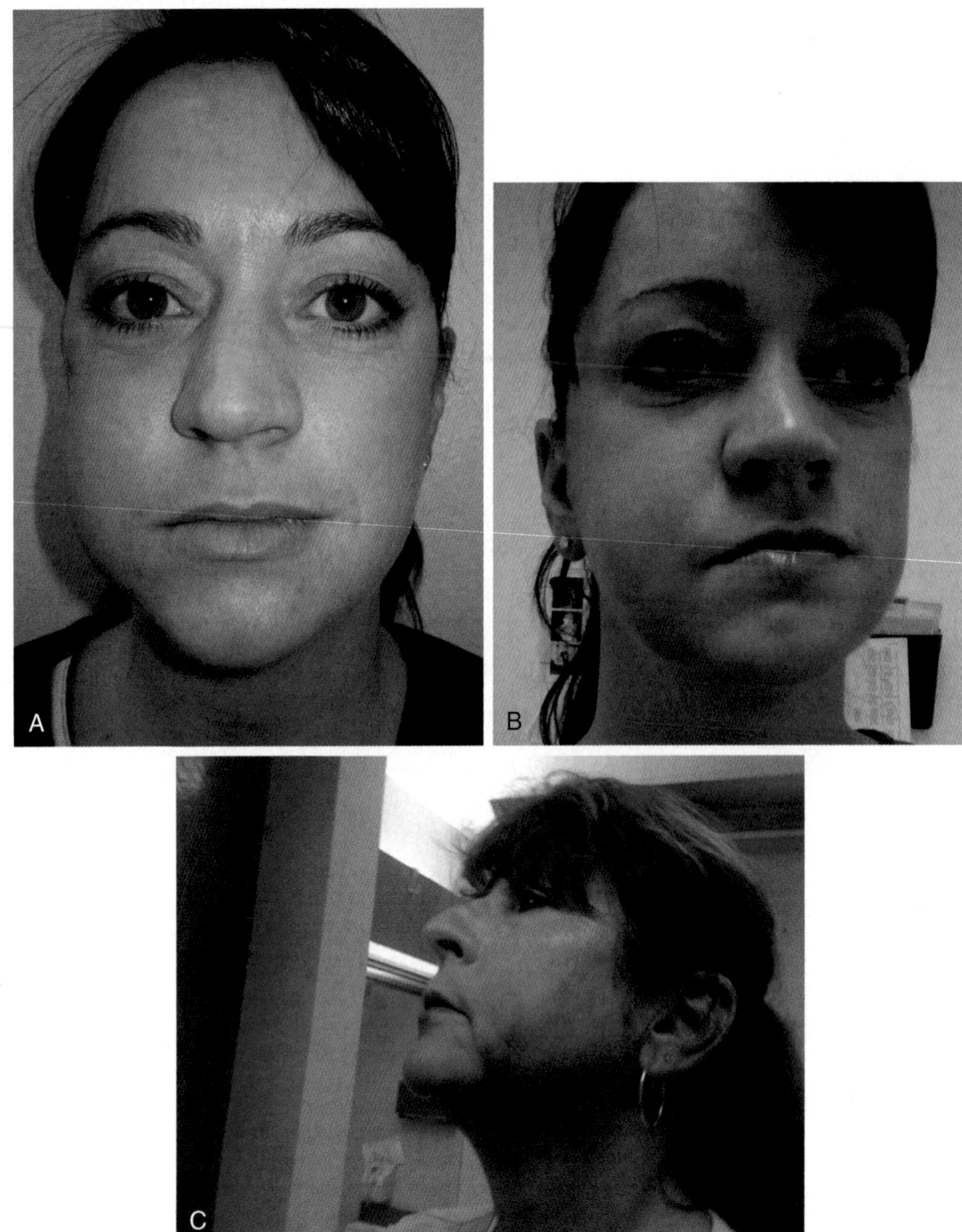

Fig. 16.2 (A) Hematoma producing initial swelling from administration of the right posterior superior alveolar block. (B) Progression of the same hematoma 1 week after initial swelling. (C) Hematoma producing extraoral bruising from the administration of an inferior alveolar block.

the posterior border of the mandibular ramus, anesthetizing the seventh cranial or facial nerve that travels through the parotid salivary gland (Fig. 16.3). This is caused by overinsertion of the needle, which then penetrates the parotid salivary gland. Shortly after the inadvertent deposition of agent into the parotid salivary gland, the patient will experience a weakening of the muscles of facial expression on the injection side and lack of anesthesia of the IA nerve. This finally produces a unilateral loss of motor function to the muscles of facial expression.

The loss of motor function is temporary and fades within a few hours once the action of the local anesthetic resolves. During this time, the patient will be unable to use these facial muscles and will have a lopsided appearance (Fig. 16.4); the corneal reflex remains functional and continues to produce tears to lubricate the eye, but the eye may need to be manually closed after any contact lenses have been removed.

Prevention of Transient Facial Paralysis

To prevent inadvertent deposition of anesthetic agent into the parotid salivary gland and to avoid transient facial paralysis, the dental hygienist should follow these guidelines for the IA block:

1. Adhere to the guidelines for administering the IA block as described in Chapter 13.
2. The needle must always contact bone at the medial surface of the mandibular ramus before the dental hygienist deposits any anesthetic agent. Thus transient facial paralysis is almost always preventable if bone is contacted because this prevents the agent from being

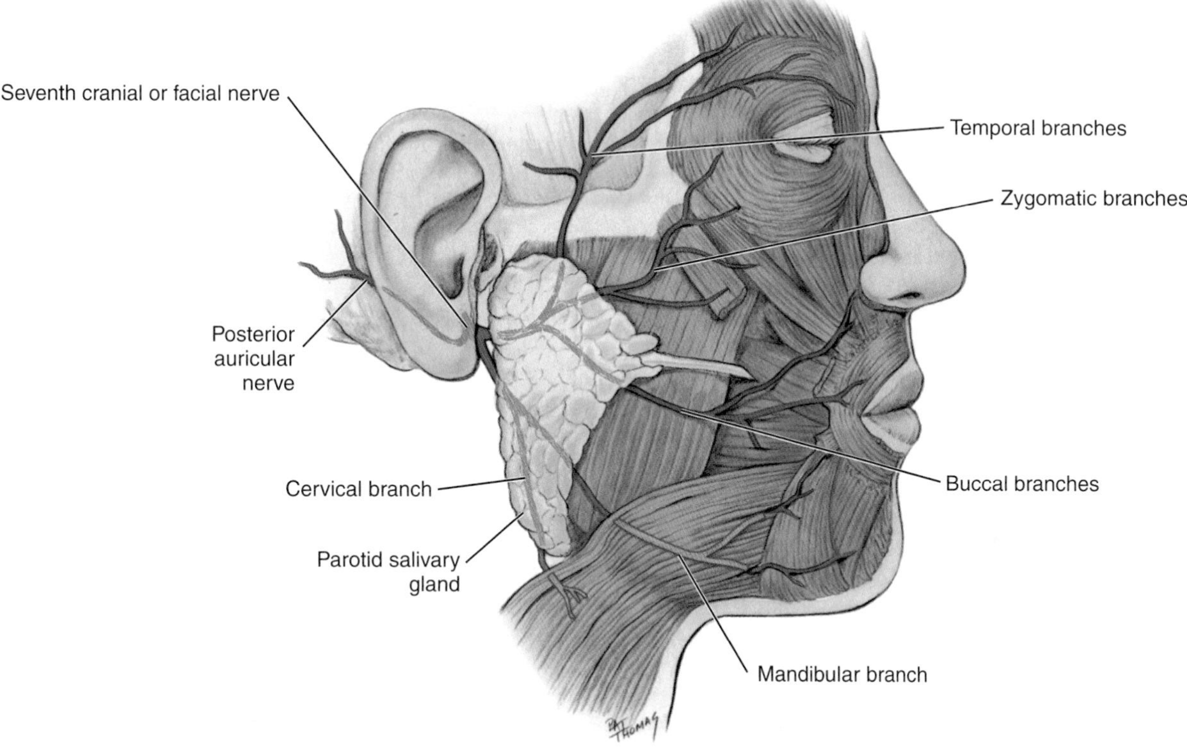

Fig. 16.3 Distribution of the facial nerve through the parotid salivary gland. (From Fehrenbach MJ, Herring SW: *Illustrated anatomy of the head and neck,* ed 6, St Louis, 2021, Saunders/Elsevier.)

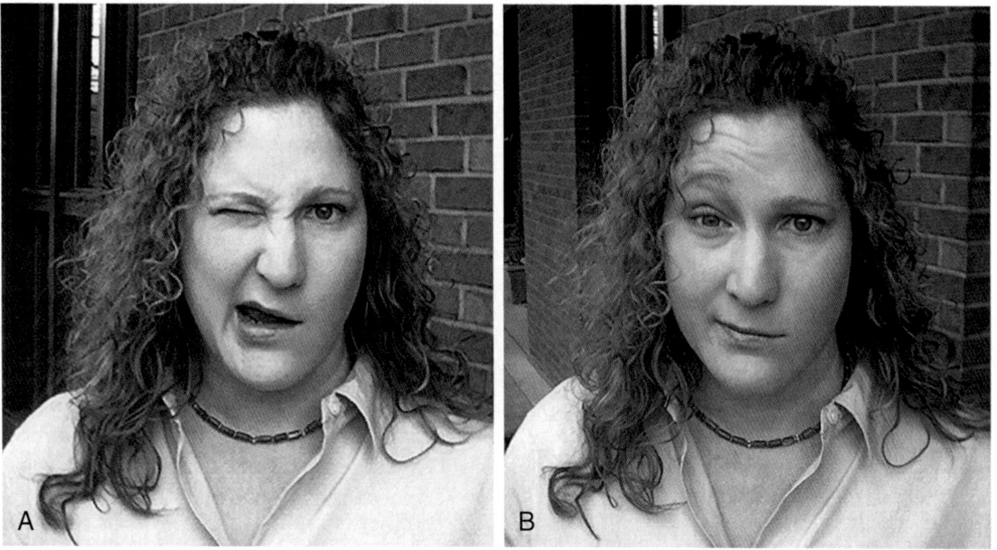

Fig. 16.4 Transient facial nerve paralysis on the patient's left side. (A) Inability to close left eyelid. (B) Drooping of ipsilateral corner of the lip on affected side (on patient's left). (From Malamed S: *Handbook of local anesthesia,* ed 7, St Louis, 2020, Elsevier.)

deposited into the deeper parotid salivary gland. However, in some rare instances, the facial nerve is located in close proximity to the IA nerve and observing the recommended depth and bony contact may still not prevent the development of facial nerve anesthesia.[3]

3. If bone is not contacted, the needle is too far posterior and there is a risk that the needle tip is located within the parotid salivary gland. To correct, the dental hygienist should withdraw the needle almost completely out of the tissue and redirect the barrel of the syringe more posteriorly over the mandibular molars. Readvance the needle into the tissue until bone is gently contacted. The agent can then be deposited after a negative aspiration (see Fig. 13.10 in Chapter 13).
4. Avoid 30-gauge needles as they are more flexible and may deflect away from the bone; instead use 25-gauge needles.

For the V-A block, the dental hygienist should follow these guidelines to prevent inadvertent deposition of anesthetic agent into the parotid salivary gland and avoid transient facial paralysis:

1. Because of the closed-mouth situation, it may be difficult to visualize the path of the needle, so depth of the needle is always a concern

and must be carefully controlled; the depth is approximately equidistant of the mesiodistal length of the mandibular ramus as measured from the maxillary tuberosity, which is approximately 25 mm or two-thirds to three-fourths of a long needle for the average-sized adult with the distance measured from the maxillary tuberosity; in smaller or larger patients, this depth of insertion should be altered to less or more.
2. Avoid 30-gauge needles as they are more flexible and may deflect; instead use 25-gauge needles.
3. No bending of the needle shank toward the lateral with the V-A block to accomplish the necessary needle and syringe barrel angulations; there should not be any change in direction of the needle within the tissue to obtain correct angulation.

Management of Transient Facial Paralysis

1. Reassure the patient. At the point of muscle weakening, the patient will be alarmed, and immediate reassurance is necessary to alleviate the patient's fears. Reassure the patient that the paralysis is only temporary and will last only a few hours. Explain that weakness in the muscles will resolve as soon as the anesthetic action fades.
2. Ask the patient to remove contact lenses if applicable and to manually close his or her eye. Although the corneal reflex remains functional, this will assist in keeping the cornea lubricated.
3. There are no contraindications to completing the scheduled treatment. However, it may be advisable to reschedule treatment for a different time. This should be determined on an individual basis and predominantly depends on the patient's reaction to the situation. If treatment is to be continued, the IA block must be completed/reinjected because the target site was missed during the first injection.
4. Arrange for patient transportation, as the patient will not be able to drive him or herself home.
5. Document the incident and the patient's reaction in the patient's chart.
6. Follow up as indicated.

Paresthesia

Paresthesia is persistent anesthesia beyond the expected duration or altered sensation, such as tingling or itching beyond the usual level with slight trauma. Paresthesia or prolonged anesthesia occurs occasionally, causing the patient to feel numbness for many hours or days after the injection. Paresthesia can also be associated with a burning sensation, and patients can experience drooling, speech impediment, loss of taste, and tongue biting.[5,6] The risk for serious complications from paresthesia occurs when the anesthesia persists for days, weeks, or months. Thankfully, this condition is rare and occasionally may be unpreventable; however, it is one of the most frequent causes of dental malpractice litigation.[3]

Paresthesia most commonly occurs with the lingual and IA nerves, with the lingual nerve being more frequently involved because of its fascicular pattern compared with the IA nerve.[7,8] In approximately 33% of individuals, the lingual nerve has been found to be unifascicular, increasing its susceptibility to paresthesia. During the administration of local anesthesia before treatment of mandibular teeth or their associated structures, the lingual or IA neurovascular bundle can be traumatized by the sharp needle tip, the movement of the needle in the tissue, extraneural or intraneural hemorrhage from trauma to the blood vessels, or neurotoxic effects of the local anesthetic.[6-9]

The local anesthetics itself can cause paresthesia as all local anesthetics are neurotoxic and can damage nerves.[10] Studies show that the primary factor in neurotoxicity of local anesthetics appears to be the concentration of the drug, with injuries increasing as concentration increases (particularly with prilocaine and articaine), when the IA block is administered.[6,11-13] Interestingly, in the United States, lidocaine has been documented as producing the greatest number of reports of paresthesia on an annual basis. However, it is important to note that lidocaine is the most used anesthetic in dentistry in the United States.[14,15]

Since the U.S. Food and Drug Administration (FDA) approval of articaine in 2000, there has been intense discussion regarding the frequent reports of paresthesia, and consequently the recommendation has surfaced that articaine should not be used for regional blocks such as the IA block.[16,17] However, this hypothesis remains controversial,[12,18] and many of those studies are anecdotal (discussed in the following paragraphs). The original source of controversy surrounding articaine seems to have stemmed from an article published by Haas and Lennon,[6] who analyzed cases of paresthesia reported to major dental malpractice carriers in Ontario, Canada. Analysis of the data indicates that articaine has a 4% higher occurrence of paresthesia than 2% or 3% local anesthetics.

A study of nonsurgical paresthesia in Ontario analogous to the Haas and Lennon study from the period of 1999 through 2008 yielded similar results.[19] A study by Garisto et al.[20] analyzed reports of paresthesia from single agents of local anesthetics after dental procedures from November 1997 through August 2008 obtained from the FDA Adverse Event Reporting System. Paresthesia in 94.5% of these cases involved the IA block, and specifically the lingual nerve in 89% of these cases. Articaine 4% was involved in 51.3% of the cases, prilocaine 4% in 42.9% of the cases, and lidocaine 2% in 4.9% of the cases. Other studies have demonstrated no additional risk. Pogrel[14] studied a total of 57 patients who demonstrated nerve damage to the IA or lingual nerve that could only have resulted from an IA block. Results on the basis of their estimated use indicated that paresthesia reports for articaine 4% were proportional to prilocaine 4% and lidocaine 2%. Baroni et.al.[21] studied the possible toxic effects of articaine and lidocaine on the mental nerve. The drugs were injected in the anterior portion of the mental nerves of 24 rats divided into three groups: 4% articaine 1:100,000 epinephrine; 2% lidocaine 1:100,000 epinephrine; and plain 1:100,000 epinephrine solution. A histopathologic analysis was then performed by using optical microscopy. An inflammatory infiltration was found around the mental nerve, but no injuries were found in the nervous structure despite the inflammatory reaction observed around the nerve. Recent studies[22-24] tested the neurotoxicity of lidocaine and articaine in SH-SY5Y cells. Results demonstrated that articaine did not produce a prolonged block of neuronal responsiveness or an increased toxicity compared with lidocaine SH-SY5Y cells.

Because of the controversy and conflicting information surrounding this issue, many clinicians are still concerned regarding articaine and the risk of paresthesia. It is important to always consider the benefits gained from the use of a drug versus the risk involved in the use of the drug, and strategies to reduce the risk of paresthesia should be considered. Pogrel[14,15] states that because most paresthesia involves the lingual nerve and with the continued debate on the role of articaine with paresthesia, it is suggested that more superiorly placed nerve blocks that avoid the more inferior located lingual nerve, such as the Gow-Gates (G-G) or the V-A nerve blocks, be administered instead of the traditional IA block when 4% drugs are used. This is a reasonable approach because no reports of paresthesia with a G-G mandibular block have been reported. Malamed[3] indicates that all reports claiming that articaine increases the risk of paresthesia are anecdotal, consisting of case reports with no scientific evidence to demonstrate this increased risk, and that articaine can be used for IA blocks. Articaine has excellent diffusion properties and is a dependable local anesthetic for maxillary and mandibular treatment. However, if clinicians are still concerned or unconvinced, 2% lidocaine with epinephrine 1:100,000 or 2% mepivacaine with levonordefrin 1:20,000 in the United States or 1:100,000 epinephrine in Canada should be used for the IA block.[3] It is essential that the dental hygienist remain abreast of the current research of all anesthetics and only administer a drug if the benefits outweigh the risks.

Paresthesia may also be a result of irritation to the nerve after the administration of a contaminated local anesthetic agent with alcohol or other disinfectants. Edema caused by the irritation places pressure on the nerve, resulting in prolonged anesthesia. Hemorrhage around the nerve sheath may also contribute to paresthesia by creating excessive pressure on the nerve. Finally, paresthesia may also be caused by trauma to the nerve sheath resulting from the needle contacting the nerve during its insertion or removal from the tissue. This occurs most commonly with the lingual nerve, producing a sensation of an electrical shock when it occurs.[2,3,5-9]

Prevention of Paresthesia

To prevent paresthesia overall with patients, the risks versus the benefits of using 4% solutions should be considered, and basic care of the cartridge should be followed. Thus local anesthetic cartridges should be stored properly in their original containers and never be placed in disinfecting solution. Finally, strict adherence to basic injection protocol should be followed as described in Chapter 11, as well as the injection techniques described in Chapters 12 and 13.

Management of Paresthesia

Most paresthesia is not serious and will typically resolve within 8 weeks. It most commonly occurs with the lingual and IA nerve and produces only minimal sensory deficit. Fortunately, permanent nerve damage rarely occurs. The dental hygienist should follow these recommendations for the management of paresthesia:

1. Reassure the patient. The patient will typically call the dental office the day after the procedure concerned about the prolonged numbness. Reassure the patient by speaking with them personally.
2. Arrange for the patient to be examined by the dentist as soon as possible to determine the extent of paresthesia. Instruct the patient that paresthesia may last up to 2 months and perhaps longer.
3. The patient should undergo an examination by their dentist every 2 months until normal sensation returns. Consultation with an oral maxillofacial surgeon is advisable if the sensation deficit persists or deteriorates.
4. Thoroughly document the incident in the patient's chart, including extent of loss of sensation and a summary of all conversations with the patient. Loss of sensation can include numbness, partial numbness, burning, tingling, loss of taste sensations, etc.
5. Dental and dental hygiene care may continue. However, avoiding injections to the already traumatized nerve is important; alternative pain control measures should be taken.

Trismus

Trismus refers to reduced opening of the jaws caused by spasm of the muscles of mastication. This can occur from spasms of the muscles of mastication, resulting in soreness and difficulty opening the mouth. Trismus is a relatively common complication associated with the administration of local anesthesia. Trismus is most frequently a result of muscle trauma in the infratemporal space after intraoral injections. Multiple needle insertions, administration of contaminated anesthetic agents, deposition of large amounts of anesthetic agent in restricted areas causing distention of the tissue, hemorrhage leading to loss of muscle function, and infection are all factors in causing trismus.

Prevention of Trismus

The following guidelines will help the dental hygienist prevent trismus:

1. Store anesthetic cartridges in a dark room in their original containers, and never place them in disinfecting solution.
2. Use sharp disposable needles and minimize the number of needle insertions.
3. Avoid contaminating the needle when not in use. Protective shields should be used to protect the needle, and the dental hygienist should know the location of an uncapped needle to avoid accidental contamination of the needle from a nonsterile surface (Fig. 16.5). Contaminated needles should not be used and should be discarded in an appropriate sharps container.
4. Inject anesthetic agent slowly.

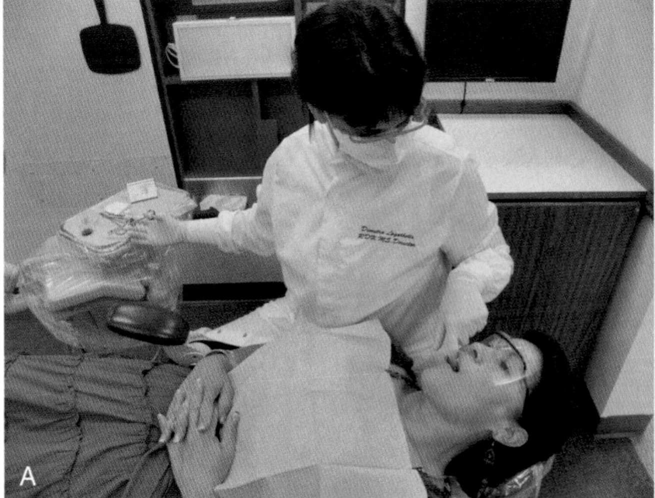

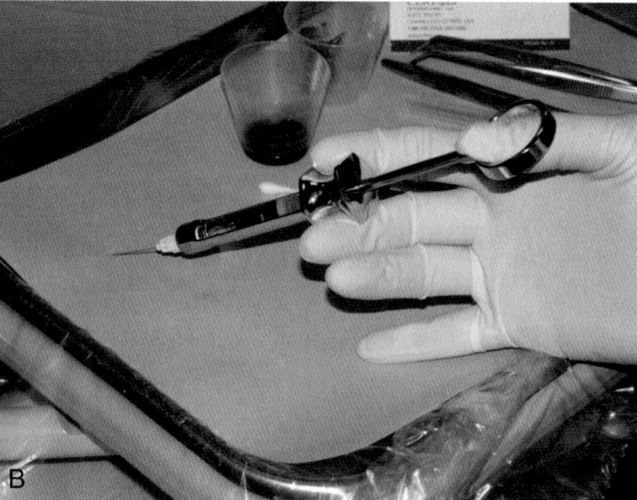

Fig. 16.5 Accidental contamination of an uncovered needle. (A) Dental hygienist uncapped the needle in preparation for the injection, and, while retracting and preparing to insert the needle, the dental hygienist does not realize that the uncovered needle is touching the tray. (B) Close-up view of needle touching the instrument tray and contaminating the needle. To prevent needle contamination from a nonsterile surface, the dental hygienist should know the location of the uncapped needle at all times.

5. Use minimal amounts of agent in restricted tissue areas.
6. Adhere to recommended anesthetic techniques as described in Chapters 11, 12, and 13. Strive to improve injection techniques to administer the most atraumatic injection possible and to decrease the necessary number of needle insertions.

Management of Trismus

Trismus is most commonly felt by the patient the day after the treatment and is typically associated with the IA or PSA blocks. Recommendations to reduce the soreness are as follows:
1. Arrange for the dentist to examine the patient if needed.
2. Instruct the patient to immediately begin heat therapy: apply warm moist towels to the affected area for 20 minutes every hour. Analgesics can be used to manage muscle soreness. If the patient experiences severe discomfort, the dentist may prescribe codeine or muscle relaxants.
3. Instruct the patient to exercise the jaw by opening and closing the mouth and by moving the mandible lateral from left to right for 5 minutes every 3 to 4 hours. Chewing sugarless gum is also a method to exercise the jaw.
4. Symptoms gradually diminish over time, typically within 48 hours after injection. Heat therapy, exercises, and analgesics should be continued until the condition resolves.
5. If pain and loss of function persist despite the recommended therapy, refer the patient to an oral and maxillofacial surgeon for consultation.
6. In the patient's chart, record the incident and a summary of all conversations and recommendations addressed with the patient.
7. Dental hygiene treatment should be avoided until all symptoms have resolved.

Infection

Infections caused by administration of local anesthetics are rare when sterile disposable needles and single-use glass cartridges are used. The most common cause of infection is the contamination of the anesthetic needle before the injection. Needle-tract contamination can introduce pathogens into deeper tissue and can spread through the blood system. In addition, dental infections can spread to deeper tissue when local anesthetics are administered through areas of dental infection.[25] Infections may also result from improper handling of the local anesthetic before injection, using contaminated agents, and/or improper tissue preparation.

Prevention of Infection

The dental hygienist should follow these guidelines to prevent infection:
1. Use sterile disposable needles.
2. Carefully sheathe and unsheathe the needle before and after the injection. The dental hygienist should be aware of the location of the uncovered needle at all times to prevent the accidental contamination of the needle from a nonsterile surface (see Fig. 16.5).
3. Store the anesthetic cartridges in their original containers. If necessary, wipe the diaphragm of the anesthetic cartridge with a disinfectant before syringe assembly.
4. Prepare the surface tissue with a topical antiseptic or wipe the injection site with a piece of gauze to reduce the surface bacteria before needle insertion.
5. Do not administer local anesthetics through areas of dental infection so as to prevent needle tract infections.

Management of Infection

Low-grade infections are very rare and often not easily recognized. The patient will express pain and discomfort to the region, and initially these symptoms should be treated as trismus. If the patient does not respond to the recommended treatment, a course of systemic antibiotics may be prescribed by the patient's dentist or physician.

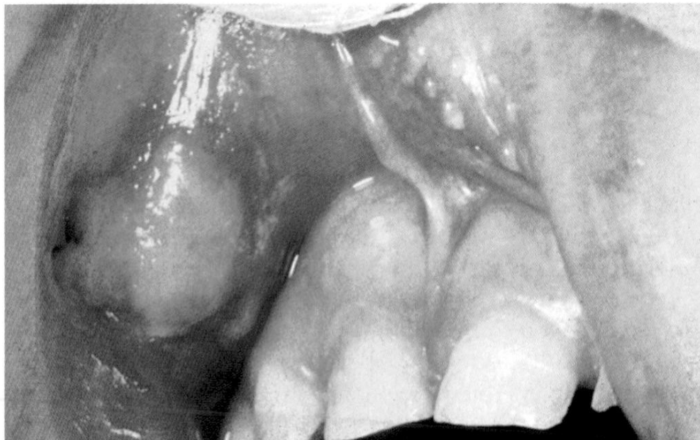

Fig. 16.6 Localized edema in response to administration of a local anesthetic agent. (From Daniel S, Harfst S, Wilder R, Francis B, Mitchell S: *Dental hygiene concepts, cases and competencies,* ed 2, St Louis, 2008, Mosby.)

Edema

Edema is an abnormal accumulation of fluid beneath the skin causing swelling of the tissue, and it describes a clinical complication[26,27] (Fig. 16.6). Edema after the administration of a local anesthetic agent may be caused by trauma during the injection, infection, administration of contaminated agents, or an allergic response. Typically edema is manifested as localized pain and loss of function. Edema associated with an allergic response is more serious and may produce airway obstruction, causing a life-threatening emergency.

Prevention of Edema

To prevent edema, the dental hygienist should follow these guidelines:
1. Conduct a thorough preanesthetic assessment.
2. Follow all recommended infection control procedures when storing or handling the local anesthetic armamentarium.
3. Follow all recommended guidelines for injection technique described in Chapters 11, 12, and 13.

Management of Edema

The cause of edema will determine its course of treatment.[3] The following management procedures are recommended.
1. *Edema produced by an allergic response:* It depends on the degree and location of swelling. If there is no airway obstruction, oral antihistamines should be administered. The patient should be referred to an allergist. If the airway is compromised, the guidelines for anaphylaxis described in Chapter 17 should be followed.
2. *Edema produced by contaminated agent or trauma:* No treatment is required; the symptoms usually subside after approximately 1 to 3 days. Recommend analgesics for discomfort.
3. *Edema produced by hemorrhage:* The tissue may be discolored and resemble a hematoma and therefore should be managed as a hematoma.
4. *Edema produced by infection:* If the edema does not resolve within 3 days and the pain and discomfort continue, antibiotics should be prescribed by the dentist or physician.

Soft Tissue Trauma

Soft tissue trauma is caused by the patient inadvertently self-inflicting damage to the tissue, such as the lips, tongue, or cheek, while

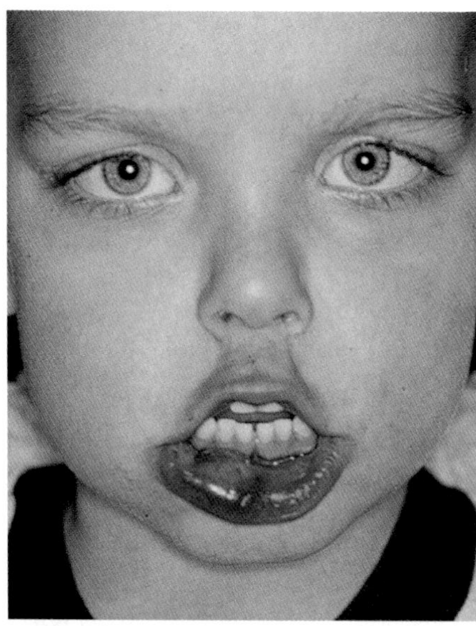

Fig. 16.7 Self-inflicted trauma caused by a child while anesthetized. (From Malamed S: *Handbook of local anesthesia*, ed 7, St Louis, 2020, Elsevier.)

anesthetized. This is most often observed in children and patients with special needs. This type of trauma can lead to swelling and significant discomfort when the anesthetic effect fades (Fig. 16.7).

Prevention of Soft Tissue Trauma

To prevent soft tissue trauma, the dental hygienist should follow these guidelines:

1. Select an anesthetic duration that is appropriate for the length of the procedure.
2. Warn the patient to not eat, drink hot fluids, or test the anesthesia area by biting until the anesthetic wears off and normal sensations have returned. The parent or guardian should also be warned about the dangers and be instructed to carefully watch young children and individuals with special needs.
3. Cotton rolls can be placed between the teeth and soft tissue to protect the lips. They can be secured with dental floss wrapped around the teeth.
4. Consider the administration of phentolamine mesylate to patients who are particularly susceptible to self-mutilation (discussed later).
5. Warning stickers are available to be placed on the patient's forehead to serve as a reminder to the parent or guardian that care should be taken while anesthetized.

Management of Soft Tissue Trauma

Management of soft tissue trauma includes the following:

1. Recommend warm saline rinses to decrease swelling and discomfort.
2. Petrolatum can be used to coat the lips to minimize discomfort.
3. Analgesics may be taken as necessary for discomfort.
4. Infection caused by soft tissue injuries is rare; however, if it occurs, a course of systemic antibiotics may be prescribed by the patient's dentist or physician.

Phentolamine Mesylate

Phentolamine mesylate (Table 16.3) is an alpha-adrenergic receptor antagonist used in dentistry to reverse the effects of local anesthetics containing vasoconstrictors. Phentolamine mesylate competes for the receptor sites of the vasoconstrictor, thus encouraging faster metabolic reuptake of the local anesthetic by way of increased vasodilation.[28,29] In May 2008, the FDA approved phentolamine mesylate (OraVerse) as a local anesthesia reversal agent for use in dentistry. It is packaged in a 1.7 mL anesthetic cartridge containing 0.4 mg of phentolamine mesylate (0.235 mg/mL) with a translucent green label and blue aluminum cap to distinguish it from local anesthetic cartridges[30] (Fig. 16.8).

Suggested clinical uses. OraVerse may be used when faster anesthetic recovery time is beneficial, such as when treating pediatric and special needs populations when the risk of self-inflicted oral trauma is increased because of lack of oral awareness or when patients prefer not to feel numb for long durations. The manufacturer claims that, when used properly, OraVerse will reduce the length of prolonged anesthesia by almost half the original duration of action when an anesthetic with epinephrine is used.[28-30]

Dosage and administration technique. OraVerse is administered by submucosal injection at a 1:1 ratio (cartridge-to-cartridge ratio) of the previously administered local anesthetic containing a vasoconstrictor. The same techniques used for the local anesthetic injection should be used when administering OraVerse.[28-30] For example, if an IA block was administered using one cartridge of local anesthetic with a vasoconstrictor, then a second IA block should be administered after treatment using one cartridge of OraVerse (see Table 16.3 for dosing guidelines).

Contraindications. OraVerse is presently contraindicated in the following patient groups:

- Patients younger than age 3 years[27]
- Patients weighing less than 15 kg or 33 lb
- Patients who are sensitive to phentolamine mesylate
- Patients with history of myocardial infarction
- Patients with angina
- Patients with coronary artery disease

Side effects. Side effects with OraVerse are rare but may include the following:

- Nausea
- Vomiting
- Diarrhea
- Weakness
- Dizziness
- Orthostatic hypotension
- Flushing
- Tachycardia
- Cardiac arrhythmias

Tissue Sloughing

Soft tissue sloughing is the loss of surface layers of epithelium that occurs after topical anesthetics are administered for extended periods. In addition, sloughing can occur from anesthetic sterile abscesses developed by prolonged ischemia caused by the inclusion of a vasoconstrictor in the anesthetic agent. Sterile abscesses are most commonly observed on the hard palate and may need to undergo incision and drainage (Fig. 16.9).

Prevention of Soft Tissue Sloughing

To prevent tissue sloughing, the dental hygienist should follow these guidelines:

1. Topical anesthetics should be minimally applied to the surface for a maximum of 1 to 2 minutes; a smaller area of use prevents tissue complications.
2. Avoid local anesthetic agents with high concentrations of vasoconstrictors unless hemostasis is required. Using epinephrine 1:50,000 is the dilution most likely to cause prolonged ischemia, increasing the likelihood of a sterile abscess.

TABLE 16.3 Phentolamine Mesylate (OraVerse)

Chemical Formula	
phenol,3-{[(4,5-dihydro-1 H-imidazol-2-yl)methyl](4-methyl-phenyl)amino}-, methanesulfonate	
Proprietary names	OraVerse
Formulations in dentistry	0.4 mg phentolamine mesylate in 1.7 mL of solution
Vasoactivity	Vasodilator
Duration of action	30–45 minutes
Toxicity	No known toxic levels
Metabolism	Liver
Excretion	Kidneys with 10% as unchanged drug
pK_a	Not available
Onset of action	Rapid
Half-life	Approximately 2–3 hours
Dosage	1:1 ratio of OraVerse cartridge to local anesthetic cartridge containing epinephrine
	Children weighing 33–66 lb: 0.2 mg (1/2 cartridge)
	Children weighing more than 66 lb and up to 12 years old: 0.4 mg (1 cartridge)
	Not recommended for children younger than 3 years old or weighing less than 15 kg (33 lb)
Pregnancy/Lactation	To be used only when risks outweigh the benefits during pregnancy. Nursing mothers should use caution because excretion in breast milk is not known.
Contraindications	Age younger than 3 years
	Weight less than 15 kg or 33 lb
	Sensitivity to phentolamine mesylate
	History of myocardial infarction
	Angina
	Coronary artery disease
Product warning	Myocardial infarction, cerebrovascular spasm, and cerebrovascular occlusion have been reported to occur after the intravenous or intramuscular administration of phentolamine, usually in association with marked hypotensive episodes or shock-like states. Tachycardia and cardiac arrhythmias may occur with the use of phentolamine or other alpha-adrenergic blocking agents. Such effects are uncommon with OraVerse (phentolamine mesylate). However, the clinician should be cognizant of the signs and symptoms, particularly in patients with a history of cardiovascular disease.

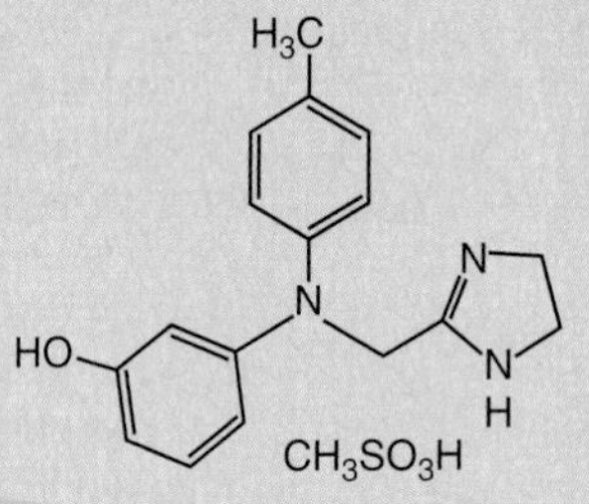

From Phentolamine. (2009). *Merck manuals: online medical library.* OraVerse (2009). *Highlights of prescribing information.* Septodont Inc. OraVerse (Phentolamine mesylate) Drug Package Insert. Louisville: Septodont Inc; 2016. OraVerse website: http://oraverse.com/dental-professionals/

Management of Soft Tissue Sloughing

Minor tissue sloughing usually requires no treatment and resolves on its own within a few days. However, soft tissue sloughing associated with sterile abscesses typically takes 7 to 10 days to resolve. Topical ointments can be used to minimize discomfort.

Postanesthetic Intraoral Lesions

Intraoral lesions are occasionally reported a couple of days after intraoral injections. These lesions typically consist of recurrent aphthous stomatitis or herpes simplex and may develop from trauma during the injection or after the administration of the anesthetic agent (Figs. 16.10 and 16.11). Lesions last approximately 7 to 10 days.

Prevention of Postanesthetic Intraoral Lesions

Prevention of such lesions is difficult in susceptible patients. Using the appropriate technique during local anesthetic administration to minimize trauma reduces the occurrence.

Management of Postanesthetic Intraoral Lesions

Topical anesthetic agents and pastes, such as triamcinolone (Kenalog in Orabase), help alleviate the discomfort associated with these lesions.

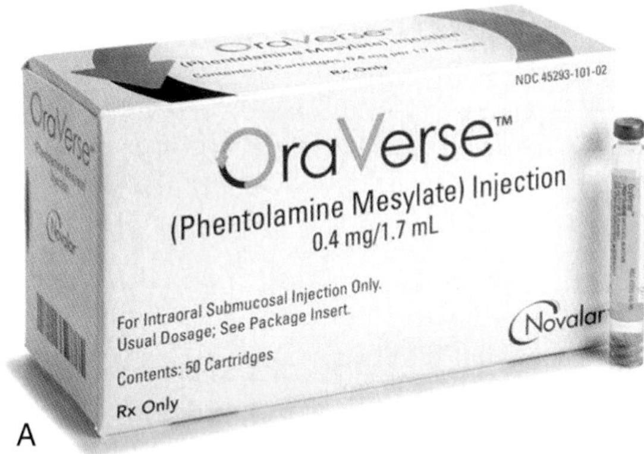

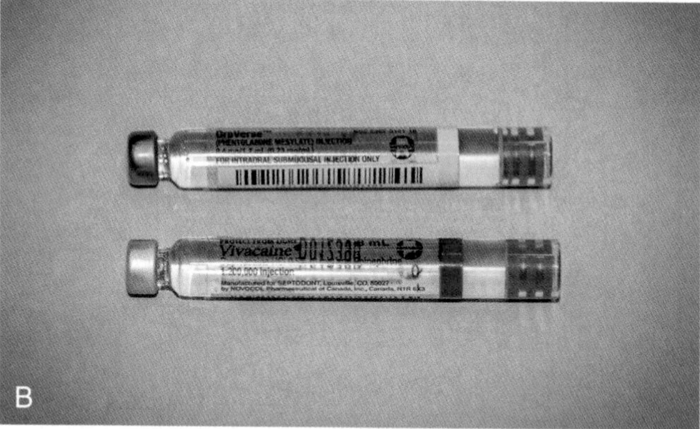

Fig. 16.8 (A) OraVerse agent used for local anesthetic reversal. (B) OraVerse (*upper cartridge*) is easily distinguished from a local anesthetic cartridge (*lower cartridge*) by its translucent green label and blue aluminum cap. (A, Image courtesy Novalar Pharmaceuticals.)

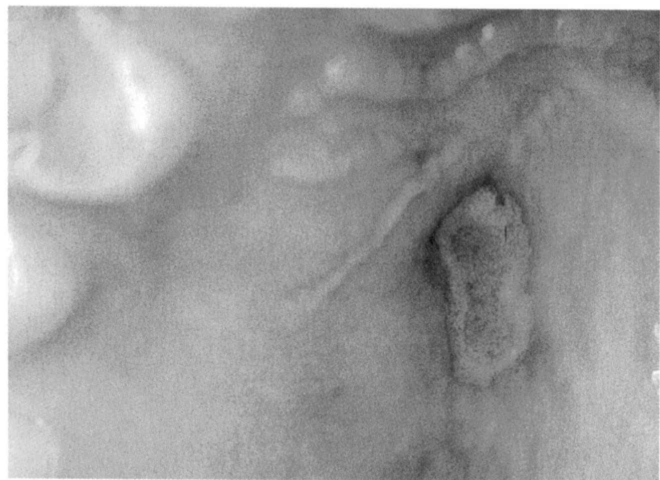

Fig. 16.9 Sloughing of tissue on the palate caused by prolonged ischemia secondary to the use of 2% lidocaine 1:50,000 epinephrine because of high concentration of vasoconstrictor. (From Malamed S: *Handbook of local anesthesia,* ed 7, St Louis, 2020, Elsevier.)

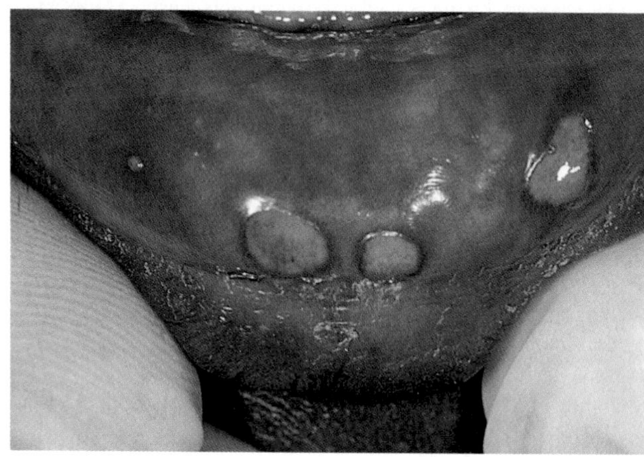

Fig. 16.10 Postinjection aphthous stomatitis. (From Eisen D, Lynch D: *The mouth: diagnosis and treatment,* St. Louis, 1998, Mosby.)

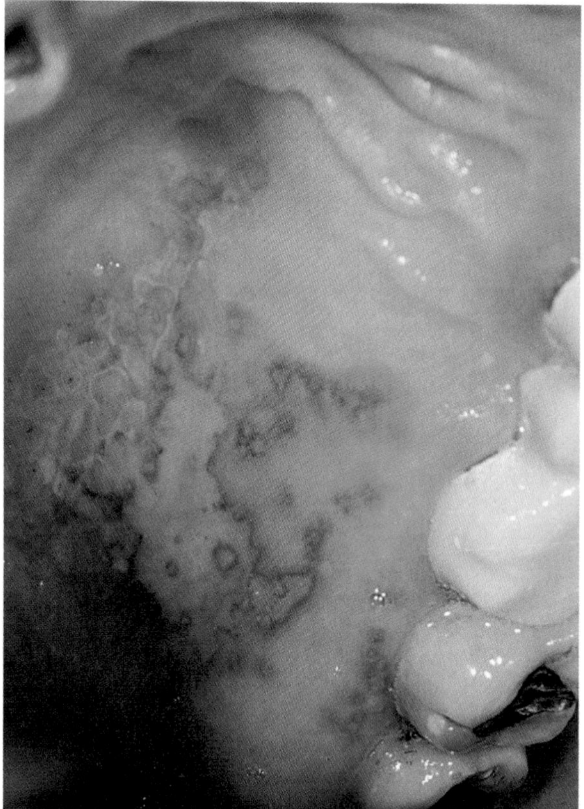

Fig. 16.11 Postinjection herpetic outbreak. (From Eisen D, Lynch D: *The mouth: diagnosis and treatment,* St. Louis, 1998, Mosby.)

DENTAL HYGIENE CONSIDERATIONS

- Most local complications associated with the administration of local anesthetics can be avoided with thorough preanesthetic assessment, proper communication, use of proper armamentarium, careful choice of local anesthetic agent, and careful injection techniques.
- Immediate appropriate management of local complications is essential. Patient referrals should be made on an individual patient basis.
- It is essential to thoroughly document local complications, including instructions to the patient and the patient's responses.
- Local complications can occur with the administration of local anesthesia even when the dental hygienist uses proper technique and risk-reduction protocol.

CASE STUDY 16.1 A Local Complication

A patient of record comes in the dental office for nonsurgical periodontal therapy of the mandibular right quadrant. The patient's medical history is reviewed, and it is determined that she is a healthy patient with no contraindications to the use of local anesthetics and vasoconstrictors. The dental hygienist decides to administer 2% lidocaine 1:100,000 epinephrine to anesthetize the quadrant. After the administration of the appropriate injections, the dental hygienist and patient notice that the right side of her face begins to droop, and the patient becomes extremely nervous about the situation.

Critical Thinking Questions

- According to the clinical symptoms described, what reaction is the patient experiencing?
- What is the cause of the symptoms described?
- Could the dental hygienist have avoided this reaction?
- If so, how?
- How should the dental hygienist respond?

CHAPTER REVIEW QUESTIONS

1. Which of the following BEST describes a localized complication?
   A. A complication that occurs in a region of the injection and is attributed to the needle or the administered anesthetic
   B. A complication that is attributed ONLY to the drug administered
   C. A complication that will resolve on its own and requires no treatment
   D. A complication that requires a definite plan of treatment
2. Which of the following BEST describes a secondary complication?
   A. A complication that occurs in a region of the injection and is attributed to the needle
   B. A complication that is experienced by the patient after the injection
   C. A complication that will resolve on its own and requires no treatment
   D. A complication that requires a definite plan of treatment
3. If needle breakage occurs and the clinician can easily retrieve the needle, what is the next step by the dental hygienist?
   A. Inform the patient
   B. Have the patient be seen by the dentist
   C. Keep one's hand in the patient's mouth and ask to open widely
   D. Take panoramic radiograph and refer to oral and maxillofacial surgeon
4. When a blood vessel is punctured or lacerated by the anesthetic needle, an asymmetric swelling and discoloration may occur. This is possibly a sign of:
   A. Hematoma
   B. Hemangioma
   C. Edema
   D. Trismus
5. What is the first step that needs to be completed by the dental hygienist when managing a hematoma?
   A. Apply heat
   B. Apply cold compress
   C. Massage soft tissue
   D. Apply pressure
6. What is soreness in the muscles of mastication caused by muscle spasms called?
   A. Trismus
   B. Nerve paralysis
   C. Hematoma
   D. Paresthesia
7. An incident of edema in patients after administration of a local anesthetic can be caused by all of the following EXCEPT one. Which one is the EXCEPTION?
   A. Trauma during injections
   B. Broken needle
   C. Contaminated agents
   D. Allergic reaction
8. Paresthesia occurs MOST commonly during which intraoral local anesthetic injection?
   A. Middle superior alveolar block
   B. Posterior superior alveolar block
   C. Inferior alveolar block
   D. Gow-Gates mandibular block
9. All of the following are ways the dental hygienist can decrease the risk of infection during a local anesthetic injection EXCEPT one. Which one is the EXCEPTION?
   A. Use sterile needles
   B. Store cartridges in original containers
   C. Use topical anesthetic
   D. Carefully sheathe and unsheathe the needle
10. Why should topical anesthetics ONLY be applied to the surface tissue for 1 to 2 minutes before administering a local anesthetic?
    A. To prevent tissue sloughing
    B. To prevent sterile abscesses
    C. To prevent soft tissue trauma
    D. A and B only
11. If nerve damage develops from an inferior alveolar block, it is considered to be which type of reaction?
    A. Mild complication
    B. Primary complication

C. Transient complication
D. Permanent complication

12. All of the following can prevent needle breakage EXCEPT one. Which one is the EXCEPTION?
A. Never bending the needle
B. Using a 30-gauge long needle
C. No sudden direction changes of the needle
D. Advancing the needle slowly

13. Which of the following is the best way to prevent pain on injection?
A. Wiping the diaphragm of the cartridge
B. Heating the cartridge of anesthetic
C. Injecting slowly
D. Placing the cartridge in a disinfectant solution

14. How many days should you tell your patient it will take for the swelling and discoloration to disappear after a hematoma?
A. 1–3 days
B. 4–5 days
C. 6–8 days
D. 7–14 days

15. Which of the following nerve blocks can produce the largest hematoma with extra oral bruising?
A. Mental/incisive block
B. Inferior alveolar block
C. Posterior superior alveolar block
D. Infraorbital block

16. In order to prevent transient facial paralysis, the dental hygienist should:
A. Use a long 25-gauge needle for the inferior alveolar block
B. Use a short 25-gauge needle for the inferior alveolar block
C. Always hit bone on the inferior alveolar block
D. Only insert the needle two-thirds the depth of a long needle for the inferior alveolar block

17. Trismus can be caused by which of the following?
A. Injecting the anesthetic slowly
B. Multiple needle insertions
C. Use of a long 25-gauge needle
D. pH of the vasoconstrictor

18. The use of phentolamine mesylate is contraindicated in which of the following?
A. A 6-year-old child
B. Patients weighing less than 15 kg or 33 lb
C. Adult patient with diabetes
D. Anxious patients

19. To prevent tissue sloughing, the dental hygienist should:
A. Apply topical anesthetic for 1 to 2 minutes
B. Avoid using epinephrine at 1:100,000 dilution
C. Avoid using topical anesthetic
D. Use Betadine prior to injection

20. Which of the following agents can be used to treat postanesthetic intraoral lesions?
A. Nystatin
B. Acyclovir
C. Kenalog in Orabase
D. Diflucan

REFERENCES

1. Bennett CR. *Monheim's local anesthesia and pain control in dental practice.* ed 7. St Louis: Mosby; 1990.
2. Jastak T, Yagiela J, Donaldson D. *Local anesthesia of the oral cavity.* St Louis: Saunders; 1995.
3. Malamed S. *Handbook of local anesthesia.* ed 7. St Louis: Elsevier; 2020.
4. Bowen DM, Pieren JA. *Darby and Walsh dental hygiene: theory and practice.* ed 5. St Louis: Saunders/Elsevier; 2020.
5. Haas DA. Localized complications from local anesthesia. *J Calif Dent.* 1998;26(9):677–682.
6. Haas DA, Lennon D. A 21-year retrospective study of reports of paresthesia following local anesthetic administration. *J Can Dent Assoc.* 1995;61(4):319–330.
7. Pogrel MA, Bryan J, Regezi J. Nerve damage associated with inferior alveolar nerve blocks. *J Am Dent Assoc.* 1995;126(8):1150–1155.
8. Pogrel MA, Thamby S. Permanent nerve involvement resulting from inferior alveolar nerve blocks. *J Am Dent Assoc.* 2000;131(7):901–907.
9. Harn SD, Durham TM. Incidence of lingual nerve trauma and postinjection complications in conventional mandibular block anesthesia. *J Am Dent Assoc.* 1990;121(4):519–523.
10. Berde CB, Strichartz GR. Local anesthetics. In: Miller RD, ed. *Miller's anesthesia.* Philadelphia: Saunders; 2015.
11. Kalichman MW, Moorhouse DF, Powell HC, Myers RR. Relative neural toxicity of local anesthetics. *J Neuropathol Exp Neurol.* 1993;52(3): 234–240.
12. Malamed SF. Local anesthetics: dentistry's most important drugs-clinical update 2006. *J Calif Dent Assoc.* 2006;34(12):971–976.
13. Hillerup S, Jensen R. Nerve injury caused by mandibular block analgesia. *Int J Oral Maxillofac Surg.* 2006;35:437–443.
14. Pogrel MA. Permanent nerve damage from inferior alveolar nerve blocks—an update to include articaine. *J Calif Dent Assoc.* 2007;35(4): 271–273.
15. Pogrel MA. Permanent nerve damage from inferior alveolar nerve blocks: a current update. *J Calif Dent Assoc.* 2012;40:795–797.
16. Oral and Dental Expert Group. *Therapeutic guidelines: oral and dental 2012, version 2.* Melbourne: Australian Dental Association; 2012; p. 116.
17. Practice alert. Paraesthesia following local anaesthetic injection. *Dispatch, Royal Coll Dent Surg Ont.* 2005;19:26.
18. Malamed SF. Articaine versus lidocaine: the author responds (comment on Dower JS Jr. Articaine vs lidocaine. *J Calif Dent Assoc.* 35[4]:240, 242, 244, 2007). *J Calif Dent Assoc.* 2007;35(6):383–385.
19. Gaffen AS, Haas DA. Retrospective review of voluntary reports of nonsurgical paresthesia in dentistry. *J Can Dent Assoc.* 2009;75(8):579.
20. Garisto GA, Gaffen AS, Lawrence HP, Tenenbaum HC, Haas DA. Occurrence of paresthesia after dental local anesthetic administration in the United States. *J Am Dent Assoc.* 2010;41(7):836–844.
21. Baroni DB, Franz-Montan M, Cogo K, Berto LA, Volpato MC, Novaes PD, Groppo FC. Effect of articaine on mental nerve anterior portion: histological analysis in rats. *Acta Odontol Scand.* 2012;71(1):82–87.
22. Albalawi F, Lim JC, DiRenzo KV, Hersh EV, Mitchell CH. Effects of lidocaine and articaine on neuronal survival and recovery. *Anesth Prog.* 2018;65:82–88.
23. Malet A, Faure MO, Deletage N, Pereira B, Haas J, Lambert G. The comparative cytotoxic effects of different local anesthetics on a human neuroblastoma cell line. *Anesth Analg.* 2015;120:589–596.
24. DiRenzo KV, Lim JL, Albalawi F, Hersh EV, Mitchell CH. Differential effects of sodium channel blockers on neural survival and responsiveness; 2% lidocaine kills more SHSY- 5Y cells and reduces cellular activity as compared to 4% articaine. *J Dent Res.* 2016;95(special issue A):0790.
25. Fehrenbach M, Herring S. Spread of dental infection. *Practical Hygiene.* September/October 1997:13–19.
26. Malamed SF. *Medical emergencies in the dental office.* ed 7. St Louis: Mosby; 2015.
27. Little JW, Falace DA, Miller CS, Rhodus NL. *Dental management of the medically compromised patient.* ed 9. St Louis: Elsevier; 2018.
28. Phentolamine. Drug monograph. ClinicalKey; 2018. https://www.clinicalkey.com.
29. Phentolamine. Merck Manuals: online medical library.
30. Septodont Inc. OraVerse (phentolamine mesylate) drug package insert. Louisville: Septodont Inc; 2016.

17

Systemic Complications and Emergency Management

Constantine N. Logothetis, MD

LEARNING OBJECTIVES

1. Discuss the predisposing factors to systemic complications.
2. Discuss the causes and prevention of local anesthetic overdose.
3. Discuss the clinical manifestations and management of local anesthetic overdose.
4. Discuss the causes and prevention of an epinephrine overdose.
5. Discuss the clinical manifestations and management of an epinephrine overdose.
6. Discuss allergic reactions derived by an immunologic reaction to an antigen, including prevention, clinical manifestations, and management of allergic reactions.
7. List and describe the signs, symptoms, and management of the following emergency situations:
   - Syncope
   - Hyperventilation
   - Bronchial asthma
   - Angina pectoris
   - Myocardial infarction
   - Cerebrovascular accident
   - Seizures
   - Hypoglycemia
   - Hyperglycemia
   - Mild allergic reaction
   - Anaphylaxis
   - Mild local anesthetic overdose
   - Severe anesthetic overdose
   - Vasoconstrictor overdose

INTRODUCTION

Systemic complications associated with the administration of local anesthetics occur less frequently than local complications (see Chapter 16). Systemic complications are attributed to the drug administered (Table 17.1) and are usually caused by high plasma concentrations of local anesthetic drugs after inadvertent intravascular injection, excessive dose or rate of injection, delayed drug clearance, or administration into vascular tissue. The dental hygienist can prevent 90% of potential life-threatening reactions caused by the administration of local anesthetics by conducting a thorough preanesthetic patient assessment and by strictly following all local anesthetic administration guidelines (see Chapters 7, 11, 12, and 13).[1]

Systemic toxicity of anesthetics involves the central nervous system (CNS), the cardiovascular system (CVS), and the immune system. In relatively rare instances (<1%), the effects on the immune system can produce an immunoglobulin E (IgE)-mediated allergic reaction. Most documented cases are associated with the use of amino esters, which are no longer available in dentistry. Some anesthetics, particularly prilocaine and benzocaine, are associated with hematologic effects, namely methemoglobinemia (see Chapter 7). Cardiovascular effects are primarily those of direct myocardial depression and bradycardia, which may lead to cardiovascular collapse.

LOCAL ANESTHETIC OVERDOSE

Unlike most medications that must be absorbed by the bloodstream to produce the desired effect, local anesthetics are chemical agents that are deposited in the area of nerve conduction to block the action potential before they are absorbed through the bloodstream. Once absorbed into the circulatory system and before biotransformation, local anesthetics will affect the CNS and the CVS. The higher the blood plasma level, the greater the effects on these systems. A drug overdose reaction is the body's response to overly high blood levels of a drug in various organs and associated tissue.[2,3] In ideal situations, local anesthetics are absorbed from the site of administration into the circulation slowly and continuously until all the anesthetic is completely removed from the injection site. Concurrently, the local anesthetic is removed from the circulation as it undergoes biotransformation by the appropriate organs. If this steady sequence of events occurs, the risk of high plasma concentrations of the drug is rare. Toxicity of anesthetics is potentiated in patients when this sequence is disrupted by predisposing factors, causing an increase in drug plasma concentrations to quantities sufficient to produce adverse effects on various organs and tissues of the body. Table 17.2 summarizes the predisposing factors related to local anesthetic overdose reactions.

Predisposing Factors Related to the Patient

Age of the Patient

Local anesthetic overdose reactions can occur in persons of any age, but children and elderly persons are more susceptible. In children, the elimination half-life of local anesthetic drugs is increased because the functions of absorption, metabolism, and excretion may be underdeveloped. This increases the risk of local anesthetic accumulation in the tissues. In elderly individuals, reduced blood flow and organ function lowers clearance, increasing the toxicity of local anesthetics. Moreover, elderly patients frequently have multiple co-morbidities (liver, renal,

TABLE 17.1 Local Anesthetic Systemic Complications

Complications Associated With the Anesthetic Agent
Overdose to local anesthetic
Overdose to vasoconstrictor
Allergic reactions
Anaphylactic reaction
Idiosyncrasy (reactions not classified as toxic or allergic)

and cardiac diseases) altering local anesthetic pharmacokinetics and pharmacodynamics.[4,5,6] All of these factors suggest there is a safety benefit in dose reduction for children and elderly patients (see Chapter 8).

Body Weight

Local anesthetics are distributed evenly throughout the body, and individuals with a greater (lean) body weight can tolerate a larger dose of a local anesthetic drug than smaller individuals. This is due to larger individuals having a greater blood volume and therefore a lower level of drug per milliliter of blood. When calculating a patient's maximum recommended dose of local anesthetic it is determined based on milligrams of drug per kilogram or pounds of body weight (see Chapter 8).

Pregnancy

During pregnancy cardiac output is increased leading to accelerated perfusion at the local anesthetic injection sites. This may cause rapid absorption and higher blood levels of the local anesthetic drug. Moreover, renal function may be disturbed, causing impaired excretion of certain drugs increasing the accumulation of the drug in the blood. For these reasons, pregnant woman are at a greater risk for a toxic overdose, and it is recommended that doses of local anesthetic be reduced for these patients.[7]

Drug/Drug Interactions

Local anesthetic drug levels may be influenced by the administration of concomitant medications. Overdose reactions may be experienced at lower administered doses because the local anesthetic drug may be competing with the concomitant drug for biotransformation. An example is the H2-histamine blocker cimetidine, which competes with lidocaine for hepatic oxidative enzymes slowing the biotransformation of lidocaine and thus leading to elevated blood levels. See Chapter 7 for local anesthetic drug/drug interactions.[8]

Presence of Disease

Virtually the entire metabolic process of lidocaine, mepivacaine, and bupivacaine occurs in the liver. The rate of biotransformation of these amide anesthetics is dependent on the liver function and hepatic perfusion. Therefore patients with lower than normal hepatic blood flow, hypotension, congestive heart failure, or significant liver disease (ASA III) such as cirrhosis and hepatitis B, may be unable to adequately biotransform the amides that are primarily metabolized in the liver, causing an interruption in the process. Interruption of the biotransformation of amides could lead to systemic toxicity.[4,5,7–9]

Predisposing Factors Related to the Drug

Vasoactivity

Local anesthetics are vasodilators and local blood vessels in the area of injection will immediately begin to absorb the anesthetic by causing vasodilation of the blood vessels, leading to increased blood flow to the site of injection and into the cardiovascular system. This will cause higher blood levels of local anesthetics, increasing the risk of systemic

TABLE 17.2 Predisposing Factors to Local Anesthetic Overdose Reaction

Patient Factors	Contributory Factors
Age	Organs involved in the biotransformation of anesthetic drugs may not be fully developed in younger patients and may be diminished in older patients, increasing the half-life of the drug and ultimately causing a higher risk of a toxic overdose.
Body weight	Lower body weight increases risk.
Drug/drug interactions	Toxicity may be influenced by the administration of concomitant medications.
Genetics	Genetic deficiencies may affect the biotransformation of certain drugs (e.g., atypical plasma cholinesterase), increasing the half-life of the drug and ultimately causing a higher risk of a toxic overdose.
Presence of disease	Presence of disease may affect the ability of the body to biotransform the drug into inactive metabolites. Hepatic or renal dysfunction impairs body's ability to breakdown and excrete the anesthetic drug, elevating blood levels. Cardiovascular disease such as heart failure decreases liver perfusion, increasing the half-life of the drug.
Pregnancy	Toxicity may be potentiated during pregnancy.
Drug Factors	**Contributory Factors**
Vasoactivity	Vasodilation increases perfusion in the area of injection causing an increased rate of absorption from the injection site into the CVS, increasing risk of overdose.
Dose	Higher administered dose increases circulating blood level of the drug, increasing risk of overdose.
Concentration of drug	Higher drug concentration (percent solution injected) causes greater circulating blood volume of the drug, increasing the risk of systemic toxicity.
Route of administration	Intravascular injection causes extremely high blood levels of the drug in a short time, increasing risk of a serious overdose, as the liver cannot metabolize the drug quick enough.
Rate of injection	Rapid injection of the drug increases risk of overdose.
Vascularity of injection site	Greater vascularity at the injection site increases rapid absorption of anesthetic into circulation, increasing risk of overdose.
Addition of vasoconstrictors	Addition of vasoconstrictor decreases perfusion of the area and a decrease in the rate of absorption, lowering the risk of an overdose.

CVS, Cardiovascular system.

toxicity. Choosing a local anesthetic with a vasoconstrictor will counteract the vasodilating properties of the local anesthetic, decreasing the risk of systemic toxicity.

Drug Concentration

Local anesthetic drug concentrations are expressed as percentages. The higher the percentage of the drug the more milligrams per milliliter of solution will be circulating in the blood, increasing the risk of systemic toxicity. For example, in a 1.8 mL cartridge of a 4% solution there is 72 mg of the local anesthetic drug; in a 2% solution, there is only 36 mg of the local anesthetic drug. For most dental hygiene procedures, the lowest concentration of a drug should be administered if it is as clinically effective as a 4% solution.[4,10,11]

Dose

Systemic toxicity attributed to local anesthetics is dose dependent. It is important to remember that the use of dental local anesthetic cartridges represents a volume of solution administered, not a dose of drug administered that is expressed in milligrams. The larger the dose of drug administered, the more circulating drug in the blood stream. The appropriate dose of local anesthetics should be the least concentrated and lowest dose that achieves the desired duration and extent of anesthesia. The maximum recommended dose (MRD) for a local anesthetic should be adhered to, especially in patients with low body weight, and presence of disease (see Chapters 7 and 8).[4,11]

Route of Administration

As discussed previously, systemic toxicity may occur from the administration of local anesthetics and is related to the serum concentration of the drug as it is absorbed into the circulation. This serum concentration is influenced by the dose, site, and method of drug administration. Local anesthetics are absorbed from the site of administration into the circulation slowly and continuously until the entire anesthetic is completely removed from the injection site allowing for biotransformation to occur at steady pace. When local anesthetics are administered directly into the bloodstream, this prevents the slow process of absorption, circulation and biotransformation increasing the risk for systemic toxicity.[4,8,10,11]

Rate of Injection

The rate of anesthetic injection is very important to the cause and prevention of local anesthetic systemic toxicity. When an anesthetic drug is injected intravascularly, the rate at which the agent was administered will determine if the drug administered will produce systemic toxicity. Slowly depositing the anesthetic agent will reduce the risk of overdose even if the anesthetic is accidentally administered intravascularly. Rapid injection of 36 mg of lidocaine in 30 seconds or less will significantly elevate serum concentrations, ensuring an overdose reaction.[12,13]

Causes and Prevention of Local Anesthetic Overdose

Biotransformation of Anesthetic Is Unusually Slow

A thorough review of the patient's medical history is important to determine the biotransformation capability of the local anesthetic agent by the patient.

1. Ester local anesthetics and the amide articaine are biotransformed in the blood by enzyme pseudocholinesterase. About 90% to 95% of articaine is metabolized in the blood and only 5% to 10% is metabolized in the liver. The ester local anesthetic drugs undergo hydrolysis to para-aminobenzoic acid. Articaine's major metabolite is articainic acid. Patients with familial history of atypical pseudocholinesterase may be unable to detoxify ester anesthetics at the usual rate. Because articaine possesses both ester and amide characteristics and is metabolized in the plasma and the liver, it can be administered safely to a patient with atypical plasma cholinesterase.
2. Biotransformation of amides occurs in the liver, with prilocaine being metabolized in the liver and the lungs. Toxicity of these anesthetics may be potentiated in patients with hepatic and lung compromise.

Elimination of Anesthetic Through the Kidneys Is Unusually Slow

Only a small percentage of both esters and amides are excreted unmetabolized through the urine. Patients who have significant loss of renal function could possibly develop a toxic level of anesthetic in their blood. However, in clinical situations this occurrence is rare and does not pose any additional risk to the administration of local anesthetics. It is always recommended to use the minimal effective dose.[4,9]

Total Dose Administered Is Too Large

1. If excessive total dose of local anesthetic is administered to a patient, toxic effects may develop.
2. Calculation of MRD is very important. Guidelines exist for the dental hygienist to determine the patient's individual MRD based on the patient's weight (see Chapter 8).
3. Age of the patient and physical status affect the anesthetic dose, which should be adjusted accordingly due to immature organ function in children or diminished organ function in the elderly.[4,7,8]

Absorption of Anesthetic From the Site of Injection Is Unusually Rapid

1. The addition of a vasoconstrictor drug in the local anesthetic agent reduces the risk of systemic toxicity of the anesthetic agent by slowing absorption into the circulatory system. Local anesthetic vasoconstrictor formulations should be used unless absolutely contraindicated by the patient's health status (see Chapters 4 and 7).
2. Limit area of use of topical anesthetics. Topical anesthetics are administered in high concentrations and are rapidly absorbed into the circulatory system. Applying topical anesthetic to large areas increases the possibility of an overdose.[1,8]

Anesthetic Is Administered Intravascularly

Inadvertent intravascular injection is the most common cause of local anesthetic toxicity even when the anesthetic was administered within the recommended dose range.[3,4] Depositing the anesthetic agent directly into the bloodstream prevents the slow process of absorption of the drug into circulation and significantly increases systemic toxicity. Although all local anesthetic injections may be administered intravascularly, they are most common during nerve blocks, such as the posterior superior alveolar (PSA), inferior alveolar (IA), and mental/incisive blocks. Overdose reactions can be avoided by following these guidelines:

1. *Know dental anatomy:* The dental hygienist must be aware of all anatomic features in the area of the anesthetic deposition.
2. *Aspirate in two planes:* Although the dental hygienist may properly aspirate, it is not always possible to avoid intravascular injection. The bevel of the needle may rest against the blood vessel during the negative pressure produced by the aspiration. This simply draws the lining of the blood vessel over the lumen of the needle, preventing access of blood into the cartridge (Fig. 17.1). Therefore it is important to aspirate in two planes, meaning to rotate the barrel of the syringe about 45 degrees and aspirate a second time. When

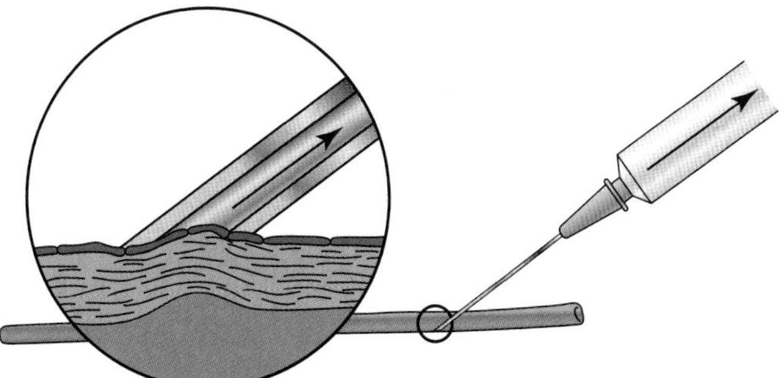

Fig. 17.1 Negative pressure during aspiration pulls the vessel wall against the bevel of the needle, giving a false-negative result.

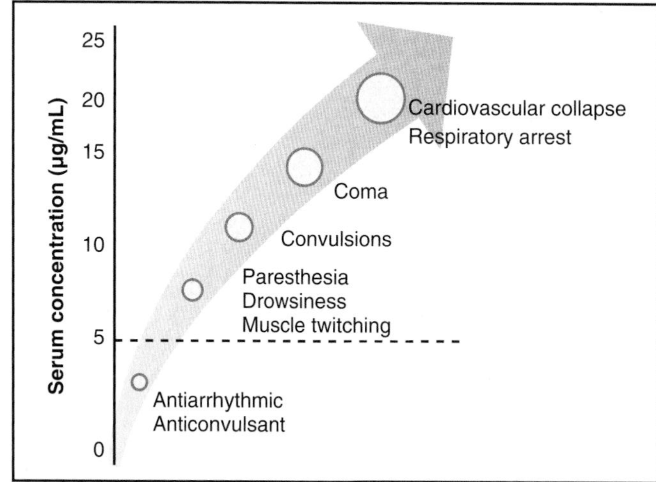

Fig. 17.2 Approximate serum concentrations and systemic influences of lidocaine. (From Becker DE, Reed KL. Local anesthetics: review of pharmacological considerations. *Anesth Prog.* 2012;59[2]:90–102.)

injecting near highly vascular areas, such as near the pterygoid venous plexus with the PSA block or with the IA block, the dental hygienist should aspirate several times during the injection in case needle movement places the needle within the blood vessel.

3. *Use a 25- or 27-gauge needle:* Larger gauge needles provide easier access for blood to enter the cartridge during the aspiration.
4. *Administer drug slowly:* An excessively rapid injection (entire anesthetic cartridge [1.8 mL] deposited in 30 seconds or less) of a local anesthetic drug into a vein or artery produces blood levels in excess of that needed for an overdose to occur.[12] The same volume of anesthetic administered within the recommended guidelines (a minimum of 60 seconds) produces blood levels lower than the blood levels needed to produce an overdose.[12] Injecting the anesthetic slowly is the most important factor in preventing an overdose.

Clinical Manifestations of Overdose

As local anesthetics are absorbed from the injection site, the serum concentration will rise, and the drug will accumulate in and affect the target organs (CNS and CVS). Because local anesthetics readily cross the blood-brain barrier, the CNS is especially sensitive to high blood levels of local anesthetics (more than any other system), and produce CNS depression. Depending on the dose administered and any predisposing factors, as discussed earlier, the degree of CNS depression will be dependent on the drug concentration in the bloodstream. At low serum concentrations, local anesthetics produce no significant effects on the CNS but may have some anticonvulsant properties. For example, lidocaine at 0.5 micrograms/milliliter (µg/mL) to 4 µg/mL is used clinically as an anticonvulsant to terminate or decrease the duration of generalized tonic clonic seizures and absence seizures. These anticonvulsant properties occur at blood levels below that which lidocaine produces seizure activity in an overdose (Fig. 17.2). Lidocaine decreases the excitability of neurons due to its depressant actions on the CNS, thus raising seizure thresholds.[4,8] Convulsive seizures that occur from high blood levels of local anesthetics are the initial life-threatening consequence of a local anesthetic overdose.[8] As serum concentrations rise, all pathways are inhibited, resulting in coma, respiratory arrest, and eventually cardiovascular collapse.[8] Lidocaine toxicity occurs at concentrations of 5 µg/mL, with convulsive seizures beginning at a concentration of 10 µg/mL (Fig. 17.2). An even greater risk is when concomitant CNS depressants, such as opioid/sedative medications, are also administered, especially in the pediatric population (see Chapter 14).[1,2,8,10,14,15]

The cardiovascular system, specifically the myocardium, is less sensitive to the actions of local anesthetics, and signs and symptoms usually do not appear until long after adverse CNS actions have appeared. Local anesthetics primarily lidocaine can be used with dosages of 1.8 µg/mL to 5 µg/mL for suppressing cardiac arrhythmias. Higher blood levels of 5 to 10 µg/mL lead to myocardial depression, decreased cardiac output, and peripheral vasodilation. Blood levels above 10 µg/mL intensify these actions that may lead to cardiac arrest (Fig. 17.2). Bupivacaine exhibits a greater potential for direct cardiac toxicity than the other amide local anesthetics. However, this is rare if the clinician does not exceed the maximum recommended dose.[8,16,17–20]

After the administration of local anesthetic agents, consider new signs or symptoms as a possible sign of toxicity when evaluating patients (Table 17.3). The manifestation of toxicity depends on the organ system or systems that are affected. The following is a list of toxicity manifestations organized by the affected system.[21]

Central Nervous System Signs

Initial symptoms

- Circumoral and/or tongue numbness
- Metallic taste
- Lightheadedness
- Dizziness
- Visual and auditory disturbances (difficulty focusing and tinnitus)
- Disorientation
- Drowsiness
- Muscle twitching

Higher-dose symptoms

- Often occur after an initial CNS excitation followed by a rapid CNS depression
- Convulsions
- Unconsciousness
- Coma
- Respiratory depression and arrest
- Cardiovascular depression and collapse

Cardiovascular Signs

Direct cardiac effects

- Toxic doses of local anesthetic agents can cause myocardial depression (tetracaine, bupivacaine), cardiac dysrhythmias (bupivacaine), and cardiotoxicity in pregnancy.
- Several anesthetics also have negative inotropic effects on cardiac muscle that lead to hypotension. Bupivacaine is especially cardiotoxic.[8,16,17–20]

Peripheral effects

- Vasoconstriction at low doses
- Vasodilation at higher doses (hypotension)

TABLE 17.3 Signs, Symptoms, and Management of a Local Anesthetic Overdose on the Central Nervous System

Signs (Observable-Objective)	Symptoms (Subjectively Felt)	Management
Low to Moderate Blood Levels		
Circumoral and/or tongue numbness	Disorientation	Terminate procedure
Metallic taste	Nervousness	Reassure patient
Excitatory-nervousness-talkativeness	Flushed skin color	Position patient in comfortable position
Slurred speech, general stutter	Apprehension	Administer oxygen
Involuntary muscular twitching or shivering	Twitching tremors	Provide basic life support
General lightheadedness, dizziness	Shivering	Monitor vital signs
Tremor or twitching in muscles	Dizziness	Activate EMS if needed
Confusion, apprehension	Lightheadedness	Allow patient to recover and discharge
Sweating	Visual disturbances	
Vomiting	Auditory disturbances	
Elevated respiration	Headache	
Elevated heart rate	Tinnitus	
Increased blood pressure	Metallic taste	
Moderate to High Blood Levels		
Convulsions, generally tonic-clonic	Muscle twitching	Terminate procedure
Respiratory depression (at high blood levels)	Seizures	Position patient supine, legs elevated
Depressed blood pressure and heart rate	Coma	Activate EMS
Unconsciousness		Manage seizure: Protect patient from injury
CNS depression—coma—death		Provide basic life support
Respiratory depression and arrest		Administer oxygen
Cardiovascular depression and collapse		Monitor vital signs
		Administer a benzodiazepine for prolonged seizures: diazepam (Valium) 5–20 mg IV or intranasal lorazepam 2–4 mg or intranasal midazolam 5 mg
		Stabilize patient's condition and transport to hospital

CNS, Central nervous system.
Modified from Little JW, Falace DA, Miller CS, Rhodus NL: *Dental management of the medically compromised patient,* ed 9, St Louis, 2018, Elsevier; Malamed SF: *Medical emergencies in the dental office,* ed 7, St Louis, 2015, Mosby.

The range of signs and symptoms of cardiovascular toxicity includes the following:

- Chest pain
- Shortness of breath
- Palpitations
- Lightheadedness
- Diaphoresis
- Hypotension
- Syncope

Management of Local Anesthetic Overdose

The onset, intensity, and severity of the local anesthetic overdose will determine how to manage the emergency. In most cases the patient's symptoms will be mild, requiring little or no treatment. For moderate to severe reactions, specific, prompt management is necessary.[1]

In patients with suspected local anesthetic toxicity, the initial step is stabilization of potential life threats. Impending airway compromise, significant hypotension, and treatment of dysrhythmias and seizures take precedence. Once other possible etiologies of the patient's new symptoms have been excluded, management of the specific symptoms can begin. Table 17.3 describes the clinical signs, symptoms, and management of mild, moderate, and severe overdose reactions[21].

EPINEPHRINE OVERDOSE

Epinephrine and levonordefrin are the two vasopressor drugs currently combined with local anesthetic agents for use in dentistry in the United States. Epinephrine is the most potent of the two and the most widely used (see Chapter 4).

Causes and Prevention of Epinephrine Overdose

An epinephrine overdose is more likely to occur when higher concentrations are administered. The use of a 1:50,000 dilution is twice as potent as the 1:100,000 dilution and is more likely to cause a toxic overdose with no added benefit to pain control. It has been stated that a dilution of 1:200,000 provides adequate duration of pain control for dental procedures with minimal risk of toxicity.[2] The only benefit to administering the 1:50,000 dilution is to increase hemostasis, which can be accomplished by infiltrating small volumes of agent to the site of excess bleeding via an intraseptal injection (see Chapters 12 and 13). An overdose in this type of administration technique is rare.

Intravascular injection may also produce an epinephrine overdose reaction. As discussed previously, it is recommended for the dental hygienist to properly aspirate on several planes and to inject the agent slowly.

Patients with cardiovascular disease are much more susceptible to an epinephrine overdose, causing more strain to an already compromised CVS. The lowest possible effective dose should always be used when administering local anesthetics with epinephrine to all patients, whether healthy or medically compromised. The MRD per visit for a healthy patient is 0.2 mg for epinephrine and 1.0 mg for levonordefrin. The MRD per visit for a cardiovascularly involved patient is 0.04 mg for epinephrine and 0.2 mg for levonordefrin. The dental hygienist should use the lowest possible concentration to achieve the desired result and follow dosage guidelines as described in Chapter 8.

TABLE 17.4 Clinical Manifestations and Management of a Patient With an Epinephrine Overdose Reaction

Signs and Symptoms	Management
Tension	Terminate procedure
Anxiety	Position patient upright
Apprehension	Reassure patient
Nervousness	Provide basic life support
Tremors	Monitor vital signs
Tension	Activate EMS if needed
Increased heart rate	Assess SpO_2 and administer oxygen at flow rate of 5–6 L/minute as needed
Increased blood pressure	
Throbbing headache	Allow patient to recover and discharge
Hyperventilation	

Modified from Little JW, Falace DA, Miller CS, Rhodus NL: *Dental management of the medically compromised patient,* ed 9, St Louis, 2018, Elsevier; Malamed SF: *Medical emergencies in the dental office,* ed 7, St Louis, 2015, Mosby.

Clinical Manifestations and Management of Epinephrine Overdose

Epinephrine overdose produces overstimulation of adrenergic receptors that can produce signs and symptoms usually observed from CNS stimulation and resemble the fight-or-flight response. Table 17.4 describes the signs, symptoms, and management of an epinephrine overdose. Because the body is very efficient at removing vasoconstrictors, these adverse effects only last about 5 to 10 minutes and typically need little or no definitive treatment. In patients who are cardiovascularly compromised, or if prolonged reactions occur, a more serious response to the overdose may be observed, and the dental hygienist must be prepared to respond to the emergency situation.

ALLERGIC MANIFESTATIONS

Allergic reactions are derived by an immunologic reaction to a noninfectious foreign substance (antigen). They comprise a series of repeat reactions to a foreign substance. These foreign substances that trigger hypersensitivity reactions are called **allergens** or **antigens**.[22]

Amino esters are derivatives of para-aminobenzoic acid (PABA) and are associated with acute allergic reactions. Previous studies indicate a 30% rate of allergic reactions to procaine, tetracaine, and chloroprocaine. Amino amides are not associated with PABA and do not produce allergic reactions with the same frequency. The incidence of a true, documented allergic reaction to an amide local anesthetic is extremely rare.[23,24] However, it is not unusual for a patient to claim they are allergic to local anesthetics.[8,25,26] Through careful investigation of the alleged allergy, one generally finds out that what the patient experienced was either a syncopal episode or an exaggerated physiologic ("fight-or-flight") response to the injected epinephrine or epinephrine released endogenously.[8] Allergic reactions associated with amides in the past were associated with the preservative methylparaben, which has since been taken out of anesthetic solutions.

Allergic reactions associated with sodium bisulfite or metabisulfite are reported frequently.[27,28] Bisulfites are antioxidants added to local anesthetic agents to prevent the oxidation of epinephrine. They are commonly used commercially in restaurants where they are sprayed on fruits and vegetables to prevent discoloration. They are also used to prevent bacterial contamination of wines, beers, and other distilled beverages.[1,29] Box 17.1 lists the common sulfite-containing agents. It is unknown whether bisulfites can trigger an anaphylactic reaction.

BOX 17.1 Sulfite-Containing Agents

Restaurant salads
Fresh fruits
Dried fruits
Wine, beer, cordials
Alcohol
All sparkling grape juices, including nonalcoholic
Potatoes including French fries, chips
Sausage meats
Cider and vinegar
Pickles
Dehydrated vegetables
Cheese and cheese mixtures
Bottled lemon and lime juice
Gelatin
Corn bread or muffin mix
Shrimp and other seafood
Fresh fish
Avocados, including guacamole
Soups (canned or dried)
Sauces and gravies (including barbecue sauce)

From Malamed SF: *Medical emergencies in the dental office,* ed 6, St Louis, 2007, Mosby.

Bisulfite allergies typically manifest as a severe respiratory allergy, commonly bronchospasm. It has been reported that 5% to 10% of people with asthma are allergic to bisulfites.[1,29]

Topical anesthetics are also possible allergens.[1] Benzocaine and tetracaine are commonly used ester topical anesthetics that can contribute to an allergic response. Lidocaine is the only amide anesthetic available topically and may contain preservatives such as parabens (including methyl, ethyl, and propyl), which could induce an allergic response. Careful consideration of the patient's potential for an allergic reaction should be determined before administering these agents.

Prevention of Allergic Reactions

The preanesthetic patient assessment is the most important measure that the dental hygienist can complete to prevent an allergic reaction. Patients who respond to questions related to asthma, hay fever, and allergies to foods have an increased potential for developing an allergic response to medications.[1] The dental hygienist should proceed with further dialogue to determine whether a true allergy exists (Box 17.2).

BOX 17.2 Questions to Evaluate an Alleged Allergic Reaction to a Local Anesthetic

When was the last time you experienced this response? Describe exactly what happened.
What position were you in during the injection?
What was the time sequence of events?
What drug was used?
What amount of drug was administered?
Did the drug contain a vasoconstrictor?
Were you taking any other medication at the time of the incident?
How was the reaction managed?
What is the name and address of the doctor who was treating you when the reaction occurred?

Modified from Pieren JA, Bowen DM: *Darby and Walsh dental hygiene: theory and practice,* ed 5, St Louis, 2020, Elsevier.

BOX 17.3 When to Refer a Patient With a History of Anesthetic Allergy to an Allergist

History shows reaction consistent with allergic response
Allergic to anesthetic that is identified
Allergic to anesthetic that cannot be identified
Allergic to several anesthetics involving both amides and esters
Skin testing not indicated because of variable results
Provocative dose testing (PDT)
Selection and recommendation of alternative local anesthetic based on result of PDT

The dental hygienist should not use the anesthetic agent in question until the allergy is disproved. If questions remain after the dialogue history, the dental hygienist should consult the dentist and the patient's physician; referral to an allergist should be considered (Box 17.3).

Clinical Manifestations and Management of Allergic Reactions

Allergic responses are either delayed or immediate. Delayed signs and symptoms of an allergic reaction are less serious, and rapid signs and symptoms of an allergic reaction are more intense and serious. The amount of time between the administration of the anesthetic agent and the signs and symptoms of the allergic response determines how the dental hygienist will manage the reaction.

Allergic manifestations of local anesthetics include rash and urticaria. If these skin reactions appear alone after considerable time following the injection (more than 60 minutes), this is most likely a delayed allergic response and is usually not life-threatening. If the skin reaction develops immediately after the injection, a more serious and generalized reaction, known as *anaphylaxis*, may occur and can be life-threatening. Anaphylaxis caused by local anesthetics is very rare but should be considered when a patient demonstrates intense itching and urticaria, as well as wheezing or respiratory distress, seconds after the administration of the local anesthetic agent.

Although allergic reactions to local anesthetics are extremely rare, these are treated by the dentist according to severity. Mild cutaneous reactions may be treated with diphenhydramine (Benadryl 25–50 mg for adult doses, 1 mg/kg for pediatric doses); treat patients with more serious reactions with 0.3 mL of epinephrine subcutaneously (1:1000), and closely monitor for further decompensation. Corticosteroids (125 mg methylprednisolone or 60 mg prednisone) should be administered to the patient with severe allergic reactions (e.g., respiratory distress, hypotension). Table 17.5 describes the signs, symptoms, and management of delayed allergic responses, as well as immediate anaphylactic reactions. The dental hygienist should also be familiar with the use of a preloaded EpiPen (Fig. 17.3).

MANAGEMENT OF MEDICAL EMERGENCIES

Life-threatening emergencies can occur during dental hygiene treatment with or without the administration of local anesthetics. Although these types of emergencies occur infrequently, the increasing number of older patients seeking dental treatment, medically compromised adults, patients taking multiple drugs, and longer dental appointments increase the likelihood of an emergency. These situations are compounded when the administration of local anesthetics is incorporated into the treatment. The best management of a dental office medical emergency is prevention. The dental hygienist should become familiar with the most common emergency situations, their management (including office procedures), and drugs used to treat such complications. The following guidelines are general measures to ensure emergency preparedness:

TABLE 17.5 Clinical Manifestations and Management of an Allergic Reaction

Delayed Allergic Response	Signs and Symptoms	Management
Skin	Erythema Urticaria (hives) Pruritus (itching) Angioedema (localized swelling of extremities, lips, tongue, pharynx, larynx)	Administer antihistamine Obtain medical consultation
Respiration	Bronchospasm Distress Dyspnea Wheezing Perspiration Flushing Cyanosis Tachycardia Anxiety	Terminate procedure Activate EMS if needed Position patient semierect Reassure patient Provide basic life support as needed Monitor vital signs Assess SpO_2 and administer oxygen at flow rate of 5–6 L/minute as needed Administer epinephrine if needed Administer antihistamine Allow patient to recover and discharge
Laryngeal edema	Swelling of vocal apparatus and subsequent obstruction of airway Respiratory distress Exaggerated chest movements High-pitched sound to no sound Cyanosis Loss of consciousness	Terminate procedure Activate EMS Position patient supine Administer epinephrine if needed Maintain airway Assess SpO_2 and administer oxygen at flow rate of 5–6 L/minute as needed Additional drug management: antihistamine, corticosteroid Cricothyrotomy if needed Transfer patient to hospital

TABLE 17.5 Clinical Manifestations and Management of an Allergic Reaction (*Cont.*)

Immediate Anaphylaxis	Signs and Symptoms	Management
Skin	Pruritus (itching) Flushing Urticaria (face and upper chest) Feeling of hair standing on end Conjunctivitis, vasomotor rhinitis	Terminate procedure Activate EMS Position the patient supine, legs elevated Provide basic life support as indicated Administer 0.3–0.5 mg 1:1000 epinephrine Assess SpO_2 and administer oxygen at flow rate of 5–6 L/minute as needed Monitor vital signs Additional drug management: antihistamine, corticosteroid if needed Transport patient to hospital
Gastrointestinal or genitourinary	Abdominal cramps Nausea, vomiting, diarrhea	Same as management of anaphylaxis related to skin
Respiratory	Substernal tightness or chest pain Cough, wheeze Dyspnea Cyanosis of mucous membranes, nail beds Laryngeal edema	Same as management of anaphylaxis related to skin
Cardiovascular	Pallor Lightheadedness Palpitations, tachycardia Hypotension Cardiac dysrhythmias Unconsciousness Cardiac arrest	Same as management of anaphylaxis related to skin

Modified from Little JW, Falace DA, Miller CS, Rhodus NL: *Dental management of the medically compromised patient,* ed 9, St Louis, 2018, Elsevier.

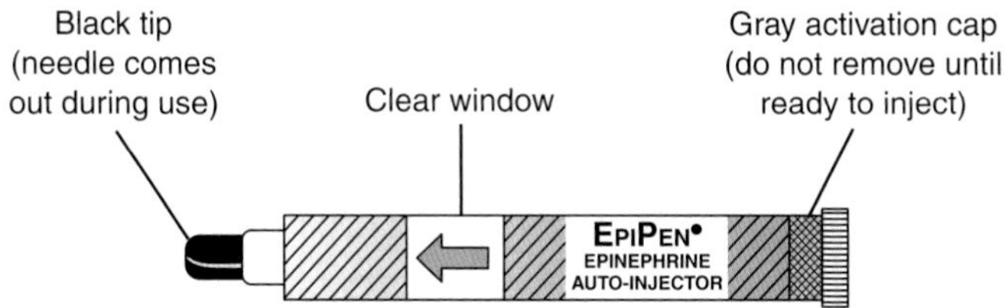

Fig. 17.3 The EpiPen is an emergency preloaded supply of epinephrine. (From Lehne R: *Pharmacology for nursing care,* ed 6, Philadelphia, 2007, Saunders.)

1. *Training:* All office personnel should be trained and retrained annually in emergency procedures. Office emergency simulations should be conducted every 6 months. Basic cardiac life support, that is, cardiopulmonary resuscitation, is required. Advanced cardiac life support training is optional unless performing conscious sedation; however, it is recommended for dental hygienists practicing local anesthesia in states allowing its use without the physical presence of a dentist.
2. *Phone number:* Telephone numbers of the closest physician, emergency department, and ambulance service should be posted and programmed for "speed dial."
3. *Emergency equipment:* Emergency equipment should include an oxygen tank, pocket mask, and automated external defibrillator (AED). All office personnel should know the location of the items, and all trained dental personnel who would use the oxygen and AED should be retrained on these devices annually.
4. *Drug kit:* Drug therapy is always secondary to basic life support. Table 17.6 describes the common dental emergency drug kit.
5. *Recognition and management of an emergency:* The dental hygienist must maintain up-to-date education on recognition and management of emergency situations. Table 17.7 describes the common medical emergencies and their management. Fig. 17.4 illustrates actions that should be taken by the dental hygienist in an emergency situation when the patient loses consciousness.

TABLE 17.6 Common Drugs in a Dental Emergency Kit

Drug	Indications	Action	Availability (Adult Doses)
Nitroglycerin Amyl-nitrite	Angina pectoris	Coronary vessel dilator	0.4 mg/metered dose
Ammonia	Syncope	Irritant: increases respiratory rate	0.3 mL/Vaporole
Atropine	Prevents vagal syncope	Parasympathetic depressant	0.5 mg/1-mL ampule
Medihaler Ventolin (albuterol)	Asthmatic attack	Bronchodilator	Two sprays 90 mcg/spray
Glucagon	Hypoglycemia (unconscious patient), or conscious patient at risk for choking (i.e., seizures or convulsions)	Elevates blood sugar	1 mg/mL ampule

(*Continued*)

TABLE 17.6 Common Drugs in a Dental Emergency Kit (*Cont.*)

Drug	Indications	Action	Availability (Adult Doses)
Orange juice, sugar, glucose paste, or dextrose	Hypoglycemia in conscious patient	Elevates blood sugar	As needed
Aspirin	Myocardial infarction	Provides a fibrinolysis effect to reduce clotting	325 mg tablet
Oxygen tank, mask, and cannula	Oxygen saturation below target peripheral capillary oxygen saturation (SpO_2)	Delivers free-flowing oxygen to patient with inadequate oxygen saturation	5–6 L/minute
Pulse oximeter	To monitor oxygen saturations to determine whether oxygen should be administered	Monitors oxygen saturation of hemoglobin in arterial blood	NA
AED	Unresponsive patient, cardiac arrest	Provides shock to the heart to allow for the connection of an irregular ineffective rhythm of heartbeat	NA
Benzodiazepine	Convulsions	Depressant	Lorazepam 2 mg intranasal or diazepam (Valium) 5–20 mg IV or midazolam 5 mg intranasal
Epinephrine	Anaphylaxis or to combat severe asthmatic attack	Bronchodilator and cardiac stimulator	0.3–0.5 mg 1:1000
Benadryl (diphenhydramine)	Mild or localized allergic reaction	Decreases the allergic response by blocking the action of histamine	25–50 mg every 6–8 hours
Aminophylline	To combat undue reactions to drugs or to combat severe asthmatic attack	Bronchodilator	250 mg/1 mL syringe
Hydrocortisone sodium succinate (Solu-Cortef)	To combat undue reactions to drugs such as penicillin or to combat severe asthmatic attack	Antiinflammatory glucocorticoid	100 mg/2 mL syringe

AED, Automatic external defibrillator; *NA,* not applicable.
From Little JW, Falace DA, Miller CS, Rhodus NL: *Dental management of the medically compromised patient,* ed 9, St Louis, 2018, Elsevier; Malamed SF: *Medical emergencies in the dental office,* ed 7, St Louis, 2015, Mosby.

TABLE 17.7 Management of Specific Medical Emergencies

Condition	Cause	Signs and Symptoms	Management (Adult Patient)
Adrenal crisis	Cortisol deficiency	Feeling of confusion, weakness, fatigue, respiratory depression, headache. Weak rapid pulse, low blood pressure, abdominal or leg pain. Possible loss of consciousness	Place patient in supine position Assess SpO_2 and administer oxygen at flow rate of 5–6 L/minute as needed Ask patient to administer his/her own corticosteroid medication Initiate BLS, if needed *If unconscious*: Place in supine position Activate EMS Assess SpO_2 and administer oxygen at flow rate of 5–6 L/minute as needed Administer hydrocortisone Initiate BLS
Syncope (fainting), the most common dental emergency	Cerebral hypoxia (reduced blood flow to brain), anxiety is a common contributing factor, especially during the administration of local anesthetics	Feeling of warmth, flushed skin, nausea, rapid heart rate, perspiration, pallor, pupillary dilation, diaphoresis Sudden, transient loss of consciousness	Place in Trendelenburg position (patient's head lower than legs) Loosen any binding clothes, ensure open airway Assess SpO_2 and administer oxygen at flow rate of 5–6 L/minute as needed Pass crushed ammonia capsule (e.g., Vaporole) under patient's nose (optional) Place cool, damp cloth on forehead, reassure Monitor and record vital signs Facilitate next steps in medical/dental care and reassure patient
Hyperventilation	Anxiety-induced rapid breathing causing excessive loss of CO_2	Abnormally prolonged rapid and shallow respirations, lightheadedness, dizziness, confusion, tingling in extremities, tightness in the chest, rapid heartbeat, lump in throat, panic-stricken appearance, cold hands, carpal-pedal spasms; can lead to seizure Impairment of problem-solving abilities, motor coordination, balance, and perceptual tasks	Terminate procedure, place patient in position of choice, usually upright Use quiet tone of voice to calm and reassure patient; encourage slow, deep breaths Maintain open airway Loosen tight clothing in neck region Work with patient to control rate of respirations Have patient count to 10 in one breath, breathe through pursed lips or nose or in cupped hands to rebreathe carbon dioxide Facilitate next steps in medical/dental care and reassure patient Do not administer oxygen

TABLE 17.7 Management of Specific Medical Emergencies (*Cont.*)

Condition	Cause	Signs and Symptoms	Management (Adult Patient)
Bronchial asthma	Can be induced by anxiety, allergy, infection, and exercise, leading to bronchial inflammation, bronchoconstriction, occlusion of bronchioles by thick mucus plugs, and bronchospasm	Coughing, shortness of breath, periodic wheezing, dyspnea, anxiety, chest tightness, increased pulse rate, sense of suffocation	Assist patient to a position that facilitates breathing (upright is usually best) Have patient self-medicate with a β_2 agonist bronchodilator (e.g., albuterol, Isuprel Mistometer) Ensure that the airway is open Encourage relaxed slow breathing Assess SpO_2 Administer oxygen as needed Monitor vital signs If patient is unresponsive, administer 0.3–0.5 mg 1:1000 epinephrine If necessary, activate EMS and initiate BLS
Angina pectoris	Blood supply to the cardiac muscle is insufficient for oxygen demand (atherosclerosis or coronary artery spasm). May be precipitated by stress, anxiety, or physical activity	Crushing, burning, or squeezing chest pain, radiating to left shoulder, arms, neck, or mandible and lasting 2–15 minutes; shortness of breath; diaphoresis (sweating), pain relieved by nitroglycerin	Terminate procedure Position patient upright Monitor and record vital signs Ensure that breathing is adequate and check circulation Assess SpO_2 and administer oxygen as needed Administer nitroglycerin sublingually (0.4 mg every 5 minutes for three doses) Activate EMS if patient's pain is not relieved, and treat as a myocardial infarction
Myocardial infarction (heart attack)	Blood supply to the heart is interrupted, most commonly caused by occlusion of coronary vessels. Anoxia, ischemia, and infarct are present.	Mild to severe chest pain (crushing, squeezing, or heavy feeling); pain in the left arm, jaw, and possibly teeth, not relieved by rest and nitroglycerin; cold, clammy skin; nausea; anxiety; shortness of breath; weakness; perspiration; burning feeling of indigestion; feeling of impending doom	Terminate procedure Activate EMS Place patient supine Initiate BLS as needed Dispense/administer aspirin 325-mg tablet in conscious patient Assess SpO_2 and administer oxygen at flow rate of 5–6 L/minute as needed Monitor and record vital signs
Cerebrovascular accident (stroke)	Interruption of blood supply and oxygen to the brain occurring as a result of ischemia or hemorrhage	Sudden weakness of one side, difficulty of speech, temporary loss of vision, dizziness (patient may fall), change in mental status, nausea, severe headache, and/or seizures	Terminate procedure Activate EMS Monitor vital signs Monitor airway Initiate BLS as needed Assess SpO_2 and administer oxygen at flow rate of 5–6 L/minute as needed
Seizures	Several causes of convulsions and seizures, including drug overdoses, syncope, hyperventilation, cerebrovascular accident, and convulsive seizure disorder	Aura (change in taste, smell, or sight preceding seizure), loss of consciousness, sudden cry, involuntary tonic-clonic muscle contractions, altered breathing	Terminate procedure, lower dental chair and clear area of all sharp and dangerous objects Make no attempt to restrain patient Protect the patient's head Assess and establish an airway Monitor vital signs Initiate BLS and activate EMS if needed If the patient's condition is stable, allow patient to rest Arrange for medical follow-up Arrange for assistance in leaving the dental facility *For status epilepticus (a seizure lasting more than 5 minutes):* Activate EMS Administer diazepam (Valium) 5–20 mg IV or intranasal lorazepam 2–4 mg or intranasal midazolam 5 mg
Hypoglycemia (insulin shock)	Lack of blood glucose to the brain; taking insulin and not eating	Mood changes, hunger, headache, perspiration, nausea, confusion irritation, dizziness and weakness, increased anxiety, rapid thread pulse, possible unconsciousness	Terminate procedure If conscious, place in upright position Administer oral sugar; give concentrated form of oral sugar (e.g., sugar packet, cake icing, concentrated orange juice, apple juice, sugar-containing sodas) If patient is unconscious, activate EMS and administer glucagon 1 mg SC or IM Monitor vital signs Assess SpO_2 and administer oxygen at flow rate of 5–6 L/minute as needed

(*Continued*)

TABLE 17.7 Management of Specific Medical Emergencies (*Cont.*)

Condition	Cause	Signs and Symptoms	Management (Adult Patient)
Hyperglycemia (ketoacidosis)	Type 1: genetic, autoimmune, and environmental factors Type 2: genetic, environmental, and aging factors	Excessive thirst, urination, and hunger; labored respirations; nausea; dry, flushed skin; low blood pressure; weak, rapid pulse; acetone breath ("fruity" smell), blurred vision, headache, unconsciousness	Terminate procedure Activate EMS Provide BLS if needed If patient is conscious, ask when he or she ate last, whether insulin was taken, and whether patient brought insulin to the appointment If able, patient should self-administer the insulin Monitor and record vital signs
Mild (delayed onset) allergic reaction	Overreactions to allergens such as drugs, pollens, or food, which cause the degranulation of mast cells and release histamine, often in skin or mucosa	Itching, skin redness, hives	Call for assistance Place patient upright Prepare an antihistamine for administration (diphenhydramine [Benadryl] 25–50 mg PO or IM [or IV if dentist has ACLS or advanced training]) Be prepared to administer BLS if needed
Anaphylaxis (immediate onset)	Overreaction to allergens such as drugs, pollens, food causing the degranulation of mast cells, which release histamine into the cardiopulmonary system	Urticaria (itchy wheals, also known as *hives*); angioedema of lips, tongue, larynx, pharynx; respiratory distress, wheezing, laryngeal edema, weak pulse, low blood pressure; may progress to unconsciousness and cardiovascular collapse	Terminate procedure and immediately activate EMS Place in upright position for conscious patient and supine position for unconscious patient Establish and maintain airway Monitor vital signs Assess SpO_2 and administer oxygen at flow rate of 5–6 L/minute as needed Administer epinephrine 0.3–0.5 mg 1:1000 epinephrine SC or IM or IV if dentist has ACLS training Initiate BLS as needed
Mild local anesthetic overdose	Too large a dose of anesthetic per patient body weight (exceeded maximum recommended dose); rapid absorption of drug; inadvertent intravascular injection; slow detoxification or elimination of the drug	Disorientation, nervousness, flushed skin color, apprehension, twitching tremors, shivering, dizziness, lightheadedness, visual disturbances, auditory disturbances, headache, tinnitus	Terminate procedure Reassure patient Position patient in comfortable position Administer oxygen Provide BLS if needed Monitor vital signs Assess SpO_2 and administer oxygen at flow rate of 5–6 L/minute as needed Activate EMS if needed Allow patient to recover and discharge
Severe local anesthetic overdose	Too large a dose of anesthetic per patient body weight (exceeded maximum recommended dose); rapid absorption of drug; inadvertent intravascular injection; slow biotransformation or elimination of the drug	Drowsiness, disorientation, convulsions, drop in blood pressure, bradycardia, apnea, unconsciousness	Terminate procedure Position patient supine, legs elevated Activate EMS Manage seizure: protect patient from injury Provide BLS if needed Assess SpO_2 and administer oxygen at flow rate of 5–6 L/minute as needed Monitor vital signs Administer an anticonvulsant (diazepam, lorazepam, or midazolam) as described under seizures for prolonged seizure Transport patient to hospital after condition is stabilized
Vasoconstrictor overdose	Too large a dose (exceeded maximum recommended dose of 0.2 mg for a healthy patient and 0.04 mg for patients with significant cardiovascular disease); inadvertent intravascular injection	Tension Anxiety Apprehension Nervousness Tremors Increased heart rate Increased blood pressure Throbbing headache Hyperventilation	Terminate procedure Position patient upright Reassure patient Provide BLS if needed Monitor vital signs Summon medical assistance if needed Assess SpO_2 and administer oxygen at flow rate of 5–6 L/minute as needed Allow patient to recover and discharge

ACLS, Advanced cardiac life support; *BLS,* basic life support; *EMS,* emergency medical system; *IM,* intramuscular; *IV,* intravenous; *PO,* oral administration (per os); *SC,* subcutaneous.

From Little JW, Falace DA, Miller CS, Rhodus NL: *Dental management of the medically compromised patient,* ed 9, St Louis, 2018, Elsevier; Malamed SF: *Medical emergencies in the dental office,* ed 7, St Louis, 2015, Mosby.

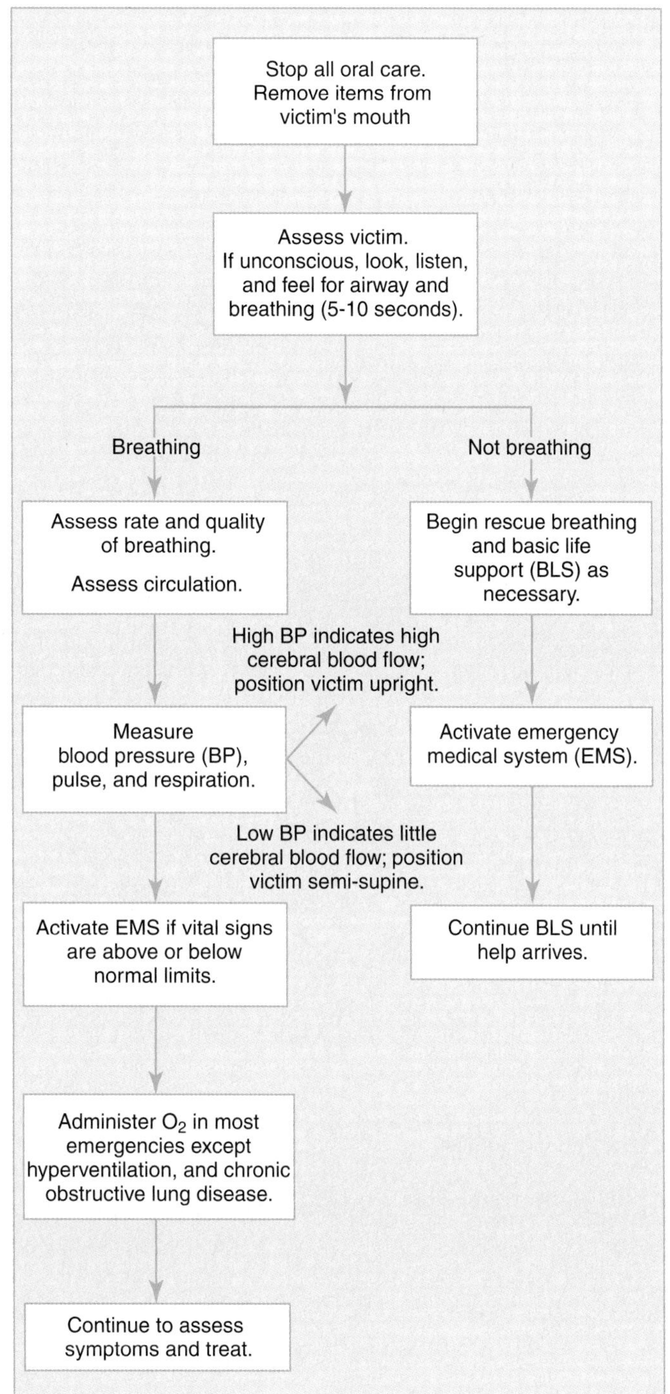

Fig. 17.4 Dental hygiene actions taken in an emergency situation when the patient loses consciousness. (From Bowen DM, Pieren JA: *Darby and Walsh dental hygiene: theory and practice,* ed 5, St Louis, 2020, Elsevier.)

DENTAL HYGIENE CONSIDERATIONS

- Most systemic reactions associated with the administration of local anesthetics can be avoided with thorough preanesthetic assessment, proper communication, careful choice of local anesthetic agent, and careful injection techniques. Conditions that place the patient at risk for an emergency should be recorded as a medical alert in the patient's medical history.
- Appropriate consultations or referrals for dental and medical considerations must be completed before administering local anesthetics.
- Baseline vital signs must be obtained before the administration of a local anesthetic. If an emergency occurs, the emergency rescue team will want to know preanesthetic vital signs.
- Always use the lowest effective dose and never exceed the maximum recommended dose (see Chapter 8).
- Always aspirate before administering the local anesthetic drug, and aspirate on two planes when injecting into highly vascular areas.
- Slowly depositing the anesthetic agent will reduce the risk of an overdose even if the anesthetic is accidentally administered intravascularly.
- Record type of drug and doses administered in milligrams in the patient's chart. If an emergency occurs, the emergency rescue team will want to know what drug was administered and how much in milligrams. Medical personnel are unfamiliar with dental cartridge doses, and all doses must be converted to milligrams for appropriate documentation in the patient's chart (see Chapter 8).
- Thorough documentation is essential, including instructions to the patient and the patient's responses.
- Office staff must be competent in the use of emergency equipment, emergency drug kits, and office emergency procedures. Emergency drills should be conducted often.
- Use stress-reduction strategies to prevent stress-related emergencies (see Chapters 1 and 7).
- Complications can occur with the administration of local anesthesia even when the dental hygienist uses proper technique and risk-reduction protocol.

CASE STUDY 17.1 A Systemic Complication

Part 1: A new patient, a 23-year-old professional baseball player, comes into the dental office for a restorative procedure on tooth #2. In this dental office, the dental hygienist is responsible for administration of all local anesthetics for the office. The patient's medical history is reviewed, and it is determined that he is a healthy patient with no contraindications to the use of local anesthetics and vasoconstrictors. In fact, during the dialogue history when the dental hygienist discusses his dental history, the patient responds by saying: "I am pretty tough and can handle any dental procedure." A few minutes after the dental hygienist's initial injection, the patient seems nervous and complains of dizziness, lightheadedness, and a racing heart. His color is ashen, and his extremities feel cold and clammy.

Critical Thinking Questions

- According to the clinical symptoms described, what reaction is the patient experiencing?
- How should the dental hygienist respond?

Part 2: Then the patient quickly recovers from this initial condition when the dental hygienist notices a faint bluish discoloration appearing on his cheek. The clinician checks intraorally and finds the same discoloration near the injection site along with some slight swelling.

Critical Thinking Questions

- According to the clinical symptoms described, what reaction is the patient experiencing?
- What is the most probable cause of the cheek discoloration?
- How should the dental hygienist respond?

CHAPTER REVIEW QUESTIONS

1. Anaphylaxis is considered to be what type of complication?
   - **A.** Localized and severe
   - **B.** Systemic and mild
   - **C.** Systemic and severe
   - **D.** Localized and mild
2. Systemic complications usually occur MORE frequently than local complications. This situation is usually caused by high plasma concentration of the local anesthetic drug.
   - **A.** Both statements are correct.
   - **B.** Both statements are NOT correct.
   - **C.** The first statement is correct; the second statement is NOT correct.
   - **D.** The first statement is NOT correct; the second statement is correct.
3. All of the following can increase the risk of local anesthetic overdose EXCEPT one. Which is the EXCEPTION?
   - **A.** Fast biotransformation
   - **B.** Rapid deposit of agent
   - **C.** Intravascular injection
   - **D.** Atypical pseudocholinesterase
4. Which of the following is a sign of a central nervous system overdose from moderate to high blood levels that can be noted in a patient after administration of a local anesthetic?
   - **A.** Dizziness
   - **B.** Hypertension
   - **C.** Excitatory-nervousness
   - **D.** Convulsions
5. The patient shows convulsions, respiratory distress, cardiovascular depression, and coma; what is occurring to the patient?
   - **A.** Heart attack
   - **B.** Cardiovascular toxicity
   - **C.** Epinephrine overdose
   - **D.** Local anesthetic overdose
6. Which of the following dilutions of local anesthetic agents has the lowest concentration of epinephrine?
   - **A.** 1:100,000 epinephrine
   - **B.** 1:200,000 epinephrine
   - **C.** 1:50,000 epinephrine
   - **D.** 1:1000 epinephrine

7. Which of the following is the appropriate treatment for a mild cutaneous reaction?
   A. Corticosteroids
   B. Diphenhydramine
   C. Nitroglycerin
   D. Aspirin
8. All of the following are signs of angina pectoris EXCEPT one. Which is the EXCEPTION?
   A. Chest pain
   B. Pain in left arm
   C. Shortness of breath
   D. Dizziness
9. If the clinician strongly suspects the patient is having a myocardial infarction, the procedure is stopped and then the clinician should immediately:
   A. Position the patient upright
   B. Administer nitroglycerin
   C. Activate emergency medical services
   D. Initiate basic life support
10. If a patient starts to experience involuntary muscle contractions and altered breathing, what should the clinician suspect?
    A. Respiratory distress
    B. Hypoglycemia
    C. Seizures
    D. Asthma attack
11. Patients with liver disease have a greater chance of developing which of the following after an administration of a local anesthetic.
    A. Delayed absorption of local anesthetic
    B. Higher blood levels of the anesthetic drug
    C. More vasoactivity at the injection site
    D. Rapid excretion of the drug by the kidneys
12. All of the following will reduce the risk of a local anesthetic overdose EXCEPT one. Which one is the EXCEPTION?
    A. Slow biotransformation
    B. Aspirating on two planes
    C. Using a vasoconstrictor
    D. Administering minimal effective dose
13. Which drug in used to treat anaphylaxis?
    A. Diphenhydramine
    B. Epinephrine
    C. Levonordefrin
    D. Lorazepam
14. Which of the following is the most common dental emergency after the administration of local anesthesia?
    A. Anesthetic overdose
    B. Epinephrine overdose
    C. Syncope
    D. Allergic reaction
15. What is the appropriate management of a patient with a delayed allergic reaction?
    A. Administer diphenhydramine
    B. Administer epinephrine
    C. Administer aminophylline
    D. Administer lorazepam
16. The dental hygienist should respond to an emergency situation in the office by first providing basic life support. Drug therapy is always secondary to basic life support.
    A. Both statements are correct.
    B. Both statements are NOT correct.
    C. The first statement is correct; the second statement is NOT correct.
    D. The first statement is NOT correct; the second statement is correct.
17. During a vasoconstrictor overdose the patient should be placed in a supine position, and the dental hygienist should provide basic life support as needed.
    A. Both statements are correct.
    B. Both statements are NOT correct.
    C. The first statement is correct; the second statement is NOT correct.
    D. The first statement is NOT correct; the second statement is correct.
18. A patient who has a sulfite allergy will have a sensitivity to which of the following?
    A. Wine
    B. Bananas
    C. Ground beef
    D. Chicken
19. Which of the following individuals have a predisposition to a local anesthetic overdose?
    A. Patients with prosthetic heart valves
    B. Elderly patients
    C. Anxious patients
    D. Patients allergic to many foods
20. What is the drug of choice for an unconscious patient with hypoglycemia?
    A. Orange juice
    B. Glucagon
    C. Glucose paste
    D. Sugar cubes

REFERENCES

1. Malamed SF. *Medical emergencies in the dental office*. ed 7. St Louis: Mosby; 2017.
2. Malamed S. *Handbook of local anesthesia*. ed 7. St Louis: Elsevier; 2020.
3. Jastak T, Yagiela J, Donaldson D. *Local anesthesia of the oral cavity*. St Louis: Saunders; 1995.
4. El-Boghdadly K, Pawa A, Chin KJ. Local anesthetic systemic toxicity: current perspectives. *Local and Regional Anesthesia*. 2018;11:35–44.
5. El-Boghdadly K, Chin KJ. Local anesthetic systemic toxicity: Continuing Professional Development. *Can J Anaesth*. 2016;63(3):330–349.
6. Gitman M, Barrington MJ. Local anesthetic systemic toxicity: a review of recent case reports and registries. *Reg Anesth Pain Med*. 2018;43(2):124–130.
7. Rosenberg PH, Verring BT, Urmey W. Maximum recommended doses of local anesthetics: a multifactorial concept. *Reg Anesth Pain Med*. 2004;29(6):564–575.
8. Becker DE, Reed KL. Local anesthetics: review of pharmacological considerations. *Anesth Prog*. 2012;59(2):90–102.
9. Pere PJ, Ekstrand A, Salonen M, et al. Pharmacokinetics of ropivacaine in patients with chronic renal failure. *Br J Anaesth*. 2011;106(4):512–521.
10. Dillane D, Finucane BT. Local anesthetic systemic toxicity. *Can J Anesth*. 2010;57(4):368–380.
11. Hogan Q. Local anesthetic toxicity: an update. *Reg Anesth*. 1996;21(6 Suppl):43–50.
12. Moore PA, Hersh EV. Local anesthesia: pharmacology and toxicity. *Dent Clin North Am*. 2010;54(4):587–599.
13. Moore PA. Preventing local anesthetic toxicity. *J Am Dent Assoc*. 1992;123:60–64.
14. Tarsitano JJ. Children, drugs, and local anesthesia. *J Am Dent Assoc*. 1965;70:1153–1158.

15. Goodson JM, Moore PA. Life-threatening reactions after pedodontic sedation: an assessment of narcotic, local anesthetic and antiemetic drug interactions. *J Am Dent Assoc.* 1983;107:239–245.
16. Bruelle P, de La Coussaye JE, Eledjam JJ. Convulsions and cardiac arrest after epidural anesthesia: prevention and treatment. *Cah Anesthesiol.* 1994;42:241–246.
17. Malagodi MH, Munson ES, Embro MJ. Relation of etidocaine and bupivacaine toxicity to rate of infusion in rhesus monkeys. *Br J Anaesth.* 1977;49:121–125.
18. Mulroy MF, Hejtmanek MR. Prevention of local anesthetic systemic toxicity. *Reg Anesth Pain Med.* 2010;27(6):556–561.
19. Mulroy MF. Systemic toxicity and cardiotoxicity from local anesthetics: incidence and preventive measures. *Reg Anesth Pain Med.* 2002;27(6):556–561.
20. Groban L. Central nervous system and cardiac effects from long-acting amide local anesthetic toxicity in the intact animal model. *Reg Anesth Pain Med.* 2003;28(1):3–11.
21. Sekimoto K, Tobe M, Saito S. Local anesthetic toxicity: acute and chronic management. *Acute Med Surg.* 2017;4(2):152–160.
22. Little JW, Falace DA, Miller CS, Rhodus NL. *Dental management of the medically compromised patient.* ed 9. St Louis: Elsevier; 2018.
23. Haas DA. An update on local anesthetics in dentistry. *J Can Dent Assoc.* 2002;68(9):546–551.
24. Yagiela JA. Injectable and topical local anesthetics. In: *ADA/PDR guide to dental therapeutics.* ed 5. Chicago: American Dental Association; 2010.
25. Jackson D, Chen AH, Bennett CR. Identifying true lidocaine allergy. *J Am Dent Assoc.* 1994;125:1362–1366.
26. Shojaei AR, Haas DA. Local anesthetic cartridges and latex allergy. *J Am Dent Assoc.* 2002;68:622–626.
27. Stevenson DD, Simon RA. Sensitivity to ingested metabisulfites in asthmatic subjects. *J Allergy Clin Immunol.* 1981;68(1):26–32.
28. Sher TH, Schwartz HJ. Bisulfite sensitivity manifesting an allergic reaction to aerosol therapy. *Ann Allergy.* 1985;54(3):224–226.
29. Borghesan F, Basso D, Chieco Bianchi F, et al. Allergy to wine. *Allergy.* 2004;59(10):1135–1136.

ADDITIONAL RESOURCES

Chen AH. Toxicity and allergy to local anesthesia. *J Calif Dent Assoc.* 1998;26(9):683–692.

Haas DA. An update on local anesthetics in dentistry. *J Can Dent Assoc.* 2002;68(9):546–551.

Katzung BG. *Basic and clinical pharmacology.* ed 14. New York: McGraw Hill; 2018; pp. 459–473.

McGee D. *Local and topical anesthesia.* In: Roberts JR, Hedges J, eds. *Clinical procedures in emergency medicine.* ed 4. Philadelphia: WB Saunders; 2004. pp. 533–551.

Wang Q, Liu Y, Lei Y, et al. Shenfu injection reduces toxicity of bupivacaine in rats. *Chin Med J (Engl).* 2003;116(9):1382–1385.

Weinberg GL, Di Gregorio G, Ripper R, et al. Resuscitation with lipid versus epinephrine in a rat model of bupivacaine overdose. *Anesthesiology.* 2008;108(5):907–913.

Weinberg GL, Ripper R, Feinstein DL, Hoffman W. Lipid emulsion infusion rescues dogs from bupivacaine-induced cardiac toxicity. *Reg Anesth Pain Med.* 2003;28(3):198–202.

Risk Management and Exposure Prevention

Demetra Daskalos Logothetis, RDH, MS

LEARNING OBJECTIVES

1. Name the primary objective of providing dental hygiene care and describe how risk management plays a role in accomplishing this objective.
2. Discuss the importance of effective dental hygienist–to-patient communication before treatment.
3. Discuss the importance of effective dental hygienist–to-employer communication.
4. Discuss the legal issues related to dental hygiene treatment and prevention strategies to reduce the risk of litigation.
5. Describe the type of information that should always be included in patient documentation for the administration of local anesthetics.
6. List and describe the three categories of prevention and management of injury in dentistry.
7. Describe the procedures to reduce the risk of accidental needle exposure.
8. Describe postexposure management.

RISK MANAGEMENT

Every great mistake has a halfway moment when it can be recalled and perhaps remedied.

—Pearl S. Buck

The primary objective of providing dental hygiene care is to assist patients in preventing disease and maintaining oral health. With the delivery of these services, the dental hygienist may experience unanticipated and problematic outcomes. For example, local anesthetics administered for pain management to effectively maximize patient comfort and treatment may bring undesirable adverse reactions. Risk management identifies preventive methods to minimize or eliminate the risk of legal action associated with the delivery of oral care. Because of the scope of practice for dentists, dentists are more at risk for litigation. However, the dental hygienist is also exposed to legal risks, and there is a greater degree of accountability when a dental hygienist is licensed to administer local anesthetics. To reduce the risk of litigation, the dental hygienist should follow these important principles for risk management.

Communication

Dental Hygienist-Patient Communication

Open and effective communication between the dental hygienist and the patient is an important risk management tool. Minimizing misunderstandings and resolving problems as they arise during the dental hygiene treatment reduce the likelihood of lawsuits. Develop a one-on-one relationship with the patient to build confidence and trust.[1,2]

Before the administration of a local anesthetic, it is essential for the dental hygienist to clearly present the benefits and risks associated with the procedure. For this type of communication to be successful, the dental hygienist should simplify technical terms to the appropriate level of the patient. Dental jargon can sound like a foreign language to most patients and should only be used with other health professionals. It is ultimately the patient's decision whether to accept the local anesthetic procedure. Usually, the patient does not fully understand the benefits of nonsurgical periodontal therapy with anesthesia, and he or she is more likely to decline the procedure. The dental hygienist must use effective communication skills to explain the procedure and the benefits for patient comfort, as well as explain the risks associated with no treatment or treatment that is difficult to effectively accomplish because the procedure is too painful. It is important for the dental hygienist to always provide a high standard of care, and to not agree to substandard care should the patient refuse local anesthesia. Box 18.1 is a sample conversation between the dental hygienist and the patient.

Dental Hygienist-Employer Communication

The dental hygienist should have an open discussion with his or her employer regarding the potential liabilities for dental hygienists and prevention strategies. Office protocols should be written and reviewed periodically by all office employees. Dental hygienists should discuss with their employers the scope of dental hygiene practice and always practice within the regulations of their license, regardless of their employer's request.

Legal Issues Related to the Dental Hygienist

A licensed dental hygienist has a contractual obligation (whether written or oral) to the patient to provide safe and thorough dental hygiene services. As a licensed practitioner, the dental hygienist is dependent on the rules and regulation laws of the state in which he or she has obtained a license. The dental hygienist must assume the legal responsibilities of his or her own actions and should never assume that the employer should be held accountable for the dental hygienist's actions. A dental hygienist may be charged with malpractice if he or she induces harm to the patient or if a breach of duty exists (Box 18.2). A dental hygienist may commit a negligent act during the administration of local anesthetics by causing paresthesia or if a needle breaks in the patient's tissue. Moreover, if a dental hygienist is unable to provide

BOX 18.1 Sample Dialogue Regarding Nonsurgical Periodontal Therapy Between the Patient and the Dental Hygienist

Hygienist: Seated in a position that allows direct eye contact and showing empathy and respect, the dental hygienist should begin the conversation outlining the treatment for the day:

Today, I will be treating the upper right quadrant (point to the upper right quadrant).

Using the periodontal chart or computerized program, discuss the periodontal involvement.

As you can see from this chart, in several areas you have "periodontal pockets," which have occurred in the past from the destruction of the supporting bone around these teeth. I will be debriding and root planing these areas with my instruments.

Patient: *Will this hurt?*

Hygienist: *As I recall from our previous visit when I was assessing the status of your teeth with my periodontal probe (show probe), it seems as if you were sensitive when I was walking the probe around your gums to determine the depth of the pocket. Is this a correct assumption?*

Patient: *Yes, it did feel uncomfortable.*

Hygienist: *Well, fortunately I can numb the area to provide you with the maximum comfort for the procedure. What are your thoughts on receiving a local anesthetic?*

Patient: *Well, gosh, I have had my teeth cleaned before at other dental offices and never had to get a shot. I don't think that is necessary.*

Hygienist: *I completely understand. Because I do not have the records from your other dental office, it is hard for me to comment on the procedures that you had in the past, or the condition of your mouth at that particular time. The type of treatment we provide is dependent on the condition of your mouth at the time of treatment. Today your condition requires me to use my instruments a little deeper under your gums than you may have experienced in the past. I want you to be as comfortable as possible, and your comfort will allow me to successfully complete the procedure for your maximum benefit.*

Patient: *Well, I do want the comfort, but I am scared of getting shots.*

Hygienist: *I understand your fear of shots; many individuals feel the same way you do. Let me explain the procedure, and then you can let me know what concerns or questions you may have.*

First, I will apply some topical anesthetic with a Q-tip to the area to numb the tissue where the injection will take place. I will then deposit the solution slowly. Once I start depositing the solution, it will only take a couple of seconds until the area begins to become numb.

Patient: *Wow, it only takes a couple of seconds?*

Hygienist: *Let me explain myself better; the injection will take longer because I will be injecting the solution slowly for better comfort to you and to increase the safety of the injection. The tissue will begin to numb even before the injection is completed, and you will only feel a pinch for a couple of seconds.*

Patient: *OK, go ahead with this procedure, and I will tell you if I am uncomfortable during the shot.*

Hygienist: *It is fine if you want me to stop during the procedure, but it is best if you do not try to talk. Instead you can raise your hand, which will signal me that you want me to stop. (This is a strategy to let the patient know that you will stop if there is a concern, and it gives them the confidence to know that they are in control of the situation). OK, before we begin, I will go over the benefits and risks associated with the treatment today and any questions you may have. If you are OK with the procedures and after you sign the informed consent, we will then begin treatment.*

Patient: *OK, that sounds good.*

BOX 18.2 Dental Hygienist Legal Case: Dental Hygienist's Unlawful Administration of Nitrous Oxide

This case[3] arises from a complaint by a dental hygienist against a former employer, Lowenberg and Lowenberg Corporation. The dental hygienist alleged that the defendant allowed dental hygienists working in their office to administer nitrous oxide to patients. Under state law, dental hygienists may not administer nitrous oxide. The Department of Education's Office of Professional Discipline investigated the complaint by using an undercover investigator. The investigator made an appointment for teeth cleaning. At the time of her appointment, she requested that nitrous oxide be administered. Agreeing to the investigator's request, the dental hygienist administered the nitrous oxide. There were no notations in the patient's chart indicating that she had been administered nitrous oxide.

A hearing panel found the involved dental hygienist guilty of administering nitrous oxide without being properly licensed. In addition, the hearing panel found that the dental hygienist had failed to record accurately in the patient's chart that she had administered nitrous oxide.

The New York Supreme Court, Appellate Division, held that the investigator's report provided sufficient evidence to support the hearing panel's determination. There is adequate evidence in the record to support a finding that the dentist's conduct was such that it could reasonably be said that he permitted the dental hygienist to perform acts that she was not licensed to perform.

thorough nonsurgical periodontal therapy because the patient refuses anesthesia, he or she may be held accountable if the patient's periodontal status declines. Whatever the situation may be, malpractice may be determined if the contractual obligations are not met by the dental hygienist. The dental hygienist should do the following to prevent litigation:[2]

1. Maintain proper licensure. Be properly licensed in all dental hygiene functions required to engage in the practice of dental hygiene. Most states require the dental hygienist to apply for an additional local anesthesia license or certificate in lieu of a regular dental hygiene license to legally administer local anesthetics. Each state has different educational and examination requirements that need to be completed by the dental hygienist before the application process for licensure. The dental hygienist can easily obtain that information from the website of the dental board for each individual state.
2. Take responsibility for lifelong learning. The dental hygienist is responsible for maintaining his or her own professional competency and credentials as determined by the licensing board. Continuing education courses are critical to maintaining dental hygiene competence.

An investment in knowledge always pays the best interest.

—Benjamin Franklin

3. Never exceed the scope of dental hygiene practice. In some states, the scope of dental hygiene practice for all dental hygiene treatment, including local anesthesia, requires the physical presence of a dentist. This means that the dentist must diagnose the patient's condition, authorize the procedures, and be physically on the premises where the dental hygienist is providing care. In other states, supervision laws do not require the physical presence of the dentist for dental hygiene treatment but do require it during the administration of local anesthesia. Because of the confusion presented by two supervision laws and the scope of dental hygiene

practice, the dentist may assume that the dental hygienist can legally administer local anesthetics without the physical presence of a dentist in this situation. It is the responsibility of the dental hygienist to know the supervision laws of the state as they pertain to the practice of dental hygiene and discuss them with the dentist. The dental hygienist should never administer local anesthetics without the physical presence of a dentist, even if requested by the supervising dentist, unless the laws of the state allow for this procedure. The dental hygienist should never administer local anesthetics unless properly licensed and should report any illegal activities by a health care provider to the responsible authorities.

In any moment of decision, the best thing you can do is the right thing. The worst thing you can do is nothing.

—***Theodore Roosevelt***

4. Obtain informed consent from the individual or parent/guardian before treatment. The process to obtain consent is an integral part of patient treatment. This process involves explaining to the patient the benefits and risks associated with all treatment, including the administration of local anesthetics, as should the risks involved in not receiving treatment. Individuals who incur a health care injury and allege that the dental hygienist did not fully inform them of the procedure to which they consented may file legal action. See Fig. 18.1 for a sample consent form.
5. Before administration of local anesthetics, make appropriate referrals and consultations regarding the patient's medical status and take vital signs.
6. Maintain patient privacy and confidentiality of information according to Health Insurance Portability and Accountability Act guidelines.
7. Always evaluate local anesthetic equipment (syringes, needles, and cartridges) prior to the administration of the local anesthetic. For instance, the syringe should be evaluated to ensure that the harpoon is sharp and functioning and the thumb ring is fitting properly. Additionally, cartridges and needles should be evaluated as described in Chapters 9 and 11. Any damage resulting from compromised equipment could result in a complication and is a breach of duty.
8. Always administer local anesthetic according to acceptable standards set by other practitioners with similar training and information described throughout this text (Box 18.3).
9. Do not experiment on a patient with new local anesthetic techniques or drugs. Dental hygienists should frequently attend continuing education courses specifically on local anesthetics. New techniques, procedures, and local anesthetic drugs will be presented in an education environment conducive to safe and effective learning.
10. Administer the appropriate volume of anesthetic for the area that can reasonably be completed during one appointment. For nonsurgical periodontal therapy for patients with advanced periodontitis, care should be taken in developing the dental hygiene care plan as to not be overly aggressive in the care. If the dental hygienist is unsure of the difficulty of the case, it is best to administer local anesthetics for just one quadrant, or even a sextant, and to complete the area in its entirety before administering more anesthetic for the next quadrant or sextant. Once one quadrant or sextant is completed, the dental hygienist can administer more anesthetic (assuming the maximum recommended dose has not been administered), if time is available.
11. Never abruptly stop treatment or abandon the patient.
12. Keep the patient informed regarding the progression of treatment and results obtained.

1. I consent to the recommended procedure or treatment ______________________________

   to be completed by Dr./Ms. ______________.
2. The procedure(s) or treatment(s) have been described to me.
3. I have been informed of the purpose of the procedure or treatment.
4. I have been informed of the alternatives to the procedure or treatment.
5. I understand that the following risk(s) may result from the procedure or treatment:

   ____
   ____
   ______________________________.
6. I understand that the following risk(s) may occur if the procedure or treatment is not completed:

   ____
   ____
   ____
   ______________________________.
7. I do—do not—consent to the administration of anesthetic.
   a. I understand that the following risks are involved in administering anesthesia:

      ____
      ____
      ____
      ______________________________.
   b. The following alternatives to anesthesia were described: ______________

      ____
      ______________________________.

All my questions have been satisfactorily answered.

Signature: ______________________________
Date

Representative: ______________________________
Date

Signature of Witness: ______________________________
Date

Fig. 18.1 Example of informed consent. (From Bowen DM, Pieren JA: *Darby and Walsh dental hygiene: theory and practice,* ed 5, St Louis, 2020, Elsevier.)

13. Keep the patient informed of any unanticipated occurrences during and after the administration of the local anesthetic.
14. Document and keep accurate records.
15. Always practice in a manner consistent with the dental hygiene code of ethics.
16. Obtain professional liability insurance. The dental hygienist as a licensed professional should maintain adequate professional liability insurance and be familiar with the policy coverage. In the event of malpractice litigation, the dental hygienist cannot rely on being covered against malpractice under the employer's insurance policy.

Documentation

Documentation in the patient's permanent record can be the dental hygienist's best defense, or worst enemy, in the event of a malpractice lawsuit.[1] In addition to the information necessary for all dental

BOX 18.3 Best Practices for the Administration of Local Anesthetics

Develop treatment plan in collaboration with the patient and confirm before treatment.
Provide open and effective communication with the patient.
Obtain informed consent.
Conduct a thorough preanesthetic patient assessment using consultations as necessary.
Obtain and document vital signs.
Select the appropriate anesthetic based on the patient's physical status, duration needed, and hemostasis.
Avoid high concentrations of vasoconstrictor.
Never exceed the patient's maximum recommended dose, and always administer the minimal clinically effective dose.
Select injections that provide minimal number of needle penetrations.
Prepare and check local anesthetic equipment.
Use personal protective equipment.
Always provide the patient with protective eyewear.
Never store or place the cartridges in disinfecting solution.
Do not use 30-gauge needles.
Never bend the needles.
Orient the bevel so that it will be toward the bone.
Obtain proper operator and patient positioning.
Prepare tissue at injection site using topical antiseptic and topical anesthesia.
Establish effective fulcrums to stabilize the syringe.
Keep the syringe out of the patient's sight.
Always know the location of the uncovered needle to prevent accidental needle contamination and needlestick exposure.
Keep the tissue taut during needle insertion and throughout the injection for the greatest visibility.
Advance the needle slowly.
Do not insert the needle through areas of infection.
Never insert the needle to the hub.
Always use long, large-gauge needles when penetrating significant tissue.
Do not change needle direction suddenly in deep tissue.
Withdraw the needle almost completely to make needle adjustments or for troubleshooting techniques.
Modify injection technique for patient size.
Always keep the large window up during local anesthetic administration.
Always aspirate and on two planes in highly vascular areas.
Always inject slowly at a rate of 1 mL per minute while providing positive communication to the patient.
Always slowly withdraw the needle in the same path as the needle insertion.
Always recap the needle using the one-handed scoop technique.
Observe the patient for possible reaction to the injection or the anesthetic.
Manage any local or systemic reactions calmly and professionally.
Document the procedure and any patient reactions.
Caution should be taken when removing the needle from the syringe.
Dispose of the needle and cartridge in an appropriate sharps container.
Always keep your knowledge and skill level up to date.

procedures, the patient record should include the following information specifically for the administration of local anesthetics:

1. Medical status of the patient including any pharmacologic history. Documentation regarding any contraindications to local anesthetics or vasoconstrictors should be included.
2. Vital signs taken before administration of the local anesthetic drug.
3. Dental history regarding the patient's psychological state as related to injections and nervousness.
4. Referrals or consultations obtained before the administration of the local anesthetic drug.
5. Any refusal of treatment by the patient and a brief statement documenting the discussion of risks associated with treatment refusal.
6. Comprehensive and chronologic documentation of treatment, including the patient's maximum recommended dose, the drug used and concentration, vasoconstrictor used if any, the amount administered in milligrams, the gauge and type of needle, the injections administered, the time of anesthetic administration, and any patient reactions or complications.
7. Any unexpected occurrences or reactions.
8. Continued care intervals or maintenance schedule.
9. Any specific postcare instructions given to the patient.

EXPOSURE PREVENTION AND MANAGEMENT

An occupational exposure in dentistry is defined by the Centers for Disease Control and Prevention as a percutaneous injury (e.g., needlestick or cut with a sharp object) or contact of mucous membrane or nonintact skin (e.g., exposed skin that is chapped, abraded, or with dermatitis) with blood, saliva, tissue, or other body fluids that are potentially infectious.[4] Exposure incidents might place dental health care personnel at risk for hepatitis B virus (HBV), hepatitis C virus (HCV), or human immunodeficiency virus (HIV) infection, and therefore should be evaluated immediately after treatment of the exposure site by a qualified health care professional.[2]

All dental facilities must have a postexposure management protocol for occupational exposures. This protocol should contain written guidelines, according to the most current guidelines from the U.S. Public Health Service (USPHS), addressing the steps for postexposure, training and education requirements for dental personnel, types of exposures that put dental personnel at risk, and procedures for prompt reporting and evaluation. Guidelines must follow the Occupational Safety and Health Administration bloodborne pathogen standards and any state or local laws or regulations.

The three categories of prevention and management of injury should be followed:

Primary prevention: The dental hygienist should strive to use all protocols to prevent the injury from occurring.
Secondary prevention: If an injury occurs, the dental hygienist should strive to contain the injury.
Tertiary prevention: The dental hygienist should strive to return the patient to a functional state and prevent future injuries.

Risk-Reduction Protocol

Avoiding occupational exposure to blood is the primary way to prevent transmission of HBV, HCV, and HIV in health care settings. Methods used to reduce such exposures in dental settings include engineering and work practice controls and the use of personal protective equipment (PPE).

Primary prevention involves the dental hygienist striving to make every effort to avoid injury during the administration of local anesthetics and throughout the dental hygiene treatment. However, in a moment of distraction during or after treatment, a needlestick injury can occur. To minimize the risk, the dental hygienist should follow these guidelines:

- Use the most currently developed medical devices with safety features designed to prevent injuries, and use the safest technique.

BOX 18.4 Summary of Postexposure Management

Wash wound and skin sites with soap and water.
Do not use bleach or other caustic agents to clean the wound.
Immediately contact the qualified health care professional.
Obtain consent for testing from the source patient.
Immediately set up testing for dental worker and source.
Incident report form should be completed and recorded in exposed person's confidential medical record.
The qualified health care professional will determine follow-up as needed.
Written report/opinion should be submitted to employer by qualified health care professional.

- Never recap the needle by hand; always use the scoop technique for capping needles. Needle-capping devices aid in effectively accomplishing this technique (see Chapter 11).
- Use disposable needle systems.
- Know the position of the uncapped needle at all times.
- Immediately after the injection, safely cap the needle before continuing with any procedure.
- Dispose of the needle in an appropriate sharps container. Caution should be taken when removing the needle from the syringe. Remember that the needle-penetrating end that is embedded in the cartridge is contaminated after the injection, and care should be taken when removing it from the syringe.
- Create a neutral zone for the sharps. The needle should not be passed between health care workers.

Postexposure Management

Postexposure management involves secondary and tertiary prevention strategies. The goal is to contain the injury to reduce the possibility of disease transmission. The exposed worker should review the most recent USPHS guidelines for postexposure. A qualified health care professional (QHCP) should be selected by the dental practice *before* the dental health care professionals are placed at risk for exposure. This QHCP should be experienced in conducting testing and providing antiretroviral therapy and should be familiar with the unique nature of dental injuries to provide appropriate guidance on the need for antiretroviral prophylaxis. The QHCP determines the source patient's disease status through testing if consent is obtained. The following steps should be conducted after the exposure (Box 18.4):

1. Wounds and skin sites that have been in contact with blood or body fluids should be cleansed with soap and water. Flush mucous membranes with water. Bleach or other caustic agents should not be used to cleanse the wound.
2. The QHCP should communicate to the source patient the incident and his or her role in the postexposure protocol. Excellent communication skills are critical at this point in the process.
3. Obtain consent for testing from the source patient if known.
4. Immediately set up testing for dental worker and source patient with the QHCP.
5. The incident report form (Fig. 18.2) should be completed and recorded in the exposed person's confidential medical record. The following information should be recorded:
   - Date and time of exposure.
   - Details of the procedure performed, including where and how the exposure occurred, whether the exposure involved a sharp device, the type of device, whether there was visible blood on the device, and how and when the exposure occurred.
   - Details of the exposure, including the type and amount of fluid or material and the severity of the exposure. For a percutaneous injury, details should include the depth of the wound, the gauge of the needle, and whether fluid was injected; for a skin or mucous membrane exposure, the estimated volume of material, the duration of contact, and the condition of the skin (e.g., chapped, abraded, or intact) should be included.
   - Details about the exposure source: (1) whether the patient was infected with HCV or HBV and the patient's hepatitis Be antigen (HBeAg) status and (2) whether the source was infected with HIV, the stage of disease, history of antiretroviral therapy, and viral load, if known.
   - Details about the exposed person (e.g., hepatitis B vaccination and vaccine-response status).
   - Details about counseling, postexposure management, and follow-up.
6. The QHCP must consider the following factors when assessing the need for follow-up of occupational exposures:

Type of exposure
- Percutaneous injury (e.g., depth, extent)
- Mucous membrane exposure
- Nonintact skin exposure
- Bites resulting in blood exposure to either person involved

Type and amount of fluid/tissue
- Blood
- Fluids containing blood

Infectious status of source
- Presence of hepatitis B surface antigen (HBsAg) and HBeAg
- Presence of HCV antibody
- Presence of HIV antibody

Susceptibility of exposed person
- Hepatitis B vaccine and vaccine response status
- HBV, HCV, or HIV immune status
- After conducting this initial evaluation of the occupational exposure, a QHCP must decide whether to conduct further follow-up on an individual basis using all of the information obtained.

7. Written report/opinion of health care provider: Within 15 days of evaluation, the qualified health care provider sends a written opinion to the employer. The report documents that the employee was informed of evaluation results and the need for further follow-up treatment, and whether the HBV vaccine was indicated and if the employee received the vaccine. All other findings are confidential and not included. The employer keeps a copy of the report in a confidential medical record and provides a copy to the exposed employee.

The most important human endeavor is the striving for morality in our actions. Our inner balance, and even our very existence depends on it. Only morality in our actions can give beauty and dignity to our lives.

—Albert Einstein

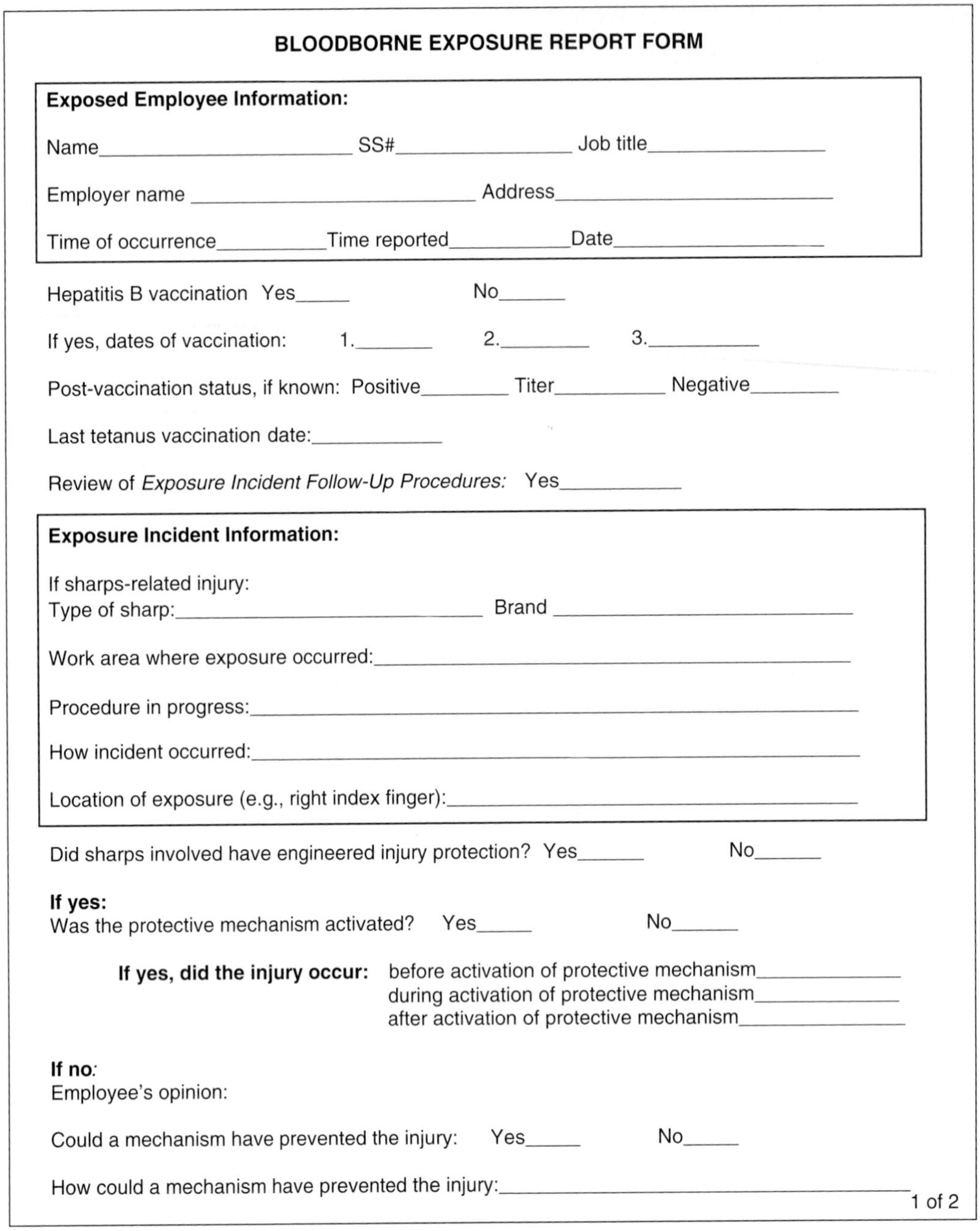

BLOODBORNE EXPOSURE REPORT FORM

Exposed Employee Information:

Name_______________________ SS#______________ Job title______________

Employer name _______________________ Address______________________

Time of occurrence_________Time reported__________Date_______________

Hepatitis B vaccination Yes_____ No______

If yes, dates of vaccination: 1._______ 2._________ 3.__________

Post-vaccination status, if known: Positive________ Titer__________ Negative________

Last tetanus vaccination date:____________

Review of *Exposure Incident Follow-Up Procedures:* Yes__________

Exposure Incident Information:

If sharps-related injury:
Type of sharp:_______________________ Brand ______________________

Work area where exposure occurred:_____________________________________

Procedure in progress:____

How incident occurred:____

Location of exposure (e.g., right index finger):_____________________________

Did sharps involved have engineered injury protection? Yes______ No______

If yes:
Was the protective mechanism activated? Yes_____ No______

If yes, did the injury occur: before activation of protective mechanism_____________
during activation of protective mechanism_____________
after activation of protective mechanism______________

If no:
Employee's opinion:

Could a mechanism have prevented the injury: Yes_____ No_____

How could a mechanism have prevented the injury:_________________________________

1 of 2

Fig. 18.2 Bloodborne exposure report form. (From Bowen DM, Pieren JA: *Darby and Walsh dental hygiene: theory and practice,* ed 5, St Louis, 2020, Elsevier.)

BLOODBORNE EXPOSURE REPORT FORM

Employee's opinion:

Could any engineering, administrative, or work practice control have prevented the injury?
Yes___ No___

Explain: ______________________________

____

Source Patient Information:

Name______________ Chart no.__________ Telephone no.__________

	Yes	No
Release of information to evaluating health care professional?	___	___

Patient's signature______________________

	Yes	No
Review of source patient medical history:	___	___
Verbally questioned regarding:		
• History of hepatitis B, hepatitis C, or HIV infection	___	___
• High-risk history associated with these diseases	___	___
• Patient consents to be tested for HIV, HCV, and HBV	___	___

If HIV-positive source patient:

List all current medications patient is taking for HIV infection:

1.________ 2.________ 3.________ 4.________

List all medications previously taken by patient to which he or she was resistant or medications that were ineffective:

1.________ 2.________ 3.________ 4.________

Provide most recent viral load: ______________ Date:__________

CD4 count if known:______________ Date:__________

Health care worker referred to: ______________________

Questionnaire completed by: ______________________

Bill for fees to: ______________________

Retain one copy in employee's confidential medical record; send one copy to evaluating health care professional. Retain copy with employee's and source patient's name removed as sharps injury log.

2 of 2

Fig. 18.2 (Continued)

DENTAL HYGIENE CONSIDERATIONS

- Ethical principles guide the conduct of the health care professions regarding moral duties and obligations to the profession, to one's self, to the employers, and to the patients.
- Dental hygienists are accountable to their patients and employers and must take responsibility for their actions.
- Obtain and maintain appropriate licensure before services are provided.
- A licensed dental hygienist has a contractual responsibility (whether written or oral) to the patient to provide safe and thorough dental hygiene services.
- A dental hygienist must meet the standard of care set by other practitioners with similar training.
- Always obtain informed consent to allow the patient to formally accept or deny services.
- Communication between the dental hygienist and the patient is an important risk management tool. Always keep the patient informed of treatment and progress.
- Confidentiality of patient records is an important responsibility of the dental hygienist.
- The dental hygienist should always identify preventable methods to minimize or eliminate risk.
- Never recap the needle by hand; always use the one-handed scoop technique for capping needles.
- Always dispose of contaminated needles in approved containers.
- The dental hygienist should know the position of the uncapped needle at all times.
- Thorough documentation of treatment and reactions to treatment are essential.
- The dental hygienist must follow the most current postexposure guidelines set by the U.S. Public Health Service (USPHS).
- The dental hygienist should stay abreast of all topics related to the administration of local anesthesia and should take continuing education courses specifically related to the administration of local anesthetics on a regular basis.

CASE STUDY 18.1 The Anxious Dental Hygienist

A dental hygienist graduated from a university dental hygiene program that did not teach the administration of local anesthetics. The dental hygienist was not concerned about not practicing this expanded function because she worked in a state where this function was not allowed for dental hygienists.

Her husband was offered a job transfer to a state where local anesthesia administration was legal for dental hygienists. The dental hygienist was thrilled to finally work in a state where she could perform that function. She was an experienced dental hygienist of 7 years and easily obtained a licensure by credentials in the state where she would soon be working. The dental hygienist took the necessary education required by the state to administer local anesthetics, passed the written and clinical examinations, and applied for her anesthesia licensure with the state's Board of Dental Health Care.

The dental hygienist received a job before her anesthesia license was sent by the board, but she was not concerned because she already had her dental hygiene license for that state. On her first day of the job, the dental hygienist was scheduled for several nonsurgical periodontal debridements requiring local anesthetics. She immediately became concerned because the dentist was scheduled to be in a continuing education class that day and would not be in the office. The dental hygienist approached the receptionist about the dentist not being in the building for the dental hygiene care. The receptionist informed the dental hygienist that the administration of local anesthesia by a dental hygienist without the physical presence of the dentist is allowed in the state, and the dentist already examined the patients and authorized the procedures.

The dental hygienist was embarrassed to reveal that she had not yet received her anesthesia license and was concerned about having to cancel the patients on her first day at work. She decided to go ahead and administer the anesthetic, because, after all, she took the appropriate education and passed all the clinical and written examinations. She convinced herself that the license was just a formality and not to be concerned with not having it in hand.

Ethical and Legal Issues

- Discuss whether or not ethical values were violated in this case.
- Describe how both ethical and legal issues are intertwined in this case.

CHAPTER REVIEW QUESTIONS

1. Before administering local anesthetics, the dental hygienist should describe the risks and benefits to the patient using which type of terms?
   A. Specific technical terms
   B. Phrases like "pokey thing" and "feels like an ouchie"
   C. Terms appropriate for the patient's education level
   D. Do not tell the patient anything; if you do not talk about it, then the patient will not be nervous.
2. Practicing within the legal scope of practice means:
   A. Practicing only within the limits set forth by your license and state's rules and regulations
   B. Practicing within the limits of your license, unless the dentist gives you permission to do expanded procedures
   C. Practicing any procedure as long the doctor is present in the office
   D. Performing procedures that the doctor has approved in the treatment plan
3. Which of the following statements is false regarding the administration of local anesthetics?
   A. Never abruptly stop treatment or abandon the patient
   B. Keep the patient informed regarding the progression of treatment and results obtained
   C. Never inform the patient of any unanticipated occurrences during and after the administration of the local anesthetic
   D. Document and keep accurate records
4. In most states the dental hygienist is not required to have malpractice insurance because the dental hygienist will be covered under the dentist's insurance.
   A. Both the statement and the reason are CORRECT and related.
   B. Both the statement and the reason are correct but NOT related.
   C. The statement is correct, but the reason is NOT correct.
   D. The statement is NOT correct, but the reason is correct.
   E. NEITHER the statement NOR the reason is correct.
5. Dental hygienists are accountable for their own actions and practice. However, the dentist is always liable for any legal actions taken against the hygienist.
   A. Both statements are correct.
   B. Both statements are NOT correct.
   C. The first statement is correct; the second statement is NOT correct.
   D. The first statement is NOT correct; the second statement is correct.
6. Dental hygienists who hold a current anesthesia license are always able to administer local anesthetics without the physical presence of a dentist, but only if the dentist authorizes the procedure.
   A. Both statements are correct.
   B. Both statements are NOT correct.
   C. The first statement is correct; the second statement is NOT correct.
   D. The first statement is NOT correct; the second statement is correct.
7. What is the appropriate amount of anesthetic to be administered during a procedure?
   A. The amount necessary to complete the area that will be treated and finished in a single appointment
   B. The amount that covers most of the area so that you do not have to give a second injection
   C. Enough for one tooth at a time; that way you can avoid the risk of toxicity
   D. Always give at least half the maximum recommended dose
8. All of the following diseases are contractible if a needlestick occurs to the dental hygienist except ONE. Which one is the EXCEPTION?
   A. Hepatitis B virus (HBV)
   B. Hepatitis C virus (HCV)
   C. Human immunodeficiency virus (HIV)
   D. Adenovirus

9. All of the following should be contained in a postexposure management protocol for occupational exposures except ONE? Which one is the EXCEPTION?
   A. Steps for postexposure
   B. Training and education requirements for dental personnel
   C. Types of exposures that put dental personnel at risk
   D. Procedures for prompt reporting and evaluation
   E. Procedures for disinfecting the operatory
10. Which statement is true regarding the handling of sharps?
    A. It is acceptable to throw unused needles in the regular trash
    B. It is acceptable to hand an uncapped needle to an assistant if you are unable to reach the cap
    C. It is acceptable to recap a needle with your hands as long as the needle has not been contaminated
    D. It is acceptable to recap a needle only using the one-handed scoop method
11. If a needlestick injury occurs, it is not necessary to report the details of what happened, only that you were possibly exposed.
    A. Both statements are correct.
    B. Both statements are NOT correct.
    C. The first statement is correct; the second statement is NOT correct.
    D. The first statement is NOT correct; the second statement is correct.
12. Secondary prevention is when there is containment of an injury after it occurs. Tertiary prevention involves the return of the patient to a functional state and the prevention of further injuries.
    A. Both statements are correct.
    B. Both statements are NOT correct.
    C. The first statement is correct; the second statement is NOT correct.
    D. The first statement is NOT correct; the second statement is correct.
13. What does PPE stand for?
    A. Patient protective equipment
    B. Personal protective equipment
    C. Person protective equipment
    D. Procedure protection equipment
14. When it comes to occupational exposure risks, a qualified health care professional should be experienced in all of the following EXCEPT one. Which one is the EXCEPTION?
    A. Conducting testing
    B. Providing antiretroviral therapy
    C. Being familiar with the unique nature of dental injuries
    D. Providing dental hygiene treatment
15. Risk management occurs when:
    A. You refuse to treat any patient with foreseeable risks
    B. You identify preventive methods to reduce or eliminate the risk of legal actions
    C. You sue the patient back if the patients sues you
    D. You make notes in the chart as general as possible to give the same treatment to every patient
16. After exposure, if there is not enough time to get tested right away, it is okay to use bleach to cleanse the exposure site. However, if you are able to get tested immediately, then you should just use soap and water.
    A. Both statements are correct.
    B. Both statements are NOT correct.
    C. The first statement is correct; the second statement is NOT correct.
    D. The first statement is NOT correct; the second statement is correct.
17. Communication, documentation, and risk-reduction protocols are all necessary elements when administering a local anesthetic. This is because they help reduce the chance of possible litigation.
    A. Both statements are correct.
    B. Both statements are NOT correct.
    C. The first statement is correct; the second statement is NOT correct.
    D. The first statement is NOT correct; the second statement is correct.
18. The qualified health care professional must take into consideration all of the following factors when determining the need for follow-up of occupational exposures except ONE. Which one is the EXCEPTION?
    A. Infectious state of source
    B. Type and amount of tissue/fluid
    C. Type of exposure
    D. Susceptibility of exposed person
    E. Blood type of the source
19. When handling a contaminated needle, it is only important to avoid being exposed to the end that penetrated the tissues or fluids. The cartridge-penetrating end of the needle is not a risk for contamination.
    A. Both statements are correct.
    B. Both statements are NOT correct.
    C. The first statement is correct; the second statement is NOT correct.
    D. The first statement is NOT correct; the second statement is correct.
20. It is the responsibility of the dental hygienist to report any illegal activities regarding the administration of local anesthesia to the proper authorities, as well as to educate the dentist about current regulations regarding the hygienist's scope of practice.
    A. Both statements are correct.
    B. Both statements are NOT correct.
    C. The first statement is correct; the second statement is NOT correct.
    D. The first statement is NOT correct; the second statement is correct.

REFERENCES

1. Bowen DM, Pieren JA. *Darby and Walsh dental hygiene: theory and practice.* ed 5. St. Louis: Elsevier; 2020.
2. Beemsterboer PL. *Ethics and law in dental hygiene.* ed 3. St Louis: Elsevier; 2017.
3. Pozgar GP. *Legal and ethical issues for health professionals.* ed 5. Sudbury: Jones and Bartlett Learning; 2020.
4. Centers for Disease Control and Prevention: www.cdc.org.

GLOSSARY

A fibers: The largest nerve fibers; can be either motor or sensory.
Absolute contraindication: The administration of the offending drug should not be administered to the individual under any circumstances.
Absolute refractory period: The interval during which a second action potential absolutely cannot be initiated to restimulate the membrane, no matter how large a stimulus is applied.
Action potential: Nerve impulse that generates an electronic signal to and from the central nervous system (CNS).
Adrenergic drugs: Drugs that stimulate the adrenergic nerves directly by mimicking the action of norepinephrine or indirectly by stimulating the release of norepinephrine.
Afferent nerves: Nerves that conduct signals from sensory neurons to the spinal cord or brain *(carry toward)*.
Allergens or antigens: Noninfectious foreign substances that trigger hypersensitivity.
All-or-none principle: The minimal threshold stimulus sends an impulse along the axon that travels the full length of the fiber without additional stimulus.
American Society of Anesthesiologists (ASA) physical status classification: American Society of Anesthesiologists' rating system is a uniform system to assess the patient's physical state before selecting an anesthetic before surgery and a means to communicate between colleagues regarding a patient's physical status.
Amide: A local anesthetic agent made from a specific class of chemical compounds that are generally broken down by the liver and are more effective and longer lasting than esters. This type of anesthetic rarely causes allergic reactions.
Analgesic: A drug that relieves pain.
Anastomosis/anastomoses: Connecting channel(s) among the blood vessels.
Anesthesiologist: A physician trained in the administration of anesthesia.
Anesthetic: A drug that produces loss of feeling or sensation generally or locally.
Anesthetic allergy: Hypersensitivity to a local agent, which is fairly common with esters but rarely occurs with amides. Allergy to bisulfites in vasoconstrictors is common.
Anesthetic cartridge: A capsule-like vessel containing the local anesthetic agent that is inserted into the syringe in preparation for an injection; older term is *carpule.*
Anion: The base form of the local anesthetic (lipid soluble and penetrates the nerve).
Anterior middle superior alveolar (AMSA) block: A type of injection that anesthetizes most of the maxillary teeth and their associated periodontium, as well as most of the facial and lingual gingival tissue in one quadrant.
Anterior superior alveolar (ASA) block: A type of injection that anesthetizes the maxillary anterior teeth and associated structures when the local anesthetic agent is deposited superior to the apex of the maxillary canine.
Armamentarium: Local anesthetic supplies, materials, and devices needed to successfully administer a local anesthetic. More generally, the equipment, pharmaceuticals, and methods used in medicine.
Arteriole: Smaller vessels of the artery.
Artery: A component of the vascular system that arises from the heart, carrying blood away from it.
Articaine: An intermediate amide local anesthetic metabolized in the blood, noted for its highly lipid characteristics.
Aspirate on two planes: The procedure of rotating the barrel of the syringe 45 degrees and aspirating after the initial aspiration test to ensure that the bevel of the needle is not abutting a blood vessel and producing a false-negative aspiration.
Aspiration test: Negative pressure placed on the anesthetic syringe before depositing the anesthetic to determine whether the tip of the needle rests within a blood vessel; observed by absence or entry of blood into the cartridge.
Asthma: A chronic inflammatory disease of the airways resulting in episodes of dyspnea coughing and wheezing commonly precipitated by stress.
Atypical pseudocholinesterase: A hereditary trait in which individuals are unable to hydrolyze ester local anesthetics and other chemically related drugs.
Autonomic nervous system (ANS): A control system (part of the peripheral nervous system) that helps people adapt to change in their environment, adjusting some functions in response to stress.
Axon: Cable-like structure of neuron.
Axon hillock: Specialized part of the neuron that emerges from the soma and connects to the axon where membrane potentials are summated before being transmitted to the axon.
B fibers: Lightly myelinated motor nerve fibers with medium diameters of less than 3 μm.
Benzocaine: A common ester topical anesthetic.
Bevel: The angled surface of the needle tip.
Biotransformation: The process by which the local anesthetic is altered within the body by the action of enzymes to produce a less toxic metabolite.
Biphasic: A process that occurs in two phases.
Blanching: A temporary whitening of the tissue because of the diffusion of anesthetic solution that decreases the blood flow in the area.
Bradycardia: Decreased heart rate.
Bradykinin: A pain mediator produced during cellular injury.
Breech-loading: The process of inserting the glass anesthetic cartridge into the syringe through the side of the barrel.
Buccal block: Type of injection that anesthetizes the buccal soft tissue of the mandibular molars.
Bupivacaine: A long-acting amide local anesthetic that is metabolized in the liver.
Butamben: An ester topical anesthetic; often combined with other topical anesthetics for use.
C fibers: Unmyelinated nerve fibers primarily responsible for dull, aching pain.
Canal: Opening in bone that is long, narrow, and tube-like.
Capillaries: Any of the fine branching blood vessels that form a network between the arterioles and venules.
Cardiac dose: Limited dose of vasoconstrictor for cardiovascularly involved patients.
Cartridge: Contains the sterile local anesthetic drug and other contents.
Cartridge-penetrating end: Part of the shaft of the needle that passes through the hub and penetrates the rubber diaphragm of the cartridge.
Catecholamine: Sympathomimetic "fight-or-flight" hormones released by the adrenal glands.
Cation: A positively charged ion, specifically the ionized portion of the anesthetic molecule that is acidic and water soluble. The active form of the molecule that binds to the receptor sites in the sodium channel.
Cell body: The nucleus-containing central part of a neuron exclusive of its axons and dendrites that is the major structural element of the gray matter of the brain and spinal cord, the ganglia, and the retina. Responsible for protein synthesis; provides metabolic support for the neuron.
Central fibers: Nerve fibers that extend from the cell body toward the CNS.
Central nervous system (CNS): The structural and functional center of the nervous system that includes the brain and the spinal cord.
Centralized nitrous oxide system: Nitrous oxide system built directly into the foundation of the dental office.
Chronic obstructive pulmonary disease (COPD): A chronic inflammatory lung disease that causes obstructed airflow from the lungs.
Clark's rule: A medical term referring to a mathematical formula used to calculate the proper dosage of medicine for children aged 2 to 17.
Cocaine: An ester local anesthetic drug with addictive properties.
Complication: An adverse reaction or event.
Computer-controlled local anesthetic delivery (C-CLAD) device: A machine that controls the amount and rate of administered anesthetic.
Concentration gradient: A ratio of different substances (ions): extracellular versus intracellular in relation to nerve conduction.
Concomitant: Two or more drugs given at the same time or in the same day.
Concomitant drugs: Having two or more drugs in the systemic circulation at the same time.
Condyle: Oval, bony prominence, usually part of a joint.
Connective tissue: A form of fibrous tissue.
Continuum: A sequence of elements that vary only by a slight difference without clearly defined points, yet the beginning and end are opposite extremes.

Core bundles: Fasciculi located in the core region (inner core).
Coronoid notch: Concavity in the anterior border of the ramus; the landmark for the inferior alveolar injection.
Crossover innervation: Overlap of terminal nerve fibers from the contralateral side.
Deflection: The deviation in the direction of the anesthetic needle from its intended path.
Demyelination: Disease of the nervous system in which the myelin sheath encompassing a neuron is damaged (e.g., multiple sclerosis).
Dendritic zone: The most distal section of the neuron that includes an arborization of nerve endings.
Dental phobia: Unfounded fear or morbid dread of dental treatment.
Dental plexus: A network of vessels or nerves.
Depolarization: The process whereby the action potential causes sodium channels to open, allowing an influx of sodium ions to change the electrochemical gradient, which in turn produces a further rise in the membrane potential.
Deposit location: The target area where local anesthetic will be deposited.
Depth of needle insertion: Needle depth covered in tissue when target area is reached.
Dialogue history: Orally communicating with the patient to gain more information regarding the patient's medical status.
Diaphoresis: Excessive sweating.
Diaphragm: Semipermeable material located at the top of the cartridge where the needle is inserted into the center of the rubber.
Dilution ratio: The strength of vasoconstrictor drug per volume of solution expressed as milligrams per milliliter (mg/mL).
Dissociation constant (pK_a): The pH at which 50% of molecules exist in the lipid-soluble tertiary form and 50% in the quaternary, water-soluble form.
Drug concentration: The strength of the local anesthetic agent in the cartridge expressed as a percentage.
Dyclonine hydrochloride: A ketone topical anesthetic.
Edema: Abnormal accumulation of fluid beneath the skin causing swelling of the tissues; describes a clinical complication.
Efferent nerves: Nerves that conduct signals away from the brain or spinal cord *(carry away).*
Electrical potential: The electrical charge across the nerve membrane.
Elimination: The process by which the kidney removes the local anesthetic drug, primarily its metabolites, from the body.
Endogenous: Originating or produced within an organism, tissue, or cell.
Endoneurium: Connective tissue that surrounds each axon by a layer of connective tissue.
Engineering controls: Devices or controls developed to provide safer administration of local anesthetics, such as safety syringes, sharps disposal containers, and recapping devices.
Epinephrine: Naturally occurring catecholamine secreted by the adrenal medulla.
Epineurium: Connective tissue that wraps the entire nerve.
Esters: Short-acting local anesthetic agents made from a specific class of chemical compounds that are broken down by blood enzymes. They are less effective than amide anesthetics and more likely to cause allergic reactions. These are no longer used as an injection in the United States but are still used as a topical agent.
Eutectic mixtures: A mixture of two elements that have a lower melting point than any of the individual components.
Exogenous: Coming from outside the body.
Extracellular: Outside the nerve membrane.
False-negative aspiration: A perceived negative aspiration where the needle tip lies within a blood vessel and is butting up against the wall of the vessel, preventing the entrance of blood into the cartridge.
Fasciculi: Nerve fibers bundled together into groups.
Felypressin: A synthetic hormone analog of vasopressin.
Fight-or-flight response: The body's primitive, automatic, inborn response that prepares the body to "fight" or "flee" from perceived attack, harm, or threat to survival.
Finger grip: Winged or wingless component of the syringe that allows the clinician to hold and control the syringe.
Foramen/foramina: Short, window-like opening in bone.
Fossa/fossae: Depression on a bony surface.
Gauge: The diameter of the needle.
General supervision: Refers to the idea that a dentist has authorized the procedures to be performed for a patient but a dentist need not be present when the procedures are performed.
Generic drug: A nonproprietary agent.
Glial cells: Nonneuronal cells that maintain homeostasis, form myelin, and provide support and protection for the brain's neurons.
Gow-Gates (G-G) mandibular block: A type of injection that anesthetizes most of the mandibular nerve.
Greater palatine (GP) block: A type of injection that anesthetizes the lingual soft tissue distal to the maxillary canine in one quadrant.
H_2 receptor antagonists: A class of drugs used to block the action of histamine on parietal cells in the stomach, decreasing the production of acid by these cells.
Half-life of drug: The period of time required to eliminate the amount of drug in the body by one-half of its strength.
Harpoon: A sharp tip attached to the internal end of the piston of an aspirating syringe that embeds into the silicone rubber stopper, allowing retraction for an aspiration test.
Hematoma: Swelling that develops when a blood vessel, particularly an artery, is punctured or lacerated by the needle.
Hemostasis: A complex process that changes blood from a fluid to a solid state.
Hemostat: An instrument used in dentistry to retrieve small items, such as broken needles.
Henderson-Hasselbalch equation: A formula that calculates the pH of a buffer solution or the concentration of acid versus base molecules in an anesthetic solution.
Hub: A plastic or metal adaptor that provides a means to attach the needle to the syringe.
Human-needs paradigm: The relationship between human needs fulfillment and human behavior.
Hydrophilic terminal amine: A portion of a local anesthetic agent's chemical structure, with strong water-attracting properties that enable the diffusion of the agent through the water portions of the tissues to the final destination in the nerves. Typically described in opposition to the lipophilic portion of a local anesthetic agent.
Hyperresponders: Individuals who overly respond to local anesthetics.
Hyperthyroidism: A condition that occurs because of excessive production of thyroid hormone by the thyroid gland.
Hyporesponders: Individuals who underrespond to local anesthetics.
Ideal body weight index: An index that shows a weight that is believed to be maximally healthful for a person, based chiefly on height but modified by factors such as gender, age, build, and degree of muscular development.
Impulse: A wave of physical and chemical excitation along a nerve fiber in response to a stimulus, accompanied by a change in electric potential in the membrane.
Incisive (I) block: A type of injection that anesthetizes the teeth and associated periodontium, as well as facial soft tissue anterior to the mental foramen.
Indirect supervision: A dentist must be physically on the premises where the dental hygienist is administering the local anesthetic.
Inferior alveolar (IA) block: A type of injection that anesthetizes the mandibular teeth and their associated periodontium and lingual soft tissue to the midline.
Infiltration injection: A type of injection that provides soft tissue anesthesia of the smaller terminal nerve endings only in the area of anesthetic deposition.
Informed consent: Written agreement from the patient consenting to treatment after a discussion of the benefits and risks associated with the treatment.
Infraorbital (IO) block: A type of injection that anesthetizes the maxillary anterior and premolar teeth and associated structures when the local anesthetic agent is deposited at the infraorbital foramen.
Injection site: The site of initial needle penetration into the tissue.
Intermediate-acting anesthetic: Anesthetics that provide pulpal anesthesia of approximately 60 minutes.
Intermediate hydrocarbon: The connector between the lipophilic and hydrophilic portions of a local anesthetic agent's chemical structure. Local anesthetic agent's classification is performed on the basis of whether the intermediate chain is made up of an ester or an amide.
Interpapillary injection: An infiltration injection depositing a small volume of local anesthetic into the buccal or lingual papilla.

Intracellular: A term meaning *within the nerve membrane.*
Intraseptal injection: A supplemental intraosseous injection that is used when there is a need for additional hemostatic control with the interdental periodontium and gingiva between adjacent teeth.
Ion channels: Membrane protein complexes that facilitate the diffusion of ions across nerve membranes.
Ionized: Cationic form of molecule.
Jet injector: Needleless syringe that delivers anesthesia to mucous membranes at high pressure.
Kilogram: The base unit of mass in the International System of Units used to calculate and record maximum recommended doses: 1 pound equals 2.2 kilograms.
Levonordefrin: A synthetic catecholamine manufactured in the United States as a 2% mepivacaine 1:20,000 levonordefrin solution.
Lidocaine: An amide local anesthetic metabolized in the liver.
Limiting drug: The drug that limits the total amount of volume of anesthetic delivered based on the patient's medical status.
Line: Straight, small ridge of bone.
Lipophilic aromatic ring: The portion of the lipophilic group that improves the lipid solubility of the molecule that facilitates the penetration of the anesthetic through the lipid-rich membrane.
Lipophilic group: A portion of a local anesthetic agent's chemical structure with its fat-attracting properties that enable the agent to pass through the lipid membrane of the tissues to reach the nerve destination. Typically described in opposition to the hydrophilic portion of the local anesthetic agent.
Localized complication: A complication that occurs in the region of the injection.
Long-acting anesthetics: Anesthetics that provide pulpal anesthesia of approximately 90 minutes.
Lumen: The inner tubular (channel) area of an anesthetic needle; the diameter size of the lumen is related to the needle gauge.
Malignant hyperthermia: An inherited syndrome triggered by exposure to certain drugs used for general anesthesia and the neuromuscular blocking agent succinylcholine.
Mandibular nerve: Third division (V3) of the trigeminal nerve.
Mantle bundles: Fasciculi located in the mantle region (outer core).
Maxillary nerve: Second division (V2) from the sensory root of the trigeminal nerve.
Maximum recommended dose (MRD): The highest amount of an anesthetic agent that can safely be administered without complication to a patient while maintaining efficacy.
Membrane expansion theory: Theory that suggests that the local anesthetic agents that are highly lipid insert themselves into the lipid bilayer of the cell membrane, affecting the nerve membrane.
Membrane potential: The difference in voltage or electrical potential between the interior and exterior of a cell.
Mental (M) block: A type of injection that anesthetizes the facial soft tissue anterior to the mental foramen.
Mepivacaine: An amide local anesthetic that provides short to intermediate duration and is metabolized in the liver.
Methemoglobinemia: A rare hereditary condition characterized by the inability of the blood to bind to oxygen that deprives oxygen being carried effectively to body tissues.
Methylparaben: A bacteriostatic agent and preservative that was added to local anesthetic agents without vasoconstrictors before 1984 to prevent bacterial growth.
Middle superior alveolar (MSA) block: A type of injection that anesthetizes the maxillary premolars and the mesial buccal root of the maxillary first molar (in 28% of the population) and associated structures when the local anesthetic agent is deposited superior to the apex of the maxillary second premolar.
Mild complication: A minor problem that will resolve without requiring treatment.
Milligram: A unit of mass equal to one one-thousandth (1/1000th) of a gram. It is used to calculate and record the maximum recommended dose.
Milliliter: A measure of volume equal to one one-thousandth (1/1000th) of a liter.
Minimal sedation: Less than 50% N_2O, and is the first stage in the continuum.
Moderate sedation: Referred to as conscious sedation and produces greater depressed consciousness.
Mucobuccal fold: The fold located in the vestibule where the labial or buccal mucosa meets the alveolar mucosa.
Myelin: Lipoprotein sheath composed of 75% lipid, 20% protein, and 5% carbohydrates.
Myelinated nerve: Lipoprotein sheath that almost completely insulates the axon from the outside.
Nasal hood: Piece of equipment that fits over the patient's nose and is essential for delivering nitrous oxide gas.
Nasopalatine nerve block: A type of injection that anesthetizes the lingual soft tissue between the maxillary right and left canines.
Needle adaptor: A threaded tip of the syringe that allows the attachment of the needle to the barrel of the syringe.
Needle insertion point: The injection site where the bevel of the needle is covered with tissue.
Needle shields: A cover that protects the needle that is inserted in the tissue, as well as the cartridge-penetrating end of the needle.
Needle tract infection: An infection that can be spread into deeper tissue along a needle pathway.
Negative aspiration: A clear air bubble entering the cartridge, or no return, after negative pressure is applied to the cartridge.
Negative pressure: Pressure produced when the thumb ring of a syringe is pulled back, causing retraction of the rubber stopper to produce an aspiration test.
Nerve: The sensitive pulp of the tooth that contains many bundles of peripheral axons.
Nerve block: An injection of local anesthetic in the vicinity of a major nerve trunk to anesthetize the nerve's area of innervations, usually at a distance from the area of treatment.
Nerve fiber: Any of the processes (as an axon or a dendrite) of a neuron that is composed of axon and myelin sheaths.
Neuron: Basic functional unit of the nervous system that manipulates information and responds to either excitation or inhibition.
Neurotransmitters: Endogenous chemicals that transmit signals from a neuron to a target cell across a synapse.
Nitrous oxide: A colorless gas used for pain control and sedation.
Nociception: The neural processes of encoding and processing noxious stimuli.
Nodes of Ranvier: Uninsulated gaps formed between myelin sheaths covering axons, allowing for the generation of electrical activity.
Nonselective beta blockers: A class of drugs used to treat hypertension and cardiac arrhythmias.
Norepinephrine: Naturally occurring catecholamine affecting primarily α receptors.
Normal responder: An individual who responds typically to the duration of local anesthesia.
Notch: An indentation at the edge of a bone.
Noxious stimulus: A mechanical, chemical, or thermal stimulus that can actually or potentially damage tissue.
Nurse anesthetist: A nurse who specializes in the administration of anesthesia.
Occupational exposure: A percutaneous injury (e.g., needlestick or cut with a sharp object) or contact of mucous membrane or nonintact skin (e.g., exposed skin that is chapped, is abraded, or has dermatitis) with blood, saliva, tissue, or other body fluids that are potentially infectious.
Oligodendrocytes: A brain cell responsible for insulating axons.
Ophthalmic nerve: First division (V1) of the sensory root of the trigeminal nerve.
Overdose: An administration of local anesthetic that results in signs and symptoms of CNS and cardiovascular system (CVS) depression.
Pain: An unpleasant sensory and emotional experience.
Pain control: The mechanism to alleviate pain.
Pain perception: Neurologic experience of pain that differs little between individuals.
Pain reaction: Personal interpretation and response to pain message; highly variable among individuals.
Pain threshold: The point at which a sensation starts to be painful and discomfort results.
Parasympathetic nervous system: Coordinates the body's normal resting activities and is known as the "rest or digest" response.
Paresthesia: Persistent anesthesia (anesthesia well beyond the expected duration) or altered sensation (tingling or itching) well beyond the expected duration of anesthesia.
Penetrating end: The part of the needle shaft that passes through the hub and penetrates the rubber diaphragm of the cartridge.
Perineurium: Connective tissue that wraps each fascicle.

Periodontal ligament injection: A supplemental injection used when pulpal anesthesia is indicated on a single tooth mainly in the mandibular arch.
Peripheral fibers: Nerve fibers that extend from the cell body away from the CNS.
Peripheral nervous system (PNS): Nerve tissues that lie in the periphery.
Permanent complication: A problem that leaves a residual effect.
Pharmacodynamics: The study of the physiologic effects of drugs on the body and the mechanisms of drug action and its relationship between drug concentration and effect.
Pharmacokinetics: The study of the action of drugs within the body.
Phentolamine mesylate: Pharmaceutical agent indicated for the reversal of soft tissue anesthesia.
Phenylephrine: A synthetic sympathomimetic amine that exerts its action predominantly on α receptors.
Piston: A solid, metallic cylinder of the anesthetic syringe attached to the thumb ring that displaces anesthetic agent when positive pressure is exerted on the thumb ring.
Polarization: Resting state; the electrical charge on the outside of the membrane is positive while the electrical charge on the inside of the membrane is negative.
Portable nitrous oxide system: Portable nitrous oxide system, which contains all the necessary components, housed together and can be moved from room to room for administration.
Positive aspiration: Blood entering the cartridge after an aspiration test, indicating the needle tip is within a blood vessel.
Posterior superior alveolar (PSA) block: A type of injection that anesthetizes the maxillary molars and associated structures when the local anesthetic agent is deposited superior to the apex of the maxillary second molar and posterior and superior to posterior border of maxilla at posterior superior alveolar foramina.
Prepuncture technique: An injection technique using the computer-controlled local anesthetic delivery device by applying pressure to the back of the needle and tissue with a cotton-tipped applicator while anesthetic is flowing to numb the tissue before needle insertion.
Pressor: An exaggerated increase in blood pressure.
Prilocaine: An intermediate amide local anesthetic that is metabolized in the lungs and the liver.
Primary complication: Experienced by the patient at the time of the injection.
Primary prevention: Using all standard protocols to prevent injury.
Procaine: An ester local anesthetic that is no longer available for use in dentistry because of its allergic potential (more commonly known as Novocaine).
Process: General term for any prominence on a bony surface.
Propagation: The process by which an action potential leaps along myelinated axons.
Proprietary drug: A drug that has a brand name that is protected by a patent.
Pterygomandibular raphe: The fibrous structure that extends from the hamulus to the posterior end of the mylohyoid line and is used as a landmark for the inferior alveolar injection.
Qualified health care professional: Designated qualified health care professional responsible for care and follow-up of occupational exposures.
Relative contraindication: A contraindication to a local anesthetic that allows the administration of the offending drug to be used judiciously (i.e., administration of a minimal effective dose).
Relative refractory period: The interval immediately after the absolute refractory period and before complete reestablishment to the resting state, during which initiation of a second action potential is possible if a larger stimulus is achieved to produce successful firing.
Repolarization: Occurs once the peak of the action potential is reached and the membrane potential begins to move back toward the resting potential (−70 mV). Results from efflux of K^+ ions.
Resting state: A neurologic term to describe the polarized nerve membrane receiving little or no stimulation.
Safety syringe: A plastic disposable syringe that decreases the risk of accidental exposure to the clinician from contaminated needles.
Saltatory conduction: The propagation of action potentials along myelinated axons from one node of Ranvier to the next node, increasing the conduction velocity of action potentials without needing to increase the diameter of an axon.
Scavenger system: Removes excess nitrous oxide gas from the immediate area, protecting the clinician.
Schwann cells: Glia cells of the peripheral nervous system (PNS).
Scoop technique: A method to safely recap contaminated needles using one hand to scoop the needle into the needle shield.
Secondary complication: Apparent after the injection is completed. The problem arises separately from and after an earlier complication.
Secondary prevention: A prevention strategy after an injury to minimize its complications.
Sedation: A continuum that ranges from minimal sedation to general anesthesia.
Severe complication: A problem that requires a definite plan of treatment to resolve the issue.
Shaft: The length of the needle, composed of long tubular metal.
Shank: Shaft.
Short-acting anesthetic: Anesthetics that provide pulpal anesthesia of approximately 30 minutes.
Sickle cell anemia: A hereditary blood disorder characterized by an abnormality in the oxygen carrying hemoglobin molecule in red blood cells.
Silicone rubber stopper: A piece of equipment located at the bottom of the anesthetic cartridge where the harpoon is embedded.
Sodium bisulfite: A preservative added by the manufacturer to a local anesthetic cartridge containing a vasoconstrictor to delay the oxidation of the vasoconstrictor. Metabisulfite and sodium bisulfite are the most commonly used antioxidants.
Soft tissue sloughing: The loss of surface layers of epithelium because of the administration of topical anesthetics for extended periods, or anesthetic sterile abscesses developed by prolonged ischemia because of the inclusion of a vasoconstrictor in the anesthetic solution.
Somatic nervous system (SNS): Subdivision of the efferent division of the PNS; controls the body's voluntary and reflex activities through somatic sensory and somatic motor components.
Specific receptor theory: The theory that explains the binding of local anesthetics to specific receptor sites on the sodium channel to prevent the depolarization phase of the nerve impulse generation.
Stress: Physical and emotional responses to particular situations.
Sulfonamides: Synthetic antimicrobial agents.
Supraperiosteal injection: A form of regional anesthesia deposited near large terminal nerve branches providing pulpal and soft tissue anesthesia of a single tooth.
Surface anesthesia: Anesthesia achieved by application of topical anesthetics to the mucosal surface by gels, creams, or sprays to block the free nerve endings.
Sympathetic nervous system: Division of ANS that prepares the body to deal with an emergency situation; involved in the fight-or-flight response.
Sympathomimetic drugs: Drugs that mimic the effects of the sympathetic nervous system.
Synapses: The junctions of nerve cells.
Syncope: Fainting; loss of consciousness resulting from insufficient blood flow to the brain.
Syringe: Metal devices used to administer local anesthetic drugs.
Syringe barrel: The part of the local anesthetic syringe that holds the glass cartridge.
Systemic complications: Complications that affect the entire body; attributed to the drug administered.
Titration: The incremental dosing of a drug until the desired effect is reached.
Topical anesthetic: A drug applied to the surface of the skin or mucosal tissues that produces local insensibility to pain.
Topical anesthetic spray: Application of an aerosol spray directly on the surface of a mucous membrane, resulting in loss of nerve conduction.
Topical antiseptic: An antimicrobial substance applied to tissue to reduce the risk of infection.
Tachycardia: Increased heart rate.
Tachyphylaxis: Increased tolerance to a drug that is administered repeatedly.
Tertiary prevention: Prevention strategy that strives to prevent disease progression and to return patient to a functional state.
Tetracaine hydrochloride: An ester anesthetic that is considered most potent and used only as a topical anesthetic.
Thumb ring: A portion of the syringe that is attached to the external end of the piston, allowing the clinician to advance or retract the piston.

Tonic-clonic seizure: A type of generalized seizure that affects the entire brain.
Topical anesthetic: An anesthetic that is applied to the body surface such as the skin or mucous membrane.
Transdermal: A route of administration delivered across the skin.
Transient complication: May appear severe at the time of its observance but eventually resolves without any residual effect.
Transoral: A route of administration delivered via oral mucosa.
Tricyclic antidepressant: Drugs used primarily to treat depression.
Trigeminal nerve: Fifth cranial nerve.
Trismus: Spasms of the muscles of mastication resulting in soreness and difficulty opening the mouth.
Tuberosity: Large, often rough prominence on the surface of bone.
Unionized: Anionic form of molecule.
Unmyelinated: A nerve that contains no myelin sheath for protection.
Vascular plexus: A large network of blood vessels.
Vasoconstrictor: An agent added to local anesthetic solutions to delay the absorption of local anesthetics.
Vasopressor: Synonym for vasoconstrictor.
Vazirani-Akinosi (V-A) mandibular block: Nerve block that has a large area of coverage of the mandibular nerve within one mandibular quadrant similar to the inferior alveolar block.
Vein: Component of the vascular system that carries blood to the heart.
Venous sinuses: Blood-filled spaces between the two layers of tissue.
Venule: A very small vein, especially one collecting blood from the capillaries.
Visual Analog Scale (VAS): A measurement instrument to measure pain.

INDEX

Page numbers followed by *b*, *t*, and *f* refer to boxes, tables, and figures respectively.

A

A fibers, 16, 17, 19*f*
Absolute contraindication, 44, 57, 101, 103*t*
Absolute maximum recommended dose, 116
Absolute refractory period, 20, 21*b*
Absorption, of local anesthetic, 37, 364
Accidental contamination of uncovered needle, 355*f*, 355
Acetylated salicylic acid, effects of, 2
Acetylcholine, 23
Acid cation form, 29
Action potential, 17*f*, 20*b*, 20. *See also* Nerve impulses
  conduction, 22
  electrophysiologic recording schematic of, 22*f*
  initiation of, 20
  propagation of, 22
  steps in, 22*t*
Adenosine triphosphate (ATP), use of, 19
Adrenalin. *See* Epinephrine
Adrenergic amines, effects on cardiovascular and respiratory systems, 46*t*
Adrenergic drugs, 43
Advance needle slowly, 348
Afferent division, 14*f*
Afferent nerve, 13
  anterior superior alveolar nerve as, 194
  auriculotemporal nerve as, 198
  buccal nerve as, 197
  incisive nerve as, 201
  inferior alveolar nerve as, 200
  infraorbital nerve as, 193
  lingual nerve as, 198
  mandibular nerve as, 195
  mental nerve as, 201
  middle superior alveolar nerve as, 193
  nasopalatine nerve as, 195
  posterior superior alveolar nerve as, 195
  sensory information and, 190
  zygomatic nerve as, 193
Afferent pathway, 12
Allergens, 367
  topical anesthetics as, 367
Allergic reaction, 367
  amino esters and, 367
  clinical manifestations/management of, 368, 368*t*
  evaluation of, 367*b*
  metabisulfite and, 367
  mild (delayed onset), management of, 370*t*
  prevention of, 367
  sodium bisulfite and, 367
Allergist, 368*b*
Allergy, 105, 106*t*
  allergist referral for, 368*b*
  manifestations of, 368
  para-aminobenzoic acid and, 38
All-or-none electrochemical pulse, 20
All-or-none firing, 23*f*
All-or-none principle, 21*b*
All-or-none response, 21*b*
Alpha (α) fiber, 17
Alveolar nerve
  anterior superior, 194
  inferior, 200
  middle superior, 195
  posterior superior, 195
Alveolar process, 185, 188
  associated structures of, 186*t*
American Dental Association (ADA), color-coded banding, 149*f*, 149, 150*t*
American Society of Anesthesiologists (ASA), 335
American Society of Anesthesiologists Physical Classification System, 102*t*
Amide, 3
Amide anesthetics, 33
Amide local anesthetics, 29, 38, 53, 58, 79
  drug/drug interactions, 106
    beta blockers, 106
    bleeding disorders, 107
    histamine H_2 receptor blockers, 106
    kidney disease, 107
    liver disease, 107
    malignant hyperthermia, 106
    methemoglobinemia, 107
    pregnancy, 107, 107*t*
  systemic toxicity and, 365
Amino esters, allergic reactions from, 367
Analgesia, local anesthetic and, 12
Anaphylaxis, 368
  immediate, clinical manifestations and management of, 368*t*
  management of, 370*t*
Anastomosis, definition of, 202
Anatomic variation, duration of anesthesia and, 55
Anesthesia
  administration technique for, 209, 210*f*
  in dental hygiene practice, 3, 6*f*
  nonsurgical periodontal therapy with, 211, 212*f*, 213*f*, 214*f*
  selection of, 211
Anesthetic
  administration, accuracy of, 55
  calculating milligrams of administered, 117*f*, 117
  individual response to, 55, 57*b*
  systemic toxicity of, 362
Anesthetic buffering, 33
Anesthetic cartridges. *See* Cartridges
Anesthetic molecule, lipid solubility of, 29
Anesthetic per cartridge, volume of, 116*b*
Anesthetics placed in disinfecting solution, 350
Anesthetic syringe. *See* Syringe
Angina
  management of, 370*t*
  vasoconstrictors and, 103*t*
Angle classification of malocclusion class III, 286
Anion, 29
Anterior middle superior alveolar block, 260, 267
  complications of, 270, 271*t*
  deposit location for, 270
  indications of clinically effective, 270
  injection site for, 270
  needle insertion point for, 268*f*, 272*f*
  procedure for, 271*b*
  review of, 268*t*
  target area for, 270
  technique errors associated with, 270
  using STA, 225
Anterior superior alveolar block, 240, 251
  complications of, 255
  deposit location for, 254
  indications of clinically effective, 255
  injection site for, 254
  procedure for, 254*b*
  review of, 252*t*
  target area for, 254
Anterior superior alveolar nerve, 194
Antigens, 367
Anxiety
  case study for, 226*b*
  clinical signs of, 100*b*
  dental care and, 6
  determining patient, 210
  moderate, clinical signs of, 8*b*
  stress reduction principles and, 6
Applicator sticks
  example of, 153*f*
  use of, 153
Armamentarium, 130, 181*b*
  components of, 131, 132*f*
  supplementary, 152
    applicator sticks, 153*f*, 153
    gauze, 153
    hemostat/cotton pliers, 153*f*, 153
    topical anesthetic, 152, 153*f*
    topical antiseptic, 152*f*, 152
Arteriole, 202
Artery, definition of, 202
Articaine, 3, 56*t*, 58*f*, 59*f*, 61, 69*t*, 70*t*, 71*t*, 72*t*, 354
  half-life of, 38*t*
  maximum recommended dose of, 115*t*
  pharmacology of, 61
  pregnancy and, 107*t*
  properties of, 55*t*
  summary of, 126*b*
Aspirating harpoon, 131
Aspirating on two planes, 220
Aspirating syringe. *See also* Syringe
  reusable breech-loading metallic cartridge-type, 134
    advantages/disadvantages of, 134*t*
  reusable breech-loading plastic cartridge-type, 135
Aspiration. *See also* Negative aspiration; Positive aspiration
  disengagement of harpoon during, 222*f*
  importance/steps for, 220
  using self-aspirating syringe, 220, 221*f*
  using standard syringe, 221*f*
Aspiration tests, 131
Aspirin, 2
Asthma, 105
  bronchial, management of, 370*t*
Atypical plasma cholinesterase, ester local anesthetics and, 106
Atypical pseudocholinesterase, 38
Auriculotemporal nerve, 198
Autonomic effector, 12
Autonomic nervous system, 12
  organizational plan of, 14*f*
Axon, 14, 15*f*, 16*f*, 18*f*
  cross section of, 18*f*
  multiple sclerosis and, 15
Axon collateral, 15*f*
Axon hillock, 14, 17*f*
Axon terminal, 25*f*
Axoplasm, 14
  electrical potential of, 17

B

Base anion form, 29
Beecher, Dr. Henry, 3
Bending the needle, 347
Benzocaine, 85, 87*f*, 87
Beta blockers
  amide local anesthetic and, 103*t*
  vasoconstrictors and, 103*t*
Beta (β) fiber, 17
Bevel
  configuration of, 142
  location of, 142
  orientation of, 215
  placement of, 143*f*
  types of, 142*f*
B fibers, 17, 19*f*
Biotransformation, of local anesthetics, 38, 363
Bi-rotational insertion technique (BRIT), 137*f*, 144, 145*f*
Bleeding disorders, 107
Blood clotting disorder, 107
Blood pressure, 98, 98*t*, 99*b*
  cuff placement for, 99*f*
  errors in, 99*b*
  vasoconstrictors and, 103*t*

Blood vessels
anastomosis and, 202
effect of epinephrine on, 47
effect of levonordefrin on, 46
vasoconstrictors and, 43
vasodilators and, 43
Bony surface, prominences and depressions on, 184
Bradycardia, 99
Breech-loading aspirating syringe
preparation of, 154*b*
unloading of, 159*b*
BRIT. *See* Bi-rotational insertion technique (BRIT)
Broken dental needle, 350*f*
Buccal artery, structures supplied, 204*t*
Buccal block, 281, 293
complications with, 294, 297*t*
indications of clinically effective, 294
injection site for, 294
procedure for, 296*b*
review of, 294*t*
target area for, 294
Buccal nerve, 197
Buffering, of local anesthetics, 33, 34*f*
process, 34
reasons, 33
Bupivacaine, 3, 58*f*, 59*f*, 69, 73*t*, 74*t*, 75*t*
half-life of, 38*t*
maximum recommended dose of, 115*t*
pregnancy and, 107*t*
properties of, 55*t*
summary of, 126*b*
Burning during injection, 351
causes of, 348*t*
prevention of, 348*t*, 351
Butamben, 87*f*, 87

C
CaineTips, 81
Calcium ions, depolarization and, 35
Canal, definition of, 184
Capillaries, 202
Cardiac dose, 101, 120
Cardiac drug, digitalis glycosides as, 104
Cardiac dysrhythmia, 99
Cardiac stimulation, 45
Cardiovascular disease, vasoconstrictors and, 103*t*
Cardiovascular system (CVS)
adrenergic amine effects on, 46*t*
effect of epinephrine on, 47
effect of levonordefrin on, 46, 49
local anesthetic and, systemic toxicity, 362
Care plan, 211, 212*f*, 213*f*, 214*f*
Carticaine, 3
Cartridge-penetrating end, 142*f*, 143
Cartridges
anesthetic, 148
blister pack of, 149, 150*f*
broken, 151
bubble in, 150, 151*f*
care and handling of, 149
color-coded bands on, 149*f*, 149
components of, 148, 149*f*
aluminum cap, 149*f*, 149
cartridge labeling, 149*f*, 149, 150*t*
diaphragm, 149*f*, 149
glass cylinder, 148, 149*f*
silicone rubber stopper, 149*f*, 149, 150*f*
corroded cap, 151
extruded stopper on, 151*f*, 151
problems with, 150
product information on, 150*f*, 150
rust on cap, 151
sticky stopper, 151
Catecholamine, 43
Catecholamine-*O*-methyltransferase inhibitors, vasoconstrictors and, 103*t*
Catecholamine-producing tumors, vasoconstrictors and, 103*t*
Cation, 29
Cavernous sinus, 205*f*
CCLAD. *See* Computer-controlled local anesthetic delivery (CCLAD)
CDC. *See* Centers for Disease Control and Prevention (CDC)
Cell body, 14, 15*f*, 17*f*
Central fibers, 12
Centralized systems, 337*f*, 337
Central nervous system (CNS)
definition of, 12
effect of epinephrine on, 48
local anesthetic and
overdose of, 366*t*
systemic toxicity, 362
organizational plan of, 14*f*
Cerebrovascular accident, management of, 370*t*
Cetacaine, 80, 84*f*
C fibers, 17, 19*f*
Chemical synapse, 23, 24*f*, 25*f*
Chloride ions, 17
Chorda tympani nerve, pathway of, 200*f*
Clarke, William, 2
Clark's rule, 120
Clinical pain, 3
CNS stimulants, vasoconstrictors and, 103*t*
Cocaine, 3
vasoconstrictors and, 103*t*
Communication, 377
dental hygienist-employer, 377
dental hygienist-patient, 377
Complications
localized, 347
needle breakage as, 347
mild, 347
permanent, 347
primary, 347
secondary, 347
severe, 347
systemic, 347, 362
local anesthetic overdose as, 362
transient, 347
CompuDent Wand System, 136*f*, 136
Computer-controlled local anesthetic delivery (C-CLAD), 136, 144
advantages and disadvantages of, 141*t*
device, example of, 137*f*
dynamic pressure sensing on, 140*f*
injection techniques for, 224
Concentration gradient, 19*f*, 20
Concomitant, 95
Conduction zone, 17*f*
Condyle, 184
Conscious sedation, 336
Constant liter flow, 340*f*, 340, 341*f*
Constant oxygen flow, 340*f*, 340, 341*f*
Continuum, 335
Core bundles, 13, 16*f*
Corneal reflex, 352
Coronary arteries
effect of epinephrine on, 47
effect of levonordefrin on, 48
Coronary bypass surgery, vasoconstrictors and, 103*t*
Coronoid notch, 189
inferior alveolar block and, 286
Coronoid process, 189
associated structures of, 186*t*
Cotton pliers (Hemostat)
example of, 153*f*
use of, 153
Cotton rolls, 357
Cotton-tipped applicator sticks
example of, 153*f*
use of, 153
Cranial nerve, facial nerve as, 201
Crossover-innervation, definition of, 195
Current Dental Terminology (CDT) code, 342

D
Deep epineurium, 16*f*
Deep temporal artery, structures supplied, 204*t*
Deflection, of needles, 142*f*, 142, 144
Delivery systems
components of, 338*f*
nitrous oxide/oxygen, 337
centralized system *versus* portable system, 337*f*, 337
equipment, 337
safety features, 338
Delta (δ) fiber, 17
Dendrite, 15*f*
Dendritic (input) zone, 14
Dental anxiety, 6
Dental care, pain and, 2
Dental emergency kit, 369*t*
Dental history, 94
Dental hygiene
considerations, 9*b*, 25*b*, 40*b*, 50*b*, 76*b*, 90*b*, 108*b*, 123*b*, 181*b*, 206*b*, 226*b*, 274*b*, 317*b*, 332*b*, 343*b*, 360*b*, 374*b*, 383*b*
human-needs paradigm and, 8*b*, 8*f*
medical emergency, actions in, 373*f*
Dental hygienist
case study for, 384*b*
communication and
with employer, 377
patient and, 377
legal issues relating to, 377
case study for, 378*b*
local anesthesia administration by, 4*t*
nonsurgical periodontal therapy, 378*b*
Dental infections, 356
Dental phobia, 6
definition of, 100
origins of, 100*b*
Dental plexus, definition of, 194
"Dental shot, " fear of, 5
DentalVibe, 220*f*, 220
Dentapen, 138, 141*f*
DentiPatch, 84
Depolarization, 20, 21*f*
Deposit location, 220
for anterior middle superior alveolar block, 270
for anterior superior alveolar block, 254
for buccal block, 294
for Gow-Gates mandibular block, 303
for greater palatine block, 260
for incisive block, 301
for inferior alveolar block, 285
for infraorbital block, 255
for mental block, 297
for middle superior alveolar block, 248
for nasopalatine block, 267
for periodontal ligament injection, 313
for posterior superior alveolar block, 242
for supraperiosteal injection, 234
for Vazirani-Akinosi mandibular block, 308
Depression, 184
Depth of needle insertion, 220
Descending palatine artery, structures supplied, 204*t*
Diabetes, vasoconstrictors and, 105*t*
Dialogue history, 94
Diaphragm, 149*f*, 149
Digitalis glycosides
use/precautions for, 104
vasoconstrictors and, 103*t*
Disposable safety syringes, 140
Dissociation constant (pK_a), 31*b*, 31
of commonly used local anesthetic drugs, 33*t*
local anesthetic and, 33*t*
Di Stefano, Francesco, 3
Distribution, of local anesthetic agents, 37
Documentation, 379
nitrous oxide/oxygen, 342
of treatment notes after, 224*t*
Drug dose, determining, 114, 123*b*
Dull needles, 350
Dyclonine hydrochloride, 86*f*, 86
Dynamic pressure-sensing (DPS), 138, 140*f*

E
Edema, 356*f*, 356
causes of, 348*t*
management of, 348*t*, 356
prevention of, 348*t*, 356
produced by an allergic response, 356
produced by contaminated agent or trauma, 356
produced by hemorrhage, 356
produced by infection, 356
Efferent division, 12, 14*f*
Efferent nerve, 13
mylohyoid nerve a, 201
Efferent pathway, 12
Electrical charge, of cell, 17
Electrical synapse, 23, 24*f*
Electric pulp tester (EPT), 33
Elimination, of local anesthetic, 364
Emergency. *See* Medical emergency

Emergency management, 362
Employer-dental hygienist communication, 377
Endogenous epinephrine, 44
 blood levels during rest, 44*f*
Endoneurium, 13, 16*f*
Endoplasmic reticulum, 15*f*
Epinephrine, 3, 44, 45*t*, 354
 actions of, in specific systems and tissue, 47
 dilution of, 46*f*, 46, 46*t*, 47*f*
 drug interactions and, 104
 maximum recommended dose, 48
 mechanism of action, 45
 pressor effects from, 102
 termination of action, 48
Epinephrine overdose, 366
 causes and prevention of, 366
 manifestations/management of, 367, 367*t*
Epineural sheath, 16*f*
Epineurium, 13, 16*f*
EpiPen, 369*f*
Ester local anesthetics, 29, 38, 53, 73, 75*t*
 atypical plasma cholinesterase and, 106
 sulfonamides and, 105
 systemic toxicity and, 364
Ether, 2
Eutectic mixtures, 87
Eutectic mixtures of local anesthetics (EMLA), 87, 88*b*
Excitatory neurotransmitters, 23
Exogenous epinephrine, 44
External carotid artery, orofacial branches of, 202, 203*f*, 204*t*
External jugular vein, 205*f*
Extraoral line, Gow-Gates mandibular block injection site and, 306*f*

F
Facial nerve, 201
 auriculotemporal nerve communicating with, 198
 pathway of
  branches, 202*f*
  trunk, 200*f*
Facial paralysis, from inferior alveolar block, 293
Facial vein, 205*f*
Fainting. *See* Syncope
Fascicles, 13
Fear
 of pain, 5
 in patient, management of, 6
Feather-light handpiece, 137*f*, 137
Felypressin, 49
Fifth cranial nerve. *See* Trigeminal nerve
Fight-or-flight response, 7, 43
 to stress, 7, 100
Finger grip, 132*f*, 132, 133*f*
Firing thresholds, depolarization and, 20
Fissure, 184
Foramen, 184
Foramen ovale, 186*t*
Foramen rotundum, 186*t*
Force, needle, 350
Fossa, 184
Free base form of local anesthetics, 31*f*
Frontal process, associated structures of, 186*t*
Fulcrum
 establishment of, 216, 217*f*
 example of, 218*f*

G
Galactocerebroside, 15
Gamma (γ) fiber, 17
Gas inhalation, 2
Gate control theory, 3
Gauge, needle, 143, 144*f*, 144*t*
30-Gauge needles, 353, 354
Gauze, 153
Generic name, 53
Glandular structures, 202
Glial cells, 15
Glycolipid, 15
Golgi apparatus, 15*f*
Gow-Gates mandibular block, 281, 303, 354
 complications with, 307, 307*t*
 indications of clinically effective, 307
 injection site for, 303
  extraoral line, 306*f*
  using needle to assess, 306*f*
 procedure for, 306*b*
 review of, 304*t*
 target area for, 303
 troubleshooting paradigm, 307
Greater palatine artery, pathways of, 204*f*
Greater palatine block, 260
 complications of, 264, 264*t*
 deposit location for, 260
 indications of clinically effective, 264
 injection site for, 260
 needle insertion point for, 263*f*, 330*f*
 procedure for, 263*b*
 review of, 260*t*
 target area for, 260
 target location for, 330*f*
Greater palatine foramen, location/contents of, 186*t*
Greater palatine nerve, 195, 196*f*
Greater petrosal nerve, pathway of, 200*f*

H
Half-life, 38
 of articaine, 69*t*
 of commonly used local anesthetics, 38*t*
 of lidocaine, 38*t*, 60*t*
 of mepivacaine, 63*t*, 64*t*, 65*t*
Halothane, 2
Halstead technique, 285
HandiCaine Stix, 81
Hard palate, view of
 inferior, 188*f*
 posteroinferior, 187*f*
Harpoon, 132*f*, 132
 disengagement of, 134, 222*f*, 222
Head, vascular system of, 202
Health history, 94
Heavy and oversedation, signs and symptoms of, 341, 343*t*
Hematoma, 351, 352*f*
 causes of, 348*t*
 management of, 348*t*, 351
 from mental block, 301, 301*t*
 posterior superior alveolar block, 351
 prevention of, 348*t*, 351
Hemostasis, 215
 epinephrine and, 48
 levonordefrin and, 49
 need for, 57
Hemostat (cotton pliers)
 example of, 153*f*
 use of, 153
Henderson-Hasselbalch equation, 31
Histamine H_2 receptor blockers, amide local anesthetic and, 106
Hub, of needle, 142*f*, 143
Human-needs paradigm, 6, 8*f*, 8*b*
HurriPak, 80, 84*f*
Hydrogen ion concentration, 33*f*
Hydrophilic terminal amine, 29
Hyperglycemia, management of, 370*t*
Hyperresponders, 55
Hyperthyroidism, vasoconstrictors and, 103*t*
Hyperventilation, management of, 370*t*
Hypoglycemia, management of, 370*t*
Hyporesponders, 55

I
Ideal body weight (IBW) index, 120
Ideal sedation, signs and symptoms of, 343*t*
Illegal drugs, 104
Immune system, systemic toxicity to, 362
Impulse propagation, 23*f*, 24*f*
Incisive artery, 204
Incisive block, 281, 297, 301
 complications with, 301, 303*t*
 indications of clinically effective, 301
 injection site for, 301
 procedure for, 303*b*
 review of, 302*t*
 target area for, 301
Incisive foramen, 186, 186*t*
Incisive nerve, 201
Infection, 356
 anesthetic administration and, 215
 in area of injection, 32
 causes of, 348*t*
 management of, 348*t*, 356
 prevention of, 348*t*, 356
Inferior alveolar arteries, structures supplied, 204*t*
Inferior alveolar block, 281, 331*f*, 347, 354
 complications with, 293*t*
 considerations following, 318*b*
 coronoid notch and, 286
 indications of clinically effective, 292
 injection site for, 285, 287*f*, 292*f*
 paresthesia from, 293
 positive aspiration and, 293
 procedure for, 286*b*
 review of, 283*t*
 target area for, 285
 troubleshooting paradigm, 289, 291*f*, 292*f*
 using STA, 225
Inferior alveolar nerve, 200
Inferior orbital fissure, 186*t*
Infiltration injections, 209
Informed consent, 212
 example of, 215*f*, 379*f*
Infraorbital artery, structures supplied, 204*t*
Infraorbital block, 240, 255
 complications of, 258, 259*t*
 correct angulation for, 273*f*
 deposit location for, 255
 incorrect angulation for, 273*f*
 indications of clinically effective, 258
 injection site for, 255
 palpation of, 258*f*
 procedure for, 258*b*
 review of, 255*t*
 target area for, 255
 technique errors associated with, 271
Infraorbital foramen and canal
 location/contents of, 186*t*
 pupil, relationship to, 259*f*
Infraorbital nerve, 193
Injecting anesthetic slowly, 351
Injection
 basic techniques in, 209, 226*b*
 burning during, 351
 burning on, 151
 leakage during, 151
 pain during. *See* Pain during injection
 selection of, 215
 steps to providing successful, 209, 210*t*
 supraperiosteal, 209
  using STA, 224
Injection site. *See* Needle insertion point
Input zone, 14, 17*f*
Insert needle to hub, 350
Insulin shock, management of, 370*t*
Intermediate-acting anesthetics, 54
Intermediate hydrocarbon chain, 29
Internal jugular vein, 205*f*
Intraosseous injections, 233
Intraseptal injection, 233
 advantages and disadvantages of, 240*t*
 complications of, 237
 indications of clinically effective, 237
 injection site for, 236
 maxillary, 236
 procedure for, 239*b*
 review of, 238*t*
 target area for, 236
Ion channels, 17*f*
Ionized, 31

J
Jet injector, example of, 136*f*, 136
Jet injector syringe, 136
Jugular vein, pathway of
 external, 205*f*
 internal, 205*f*

K
Ketoacidosis, management of, 370*t*
Kidney disease, 107
Kidneys, 38
Koller, Karl, 3

L
Laughing gas. *See* Nitrous oxide
"Laughing gas" parties, 2

Length, needle, 145, 146*f*
Lesion formation, considerations with, case study for, 274*b*
Lesser palatine artery, pathways of, 204*f*
Lesser palatine foramen, location/contents of, 186*t*
Lesser palatine nerve, 195, 196*f*
Levarterenol. *See* Norepinephrine
Levonordefrin, 43, 48, 48*t*, 57, 59
  actions of, in specific systems and tissues, 48
  maximum recommended dose, 49
  pressor effects from, 102
  termination of action, 49
Lidocaine, 3, 58*f*, 58, 59*f*, 60*t*, 61*t*, 62*t*, 63*t*, 86*f*, 86, 354
  half-life of, 38*t*
  maximum recommended dose of, 115*t*
  pregnancy and, 107*t*
  properties of, 55*t*
  summary of, 126*b*
Life-threatening emergency. *See* Medical emergency
Limiting drug, 114, 115*b*, 123
Line, 184
Linear insertion technique, 144
Lingual artery, 202
  structures supplied, 204*t*
Lingual nerve, 198
Lingual shock, 292
Lipid solubility, local anesthetic and, 32*t*
Lip, masticatory trauma of, 327*f*
Lipophilic aromatic ring, 29
Liver disease, 107
Local anesthesia
  administration, anatomic considerations for, 184, 206*b*
  case study for, 332*b*
  for child and adolescent, 326, 327*f*
  definition of, 2
  delivery techniques, 328
  in dental hygiene practice, 1
  dental hygienist administering, 3, 4*t*
  patient perception of, 3
  programs, 3
  synopsis of, 7*t*
Local anesthetic agents, 53, 76*b*
  absorption of, 37, 364
  action, 32*t*
  administered intravascularly, 364
  administration of, 380*b*
    fulcrum during, 218*f*
    needle insertion during, 220
    patient communication during, 216
    technique for, 209, 210*f*
  administration protocol, 328
    applying topical anesthetic, 328
    maxillary anesthesia, 329, 330*f*
    positioning patient in dental chair, 328, 329*f*
    stabilization and communication, 328
  for anxious patient, 101
  armamentarium for, 132*f*
  aspiration of, 220
  biotransformation of, 362
  buffering of, 33, 34*f*
  case study for, 181*b*, 360*b*, 374*b*
    patient anxiety, 226*b*
  characteristics affecting induction and action of, 32*t*
  chemistry of, 29, 30*f*
  composition of, 53
  contraindications to, 104
  deposit of solution, 222, 223*b*
  distribution of, 37
  documentation of, 224
  duration of, 37
  effects of
    on cardiovascular system, 39, 40*t*
    on central nervous system, 39, 39*t*
  elimination of, 364
  equipment
    checking of, 215
    preparation of, 215*f*, 216*f*
  ester, 73, 75*t*
  ester derivative, interactions, 105
  excretion of, 38
  fulcrum, establishing, 216, 217*f*
  history of, 3*b*, 3
  induction of, 36*f*, 36
  induction time for, 37
  infection in the area of injection, 32
  informed consent and, 212
  local complications associated with administration of, 348*t*
  maximum recommended doses of, 114, 127*b*, 128*t*, 129*t*
    calculation of, 327
  mechanism of action of, 34, 35*b*
  metabolism of, 38, 38*t*
  mode of action of, 25*b*, 25
  needle, fear of, 101
  observation of patient's reaction to, 223
  onset of action of, 35
  patient anxiety, case study for, 226*b*
  patient assessment before, 209
  patient communication during, 216
  patient positioning for, 216*f*, 216
  patient preparation, 328*b*, 328
  penetration site, palpation of, 216
  pharmacodynamics of, 30, 31*f*, 31*b*, 32*f*, 32*t*
  pharmacokinetics of, 35
  pharmacology of, 28, 30*b*, 40*b*
  physical properties of, 55*t*
  reinjection of, 37
  routes of delivery, 30
  selection of, 53, 211
    for children, 327
    duration of action and operative pain control, 54, 56*t*
    local anesthetic allergy and, 57, 58*t*
    metabisulfite allergy and, 57, 58*t*
    need for hemostasis, 57
    patient health assessment and current patient medications, 57
    posttreatment pain control, 56, 56*t*
    sodium bisulfite allergy and, 57, 58*t*
  skull bones and, 184
  steps for, 209, 210*t*
  summary of, 126*b*, 127*b*
  systemic effects of, 38
  systemic toxicity from, 326
  tissue preparation for, 216, 217*f*
  tissue taut on, 218, 219*f*, 220
  total dose administered, 364
  training needles, 148
  use of, 3
  vasodepressor syncope from, 209
  withdrawing syringe/needle capping after, 223
Local anesthetic block, 240*f*
  recovery from, 37
Local anesthetic overdose
  cardiovascular system and, signs of, 365
  causes/prevention of, 364
  central nervous system and
    signs of, 365
  clinical manifestations of, 365
  management of, 366, 370*t*
  predisposing factors for, 363
  signs/symptoms/management of, 367*t*
  as systemic complication, 362
Local anesthetic pool, 16*f*
Local anesthetic syringes, types of, 133, 134*f*
Localized complications, 347, 348*t*
  burning during injection, 351
  edema, 356
  hematoma, 351
  infection. *See* Infections
  needle breakage, 347
    management of, 348*t*, 350
    prevention of, 347, 348*t*
  pain during injection. *See* Pain during injection
  paresthesia, 354
  postanesthetic intraoral lesions, 358
  prevention, and management, 348*t*
  primary complication, 347
  secondary complication, 347
  soft tissue trauma, 356
  systemic complications, 347
  tissue sloughing, 357
  transient complications, 347
  transient facial paralysis, 351
  trismus, 355
Local infiltration, 209
Localized complications, 347
Lofgren, Nils, 3
Long-acting anesthetics, 54
Long buccal block, 293, 331*f*
  target location of, 331*f*
Long, large-gauge needle, 347
Loss of motor function, 352
Low-grade infections, 356
Luer-Lok needles, for Wand STA handpiece, 145, 146*f*
Lumen, 143

M

Malignant hyperthermia, 106
Malocclusion class III, Angle classification of, 286
Mandible, 187
  landmarks of, 189*f*, 190*f*
  processes of, 186*t*
  supraperiosteal injection of, 292*f*
  view of
    anterior, 189*f*
    medial, 191*f*, 199*f*
    oblique lateral, 189*f*
Mandibular anesthesia, 280, 329
Mandibular block, 281
Mandibular foramen, 186*t*, 331*f*
Mandibular intraseptal injection, 313, 314*f*
Mandibular nerve, 195
  branches to oral cavity, 197*f*
  dissection of, 197*f*
  pathway of, 197*f*
    anterior trunk of, 197*f*
    posterior trunk of, 199*f*
Mandibular nerve blocks, 281
Mandibular supplemental injections, 312, 313*f*
Mandibular supraperiosteal injection, 313*f*, 313
Mandibular teeth
  average root length, 314*t*
  nerve blocks for, 282*t*
Mantle bundles, 13, 16*f*
Masseteric artery, structures supplied, 204*t*
Masticatory trauma, of lip, 327*f*
Maxillae, 184
  processes of, 186*t*
  sutures of, 187*t*
  view of
    anterior, 185*f*
    cutaway, 187*f*
    lateral, 188*f*
    panoramic, 185*f*, 188*f*
    posteroinferior, 187*f*
Maxillary anesthesia, 233, 329, 330*f*
Maxillary arch, facial surface of, 242*f*
Maxillary artery, 203
  orofacial branches, 204*t*
Maxillary facial nerve blocks, 239
Maxillary injection
  summary of, 277*b*
  technique errors associated with, 270
Maxillary nerve, 192
  branches to oral cavity, 194*f*
  pathway of, 193*f*
Maxillary supplemental injections, 233
Maxillary teeth, 236*t*
  nerve blocks for, 241*t*
Maxillary tuberosity, 185
Maxillary vein, 205*f*, 206
Maximum recommended dose (MRD), 44, 57, 114, 115*t*, 126*b*, 127*b*, 128*t*, 129*t*
  calculation of, 115, 116*t*, 117*b*, 327
    additional doses of different drugs, 118, 118*t*
    additional doses of the same drug, 118
    anesthetic administered, 117*f*, 117
    converting MRD to cartridges, 116, 117*f*
    converting MRD to milliliters, 117*b*, 117
    convert maximum recommended dose of vasoconstrictor cartridges, 122, 122*t*
    for lidocaine, 117*b*
    for medically compromised patients and elderly patients, 119
    in mg, 115*t*, 116, 118*t*
    milligrams of selected anesthetic in one cartridge, 115, 116*b*, 116*t*
    patient information, obtaining, 115
    pediatric doses, 120, 120*t*
    for pediatric patients, 119
    for vasoconstrictor drugs, 121*b*, 121, 121*t*
  cardiac dose and, 101
  definition of, 114
  weight of patient and, 100
Median palatine suture, 185, 187*t*
Medical emergency
  dental emergency kit, 369*t*

dental hygiene actions in, 373*f*
management of, 368, 370*t*
Medical history, 94
case study for, 108*b*
Membrane channels, 19
Membrane expansion theory, 35, 36*f*
Membrane potential, 17
Mental artery, 203
Mental block, 281, 297
complications with, 301, 301*t*
hematoma from, 301, 301*t*
indications of clinically effective, 301
injection site for, 297, 300*f*
procedure for, 300*b*
review of, 297*t*
target area for, 297
Mental foramen, 186*t*, 301
radiographs in locating, 300*f*
Mental nerve, 201
Mepivacaine, 3, 58*f*, 59*f*, 59, 63*t*, 64*t*, 65*t*
half-life of, 38*t*
maximum recommended dose of, 115*t*
pregnancy and, 107*t*
properties of, 55*t*
summary of, 126*b*
Metabisulfite allergy, 57, 58*t*
Metabolic system
effect of epinephrine on, 47
effect of levonordefrin on, 48
Methamphetamine, vasoconstrictors and, 103*t*
Methemoglobinemia, 60, 107
Methylparaben, 53
Middle superior alveolar block, 240, 247
complications of, 250, 251*t*
deposit location for, 248
indications of clinically effective, 250
injection site for, 248
needle insertion point for, 251*f*, 272*f*
procedure for, 251*b*
review of, 248*t*
target area for, 248
technique errors associated with, 270
Middle superior alveolar nerve, 195
Mild complications, 347
Minimal sedation, 336, 341
Minor tissue sloughing, 358
Minute volume, 338
Mitochondrion, 15*f*
Mixed nerves, 13
Morphine, 2
Motor pathway, 12
MRD. *See* Maximum recommended dose (MRD)
Muscular branches, 198
Myelin, 15, 18*f*, 18*b*
Myelinated nerve, 15
Myelin sheath, 15*f*
Mylohyoid artery, 203
Mylohyoid nerve, 201
Myocardial infarction
management of, 370*t*
vasoconstrictors and, 103*t*
Myocardium
effect of epinephrine on, 47
effect of levonordefrin on, 48

N

Narcotics, 2, 3*b*
Nasal hoods, 338*f*, 338, 340*f*
Nasopalatine block, 260, 264
complications of, 267, 268*t*
deposit location for, 267*f*, 267
indications of clinically effective, 267
injection site for, 267
procedure for, 266*b*
review of, 264*t*
target area for, 267
target location for, 330*f*
Nasopalatine nerve, 195
Neck, vascular system of, 202
Needle
care and handling of, 146
components of, 142
bevel, 142*f*, 142
cartridge-penetrating end, 142*f*, 143
hub, 142*f*, 143
needle shields, 143, 144*f*
shaft, 142*f*, 142
deflection of, 142*f*, 142, 144
dental, average length of, 146*f*
disposal of, 147*f*
insertion of, 220*f*
Luer-Lok, 145, 146*f*
problems with, 147
recapping techniques, safe and unsafe, 230
use of, 142
Needle adaptor, 131, 132*f*, 133*f*
Needle breakage, 142, 147, 347, 350*f*
causes of, 348*t*
management of, 348*t*, 350
needle fragment not visible, 350
needle fragment visible, 350
prevention of, 347, 348*t*
advance needle slowly, 348
do not bend needle, 347
long, large-gauge needle, 347
never force needle, 350
never insert needle to hub, 350
no sudden direction changes, 350
patient communication, 347
Needle capping
devices for, 147*f*, 223*f*
procedures for, 223*f*
scoop method of, 147*f*
Needle fragment
not visible, 350
visible, 350
Needle gauge, 143, 144*f*, 144*t*
color-coding by, 144*f*
for intraoral injections, 144*t*
large *versus* small, 145*b*
selection of, 143
Needle insertion point, 220
for anterior superior alveolar block, 268*f*, 272*f*
for buccal block, 294
for Gow-Gates mandibular block, 301
for greater palatine block, 263*f*, 330*f*
for incisive block, 301
for inferior alveolar block, 285, 287*f*, 292*f*
for infraorbital block, 255
for mental block, 300*f*, 301
for middle superior alveolar block, 251*f*, 272*f*
for nasopalatine block, 267
for periodontal ligament injection, 313
for posterior superior alveolar block, 247*f*
for supraperiosteal injection, 272*f*
for Vazirani-Akinosi mandibular block, 309, 311*f*
Needle length, 145, 146*f*
Needle shields, 143, 144*f*
Needlestick exposure, to clinician, 147
Needle-tract contamination, 356
Negative aspiration, 220, 222*f*
Negative pressure
aspiration test and, 131, 365*f*
harpoon and, 132
Neo-cobefrin. *See* Levonordefrin
Neo-Synephrine. *See* Phenylephrine
Nerve, 13, 16*f*
Nerve block, 55, 209
for mandibular teeth, 282*t*
for maxillary teeth and associated structures, 241*t*
Nerve cells. *See* Neurons
Nerve fibers, 13, 16*f*
classification of, 15
Nerve impulses. *See also* Action potential
generation and conduction, 17
Nervous system, organization of, 12, 14*f*
Neuroanatomy, 13
Neurons, 13, 15*f*
classification of, 13, 17*f*
structure of, 13
Neurophysiology, 12, 19*f*, 20*f*, 21*b*
Neurotransmitters, 23, 24*f*
Niemann, Albert, 3
Nitrous oxide/oxygen, 3, 335
administration, 338, 339*b*, 340*f*
calculations, 341
constant liter flow *versus* constant oxygen flow, 340
case study, 344*b*
characteristics of, 335
sedation continuum, 335, 336*t*
concentration of, 343*f*
delivery systems, 337
centralized system *versus* portable system, 337*f*, 337
components of, 338*f*
equipment, 337
safety features, 338
effects, 341
physiology and pharmacology, 341
signs and symptoms, 341
history of, 335
molecule, 336*f*
professional consideration, 342
documentation, 342
rules and regulations, 343
scope of practice, 343
respiratory anatomy, 342*f*
role in pain management, 336
advantages *versus* disadvantages, 336, 336*t*
indications *versus* contraindications, 336
safety feature, 335*b*
treatment note after the administration of, 343*t*
Nodes of Ranvier, 15*f*, 15, 18*f*, 18*b*
Nonmyelinated nerve, 15, 18*f*
Nonnervous tissue diffusibility, 32*t*
Nonselective beta blockers, 102
Nonsurgical paresthesia, 354
Nonsurgical periodontal therapy (NSPT), 114, 211, 212*f*, 213*f*, 214*f*, 378*b*
Norepinephrine, 23, 43, 49*f*, 49
Normal responder, 55
Notch, 184
Novocaine, 3
Nucleus, 15*f*

O

Occupational exposure, 380
exposure prevention and management, 380
postexposure management of, 381*b*, 381
primary prevention and, 380
qualified healthcare professional and, 381
risk reduction protocol for, 380
secondary prevention and, 380
tertiary prevention and, 380
Oligodendrocyte, 15
myelin sheath formation by, 18*f*
Onset Cartridge Connector, 151, 152*f*
Onset Mixing Pen, 151, 152*f*
Operation, on unconscious patient, 2
Ophthalmic nerve, 191, 193*f*
of facial region, 193*f*
Opium, 2
Oral cavity
mandibular nerve to, 197*f*
maxillary nerve to, 194*f*
Oraqix, 87, 88*f*
OraVerse. *See* Phentolamine mesylate (OraVerse)
Orofacial skull bones, 184
Orofacial structures, 192*t*
Orthotoluidine, 107
Output zone, 15, 17*f*
Overdose, of local anesthetic, 362
signs, symptoms, and management of, 367*t*
Oxygen saturation, 340*f*

P

Pacemaker cells
effect of epinephrine on, 47
effect of levonordefrin on, 48
Pain, 350
anesthetics placed in disinfecting solution, 350
definition of, 2
drugs used in the past to reduce, 2*b*
fear of, 5
inject slowly, 351
on needle insertion, 147
on needle withdrawal, 147
proper technique, 350
room temperature agents, 351
sharp needles, 350
topical anesthetic, 350
Pain control
benefits of, 101*b*
definition of, 2
hemostatic, 202
history of, 2
needle, fear of, 101
posttreatment, 56

Pain management
with hemostatic control, 184
nitrous oxide role in, 336
advantages *versus* disadvantages, 336
indications *versus* contraindications
Pain perception, 3
Pain reaction, 3
Pain reaction threshold
definition of, 3
influences of, 7*t*
Pain scales, 5
Pain threshold, definition of, 3
Palatal nerve blocks, 259
Palatine bones
components of, 186
sutures of, 187*t*
view of
inferior view, 188*f*
posterior view, 187*f*
Palatine process, 185
associated structures of, 186*t*
Para-aminobenzoic acid (PABA)
allergy and, 38
ester, 75*t*
Parasympathetic division, 12
Paresthesia, 354
causes of, 348*t*
complications, 354
definition of, 354
from inferior alveolar block, 293
local anesthetics and, 354
management of, 348*t*, 355
prevention of, 348*t*, 355
Patient communication, 347
Patient-dental hygienist communication, 377
Patient health assessment
physical examination for, 98
risk assessment and, 101
Pediatric dose, calculating, 120, 120*t*
Perineurium, 13, 16*f*
Perineurium thickness, 32*t*
Periodontal ligament injection, 233, 313
advantages and disadvantages of, 317*t*
complications of, 315
indications of clinically effective, 315
injection site for, 313
maxillary, 237
procedure for, 316*b*
review of, 315*t*
target area for, 313
Peripheral fibers, 12
Peripheral nerve anatomy, 15
Peripheral nervous system
definition of, 12
myelinated axon of, 16*f*
organizational plan of, 14*f*
Permanent complications, 347
Petite syringe, 134*f*
Pharmacodynamics, definition of, 30
Pharmacology
of nitrous oxide/oxygen, 341
of vasoconstrictors, 43
Phenothiazines, vasoconstrictors and, 106*t*
Phentolamine mesylate (OraVerse), 328, 357, 358*t*, 359*f*
contraindications, 357
dosage and administration technique, 357
side effects, 357
suggested clinical uses, 357
Phenylephrine, 49
Pheochromocytoma, 103*t*
Physical examination
blood pressure, 98
cuff placement for, 99*f*
guidelines for, 98*t*
pulse and
acceptable ranges for, 99*t*
factors influencing, 100*t*
procedure for, 99*f*, 99
respiration and, 99
acceptable ranges for, 100*t*
visual examination, 98
vital signs and, 98
weight of patient and, 100
Physicians' Desk Reference (PDR), 95
Physiology, of nitrous oxide/oxygen, 341
"Pins-and-needles" feeling, 293
Piston, 132*f*, 132
Polarization, 17, 19*f*, 20*f*
Portable delivery systems, 337*f*, 337
Positive aspiration, 132, 220, 222*f*
inferior alveolar block and, 293
Postanesthetic intraoral lesions, 358, 359*f*
causes of, 348*t*
management of, 348*t*, 358
prevention of, 348*t*, 358
Posterior superior alveolar artery, structures supplied, 204*t*
Posterior superior alveolar block, 241, 330*f*, 351
complications of, 246, 248*t*
deposit location for, 242
hematoma and, 351
indications of clinically effective, 246
injection site for, 242, 246*f*
needle insertion point for, 247*f*
procedure for, 245*b*
review of, 243*t*
syringe barrel angulation of, 273*f*
target area for, 242, 246*f*
technique errors associated with, 271
Posterior superior alveolar nerve, 195
view of, 194*f*
Postinjection aphthous stomatitis, 359*f*
Postinjection herpetic outbreak, 359*f*
Preanesthetic assessment, 93, 108*b*
dental history, 94
dialogue history, 94
medical history, 94, 95*t*
physical examination, 98
Pregnancy, 107
Prepuncture technique, 224*f*, 225
Pressor, 102. *See also* Blood pressure
Pressure-type syringes, 135
example of, 136*f*
Prevention of, needle breakage, 347
advance needle slowly, 348
do not bend needle, 347
long, large-gauge needle, 347
never force needle, 350
never insert needle to hub, 350
no sudden direction changes, 350
patient communication, 347
Prilocaine, 3, 56*t*, 58*f*, 59, 59*f*, 66*t*, 67*t*, 68*t*, 69*t*
duration of, 56*f*, 57*f*
half-life of, 38*t*
maximum recommended dose of, 115*t*
pregnancy and, 107*t*
properties of, 55*t*
summary of, 126*b*
Primary complication, 347
Primary prevention, 380
Procaine, 3, 75
Process, definition of, 184
Propagation of action potential, 22
Proprietary name, 53
Protein binding, local anesthetic and, 32*t*
Psychological evaluation, dental phobia and, 100
Pterygoid, 204*t*
Pterygoid plexus of veins, 205*f*, 205
Pterygomandibular raphe, 190
Pterygomandibular space, 190, 285, 287, 291*f*
needle insertion into, 291*f*, 312*f*
oral view of, 288*f*
Pterygopalatine fossa, 187, 205
Pterygotemporal depression, 190
Pulpal anesthesia, 3, 33, 281
of mandibular first molar, 292*f*
Pulse, 99
acceptable ranges for, 99*t*
factors influencing, 100*t*
procedure for, 99*f*, 99
Pulse oximeter, 338*b*, 338, 340*f*

Q

Quadrant dental hygiene treatment
on mandible, 281
on maxillary arch, 240, 260
Qualified healthcare professional, occupational exposure and, 381
Quaternary amine, 30*f*

R

Ramus, 189
Rapid depolarization, 20
Reanesthetization, 40*b*
α receptors, 45
stimulation of, 46
β receptors, 45
Recapping techniques for needles, safe and unsafe, 230
Recovery, from local anesthetic block, 37
Refractory periods, 20, 21*b*, 22*f*
Regional local anesthesia board examinations requiring calculations based on 1.7 mL of solutions, dosing information for, 116*b*, 128*b*, 128*t*, 129*t*
Relative contraindication, 44, 57, 102
Relative refractory period, 20, 21*b*
Remain calm, 350
Repolarization, 20, 21*f*, 21*b*
Respiration, 99
acceptable ranges for, 100*t*
Respiratory system
adrenergic amine effects on, 46*t*
effect of epinephrine on, 47
effect of levonordefrin on, 49
Resting membrane potential (RMP), 17, 19*f*
ions in, 17
role of ion channels in maintaining, 19*f*
Resting state, 17, 20*f*, 22*t*. *See also* Resting membrane potential (RMP)
"Rest or digest" response, 12
Retromandibular vein, 205*f*
Reusable breech-loading metallic cartridge-type aspirating syringe, 134
advantages/disadvantages of, 134*t*
Reusable breech-loading metallic cartridge-type self-aspirating syringe, 134
advantages and disadvantages of, 135*t*
Reusable breech-loading plastic cartridge-type aspirating syringe, 135
advantages and disadvantages of, 136*t*
Reusable syringes, routine maintenance of, 141
Risk assessment, 101, 102*t*
ABCs of, 102*t*
Risk management, 377
communication and, 377
dental hygienist-employer, 377
dental hygienist-patient, 377
documentation as, 379
and legal considerations, 377
RMP. *See* Resting membrane potential (RMP)
Room temperature agents, 351

S

Safe-D-Needle, 148*f*, 148
Safety syringe, disposable, 140
Saltatory conduction, 22, 23*f*, 23*b*
Salt form of local anesthetics, 31*f*
Scavenger system, 338*f*, 338
Schwann cell, 15*f*, 16*f*
Scoop method, 147*f*, 223*f*
Secondary complication, 347
Secondary prevention, 380
Sedation continuum, 335, 336*f*, 336*t*
Seizures, management of, 370*t*
Self-aspirating syringe
aspiration using, 220, 221*f*
example of, 135*f*
reusable breech-loading metallic cartridge-type, 134
Sensory neuron, functional regions of, 14, 17*f*
Sensory pathway, 12
Sensory root, divisions of, 191
maxillary nerve, 192
ophthalmic nerve, 191
zygomatic nerve, 193
Severe complications, 347
Shaft, of needle, 142*f*, 142
Sharp needles, 350
Sharps, management of, 229
Short-acting anesthetics, 2, 54
SH-SY5Y cells, 354
Sickle cell anemia, 105*t*
Silicone rubber stopper, 134, 149*f*, 149, 150*f*
harpoon in, 134
Single tooth anesthesia (STA) system, 224, 225*f*
Single unit-dose applicator, 80, 85*f*
Skull

bony openings in, 186*t*
lateral view of, 194*f*
parts of
mandible, 187
maxillae, 184
palatine bones, 186
Sloughing. *See* Soft tissue sloughing
Sodium bisulfite, 53
allergy, 57, 58*t*
Sodium bisulfite preservative, 47
Sodium chloride, 53
Sodium hydroxide, 53
Soft tissue anesthesia, local infiltration and, 209
Soft tissue injury
management of, 328
postoperative, 328
preventive measures of, 328
Soft tissue sloughing, 357, 359*f*
causes of, 348*t*
management of, 348*t*, 358
prevention of, 348*t*, 357
Soft tissue trauma, 356, 357*f*
causes of, 348*t*
management of, 348*t*, 357
phentolamine mesylate, 357, 358*t*
prevention of, 348*t*, 357
Somatic nervous system, 12
organizational plan of, 14*f*
Specific protein receptor theory, 34, 35*f*, 36*f*
Sphenopalatine artery, structures supplied, 204*t*
Sterile abscesses, 357
Stress
cardiovascular disease and, 104
definition of, 7
effects of, 101*b*
fight-or-flight, 7, 100
reduction protocol for, 101*b*
signs of, 100*b*
Stress reduction, principles of, 8
Stroke, management of, 370*t*
Sublingual artery, structures supplied, 204*t*
Sulcus, 184
Sulfite allergies, vasoconstrictors and, 103*t*
Sulfite-containing agents, 367*b*
Sulfonamides, ester local anesthetics and, 105
Summation zone, 14, 15*f*
Superficial epineurium, 16*f*
Superior alveolar nerve
anterior, 194
middle, 195
posterior, 195
Superior orbital fissure, 186*t*
Supraperiosteal injection, 55, 209, 234
complications of, 236, 237*t*
deposit location for, 234
indications of clinically effective, 236
injection site for, 234
of mandibular first molar, 292*f*
maxillary, 234, 237*f*
needle insertion point for, 272*f*
procedure for, 234*b*
review of, 235*t*
target area for, 234
technique errors associated with, 270
Surface anesthesia, use of, 209
Sympathetic division, 12, 14*f*
Sympathomimetic amines, 44*f*
Sympathomimetic drugs, 43
Synaptic knobs, 17*f*
Synaptic transmission, 23
Syncope, management of, 370*t*
Syringe
anesthetic
components of, 131
example of, 133*f*
types of, 133, 134*f*
aspiration using, 221*f*
disposable safety, 140
history of, 131
jet injector, 136*f*, 136
keeping syringe out of patient's sight, 219*f*, 219
maintenance of, 141
petite, 134*f*
preparation of, 130, 181*b*
pressure-type, 135
reusable breech-loading metallic cartridge-type aspirating, 134
reusable breech-loading metallic cartridge-type self-aspirating, 134
reusable breech-loading plastic cartridge-type aspirating, 135
selection of, 215
types of, 133
withdrawing after local anesthesia, 223
Syringe adaptor, 143
Syringe barrel, 131, 132*f*
Systemic complications, 347, 362
epinephrine overdose as, 366
local anesthetic overdose as, 362
Systemic toxicity, 362, 364

T
Tachycardia, 99
Tachyphylaxis, 37
Target area. *See* Deposit location
Tertiary amine, 30*f*
Tertiary prevention, 380
Tetracaine, 87*f*, 87
Tetracaine hydrochloride, 86
Thiophene, 3
Thumb ring, 132*f*, 133*f*, 133
Thyroid hormones, vasoconstrictors and, 103*t*
Thyroid storm, 104
Tidal volume, 338
Tissue sloughing. *See* Soft tissue sloughing
Titration, 340
Topical anesthetic agents, 80, 81*b*, 81*t*, 82*f*, 328, 350
application of, 216, 217*f*
combinations of, 86
forms and methods of delivery, 80, 82*f*, 85*f*
mechanism of action of, 80
special considerations, 88, 90*b*
used in dentistry, 85
use of, 3, 152
Topical antiseptic
application of, 217*f*
example of, 152*f*
purpose of, 216
use of, 152
Tracts, 13
Transdermal patches, 83
Transient complications, 347
Transient facial paralysis, 351, 353*f*
causes of, 348*t*
prevention of, 348*t*, 352
Transoral anesthetic patch, 84, 85*f*
Trauma
edema caused by, 356
soft tissue, 348*t*
Treatment notes, 224*t*
Tricyclic antidepressant
indication for, 102
types of, 104*b*
vasoconstrictors and, 103*t*
Trigeminal ganglion, 192*f*
Trigeminal nerve, 190
innervation of, 192*t*
pathway of, 192*f*
Trismus, 355
causes of, 348*t*
management of, 348*t*, 356
prevention of, 348*t*, 355
Tuberosity, 184

U
Ultra Safety Plus XL, 140
example of, 141*f*
Unconscious patient, operating on, 2
Unionized, 31
Unmyelinated fiber, 15, 22
Unmyelinated peripheral nervous system axon, 18*f*
Urine, local anesthetic excretion in, 38

V
VAS. *See* Visual analog scale (VAS)
Vascularity of tissue, anesthesia duration and, 55
Vascular structures, 202
Vascular system
arteries of, 202
veins of, 202
Vasculature
effect of epinephrine on, 47
effect of levonordefrin on, 48
Vasoconstriction, 46
Vasoconstrictor dilutions, 120, 120*t*
Vasoconstrictor doses, 115*b*, 120
Vasoconstrictors
administered, calculating milligrams of, 120*t*, 123
calculation of, 120
additional doses of the same vasoconstrictor, 123
convert maximum recommended dose of vasoconstrictor cartridges, 122, 122*t*
milligrams of vasoconstrictor in one cartridge of anesthetic, 121
obtaining maximum recommended dose of vasoconstrictor, 121, 121*t*
cardiac dose and, 104
chemistry of, 43
contraindications for, 104
definition of, 43
dosing facts for, 121*b*
drug interactions and, 104
maximum recommended dose for, 120, 121*b*, 129*t*
overdose, management of, 370*t*
patient's information, obtain, 121
pharmacology of, 43, 50*b*, 50*t*
side effects and overdose of, 49, 49*t*, 50*t*
summary of, 126*b*, 127*b*
and systemic disease interactions, 104
use of
in dentistry, 44*f*, 44, 45*f*
modifications to, 105*t*
volume of, 129*t*
Vasodepressor syncope, 209
Vasodilator
local anesthetic as, 43
vasoconstrictor and, 53
Vasodilator activity, local anesthetic and, 32*t*
Vazirani-Akinosi mandibular block, 281, 308, 351
complications with, 312, 312*t*
indications of clinically effective, 312
injection site for, 308, 311*f*
procedure for, 311*b*
review of, 308*t*
target area for, 308
troubleshooting paradigm, 311
Vein, definition of, 202
Venous plexuses, 202
Venous sinuses, definition of, 202
Venule, 202
Vessel, 16*f*
VibraJect, 220*f*, 220
Visceral effector, 12
Visual analog scale (VAS), 7*f*, 33, 210, 211*f*
definition of, 5
Visual examination, 98
Vital signs, 98
Voltage-gated sodium channels, 25
blockade of, 35*b*
Volume indicator label, 117*f*
example of, 149, 150*f*
Volume, of anesthetic per cartridge, 116*b*

W
Wand Compudent, 136*f*, 138
Wand handpiece
example of, 140*f*
modification of, 138*b*
Wand STA, 137, 140*f*
computer-controlled local anesthetic delivery system
assembly of, 169*b*
disassembly of, 173*b*
foot control of, 140*f*
handpiece needle lengths, 146*f*
Luer-Lok needles for, 145, 146*f*
Warning stickers, 357
Weight of patient, MRD and, 100
White fibers, 15

Z
Zygomatic nerve, 193*f*, 193
Zygomaticofacial nerve, 193*f*, 193
Zygomaticomaxillary suture, 259*f*
Zygomaticotemporal nerve, 193*f*, 193
Zygomatic process, 185
associated structures of, 186*t*